Living with Chronic Illness and Disability

4TH EDITION

Living with Chronic Illness and Disability

Principles for Nursing Practice

4TH EDITION

EDITED BY

ESTHER CHANG

AMANDA JOHNSON

ELSEVIER

ELSEVIER

Elsevier Australia. ACN 001 002 357
(a division of Reed International Books Australia Pty Ltd)
Tower 1, 475 Victoria Avenue, Chatswood, NSW 2067

ISBN: 978-0-7295-4358-3

Notice

National Library of Australia Cataloguing-in-Publication Data

---

A catalogue record for this book is available from the National Library of Australia

---

Content Strategist: Natalie Hunt
Content Project Manager: Fariha Nadeem
Copy edited by Margaret Trudgeon
Proofread by Annabel Adair
Cover by Georgette Hall
Index by Straive™
Typeset by GW Tech
Printed in Singapore by KHL Printing Co Pte Ltd

Last digit is the print number: 9 8 7 6 5 4 3 2 1

Contributors

Jeffery Adams, PhD
Senior Research Officer, SHORE and Whariki Research Centre, Massey University, Auckland, New Zealand

Charlotte Allen, RN, BSC, DipPaedRespir(UK)
Credentialed Clinical Nurse Specialist, Department of General Paediatrics, Perth Children's Hospital, Perth, WA, Australia

Michael Baker, GradCert(HEd), MAppSc(Ex&SpSc), PhD, FESSA
Associate Professor and Director of Research Services, Australian Catholic University, NSW, Australia

Robert Batterbee, RN, BSc(Hons), GDip(CBT), CMHN
Lecturer, Generalist and Mental Health Nursing, College of Science, Health, Engineering and Education Professions, Murdoch University, WA, Australia

Michelle Bissett, BAppSc(Hons)(OccTherapy), GCertBiostat, PhD
Senior Lecturer, Discipline of Occupational Therapy, Griffith University, QLD, Australia

Ann Bonner, RN, BAppSc(Nurs), MA, PhD, MRCNA
Professor and Head of School, School of Nursing & Midwifery, Griffith University, QLD, Australia
Visiting Research Fellow, Kidney Health Service, Metro North Hospital and Health Service, QLD, Australia

Melissa Bonser, RN, DipAppSc(Nurs), GCertNeurosciNurs, GCertRehabNurs
Clinical Nurse Consultant, Rapid Response Rehabilitation Team, Liverpool Hospital, NSW, Australia

Leanne Brown, RN, GCertHMgt, GDipAppSc(Nephrology), GDipAppSc(Nurs), MNSc(NP), PhD
Nephrology Nurse Practitioner, Cape York Kidney Care, Torres and Cape Hospital and Health Service, Cairns, QLD, Australia

Niels Buus, RN, MNurs, PhD
Honorary Professor, Faculty of Medicine and Health, The University of Sydney, NSW, Australia
Adjunct Professor, University of Southern Denmark, Faculty of Health, Odense, Denmark

Keryln Carville, RN, PhD
Professor Primary Health Care and Community Nursing, Silver Chain and Curtin University, Perth, WA, Australia

Esther Chang, RN, CM, DNE, BAppSc(AdvNurs), MEdAdmin, PhD, FRCNA
Professor of Aged and Palliative Care, School of Nursing and Midwifery, Western Sydney University, NSW, Australia

David Charnock, DipAdvEd, MSc, PhD, RNLD
Assistant Professor, University of Nottingham, Nottingham, United Kingdom

Christine Chisengantambu, RN, DNE, PGCertDE, PGCommH, MPubH, PhD
Lecturer, Australian Catholic University, NSW, Australia

Sharon Croxford, GCertAcademicPractice, APD, PhD
Associate Professor, Nutrition and Dietetics, Faculty of Health Sciences, Australian Catholic University, Melbourne, VIC, Australia

Patricia M. Davidson, RN, MEd, PhD, FAAN
Dean & Professor, John Hopkins School of Nursing,
  Baltimore, Maryland, USA

Colleen Doyle, PhD
Senior Principal Research Fellow, Aged Care Division,
  National Ageing Research Institute, VIC, Australia
Honorary Professor, School of Nursing and Midwifery,
  Deakin University, VIC, Australia
Honorary Professor, School of Health Sciences,
  Swinburne University, VIC, Australia

**Vicki Drury, RN, CertMensHlth, MCINurs,
PGCertNurs(Psych), PhD, RMHN, OND**
Independent Scholar, Educare Consulting, Australia
Adjunct Associate Professor, Curtin University, Perth,
  WA, Australia

Tinashe M. Dune, MPH, PhD
Senior Lecturer in Interprofessional Health Sciences,
  School of Health Sciences; Translational Health
  Research Institute; Diabetes Obesity and
  Metabolism Translational Research Unit, Western
  Sydney University, NSW, Australia

Trisha Dunning, RN, MEd, PhD, AM, CDE
Chair in Nursing (Retired), Centre for Quality and
  Patient Safety Research, Deakin University and
  Barwon Health Partnership, VIC, Australia

**Caleb Ferguson, RN, MHlth, PhD, FACN, FESC,
FCSANZ**
Senior Research Fellow, Western Sydney Nursing &
  Midwifery Research Centre, Western Sydney
  University & Western Sydney Local Health District,
  Blacktown, NSW, Australia

Claire Fraser, MSc(PallCare)
PhD candidate, Centre for Improving Palliative,
  Aged and Chronic Care through Clinical Research
  and Translation (IMPACCT), Faculty of Health,
  University of Technology Sydney, NSW, Australia

Steven A. Frost, RN, ICU Cert, MPH, PhD
Deputy Director Nursing and Midwifery Research
  South Western NSW Local Health District, Ingham
  Institute of Applied Medical Research and Western
  Sydney University, Sydney, NSW, Australia

Hilary Gallagher, MSocWk
Lecturer, Griffith University, QLD, Australia

Gisselle Gallego, PhD
Senior Research Fellow, Auburn Clinical School,
  School of Medicine, The University of Notre Dame
  Australia, NSW, Australia

**Gillian Garrett, RN, CertNeurosci,
GradCertChangeMgt, GradCertNurs(Rehab)**
Spinal Cord Injury Clinical Nurse Consultant, Royal
  Rehab, NSW, Australia

Lynne S. Giddings, RN, RM, PhD
Associate Professor (retired), School of Clinical
  Sciences, Faculty of Health and Environmental
  Sciences, AUT University, Auckland, New Zealand

Mark Hughes, BSW(Hons), PhD
Professor of Social Work, Faculty of Health, Southern
  Cross University, QLD, Australia

Serra E. Ivynian, PhD
Research Fellow, IMPACCT – Improving Palliative,
  Aged and Chronic Care through Clinical Research
  and Translation, Faculty of Health, University of
  Technology, Sydney, NSW, Australia

**Jacqueline Jauncey-Cooke, RN, GDipCritCare,
GCertHlthProfEd, PhD**
Lecturer, School of Nursing, Midwifery & Social Work,
  The University of Queensland, QLD, Australia

Sunita R. Jha, BMedSci(Hons)
Casual Academic, Faculty of Health, University of
  Technology Sydney, NSW, Australia

**Amanda Johnson, RN, DipT(Nurs), MSc(HEd),
PhD**
Head of School and Dean of Nursing and Midwifery,
  College of Health Medicine and Wellbeing, School
  of Nursing and Midwifery, University of Newcastle,
  Gosford, NSW, Australia

Belinda Kenny, PhD, FSPAA
Director Academic Program, Speech Pathology, Health
  Sciences, Western Sydney University, NSW,
  Australia

Liam Langford, BHSc(Paramedic), MPH
Lecturer of Paramedicine, Faculty of Nursing,
  Midwifery and Paramedicine, Australian Catholic
  University, Canberra, ACT, Australia
Intensive Care Paramedic, ACT, Australia
Ambulance Service, Canberra, ACT, Australia

Sonia Matiuk, RN, GCertNeuroscNurs, MNurs
Lecturer in Nursing, School of Nursing and Midwifery, University of Technology Sydney, NSW, Australia

Andrea McCloughen, RN, MN(Mental Health), PhD, FACMHN, CMHN
Associate Professor of Mental Health Nursing, Susan Wakil School of Nursing and Midwifery, Faculty of Medicine and Health, The University of Sydney, NSW, Australia

Paul McDonald, RN, RGeriN, ROncN, MNurs(Clinical), MPET, GCHE
Lecturer, School of Nursing, Midwifery and Paramedicine, Australian Catholic University, NSW, Australia

Duncan McKechnie, RN, DipPublicSafety, GradCertNurs(Rehab), PhD
Brain Injury Clinical Nurse Consultant, Royal Rehab, Ryde, NSW, Australia

Geoffrey Mitchell, MBBS, PhD, FRACGP, FAChPM
Emeritus Professor, Faculty of Medicine, The University of Queensland, Brisbane, QLD, Australia

Graham Munro, GCertEmerHlth, MHSM
Senior Lecturer/Course Coordinator, School of Nursing, Midwifery and Paramedicine, Australian Catholic University, North Sydney, NSW, Australia

Stephen Neville, RN, PhD, FCNZ(NZ)
Professor of Wellbeing and Ageing, Head of Nursing, School of Clinical Sciences, Auckland University of Technology, Auckland, New Zealand

Phillip J. Newton, RN, PhD, FCSANZ, FESC, FAHA
Associate Professor, University of Technology Sydney, NSW, Australia

Tiffany Northall, RN, GCertClinEd, MNR(Distinction), PhD
Lecturer, School of Nursing and Midwifery, Western Sydney University, NSW, Australia

Kate O'Reilly, RN, GCertNurs(Community), MClinRehab(Research)
Director International (Programs and Engagement), Lecturer, School of Nursing and Midwifery, Western Sydney University, NSW, Australia

Jane Phillips, PhD, RN, FACN
Head, Faculty of Health, School of Nursing, Queensland University of Technology, Brisbane, QLD, Australia
Emeritus Professor Palliative Nursing, University of Technology Sydney, NSW, Australia

Julie Pryor, RN, GCertRemoteHlthPrac, MNurs, PhD, FACN
Director Research and Innovation, Royal Rehab, NSW, Australia
Clinical Associate Professor, University of Sydney, NSW, Australia

Sue Randall, RN, RHV, MSc(HealthStud), PhD, SFHEA
Associate Professor Primary Health Care and Rural/Remote Nursing, Susan Wakil School of Nursing and Midwifery, The University of Sydney, NSW, Australia

Dianne Reidlinger, GCert(Academic Practice), PhD, APD, RD(UK)
Associate Professor, Master of Nutrition and Dietetic Practice, Faculty of Health Sciences and Medicine, Bond University, QLD, Australia

Joel Rhee, MBBS(Hons), GCULT, PhD, FRACGP
Associate Professor of General Practice, General Practice Academic Unit, Graduate Medicine, University of Wollongong, NSW, Australia

Vanessa J. Rice, BS(Health Science), PhD, AEP, AES, ESSAM
Senior Lecturer (Retired), School of Exercise Science, Australian Catholic University, VIC, Australia

Gail Roberts, RN, GDipCouns, CertIV TAE, MA(SocSci)
Senior Project Officer, Research and Ethics Officer, Foundation and Research, Royal Australian College of General Practitioners, Melbourne, VIC, Australia
Academic staff, School of Nursing and Midwifery, Faculty of Medicine Nursing and Health Science, Monash University, Clayton, VIC, Australia

John Xavier Rolley, RN, PhD, FACN
Associate Professor, School of Nursing and Midwifery, University of Canberra, ACT, Australia

Dianne E. Roy, RN, PhD, FCNA(NZ)
Associate Professor, Nursing, School of Healthcare
and Social Practice, Unitec Institute of Technology,
Auckland, New Zealand

Isabelle Skinner, RN, RM, MPHTM, MBA, PhD
Professor, Charles Darwin University, NT, Australia

Karen Strickland, RN, PGCert, MSc, PhD, FHEA, FEANS
Professor of Nursing and Head of School, School of
Nursing, Midwifery and Public Health, University
of Canberra, ACT, Australia
Adjunct Professor of Nursing, School of Clinical
Sciences, Faculty of Health and Environmental
Sciences, AUT, Auckland, New Zealand
Visiting Professor of Nursing, Robert Gordon
University, Aberdeen, Scotland

Angelica G. Thompson-Butel, BSc(Ex&SpSc), PhD, AEP, AES, ESSAM
National Course Coordinator of Exercise
Physiology, School of Behavioural and Health
Sciences, Australian Catholic University, NSW,
Australia

Claudia Virdun, RN, BN(Hons), MSc, PhD, MACN
Senior Research Fellow, Cancer and Palliative Care
Outcomes Centre, School of Nursing, Centre for
Healthcare Transformation, Faculty of Health,
Queensland University of Technology, QLD,
Australia

Sandy Mary Ward, MEduc Adv Dip Business Management and Human Resources
Retirement Living, Kirkbrae Presbyterian Homes,
Kilsyth, VIC, Australia

Nathan J. Wilson, MSc, PhD
Senior Lecturer, School of Nursing and Midwifery,
Western Sydney University, NSW, Australia

Michelle Woods, RN, GradDipHlthEd, MSN-NP, DNSc
Nurse Practitioner, Tasmanian Health Service, TAS,
Australia

Anthony Wright, PhD
Adjunct Professor, Curtin University, WA, Australia

Patsy Yates, RN, MSocSci, PhD, FACN, FAAN
Distinguished Professor, Faculty of Health,
Queensland University of Technology, QLD,
Australia

Lee Zakrzewski, BAppSc(OccTherapy), HScD
Previously Senior Lecturer, Occupational Therapy,
Western Sydney University, NSW, Australia

Reviewers

Aaisha Syed, RN, MSN
Head of Discipline, Nursing, Partners in Training
Australia, Melbourne, VIC, Australia

Lyn Taylor, GDipNurs(Perioperative), GCert(HEd), MEd(AVET)
Lecturer in Nursing and Course Coordinator
(Melbourne), Bachelor of Nursing, School of
Nursing, Midwifery and Paramedicine, Australian
Catholic University, Melbourne, VIC, Australia

Colleen Van Lochem, MNurs
Lecturer/Course Coordinator, University of Notre
Dame, Werribee, VIC, Australia

Cecilia Yeboah, PhD
Lecturer in Nursing, Australian Catholic University,
Melbourne, VIC, Australia

Preface

The Coronavirus disease 2019 (COVID-19) pandemic is a human, social and economic crisis that has impacted on everyone in a small or large way. No doubt it has impacted on you too. Public health actions, such as social distancing, can make people feel isolated and increase stress and anxiety. Academics had to change their teaching to online. You had to change your way of learning. The onset of COVID-19 has also intensified the pressure on the healthcare workforce. The clinicians and academic authors of this book, despite their heavy workload, contributed to the writing of the chapters as they saw the importance of getting this textbook out to you.

We hope you enjoy using the fourth edition of this text, and that it inspires and encourages you to give the best quality of care for people living with chronic illness and disability. We also hope that this text will improve your knowledge and the development of your skills, and at the same time enhance your confidence when caring for people with chronic illness and disability.

This book has been developed for undergraduate nursing students, students in the TAFE sector, newly registered nurses and other health professionals who share our commitment to providing quality of care to people living with chronic illness and disability. This book continues to champion the principles for practice supported by evidence from Australian and international literature to enhance the understanding of some of the issues and challenges of caring for a person living with chronic illness and disability. Across all chapters, the text illustrates a holistic approach, highlighting quality of life in all aspects of care for chronic illnesses and disability. Concepts essential for underpinning best practice in self-management of chronic illness and disability are included, such as spirituality, individual education strategies, valuing the person's expertise, resources, culture, minimising socially stigmatising processes and social isolation. Issues affecting carers and family are also addressed. Attention to these concepts recognises the important shift nurses and other health professionals are making towards working in partnership with individuals, their family and carers.

Through education and empowerment, individuals, their family and carers are supported in their adjustment and adaptation to chronic illness and disability to achieve optimal outcomes.

This fourth edition provides extra media resources that will enhance your learning. With this book comes the case studies and reflective questions on chronic illness and disability for discussion. Where relevant, the text is supported by current statistics to illustrate key aspects of the discussion. Acquiring the knowledge and skills for people living with a chronic illness and/or disability is vital in giving competent care. You will find viewpoints that are challenging, but at the same time motivating and thought-provoking. The exercises and learning activities that are presented throughout the text offer a range of helpful suggestions in understanding the context. Chapter 2 of this edition also includes the roles of nurse, dietitian, exercise physiologist, medical practitioner, occupational therapist, paramedic, pharmacist, physiotherapist, social worker and speech pathologist, and their responsibilities in the interdisciplinary/multidisciplinary team. In addition, each chapter has case studies, recommended readings and online resources for further exploration.

Nurses and other health professionals in clinical practice and academic roles have been involved in producing this text resource. We hope that you will find the text scholarly, accessible, reality-based and practically useful. It is a resource intended for every student, practising nurse, educator and administrator in understanding the issues of caring for people living with chronic illness and disability. By reading the text, reflecting on the issues and composing possible answers, you should be able to gain a comprehensive view of the issues, challenges and opportunities that lie ahead of you in your practice.

We gratefully acknowledge several key people who have contributed and assisted us in preparing this fourth edition for publication. The authors took time to finish their chapters even though their workloads were heavy in the climate that they are in. We wish to extend our heartfelt thankfulness and appreciation to the contributors for their shared interest and concern in the issues and challenges of caring for people and their families in nursing. **This book would not be possible without them. Our grateful and sincere thanks.** We would like to extend our special appreciation to members of the Elsevier team: Natalie Hunt, Fariha Nadeem, Margaret Trudgeon and Annabel Adair for their encouragement and support. Elsevier Australia joins us in thanking all the reviewers who were involved in providing invaluable feedback during the development process (listed on page xiii). Finally, we would also like to thank our husbands and children for their endless support and encouragement through the years.

Esther Chang and Amanda Johnson

Contents

CHAPTER 1

Chronic Illness and Disability: An Overview

AMANDA JOHNSON • ESTHER CHANG

LEARNING OBJECTIVES

When you have completed this chapter, you will be able to:
- describe the global and local contexts of chronic disease and disability
- describe the key terms used in relation to chronic disease and disability
- understand the role of modifiable risk factors and their prevention in reducing the presence of chronic disease and disability in the community
- develop an understanding of the impact that living with a chronic disease and/or disability poses for the individual and their family, health system and wider community
- appreciate the need for the implementation of holistic care, inclusive of a multidisciplinary approach to promote self-management and optimal functioning.

KEY WORDS

chronic disease	nurse
chronic illness	risk factors
disability	

INTRODUCTION

Worldwide the global health status of all countries remains challenged by the continued rise in chronic disease, the impact this burden poses on communities and healthcare systems, and the subsequent disabilities which may emerge as a consequence of the disease and/or treatments (World Health Organization [WHO] 2020). Chronic disease is no longer exclusive to high-income countries but is now encompassing middle- or low-income countries, with significant increases in premature deaths associated with chronic disease. WHO (2020) reports 41 million people die prematurely across the world with links to chronic disease, and their monitoring of the Global Action Plan (2013–2020)

suggests that less than 50% of countries are meeting targets to mitigate the risks of chronic disease in their country (WHO 2020). The term chronic disease may be used interchangeably in the literature with non-communicable diseases (NCDs), chronic illness, chronic conditions and long-term health conditions (Australian Institute of Health and Welfare [AIHW] 2020). Collectively these terms represent a group of diseases that are long-lasting with persistent effects that frequently lead to disabilities, ultimately impacting on the person's quality of life (AIHW 2020). These diseases are: arthritis, asthma, back pain, cancer, cardiovascular disease, chronic obstructive pulmonary disease, diabetes, chronic kidney disease, mental health

1

conditions and osteoporosis (AIHW 2020). Importantly, the rising prevalence of chronic disease can be reversed if individuals take responsibility for their health and modify risk factors (and governments institute healthcare policy focused primarily on prevention rather than intervention).

Globally, nurses hold a pivotal role in coordinating care and acting as educators, advocators and health promoters to optimise an individual's capacity for quality of life. In this context, the role requires nurses to possess an empathetic attitude, have knowledge of, and the skills in, the principles of nursing practice to provide optimal care to individuals, their family and the wider community. Subsequent chapters in this text use key chronic diseases and/or disabilities to illustrate the nurse's role and explain how it contributes to an individual self-managing and achieving optimal functioning.

The use of a multidisciplinary approach to care has been reported as making significant improvements in the health outcomes for people with chronic diseases (McDonald et al 2006). Frequently the care coordination role in the multidisciplinary team is undertaken by the nurse (Parker & Fuller 2016); however, it is not exclusive to the nursing profession, and other health professionals in some settings may take on the role. Chapter 2 explores the nurse's role with other health professionals to illustrate the role they play when managing people with chronic disease, within a multidisciplinary approach. Understanding what it means for individuals, families and the wider community to live with a chronic disease and/or disability is as important as having the knowledge and skills to practise in this context.

The chapters are constructed to reflect this emphasis through the case studies presented and the media resources identified, highlighting that the person and their family are central to the nurse's understanding of their needs, as they commence the illness trajectory related to chronic disease and associated disability.

What follows in this chapter is a discussion on the key terms used throughout the text; an overview of the global context of chronic disease and disability followed by information specific to the Australian and New Zealand contexts.

UNDERSTANDING KEY TERMS

To support your engagement in the reading of this text it is important to understand what is meant by a number of key terms to aid your understanding and application within the case studies.

Chronic Disease

Chronic disease is often difficult to define and frequently several terms are used interchangeably across the world and within countries. When chronic disease is referred to in a global context and reported on by the World Health Organization (WHO), the term used is 'non-communicable diseases' (NCD) (WHO 2014). NCDs are considered to be long term in nature, not acquired by transmission between people, but share many common lifestyle-related risk factors (WHO 2014). In Australia, the term 'chronic disease' is more frequently used and relates to a group of diseases which cause substantial ill-health, disability and premature death (AIHW 2020). The New Zealand literature is most likely to report on chronic disease using the term 'long-term conditions' (Ministry of Health [MoH] NZ 2016b), which are described in the New Zealand context to be ongoing, long-term or recurring conditions that have a significant impact on people's lives. Importantly, however, named chronic diseases are complex, with multiple causes, usually not life threatening but rather develop gradually, requiring long-term management and become more common with ageing (AIHW 2020).

Risk Factors

Risk factors constitute determinants of health that impact on our health negatively. They may be demographic, behavioural, biomedical, genetic, environmental, social or other factors, acting independently or in combination (AIHW 2016). Initially, it was thought that risk factors were exclusively adult behaviours; however, we now understand their importance from the period of gestation until death. For example, the increased numbers of overweight and obese children and the increasing incidence of type 2 diabetes found in the younger generation (WHO 2014). In relation to chronic disease, they can affect the onset, maintenance and prognosis of chronic disease. The risk factors associated with chronic disease are:

- poor nutrition
- physical inactivity
- smoking
- risky alcohol consumption and illicit drug use
- high blood pressure
- high blood lipids
- overweight and obesity
- impaired fasting glucose (AIHW 2016, 2020).

Significantly, the vast majority of these risk factors are modifiable to prevent chronic disease from occurring. The lifestyles engaged in by the populations of developed countries have seen an increasing rise in the prevalence of chronic disease, while those who are vulnerable and poor in our communities tend to have one or more of these risk factors present. As you read over the chapters about specific chronic diseases, you will learn about the identification of risk factors in relation to disease and how these are best prevented and/or managed to prevent development of the chronic disease in the first instance.

Risk factors in the development of chronic disease

Controlling body weight, eating nutritious foods, avoiding tobacco use, controlling alcohol consumption and increasing physical activity may lead to the prevention or delay of many chronic diseases (AIHW 2020).

Controlling some risk factors and effectively managing others through initiatives such as screening and early intervention programs (AIHW 2020; National Public Health Partnership [NPHP] 2006) can significantly reduce the presence of chronic disease within communities. In Australia, health promotion is acknowledged as the key to preventing chronic disease via prevention and management of risk factors (AIHW 2020). The most common modifiable risk factors contributing to chronic disease are unhealthy diet, which leads to raised glucose levels, increased body mass and abnormal blood lipids; physical inactivity, which leads to increased body mass, increased blood pressure and increased blood lipids; and tobacco use, which leads to raised blood pressure (AIHW 2020; WHO 2017). These risk factors are said to be modifiable because chronic disease can be prevented by the person changing their behaviour and/or medical intervention (AIHW 2020). The two key non-modifiable risk factors contributing to the development of chronic disease are age and heredity (WHO 2005, p. 48). Identification of these factors within population groups allows for the development of prevention and management strategies that may be constructed to meet the cultural and linguistic needs of the group (AIHW 2020).

Chronic Illness

In this text, the editors have selected chronic illness as the form of expression. This has been chosen for this book because it emphasises the human experience of the disease, as experienced by the person. Larsen (2016) describes chronic illness as: 'the lived experience of the individual and family diagnosed with a chronic disease' (pp. 5–6). 'It constitutes how the disease is perceived; lived with; responded to by the individual, family and health care professionals' (Larsen 2019, p. 4). The expression takes account of the impact on all aspects of the person's life, inclusive of the physical without negating the spiritual or the key role held by healthcare professionals to address the individual's and family's needs holistically (Larsen 2019).

Disability

Globally, the International Classification of Functioning, Disability and Health (2001) (Fifty-Fourth World Health Assembly 2001) defines a person as being disabled when a level of difficulty is experienced in one or more of the following interconnecting areas. The first area is that of impairment. A person with an impairment experiences issues related to body function or alteration to body structure (WHO 2011). The second area is activity limitations. In this area the person faces challenges in carrying out everyday activities (WHO 2011). The final area identified is participation restrictions. In this area an individual faces problems in any area of their life, not just health related (WHO 2011). Further, disability arises from several contextual elements: those of health conditions (diseases or disorders), along with environmental and personal factors that can influence an individual's capacity to live in society. This means that interventions need to be much broader than just medical, and frequently involve education and welfare support (WHO 2011). In relation to chronic disease, a person may experience disability independent of the disease state, for example, a person who has arthritis but develops cardiovascular disease; or disability may be a consequence of the disease, for example, a person with diabetes who develops blindness; or disability may be present as a side effect to treatment, for example, a person who recovers from cancer but has reduced hearing due to ototoxicity related to the chemotherapy drugs. It is important to understand that in some contexts the terms 'disability', 'chronic disease' and 'impairments' are used interchangeably within the literature and may mean the same thing.

Co-morbidity

The term co-morbidity describes the presence of two diseases occurring simultaneously in a person (AIHW 2020). Frequently because of shared risk factors, there is a relationship between the original disease and the second disease that emanates; for example, a person who has diabetes can go on to develop cardiovascular disease. Getting older is also a factor, as with increased life expectancy there is greater opportunity for other conditions to emerge; for example, an older person who has cancer but also has the presence of arthritis experiences severe limitations with mobility.

Multimorbidity

Since our first edition (Chang & Johnson 2008), the term co-morbidity has now been replaced by the term multimorbidity, illustrating how expansive chronic disease has become. The term multimorbidity is where an individual experiences more than three conditions concurrently (Johnston et al 2019). Multimorbidity is becoming more prevalent as life expectancy is prolonged and people acquire other diseases and disabilities across the lifespan. In Australia, in the 2017–18 reporting period, 20% of Australians were reported as having two or more of the 10 chronic conditions (ABS 2019). Concurrently, in New Zealand one in four adults reported two or more long-term conditions (MoH NZ 2016b).

THE GLOBAL PERSPECTIVE OF CHRONIC DISEASE

Now, more than ever, there is a need to globally prevent and control the rise of chronic disease. The world and individual countries, whether low-, middle- or high-income, can no longer sustain the human, social, economic and health impacts of chronic disease either now or into the future. Importantly, recognising that health disparities exist across populations because of socioeconomic status; educational attainment; employment opportunities; disability; access to health services; social supports; and built and natural environments (AIHW 2020) is critical to our understanding of the how and why chronic disease is present in our communities. In particular, it is the poor and vulnerable populations who are most at risk (WHO 2014). By 2030, it is projected that chronic disease will account for 82% (55 million) of all deaths worldwide; this projection is an increase of 17 million from 38 million in 2012 (WHO 2013). Of the 56 million deaths reported in 2012, 68% (38 million) were attributed to chronic disease; more than 40% (16 million) were premature deaths under 70 years of age, and 48% of them occurred in low- to middle-income countries (WHO 2014). Of concern is the projected increase in these deaths underpinned by four risk factors: tobacco use, unhealthy diet, physical inactivity and harmful use of alcohol (WHO 2013), all of which are directly preventable. The leading deaths specifically attributable to these risk factors are: cardiovascular disease; cancers; chronic respiratory disease; and diabetes (WHO 2013). These deaths, and the resultant co-morbidities, multimorbidities and disability, evoke much human suffering, impacting at social, economic and public health levels on the individual, their family and the wider community. Individual behavioural change is important; however, the effects of globalisation on marketing and

trade, rapid urbanisation and population ageing (WHO 2014, p. vii) are also significant contributing influences that no one person can control, but where governments need to provide leadership.

To support countries in the leadership of preventing and controlling chronic disease, the World Health Assembly endorsed the *WHO Global Action Plan for the Prevention and Control of NCDs 2013–2020* (WHO 2013). The Action Plan offers a means by which to guide countries in establishing multi-sectoral action plans and policies to achieve a reduction in premature deaths by 25% (WHO 2013). The plan articulates nine voluntary global targets for attainment by 2025:

1. a 25% reduction in overall mortality from cardiovascular diseases, cancer, diabetes or chronic respiratory diseases
2. a 10% reduction in the harmful use of alcohol
3. a 10% reduction in prevalence of insufficient physical activity
4. a 30% reduction in intake of salt/sodium
5. a 30% reduction in the prevalence of tobacco use
6. a 25% reduction in the prevalence of high blood pressure
7. a halt in the rise of diabetes and obesity
8. at least 50% of people receiving drug therapy and counselling (glycemic control) to prevent heart attacks and strokes
9. an availability of the affordable basic technologies and essential medicines to treat NCDs (WHO 2013, p. 5).

In 2014, WHO conducted a review on the progress of these targets, documenting varying degrees of success by different countries against the targets. It is evident from the 2014 WHO report that the majority of countries are off-course to meet their global targets and as an imperative need to set national targets and a monitoring framework to track progress towards the 2025 date. The burden of disease for OECD countries (including Australia and New Zealand) is similar; however, the rates for both ischemic heart disease and lung cancer in Australia are significantly lower than in other OECD countries (WHO 2013). This reduction has been directly attributed to the health promotion educational activities Australia implemented.

Australian and New Zealand Context

Australia and New Zealand are both fortunate countries as the vast majority of their population have an increased life expectancy and consider themselves to be in 'good' health (AIHW 2016; MoH NZ 2016a). However, both countries also report chronic disease as a growing problem, which is exerting significant pressure on an already strained healthcare system and is a burden on the community (AIHW 2016; MoH 2016b). In Australia, one in two people reported they had one or more of the 10 conditions monitored by the Australian Government (arthritis, asthma, back pain, cancer, cardiovascular disease, chronic obstructive pulmonary disease, diabetes, chronic kidney disease, mental health conditions and osteoporosis), equating to 47% of the population with a chronic disease (AIHW 2020). This was also reflected in the number of hospitalisations which saw one in two hospitalisations (51%) involving chronic disease (AIHW 2020). Both countries have recognised that to meet the health challenges they face now and into the future, the health system will need to adapt and be responsive to the changing care needs and the level of complexity presented by chronic disease. Currently in New Zealand, health spending represents 22% of the overall budget in line with other developed countries. However, this current funding level is not sustainable (MoH 2016b). An increased life expectancy and greater percentage of the population with long-term health conditions necessitates a model of care that is different to current practice. The model needs a focus on prevention of long-term conditions or slowing down the development of chronic disease and related multimorbidities and disabilities. Further discussion on models of care can be found in Chapter 3.

Australian profile

Successive Australian governments have been informed by the WHO's strategic directions on chronic disease and prevention (WHO 2005). This led to a series of National Health Priority Areas (NHPAs) being identified in 1996 for the first time. These priorities are promoted as being areas where personal and community action can be taken to modify or reduce their prevalence. There are nine NHPAs currently, listed below.

The nine priorities are:
1. cancer control (first set of conditions, 1996)
2. cardiovascular health (first set of conditions, 1996)
3. injury prevention and control (first set of conditions, 1996)
4. mental health (first set of conditions, 1996)
5. diabetes mellitus (added 1997)
6. asthma (added 1999)
7. arthritis and musculoskeletal conditions (added 2002)
8. obesity (added 2008)
9. dementia (added 2012) (AIHW 2017b).

In 2017–18 one in two Australians had at least one of the ten selected chronic diseases, and nine in ten (89%) of all deaths were related to chronic disease (AIHW

2020). Many of these diseases also share common risk factors that are preventable or modifiable. One in five (20%) Australians had two or more of the 10 selected diseases (AIHW 2020), the most common co-morbidities being cardiovascular disease (7.4%) or arthritis (5.1%). Of growing concern is the emergence of the population group with multimorbidities, which places even more pressure on the healthcare system. The most commonly occurring chronic diseases are: cancer, cardiovascular disease, arthritis, asthma, diabetes, chronic kidney disease, mental and behavioural conditions, musculoskeletal disorders and injuries (AIHW 2020). In 2017–18 almost half the Australian population had one or more of these chronic diseases (AIHW 2020). Furthermore, the AIHW reports that people living in rural and remote areas, or who come from low socioeconomic situations or people with disability who are also Aboriginal and Torres Strait Islander people, were more likely to experience higher rates of illness, hospitalisation and premature death, as compared to the rest of the population. Examples of people with multimorbidities are: the one-third of Australian people (31.8%) who experience a psychotic disorder, who also experience chronic pain; one-fifth (20.8%) also have diabetes and just over one-quarter (26.8%) also have a heart or circulatory problem (AIHW 2016). By targeting specific areas that impose high social and financial costs on Australian society, collaborative action can achieve significant and cost-effective advances in improving the health status of Australians. Of the modifiable risk factors previously discussed, the AIHW 2016 report identifies that 31% of chronic disease in Australia could have been prevented by reducing exposure to tobacco use, harmful alcohol use, high body mass, physical inactivity and high blood pressure.

In addition to the NHPAs, the Commonwealth Government, through the Department of Health, has sought to establish a National Strategic Framework for Chronic Conditions in conjunction with the six states and two territories of Australia. The framework is still under development, but will seek to provide a national approach to guide planning, design, delivery of policies, strategies, actions and services to reduce the impact of chronic conditions in Australia (Australian Government Department of Health 2017). It will move away from the more traditional approach of managing diseases specifically to generating principles that can be applied more broadly. Another element to the framework will be how best to provide care through a coordinated approach drawing on a diversity of health and care providers to deliver services. Once completed, it will replace the National Chronic Disease Strategy 2005 (NHPAC 2006). This strategy emerged in response to the growing impact of chronic disease and was aimed at encouraging a coordinated approach.

In 2014–15, more than 50% (11 million) of the Australian population experienced a chronic disease (AIHW 2016). Specifically, those aged 65 and over constituted 87% of the 11 million experiencing a chronic disease, reflecting the ageing population. The AIHW 2016 report also demonstrates that 55% of those with a chronic disease come from the lowest socioeconomic areas in Australia, predominantly in regional and remote areas (54%), compared to the major cities (48%). This is an important statistical fact to consider in understanding how services are planned to promote access and uptake in regional and remote areas. The AIHW report (2016), on the self-reported data, showed that the most commonly reported chronic diseases for the period 2014–15 were: cardiovascular and mental health conditions (18% each), followed by back pain (16%). In the age group 45–64 and those 65 years or older, cardiovascular disease (27%) and arthritis (26%) were most commonly identified.

New Zealand profile

New Zealanders are living just as long as Australians, with 88% of the population experiencing some form of health loss as a consequence of long-term mental and physical disease (MoH NZ 2016a). In 2013, the Ministry of Health reported over half of the health loss (52%) was attributable to a disability. Furthermore, mental health and dementia are the leading causes of health loss (19%), two areas of practice that are providing the biggest challenges (MoH NZ 2016a). Another emerging area contributing to health loss is the rise of musculoskeletal disorders (13%) due to a higher incidence of obesity (MoH NZ 2016a). As is the case for Indigenous Australians, Māori and Pacific Islanders experience serious inequalities in health outcomes relative to the total population (MoH NZ 2016a). For example, high smoking rates continue to be present in Māori adults, especially for those living in the most deprived areas, and Pacific Islander adults experience higher rates of diabetes than any other ethnic group in New Zealand (MoH NZ 2019).

Indigenous Populations

Worldwide, there are vast disparities in the health of Indigenous people and their subsequent experiences of chronic illness and/or disability, as compared to non-Indigenous people (WHO 2008). This disparity is attributable to a life expectancy that is 10–20 years less than for the main population; infant mortality 1.5 to 3 times greater than the national average; and a large proportion of Indigenous people who suffer from malnutrition and communicable diseases (WHO 2008). Indigenous peoples' ill-health is further exacerbated by damage to their habitat and resource base (WHO 2008). In its 2008 report, *Primary health care: now more than ever*, WHO made it explicit that health service providers need to take better account of the lack of services and the disadvantage that remoteness plays in Indigenous people accessing and achieving the same health status as non-Indigenous people.

The health disparity presented worldwide continues to also be true for both Australian and New Zealand Indigenous populations. They are more likely to have an increased presence of chronic disease; to be less healthy; to die at a much younger age; and to have a lower quality of life than non-Indigenous people (AIHW 2020; MoH NZ 2012). At the present time, Australian Indigenous people experience 80% mortality directly linked to chronic disease (AIHW 2017a), with 64% of the burden of disease attributable to chronic disease (AIHW 2020). Australia is not on track to meet Closing the Gap targets (AIHW 2020).

With respect to long-term conditions (in the reporting period 2018–19), 67% of Indigenous Australians have at least one chronic disease; 38% have an eye or hearing disability; and 24% have a mental health or behavioural condition (AIHW 2020). Of significance, not only do Indigenous Australians experience more chronic disease than non-Indigenous Australians, but they also experience it at a much younger age – 35 years onwards as compared to 45–55 years depending on the disease (AIHW 2020). Four in 10 Indigenous people are obese, a level that is one and a half times more than for the non-Indigenous population, and which is considered a key underlying factor in many chronic diseases; for example, heart disease, diabetes, high blood pressure and some forms of cancer (AHIW 2020). The prevalence of disability in the Australian Indigenous people is 23.9%, representing one-quarter of their community and they are more than 1.8 times more likely than non-Indigenous people to acquire a disability (ABS 2015). In New Zealand, the most recently reported figures (2006) show life expectancy for Pacific Islander males as 6.7 years less than total males, and for Pacific Islander females it was 6.1 years less than total females (MoH NZ 2012, p. 25). In New Zealand, it is estimated that 18 700 Pacific Islander adults have a disability. For 43% (n = 8100), the most common cause of their disability was most likely attributed to chronic disease or illness (MoH NZ 2012, p. 27).

By way of illustrating the disparity, in 2011 Australian Indigenous peoples were 12% more likely than non-Indigenous Australians to experience cardiovascular disease; were 3.4 times more likely to report some form of diabetes, and had a 27% increased risk of having a respiratory disease (Thomson et al 2011). In New Zealand, the rate of diagnosed diabetes was significantly higher for Pacific Islander men and women (45–64 years age group) than men and women in the total population by approximately 20% and 12% respectively (MoH NZ 2012, p. 43). In terms of respiratory disease, the Ministry of Health (2012) reported Pacific Islander men as being three times more likely to present for hospitalisations and Pacific Islander women five times more likely than the total population.

The factors identified which contribute to Indigenous health are: nutrition; physical activity; body weight; immunisation; breastfeeding; tobacco smoking; alcohol use; and illicit drug use (MoH NZ 2012; Thomson et al 2011). Indigenous peoples have and continue to experience substantial social disadvantage in relation to their health through limited education; reduced employment opportunities; lower than national average income; higher levels of poverty; poorer housing; greater exposure to violence; limited access to services; underdeveloped social networks; connection with land; racism and incarceration; and impaired communication when English is a second language (McMurray & Clendon 2011; MoH NZ 2012; Thomson et al 2011). It is important to recognise that for Indigenous populations both the social determinants of health and the cultural concepts of Indigenous health strongly influence the health status of their communities (McMurray & Clendon 2011; MoH NZ 2012; Thomson et al 2011). The presence of these risk factors, either singly or in combination, leads to a higher proportion of the Indigenous population developing chronic disease and/or disability as compared to the non-Indigenous population.

As a consequence, Indigenous Australians suffer much more ill-health than non-Indigenous Australians (AIHW 2012). Indigenous Australians experience higher levels of disability when compared to the general population (36%): 8% experience a severe limitation of a core activity (AIHW 2006, p. 56), which is twice that experienced by non-Indigenous Australians (AIHW 2006, p. 56). In terms of chronic disease, Indigenous Australians experience a higher mortality rate from diabetes (14 times higher than the general population), chronic kidney disease (eight times) and heart disease (five times) (AIHW 2006, p. ix). The resulting outcome for Indigenous Australians is that they are four times more likely to experience death as compared to non-Indigenous Australians (AIHW 2006).

In New Zealand, 24% of Māori experience disability, followed by 18% of Europeans, and 17% of Pacific Islander peoples (MoH NZ 2005, p. 8). As a consequence, Māori and Pacific Islander peoples have a life expectancy decreased by 8.5 years compared with the European population, largely attributable to the increased incidence of chronic disease in these population groups (McMurray & Clendon 2011; National Health Committee 2007, p. 10).

GLOBAL PERSPECTIVE ON DISABILITY

Globally, 15% of the world's population experience some form of disability and it continues to rise (WHO 2011). Reasons for this continued rise relate to more people getting diseases which can cause disability; people who are unable to get timely access to healthcare; people who are disabled by war, and natural disasters. The 15% equates to 15 out of every 100 people being disabled, with two to four of those people having severe disability, preventing their productive participation in society (WHO 2011). WHO reports several factors that have contributed to this increase: an increasingly ageing population; the rapid spread of chronic disease; and better ways of reporting on disability (2011). It is also recognised that there are more vulnerable groups within our communities, for example, the poor; women; older people; those with no employment; those with low levels of education qualification; and minority ethnic groups, all of whom are more likely to experience higher rates of disability within their group (WHO 2011). This figure is expected to rise as a result of the world's ageing populations and the higher presence of disability in older people, as well as the global rise of chronic diseases (WHO 2011, p. xi).

The global impact of disability on communities has only been acknowledged in the last decade by the first world report on disability, *The world report on disabilities* (WHO 2011). This report demonstrates the attitudinal, physical and financial burdens a person experiences every day with a disability. Further, this report shows the need for governments to remove the barriers to participation and to provide sufficient funds to allow people with disability access to health, rehabilitation, support, education and employment (WHO 2011, p. ix). Finally, the report concludes by illustrating the need for policymakers, researchers, practitioners, advocates and volunteers in disability to work together at local, national and international levels. This is necessary to bring about a reduction of the burden of disabilities to society, to bring about changes to practices and to value more explicitly the contribution that people with disability can make to the productivity of the community.

AUSTRALIAN PROFILE OF DISABILITY

The National Disability Strategy 2010–2020 has as one of its six priority areas: 'People with disability attain the highest possible health and wellbeing outcomes throughout their lives' (Australian Government Department of Social Services 2014). It is telling, however, that the health outcomes for people who are disabled are not well featured as part of the national health report (AIHW 2016). In 2015, nearly one in five Australians (18.3% or 4.3 million) experienced some form of disability (ABS 2015). This figure increased significantly for those aged 65 years or older, with 50.7% reporting a disability (ABS 2015). This is important to understand in the context of Australia, where the portion of its total population aged 65 years or older is growing faster than any other age group. The result is one in seven, or 15.1%, of the population being in this age group (ABS 2015). Such a result plays a role in the determination of healthcare services into the future. The most common disability people experience is impairment to communication, mobility and/or self-care. In 2015, 5.8% (1.4 million) of the population experienced this form of disability, requiring the greatest assistance. More than half those aged 65 years or older were affected (ABS 2015). It is also important to understand that those with a disability were also 3.3 times more likely to have a long-term health condition (AIHW 2016). Two illustrations of why this is the scenario are: 1) in adults with a profound to severe disability they were 70% more likely to be overweight or obese as compared to a person without a disability, and 2) those who are profoundly or severely disabled are twice as likely to smoke than those without a disability (AIHW 2016). Services to support Australians who are disabled have fallen under the National Disability Agreement (NDA) with over half the users (55%) in 2013–14 having an intellectual or learning disability (AIHW 2014a). The most commonly reported conditions were mental and behavioural problems, followed by back problems, deafness, arthritis, cardiovascular diseases, asthma and migraine (AIHW 2016). It is also evident that co-morbidity between mental and physical disability exists and is expanding. For example, people with a disability and depression are more likely to develop diabetes (AIHW 2016) as a consequence to changes in lifestyle.

Aboriginal and Torres Strait Islander people with a disability

A large disparity exists between Aboriginal and Torres Strait Islander (ATSI) people and non-Indigenous populations of Australia. Of ATSI people, 38% had some

form of disability restricting their everyday activities (AIHW 2020). This disparity exists because of the difference in socioeconomic circumstances and access to healthcare services between these two populations. Indigenous Australians report a disability 1.8 times the rate for non-Indigenous Australians and this is likely to be higher because of the lack of reporting from very remote areas on disability (ABS 2019). It was also noted that 8.1% of ATSI people had a profound or severe disability impacting on their capacity to communicate, be mobile and/or self-care (ABS 2019).

NEW ZEALAND PROFILE OF DISABILITY

In 2013, the total New Zealand population had a disability rate of 24%, partially explained by an increase in the age of the population (Statistics New Zealand 2015) and reflecting a similar pattern to the Australian and worldwide context. Those aged 65 years or older were more likely to be disabled (59%), with physical limitations being the main form of impairment (Statistics New Zealand 2015). New Zealand has recognised the disparity in the levels of care for its population groups. A systems review of health and disability was conducted and reported on in March 2020 to promote equity and a sustainable approach to the delivery of services (Health and Disability System Review 2020).

Māori People With Disability

New Zealand's Indigenous population suffers a similar health disparity to Indigenous Australians. In 2013, 26% (176,000) of the Māori population identified as being disabled in a younger age group, an increase of 6% since 2001 (Statistics New Zealand 2015). This equates to one in four Māori who are disabled with an impairment, mostly related to mobility. Impairments for Māori stem primarily (40%) from disease or illness (Statistics New Zealand 2015). Low socioeconomics, ethnicity, poor housing and limited education combine to contribute to the Māori population experiencing a higher percentage of disability than the non-Māori population (Statistics New Zealand 2015).

IMPACT AND CHALLENGES OF CHRONIC ILLNESS AND DISABILITY

It is difficult to quantify the impact of chronic illness and disability experienced by the individual, family and community, as many of the costs are invisible. For example, in Australia 65% of people who experienced a severe or profound core activity limitation relied on informal carers for such activities as self-care, mobility and communication (AIHW 2006, p. 49). The difficulty arises due to the nature of the chronic illness and/or disability, and the resources available to manage the condition are highly variable, largely determined by each person's individual situation (Guillett 2004).

Chronic disease is often thought of as a disease of the aged, and while it is more prevalent in that age group, we are now seeing evidence of chronic disease in younger generations, which are directly attributable to lifestyle risk factors; for example, children who are overweight and obese (AIHW 2020). The implications of this are that individuals who acquire a chronic disease early on in life will need to live and adapt to their illness and sequelae for the rest of their life, placing a significant burden on the community. People living with a chronic illness are more likely than the general population to experience periods of hospitalisation as a consequence of acute flare-ups of their underlying chronic disease (AIHW 2020). What is emerging is that due to the increasing prevalence of chronic disease, many admissions to hospital now constitute the underlying pathology of chronic disease.

The challenges presented to health professionals by chronic illnesses and disabilities are vast. Consideration must be given to finding new ways of prevention to control the prevalence of chronic disease within our community. Controlling the prevalence of chronic disease is not the sole responsibility of government or health services, but must emanate from individuals taking ownership of their health behaviours, working in collaboration with government and health services to eradicate the increasing presence of chronic disease in our communities (WHO 2014). Some challenges that have been articulated are the rising costs of care, the number of people needing to access chronic disease care, inequities between the Indigenous and general populations, the changing composition of the population experiencing chronic disease and/or disability, ethical issues, providing culturally competent care, caregiver issues (AIHW 2016; MoH NZ 2016; Remsburg & Carson 2006, pp. 591–599), and the mismatch between the needs of people with a chronic condition and what the health system offers (NHC 2007, p. 13).

Other ways in which these challenges can be addressed include improving the health experiences of various disadvantaged groups in Australia and New Zealand; providing public health programs in a more cohesive and non-fragmented manner; adopting a model of practice that recognises the importance of early life factors and their contribution to creating chronic disease in adulthood; using a multifaceted approach involving others outside the healthcare area to

TABLE 1.1
Comparison Between Acute and Chronic Care Models

Acute Model	Chronic Care Model
Disease-centred	Person-centred
Doctor-centred	Team-centred
Focus on individuals	Population health approach
Secondary care emphasis	Primary care emphasis
Reactive, symptom-driven	Proactive, planned intervention
Episodic care	Ongoing care
Cure focus	Prevention/management focus
Single setting: hospital, specialist centres, general practice	Community setting, collaboration across primary and secondary care
1:1 contact through visit by patient	1:1 or group contact through visit by patient or health professional, email, phone or Web contact
Diagnostic information provided	Support for self-management

National Health Committee 2007.

reduce the prevalence of conditions such as obesity and depression to foster social norms of active living; acknowledging the contribution of psychosocial factors, such as resilience and family environment, to chronic disease and the need for multiple strategies to address these factors; and adopting a holistic approach in developing prevention and management strategies (NPHP 2001, p. 2) (Table 1.1).

PRINCIPLES OF PRACTICE

To provide optimal care to a person and their family experiencing a chronic illness and/or disability that ensures all needs are met, a number of key principles of practice must be implemented by nurses in conjunction with other members of the multidisciplinary healthcare team. These principles are to:

- recognise that chronic illness and/or disability affects all dimensions of personhood: physical, psychosocial, emotional, cognitive and spiritual (Guillett 2004; Larsen 2019)
- recognise that cultural responses to illness are important when providing care (Larsen 2019)

- provide holistic care by incorporating a team approach to providing care that is relevant to the needs of the person experiencing the chronic illness and their family (Guillett 2004, p. 19)
- adopt a 'whole of life' approach, recognising that risk factors occur across the lifespan and play a significant role in the development of chronic disease (NPHP 2001, p. 4)
- provide care that is person-centred and inclusive of the family, however the person defines this for themselves (Morris & Edwards 2006).

As you read through the following chapters you will see further expansion and application of these principles that will assist you in your understanding of chronic illness and disability, as applied to the Australian and New Zealand context. The authors discuss critical components related to understanding the experience of chronic illness, such as behaviours that contribute to the development of the condition; the relationship between chronic illness and activities of daily living (ADLs); the impact of body image and identity on the person and their family or carers; issues concerning quality of life; a range of interventions to support restorative function and quality of life; the role of family and carers; and education of the person and family. Case studies are included to support your understanding and cover issues such as culture; complementary and alternative therapies; rehabilitation/facilitation; financial considerations and their impact on the person's life; aspects of stigma; self-efficacy and social isolation; sexuality; the impact of psychosocial dimensions of disease, disability and treatments; spirituality; chronic pain; powerlessness; and the nurse's role in advocacy.

CONCLUSION

This chapter has provided an overview of the gravity of our health needs from a global, Australian and New Zealand perspective. The burden that chronic illness and/or disability currently places, and will continue to place, on our communities is significant. It is important to recognise that with the projected ageing population figures for both countries and the increasing prevalence of modifiable risk factors within our lifestyles and increased survival rates from potentially fatal diseases, chronic disease will emerge as the new epidemic of the twenty-first century. It is unlikely that our communities will be able to sustain health service provision to meet this growing demand. The resources (informal carers, equipment, qualified personnel and finance) required for the management of chronic illness and/or disability

are not found in an endless supply. The challenge for nurses and other health professionals is to provide models of care aimed at preventing, reducing or eliminating modifiable risk factors from their communities' lifestyle in order to halt the growth of this cancer-like phenomenon and to promote sustainable, healthy communities.

Reflective Questions

1. What challenges does the presence of multimorbidity conditions pose when caring for people with chronic disease and/or disability in your nursing practice?

2. How does Australia's NCDs report card compare to the other 194 countries in the WHO 2013–2020 Global Action Plan for the Prevention and Control of NCDs? https://apps.who.int/iris/handle/10665/330805

3. How do you see your role as educator, health promoter and advocator to support people to self-manage their disease and/or disability?

RECOMMENDED READING

Australian Institute of Health and Welfare (AIHW) 2020. Australia's health 2020. Cat. no. AUS 232. AIHW, Canberra.

Ministry of Health NZ 2020. Annual update of key results 2019/2020 New Zealand Health Survey. Online. Available: www.health.govt.nz/publication/annual-update-key-results-2019-20-new-zealand-health-survey

Australian Bureau of Statistics (ABS) 2018. National health survey: first results 2017–18 financial year. Online. Available: www.abs.gov.au

REFERENCES

Australian Bureau of Statistics (ABS) 2019. Microdata: national health survey 2017–18. Cat. no. 4324.0.55.001. ABS, Canberra. Online. Available: www.abs.gov.au/ausstats/abs@.nsf/Lookup/4324.0.55.001main+features12017-18

Australian Bureau of Statistics (ABS) 2015. Disability, ageing and carers, Australia. Cat. no. 4430.0. ABS, Canberra. Online. Available: www.abs.gov.au/ausstats/abs@.nsf/Lookup/4430.0main+features202015

Australian Bureau of Statistics (ABS) 2012. Aboriginal and Torres Strait Islander people with a disability 2012. Cat. no. 4433.0.55.005. ABS, Canberra. Online. Available: www.abs.gov.au/ausstats/abs@.nsf/mf/4433.0.55.005

Australian Government, Department of Health 2017. National Strategic Framework for Chronic Conditions. Online. Available: www.health.gov.au/resources/publications/national-strategic-framework-for-chronic-conditions?utm_source=health.gov.au&utm_medium=callout-auto-custom&utm_campaign=digital_transformation.

Australian Government, Department of Social Services 2014. National Disability Strategy 2010–2020. Online. Available: www.dss.gov.au/our-responsibilities/disability-and-carers/publications-articles/policy-research/national-disability-strategy-2010-2020

Australian Institute of Health and Welfare (AIHW) 2020. Australia's health 2020. Cat. no. Aus 232. AIHW, Canberra. Online. Available: www.aihw.gov.au/australias-health/

Australian Institute of Health and Welfare (AIHW) 2017a. Indigenous observatory: chronic disease. Online. Available: www.aihw.gov.au/indigenous-observatory-chronic-disease/.

Australian Institute of Health and Welfare (AIHW) 2017b. National health priority areas. Online. Available: www.aihw.gov.au/national-health-priority-areas/.

Australian Institute of Health and Welfare (AIHW) 2016. Australia's health 2016. Online. Available: www.aihw.gov.au/australias-health/.

Australian Institute of Health and Welfare (AIHW) 2012. Australia's health 2012. Cat. no. AUS 157. AIHW, Canberra.

Australian Institute of Health and Welfare (AIHW) 2006. Chronic diseases and associated risk factors in Australia 2006. Cat. no. PHE 81. AIHW, Canberra.

Chang E, Johnson A 2008. Chronic illness and disability: principles for practice, 1st edn. Elsevier, Sydney.

Fifty-Fourth World Health Assembly 2001. International classification of functioning, disability and health. Online. Available: http://apps.who.int/gb/archive/pdf_files/WHA54/ea54r21.pdf?ua=1.

Guillett S 2004. Understanding chronic illness and disability. In: LJ Neal, SE Guillett (eds), Care of the adult with a chronic illness or disability: a team approach. Elsevier, St Louis.

Health and Disability System Review 2020. Health and Disability System Review – Final Report – Pūrongo Whakamutunga. HDSR, Wellington. Online. Available: https://systemreview.health.govt.nz/final-report/download-the-final-report/

Johnston M, Crilly M, Black C et al 2019. Defining and measuring multimorbidity: a systematic review of systematic reviews. European Journal of Public Health 29(1), 182–189.

Larsen P 2019. Chronicity. In: PD Larsen (ed.), Lubkin's chronic illness: impact and interventions, 10th edn. Jones and Bartlett Learning, Burlington, MA.

Larsen P 2016. Chronicity. In: PD Larsen (ed.), Lubkin's chronic illness: impact and interventions, 9th edn. Jones and Bartlett Learning, Burlington, MA.

McDonald J, Cumming J, Harris M et al 2006. Systematic review of comprehensive primary care models. Australian Primary Health Care Research Institute, Sydney.

McMurray A, Clendon J 2011. Community health and wellness. Primary health care in practice, 4th edn. Elsevier, Chatswood, NSW.

Ministry of Health (MoH) NZ 2020. Health and disability system review. MoH, Wellington. Online. Available: https://systemreview.health.govt.nz/

Ministry of Health (MoH) NZ 2019. Wai 2575 Māori health trends report. MoH, Wellington.

Ministry of Health (MoH) NZ 2016a. Health loss in New Zealand 1990–2013. Online. Available: www.health.govt.nz/publication/health-loss-new-zealand-1990-2013.

Ministry of Health (MoH) NZ 2016b. Self management support for people with long term conditions, 2nd ed. MoH, Wellington.

Ministry of Health (MoH) NZ 2012. Implementing the New Zealand health strategy 2011. MoH, Wellington. Online. Available: www.health.govt.nz.

Ministry of Health (MoH) NZ 2005. Living with disability in New Zealand: summary. MoH, Wellington. Online. Available: www.moh.govt.nz.

Morris TL, Edwards LD 2006. Family caregivers. In: IM Lubkin, PD Larsen (eds), Chronic illness: impact and interventions, 6th edn. Jones and Bartlett Learning, Sudbury, MA.

National Health Committee 2007. Meeting the needs of people with chronic conditions. Hapai te whanau mo ake ake tonu. National Advisory Committee on Health and Disability, Wellington.

National Health Priority Action Council (NHPAC) 2006. National chronic disease strategy. Australian Government Department of Health and Ageing, Canberra.

National Public Health Partnership (NPHP) 2006. Blueprint for nation-wide surveillance of chronic diseases and associated determinants. NPHP, Melbourne.

National Public Health Partnership (NPHP) 2001. Preventing chronic disease: a strategic framework. Background paper. NPHP, Melbourne.

Parker S, Fuller J 2016. Are nurses well placed as care coordinators in primary care and what is needed to develop their role: a rapid review? Health and Social Care in the Community 24(2), 113–122.

Remsburg RE, Carson B 2006. Rehabilitation. In: IM Lubkin, PD Larsen (eds), Chronic illness: impact and interventions, 6th edn. Jones and Bartlett Learning, Sudbury, MA.

Statistics New Zealand 2015. He hauā Māori: findings from the 2013 Disability Survey. Online. Available: www.stats.govt.nz/browse_for_stats/health/disabilities/He-haua-maori-findings-from-2013-disability-survey/disability-amongst-maori.aspx.

Thomson N, MacRae A, Brankovich J et al 2011. Overview of Australian Indigenous health status 2011. Australian Indigenous HealthInfoNet. Online. Available: www.healthinfonet.ecu.edu.au.

World Health Organization 2020. Noncommunicable diseases: progress monitor 2020. WHO, Geneva. https://apps.who.int/iris/handle/10665/330805.

World Health Organization (WHO) 2017. Integrated chronic disease prevention and control. Online. Available: www.who.int/chp/about/integrated_cd/en/.

World Health Organization (WHO) 2014. WHO Global Status report on non-communicable diseases. Online. Available: http://whqlibdoc.who.int/publications/2011/9789240686458_eng.pdf.

World Health Organization (WHO) 2013. Global action plan

for the prevention and control of non communicable diseases 2013–2020. Online. Available: www.who.int/nmh/publications/ncd-action-plan/en/.

World Health Organization (WHO) 2011. World report on disability. Online. Available: www.who.int/disabilities/world_report/2011/report.pdf.

World Health Organization (WHO) 2008. 2008–2013 action plan for the global strategy for the prevention and control of noncommunicable diseases. Online. Available: www.who.int/nmh/publications/ncd_action_plan_en.pdf.

World Health Organization (WHO) 2005. Preparing a health-care workforce for the 21st century. The challenge of chronic conditions. Online. Available: www.who.int/chp/chronic-disease-report/en/index.html.

CHAPTER 2

Partnerships in Collaborative Care

SUE RANDALL • SHARON CROXFORD • VANESSA J. RICE • MICHAEL K. BAKER
• ANGELICA G. THOMPSON-BUTEL • GEOFFREY MITCHELL • JOEL RHEE
• MICHELLE BISSETT • LEE ZAKRZEWSKI • LIAM LANGFORD
• GRAHAM MUNRO • GISSELLE GALLEGO • ANTHONY WRIGHT
• MARK HUGHES • HILARY GALLAGHER • BELINDA KENNY

LEARNING OBJECTIVES

When you have completed this chapter you will be able to:

- appreciate the roles and scope of practice offered by health professionals and other agencies and services, in the provision of evidence-based care
- recognise the central presence of the individual and their family in the determination of care priorities in conjunction with the team
- comprehend the importance of a team approach and the need for change in response to an individual's needs
- understand the nature of collaborative partnerships and effective communication to provide care to people with complex needs and achieve optimal outcomes
- reflect on the nurse's scope of practice in managing chronic disease and disability across a range of settings.

KEY WORDS

collaboration	partnerships
goal setting	team
nurse's role	

INTRODUCTION

This chapter describes frequently encountered roles that are required to support the delivery of contemporary practice in the care of individuals with a chronic illness and/or disability. The provision of contemporary practice necessitates the adoption of a team approach, which brings together in partnership a range of health professionals and other agencies and services. The nature of this partnership is one of collaboration and goal setting to see that optimal outcomes are achieved for the individual and their family. Determination of these outcomes is based on the use of evidence-based practice and the collective learnings of each of the team members to see what might be possible; to consider new ways of doing or set up innovative

ways to manage. The complexity of need that exists for many people experiencing a chronic illness or disability is significant and changing. This may mean that the leader of the team changes and that it is not necessarily medically driven. However, it is recognised that most care in this context is coordinated through the nurse, who is frequently the constant in the lives of the individual. Young and colleagues (2016) identified key themes for how nurses engage with individuals, which are highly translatable to multiple settings. The themes are: time, ambiance and the dimensions of therapeutic relationships; education and clinical knowledge (pp. 912–916). It is also recognised that the composition of the 'team' may need to change as the needs of individuals with a chronic illness and/or disability also change, requiring different professionals, agencies or services to be involved.

Working collaboratively and drawing on the skills and expertise of others offers the capacity to respond to the changing needs of a person with chronic illness and/or disability and their family. The partnerships created between the person and their family with the various members of the team enable the person and their health needs to be the central priority. The team seeks to resolve issues for the person and their family by determining a shared goal of care, involving a number of strategies that are not discipline-specific, but rather conceptualised from knowledge and experience to best suit the needs of the individual.

The delivery of high-quality care uses team meetings and patient/family conferences to share information and discuss possible ways of achieving an optimal outcome for the person requiring care and their family (ACN 2019; Pierce & Lutz 2013).

Effective communication is key to achieving the goals determined by the team in collaboration with the person. The nurse is equal to all other members of the interdisciplinary/multidisciplinary team and is most likely to be the primary carer in the majority of health or home settings (ACN 2019). As a result, the nurse will often assume a coordination role within the team to bring together the other health professionals. Having the primary carer assume this coordination role directly benefits the person and their family by bringing together the wealth of knowledge, experience and skills in the planning of a range of interventions to manage the issues arising for people with chronic illness and/or disability. This role is also pivotal in ensuring that the interventions and solutions implemented are evaluated on an ongoing basis and to recognise that as people's needs change so does the plan of care.

This chapter aims to describe the scope of practice undertaken by these frequently encountered roles and their contribution to supporting a person with a chronic illness and/or disability.

This chapter begins with a description of the nurse's role followed by the dietitian, exercise physiologist, general practitioner, occupational therapist, paramedic, pharmacist, physiotherapist, social worker and speech pathologist.

In this chapter the terms 'interdisciplinary' and 'multidisciplinary' are used interchangeably by the various authors to enable both approaches to care to be illustrated and contextualised, depending upon the needs of the person and their family.

REFERENCES

Australian College of Nursing (ACN) 2019. The role of nurses in chronic disease prevention and management in rural and remote areas – position statement. ACN, Canberra.

Pierce LL, Lutz BJ 2013. Family caregivers. In: IM Lubkin, PD Larsen (eds), Chronic illness, impact and interventions, 8th edn. Mass Jones and Bartlett Learning, Burlington.

Young J, Eley D, Patterson E et al 2016. A nurse-led model of chronic disease management in general practice. Patient's Perspectives 45(12), 912–916.

Role of the Nurse

Sue Randall

The importance of managing people who live with chronic illness or disability has become the focus of public health internationally as rates of both have risen (Askerud & Conder 2017). The role of the nurse is central for successful management across any healthcare setting. The Australian College of Nursing (2019) describes nurses as integral in both prevention and management of chronic disease, thus ensuring optimal health outcomes for people across the lifespan.

Focusing on management of people, there are many models of care that exist. Some models place a greater emphasis on the role of the nurse and include care coordination, case management and nurse-led clinics (Randall, Daly et al 2014; Randall, Crawford et al 2017). Other models have a multidisciplinary approach, in which the nurse is a member of a wider team: shared care, integrated care, chronic care model, collaborative care. Typically the nurse will have a coordination role. Care coordination helps people to access care that integrates across all providers with the goal of improving health outcomes while containing health costs (Centre for Primary Care and Equity 2017). Coordination requires effective communication, a knowledge of local systems and an understanding of the local community (Centre for Primary Care and Equity 2017). Coordination draws on collaborative partnerships across disciplines and teams, including with the person living with a chronic condition and/or family as well as other healthcare professionals and organisations outside of health. Successful coordination requires a nurse to have core skills which are transferable between people living with a chronic illness or disability, regardless of the specific nature of the disease or disability. Focusing on the person living with a chronic condition is central to achieving optimal health outcomes that focus on goals that matter to the person (National Voices UK 2013).

The Chronic Care Model (Wagner et al 1996) advocated moving away from the traditional model of acute care to one that focused on the long-term episodic nature of chronic conditions. The nurse's role in coordination fits this model. While a nurse can take the title of care coordinator they can also be referred to as a care navigator. Hudson and colleagues (2019) describe a care navigator as a nurse who understands the complex health system, which, added to their knowledge of patients and carers, allows a clear sense of direction in care to be developed. A nurse with a coordinator role can also be named a community matron or a case/care manager. In a meta-synthesis of 15 qualitative studies on patients' experiences of case management, Askerud and Conder (2017) reported that good communication was important to patients and continuity of care provided by the nurse case manager was highly valued. The ability of the nurse case manager to coordinate care from other professionals, in health and beyond, was seen as making all the involved services more useful to the user with chronic conditions.

Effective communication enables successful care coordination and can result in improved equity and access to services in line with principles of primary healthcare (World Health Organization [WHO] 2003). Communication, in part, relies on assessment of a patient's health literacy. Health literacy is about how people understand information about health and healthcare and how they apply that information to their lives by using it to make and act on decisions (Australian Commission on Safety and Quality in Health Care [ACSQHC] 2019). It forms part of the role of the nurse to work with patients to develop health literacy and to assume poor health literacy in all and to deploy universal precautions. Treating everyone as having poor health literacy offers a safety net to catch those in need of more help, because even people with good education and general literacy can be challenged by healthcare information (Cornett 2019). Strategies the nurse can employ include: using plain language about information in a format that is easy to understand; speaking clearly and at a moderate pace; and offering help to all patients who need to fill in forms (Cornett 2019). A specific and successful strategy for managing appointment non-attendance in patients from culturally and linguistically diverse (CALD) backgrounds is reported by Randall, Thunhurst and Furze (2016). A case manager liaised with agencies to place an 'x' on the back of appointment letters. On receipt, the patient knew to contact the case manager, who, with consent, would read the letter, explain and help them to make any arrangements as needed (Randall, Thunhurst et al 2016). The case manager was noted as engendering high levels of confidence and trust in patients and their carers.

Improving levels of confidence in people living with long-term conditions is an important nursing skill as confidence is critical to a person's ability to self-manage their condition(s). The importance of confidence, also known as self-efficacy, is the basis of Bandura's social learning theory (Bandura 1977, 1986, 1985). In essence, the majority of people will avoid taking on tasks such as self-management of their chronic condition(s) if they believe it is beyond their capabilities, or if the expected outcome does not provide sufficient reward for the amount of effort they put in. Part of the role of the nurse in managing people with chronic conditions or disability is to work with them to build self-efficacy. The development of mutually agreed goals that pool the expertise of nurse and patient in concordance (defined as 'the process of developing a mutually agreed care plan [Snowden & Marland, 2013]') is evidence of true partnership working (Randall & Neubeck 2016). To achieve concordance, language choice by nurses is another important factor to defuse power imbalances and create active partnerships (Randall & Neubeck 2016). Furthermore, Bodenheimer and colleagues (2002), in their seminal work, state the importance of healthcare professionals acknowledging individuality, and the unique circumstances that make up patients' lives as requirements for developing partnerships that lead to optimum health outcomes. After all, it is a fundamental human right for a person to participate in their own healthcare (WHO 1986).

REFERENCES

Askerud A, Conder J 2017. Patients' experiences of nurse case management in primary care: a meta-synthesis. Australian Journal of Primary Health 23, 420–428.

Australian College of Nursing 2019. The role of nurses in chronic disease prevention and management in rural and remote areas. Collegian 26(5), 605–606.

Australian Commission on Safety and Quality in Health Care (ACSQHC) 2019. Health literacy. Online. Available: www.safetyandquality.gov.au/our-work/patient-and-consumer-centred-care/health-literacy

Bandura A (ed.) 1995. Self-efficacy in changing societies. Cambridge University Press, NY.

Bandura A 1986. Social foundations of thought and action: a social cognitive theory. Prentice Hall, Englewood Cliffs.

Bandura A 1977. Self-efficacy: toward a unifying theory of behavioural change. Psychological Review 84, 191–215.

Bodenheimer T, Lorig, K Holman H et al 2002. Patient self-management of chronic disease in primary care. Journal of American Medical Association (JAMA) 288(19), 2469–2475.

Centre for Primary Health Care and Equity, University of NSW 2017. Rapid review: integrated care interventions: final report. NSW Ministry of Health, Sydney.

Cornett S 2019. Assessing and addressing health literacy. OJIN: The Online Journal of Issues in Nursing 14(3) manuscript 2. DOI: 10.3912/OIJN.Vol14No03Man2

Hudson A, Spooner A, Booth N et al 2019. Qualitative insights of parents and carers under the care of nurse navigators. Collegian 26, 110–117.

National Voices UK 2013. A narrative for person-centred coordinated care. Online. Available: www.england.nhs.uk/wp-content/uploads/2013/05/nv-narrative-cc.pdf.

Randall S, Crawford T, Currie J et al 2017. Impact of community based nurse-led clinics on patient outcomes, patient satisfaction, patient access and cost effectiveness: a systematic review. International Journal of Nursing Studies 73, 24–33.

Randall S, Daly G, Thunhurst C et al 2014. Case management of individuals with long-term conditions by community matrons: report of qualitative findings of a mixed methods evaluation. Primary Health Care and Research 15(1), 26–37.

Randall S, Neubeck L 2016. What's in a name? Concordance is better than adherence for promoting partnership and self-management of chronic disease. Australian Journal of Primary Health 22(3), 181–184.

Randall S, Thunhurst C, Furze G 2016. Community matrons as problem-solvers for people living with co-morbid disease. British Journal of Community Nursing 21(12), 563–567.

Snowden A, Marland G 2013. No decision about me without me: concordance operationalized. Journal of Clinical Nursing 22, 1353–1360.

Wagner E, Austin B, Von Korff M. Organizing care for patients with chronic illness. Millbank Quarterly 1996 (74), 511–544.

World Health Organization (WHO) 2003. The World Health Report: the core principles of primary health care. Online. Available: www.who.int/whr/2003/chapter7/en/index1.html.

World Health Organization (WHO) 1986. Ottawa Charter for Health Promotion: First International Conference on Health Promotion Ottawa, 21 November 1986. Online. Available: www.healthpromotion.org.au/images/ottawa_charter_hp.pdf.

Role of the Dietitian

Sharon Croxford

Effective interdisciplinary/multidisciplinary teams understand the roles of other disciplines, provide appropriate screening and assessment, and know when to refer and how to best work together with other healthcare professionals to improve health outcomes for people. In both acute and community settings the dietitian is part of a professional interdisciplinary/multidisciplinary team that aims to prevent, treat, manage and improve population, community and individual health. Dietitians are specialists in human nutrition, the metabolic, physiological and psychological responses to food, and the impact of food intake and nutritional status on health and wellbeing.

In Australia, the Accredited Practising Dietitian (APD) credential is recognised by Dietitians Australia (DA). A graduate of a DA-accredited university course can apply to become a member of the DA and an APD. In New Zealand, dietitians who hold a current certificate under the *Health Practitioners Competence Assurance Act* (2003) are eligible to become professional members of Dietitians NZ.

All dietitians are nutritionists; however, nutritionists without a dietetics qualification cannot take on the expert role of a dietitian (DA 2020a). A dietitian's primary aim is to improve individual, community and population health and wellbeing through food. They assist people to understand the relationship between food and health, and how to make beneficial food choices. Nutrition advice is in strong demand, given the increase in the incidence of diet-related diseases, which often lead to chronic illness and disability (Wahlqvist 2011). A dietitian uses a range of skills to assess nutrition status, identify specific food and nutrition-related problems, determine a nutrition diagnosis, and plan, counsel, motivate and support individuals and communities to achieve better health outcomes.

Dietitians work in a range of settings and with people of all ages. They may work in clinical nutrition, community and public health nutrition, nutrition and food service management, sports nutrition, nutrition education and advocacy, nutrition research, government policy, the food industry and hospitality sector, or as private practitioners. Dietetic practice will vary with each setting and often includes individual assessment, education and prevention. Dietitians have to deal with a range of scenarios from developmental anomalies to acute care, the ongoing management of chronic and debilitating conditions, through to peak athletic performance and improving quality of life and physical function in older adults. With the rise in diet-related diseases, dietitians are often engaged as public health nutritionists, working at the local community level or at national or international level to design and implement health improvement programs aimed at decreasing the risk factors associated with diet-related chronic and preventable diseases.

A clinical dietitian works with people with particular medical conditions and is responsible for all aspects of nutrition care and nutrition intervention. This may include assessing the need for a therapeutic or special diet, such as a gluten-free diet for coeliac disease, or modified texture for clients experiencing dysphagia. It may also include making recommendations to medical staff for biochemical tests, nutrition supplements and modes of feeding such as enteral feeding and total parenteral nutrition (TPN). Dietitians are great resources for other disciplines, organisations, patients/clients and caregivers. In a clinical setting, they provide appropriate advice on food and nutrition for the interdisciplinary/multidisciplinary team, the patient and their family, and this may include enteral and parental, as well as oral nutrition. Dietitians help translate technical information into practical advice on food and eating (DA 2020b).

Nutrition challenges tend to fall into two areas: (1) malnutrition risk and undernutrition, such as failure to thrive, growth retardation, significant weight loss in the elderly; and (2) obesity, metabolic disorders and chronic disease. Poor nutrition-related health habits, limited access to services, and long-term use of multiple medications are considered health risk factors in individuals with disability and/or chronic disease (Academy of Nutrition and Dietetics 2015).

Nurses play a key role in screening for nutrition risk factors. There are several valid and reliable tools for identifying undernutrition such as the Malnutrition Screening Tool (MST) (Ferguson et al 1999) and the Malnutrition Universal Screening Tool (MUST) (Malnutrition Advisory Group 2003). Consider a referral to a dietitian if your patients/clients require assistance with any of the following:

- mealtime support, cutting up food
- dysphasia, difficulty chewing, ill-fitting dentures
- food–medicine interactions
- poor appetite, taste or smell changes, nausea, vomiting
- enteral or parenteral feeding.
  A dietitian will undertake a nutritional assessment by:
- assessing anthropometrical measures, e.g. height, weight, waist circumference
- interpreting biochemical and haematological indicators
- conducting a clinical and physical assessment
- determining dietary intake, e.g. diet history
- assessing environmental factors that affect food intake and nutritional status.

Integration of all this information will determine an individual, community or population's nutrition status. For individuals, the dietitian makes a nutrition diagnosis following the assessment and works with the client/patient (and/or their carer) to formulate a plan of management. The client/patient will receive personalised advice tailored to their specific health and food requirements. The dietitian will assist with meal and menu planning, recipe modification, referral to cooking classes, reading food labels and communicating important health promotion messages to assist optimisation of individual health. Timely and cost-effective nutrition interventions can promote health maintenance and reduce the risk and cost of co-morbidities and complications (Academy of Nutrition and Dietetics 2015).

As part of the dietetic care process, dietitians use a range of reference standards to analyse, modify and plan individual diets and food service menus to treat specific diet-related conditions and promote healthy eating.

NUTRITIONAL ANTHROPOMETRIC REFERENCE VALUES

Height-for-age, weight-for-age, weight-for-height ratios and body mass index (BMI) are the most common anthropometric tools used to assess growth and fat mass. In children there is an expected range in variation, often referred to as a percentile. For example, the 50th percentile represents the median weight (or height) as the value below which the heights and weights of 50% of healthy children are expected to fall. BMI (weight in kg divided by the square of height in metres) is used as a measure of fat mass. It is the most common indicator to assess nutritional status (Wahlqvist 2011) in adults. BMI-for-age percentiles are now commonly used to predict body fat in children over 2 years of age.

BIOCHEMICAL VALUES

Serum biochemical assessments can be useful indicators of nutritional status and often signify the degree and severity of the disease process. Analysis of biochemical values is used in conjunction with clinical, medical and dietary histories, nutrition impact symptoms, such as nausea and vomiting, and body composition, to help monitor management and progress in specific conditions.

FOOD COMPOSITION DATABASES

Food composition tables are used to convert information about food intake to nutrient intake (Wahlqvist 2011). In Australia, the reference database is the Australian Food Composition Database (formerly known as

NUTTAB), where much of the data comes from analysis of over 1500 foods available in Australia. The New Zealand Food Composition Database contains food composition data on 2700 commonly prepared and eaten foods in New Zealand. Both databases provide useful summaries of nutrient data for commonly consumed foods (FSANZ 2019; New Zealand Institute for Plant and Food Research Ltd, Ministry of Health (NZ) 2019).

NUTRIENT REFERENCE VALUE

Nutrient reference values (NRVs) are recommendations for nutrient intake, published by the National Health and Medical Research Council for Australia and New Zealand (NHMRC 2017). NRVs are determined for healthy populations and consist of a range of reference terms, including estimated energy requirement, estimated average requirement (EAR); a nutrient level estimated to meet the daily requirements of 50% of the population, and recommended dietary intake (RDI); and an average nutrient intake that would meet the daily requirements of 97–98% of the population. NRVs also include guidance on the upper level of intake (UL) for nutrients, where intake above the UL increases the potential risk of adverse health effects (NHMRC 2017). NRVs are particular to life stage and gender.

When working with individuals, dietitians will use this information to develop and implement plans for the nutritional care of individuals during acute and chronic illness. In residential food service settings, menus are designed to meet the NRVs of the people with the greatest nutrient needs, at the same time as sensory appealing and safe food. When working at a population level, dietitians assess nutrient requirements and influence policy regarding food supply.

AUSTRALIAN DIETARY GUIDELINES

Dietitians also use the Australian Dietary Guidelines as a practical way of educating people about the general principles of healthy eating. The Australian Dietary Guidelines and the user-friendly resource *Australian Guide to Healthy Eating* apply to healthy people and those with common diet-related conditions, such as being overweight (NHMRC 2013). They are based on good-quality research and provide useful information on the types and quantities of food that will promote health and wellbeing, for use by health professionals and educators (NHMRC 2013).

CONCLUSION

As the largest health professional group in Australia, nurses play a key role in delivering healthcare services to people with disabilities, including disease prevention, detection and treatment (Academy of Nutrition and Dietetics 2015; Trollor et al 2016). Working alongside dietitians as part of the interdisciplinary/multidisciplinary team, solutions to food and nutrition-related problems can be developed to achieve the best possible health outcomes for every individual. All team members play an important role in observing and communicating with one another when determining priorities and plans, assessing signs of progress or complications and therefore working together towards maximising health outcomes for all.

Acknowledgements

The author would like to acknowledge the work of Liz Isenring and Annette James, who contributed to the previous edition.

RECOMMENDED READING

Mann J, Truswell AS 2017. Essentials of human nutrition, 5th edn. Oxford University Press, Oxford.
Whitney E, Rolfes S R, Crowe T et al 2019. Understanding nutrition: Australian and New Zealand edition. 4th edn Cengage Learning, Melbourne.

REFERENCES

Academy of Nutrition and Dietetics 2015. Position of the Academy of Nutrition and Dietetics: nutrition services for individuals with intellectual and developmental disabilities and special health care needs. Journal of the Academy of Nutrition and Dietetics 115, 593–608.
Dietitians Australia (DA) 2020a. Dietitian or nutritionist? Online. Available: https://dietitiansaustralia.org.au/what-dietitans-do/dietitian-or-nutritionist/.
Dietitians Australia (DA) 2020b. National competency standards for dietitians. Online. Available: https://dietitiansaustralia.org.au/maintaining-professional-standards/.
Ferguson M, Capra S, Bauer J et al 1999. Development of a valid and reliable malnutrition screening tool for adult acute hospital patients. Nutrition 15, 458–464.
Food Standards Australia New Zealand (FSANZ) 2013. Australian food composition database. Online. Available: www.foodstandards.gov.au/science/monitoringnutrients/afcd/Pages/default.aspx.
Malnutrition Advisory Group (MAG): A Standing Committee of the British Association for Parenteral and Enteral Nutrition (BAPEN) 2003. The 'MUST' explanatory booklet. A guide to the 'Malnutrition Universal Screening Tool' ('MUST') for adults: BAPEN.

National Health and Medical Research Council (NHMRC) 2013. Australian dietary guidelines. Online. Available: www.nhmrc.gov.au/guidelines-publications/n55.

National Health and Medical Research Council (NHMRC) 2017. What are nutrient reference values? Online. Available: www.nrv.gov.au/node/50.

New Zealand Institute for Plant and Food Research, Ministry of Health NZ 2019. New Zealand food composition data. Online. Available: www.foodcomposition.co.nz.

Trollor JN, Eagleson C, Turner B et al 2016. Intellectual disability health content within nursing curriculum: an audit of what our future nurses are taught. Nurse Education Today 45, 72–79.

Wahlqvist M (ed.) 2011. Food and nutrition: food and health systems in Australia and New Zealand, 3rd edn. Allen & Unwin, Crows Nest, NSW.

Role of the Exercise Physiologist

Vanessa J. Rice, Michael K. Baker and Angelica G. Thompson-Butel

ACCREDITED EXERCISE PHYSIOLOGISTS

An accredited exercise physiologist (AEP) is an allied health professional who specialises in the delivery of exercise for the prevention and management of chronic diseases and injuries (ESSA 2018). AEPs are university qualified and accredited by Exercise and Sports Science Australia (ESSA). They provide support for clients with conditions such as cardiovascular disease; metabolic disease; mental health conditions; cancer; bone, muscle and joint conditions; pulmonary disease and more. AEPs are eligible to register and work in the compensable healthcare systems, including Medicare, Department of Veterans' Affairs, most private health insurance companies, as well as workers' compensation regulatory bodies.

AEPs incorporate other disciplines such as anatomy, motor control, biomechanics, biochemistry, molecular biology and biophysics into this study. This knowledge is needed to understand the natural laws of structure and function of the body and the interrelationship of these disciplines. Furthermore, AEPs use their knowledge of frequency, intensity and duration, as well as environmental factors, nutrition and the physiological status of the individual, to guide their clinical decision-making for the most effective exercise prescription to achieve the expected body's response to exercise. It is this physiological understanding that positions the AEP as an expert in exercise prescription.

CLINICAL ROLE

AEPs use their knowledge of pathophysiology and timeline of disease, contraindications, special considerations and safety precautions to implement safe, effective and individualised exercise programs and lifestyle interventions for clients, using the best available evidence for chronic and complex conditions. When working with these populations, an AEP's focus is on the specific needs of each individual with the aim to empower them to become more independent and manage their own health and wellbeing. In the healthcare system, the AEP's main roles of assessment, exercise prescription, education, physical activity advice, self-management support and referral, are driven by strong clinical decision-making and clinical expertise. They maintain an important role within multidisciplinary teams (e.g. nurses, physicians and other allied health team members) to provide individualised, effective and safe patient-centred care.

The role of the AEP in working with all patients is to provide expertise in various aspects of exercise prescription. This process includes a comprehensive assessment of cardiovascular fitness and functional capacity, tailoring exercise prescription to prevent cardiovascular events, secondary complications, manage symptoms, improve function, enhance independence and promote reintegration into society (return to work, study, travel, social, and everyday activities). These programs also include strength and conditioning, balance/fall prevention, gait re-training, as well as recreational/sport skills re-training. They can be part of community-based programs, ongoing lifestyle management programs, prevention programs and hospital-based programs. AEPs also utilise lifestyle change strategies and behaviour modification strategies to support an individual to incorporate exercise as part of a healthy lifestyle.

WHERE DO AEPS WORK?

AEPs practise in a wide variety of settings. They work in public and private hospitals, primary, secondary and tertiary healthcare, private and multidisciplinary clinics, occupational rehabilitation settings, workplace health and rehabilitation, GP clinics, residential aged care and retirement facilities, research institutes and sport settings. They work across the lifespan, prescribing individualised programs for clients ranging from paediatric to elderly patients. With more demands on healthcare expenditure, innovative roles (e.g. AEPs working as conduits to assist cardiopulmonary clients to transition into community gym settings) can be a cost- and time-efficient way to improve health outcomes of clients. Such programs can reduce waiting lists for hospital-based programs, improve physical health outcomes beyond those gains in hospital outpatient programs, reduce depression signs and symptoms, and reduce emergency department attendance and hospital presentation (Deloitte Access Economics 2015, 2016).

COMMON CONDITIONS

If exercise could be packed into a pill, it would be the single most widely prescribed and beneficial medicine in the nation.

Dr Robert Butler, National Institute on Aging 2005

Decades of research have revealed exercise to be a potent medicine for the prevention and management of chronic disease, with new evidence constantly emerging. Exercise improves blood glucose control in both those with, or at risk of, type 2 diabetes (Hordern et al 2012; Jadhav et al 2017; Yanai et al 2018). There is a wealth of evidence about the effect of exercise on cardiovascular conditions, cutting the risk of heart disease in half (Nocon et al 2008; Zachariah, Alex 2017). There is a growing body of evidence to support the use of exercise in the management of mental health conditions (Rethorst 2019; Rosenbaum, Tiedemann, Sherrington et al 2014; Rosenbaum, Tiedemann, Stanton et al 2016). Guidelines for hip and knee osteoarthritis recommend exercise and weight management as the best non-pharmacological and non-surgical practice options in the long term and for cost-effectiveness (McAlindon et al 2014; Roos & Juhl 2012). Exercise is considered a safe and effective treatment for people with cancer, counteracting many of the adverse treatment-related side effects (Hayes et al 2019; Segal et al 2017). Exercise and regular physical activity are the most effective strategies to maximise peak bone mass and to reduce the risk of falls and fractures later in life (Sherrington et al 2017; Tiedeman et al 2011).

CONCLUSION

The importance of prevention for chronic disease management should not be overlooked. There is in-depth research to support a strong inverse relationship between all-cause mortality and exercise (Gebel et al 2015;

Kodama et al 2009; Lear et al 2017). The Australian physical activity guidelines recommend 150–300 minutes of moderate or 75–150 minutes of vigorous activity each week (Brown et al 2012). The role of the AEP to engage with individuals through education and exercise uptake should be espoused. Engagement of an AEP at first signs of risk factors (i.e. hypertension, hypercholesterolemia or overweight) should be part of the healthcare plan.

The management of complex and chronic disease is a challenge and burden on the healthcare system. Engaging and supporting patients through self-managed care will provide better outcomes for the individual. The use of a multidisciplinary team with expertise, evidence-based practice and a patient focus will offer the best outcomes for an individual. AEPs are an integral part of the multidisciplinary team to provide targeted exercise prescription and achieve the best possible outcomes needed for chronic disease management and/or injury.

RECOMMENDED READING

American College of Sports Medicine 2017. ACSM's guidelines for exercise testing and prescription, 10th edn. Wolters Kluwer, Philadelphia.

American College of Sports Medicine 2016. ACSM's exercise management for persons with chronic disease and disabilities, 4th edn. Human Kinetics, Champaign, IL.

Ehrman JK, Gordon PM, Visich PS et al 2018. Clinical exercise physiology, 4th ed. Human Kinetics, Champaign, IL.

Exercise is Medicine Australia. Online. Available: www.exerciseismedicine.org.au.

REFERENCES

Brown WJ, Bauman AE, Burton NW 2012. Development of evidence-based physical activity recommendations for adults (18–64 years). Australian Government, Department of Health, Canberra.

Deloitte Access Economics 2016. The value of accredited exercise physiologists to consumers in Australia. Report for Exercise and Sport Science Australia, Canberra.

Deloitte Access Economics 2015. Value of accredited exercise physiologists in Australia. Report for Exercise and Sport Science Australia, Canberra.

Exercise and Sports Science Australia 2018. Accredited exercise physiologist scope of practice. Online. Available: www.essa.org.au/wp-content/uploads/2018/04/AEP-scope-of-practice_2018.pdf

Gebel K, Ding D, Chey T et al 2015. Effect of moderate to vigorous physical activity on all-cause mortality in middle-aged and older Australians. Journal of the American Medical Association 175(6), 970–977.

Hayes SC, Newton RU, Spence RR et al 2019. The Exercise and Sport Science Australia position statement: exercise medicine in cancer management. Journal of Science and Medicine in Sport 22(11), 1175–1199.

Hordern MD, Dustan DW, Prins JB et al 2012. Exercise prescription for patients with type 2 diabetes and pre-diabetes: a position statement from Exercise and Sport Science Australia. Journal of Science and Medicine in Sport 15(1), 25–31.

Jadhav RA, Hazari A, Monterio A et al 2017. Effect of physical activity intervention in prediabetes: a systematic review with meta-analysis. Journal of Physical Activity and Health 14, 745–755.

Kodama S, Saito K, Tanaka S et al 2009. Cardiorespiratory fitness as a quantitative predictor of all-cause mortality and cardiovascular events in healthy men and women: a meta-analysis. JAMA 301(19), 2024–2035.

Lear SA, Hu W, Rangarjan S et al 2017. The effect of physical activity on mortality and cardiovascular disease in 130 000 people from 17 high-income, middle-income, and low-income countries: the PURE study. Lancet 390(10113), 2643–2654.

McAlindon TE, Bannuru RR, Sullivan MC et al 2014. OARSI guidelines for the non-surgical management of knee osteoarthritis. Osteoarthritis and Cartilage 22(3), 363–388.

Nocon M, Hiemann T, Muller-Riemenschneider F et al 2008. Association of physical activity with all-cause and cardiovascular mortality: a systematic review and meta-analysis. European Journal of Cardiovascular Prevention and Rehabilitation 15, 239–246.

Rethorst CD 2019. Effects of exercise on depression and other mental disorders. In: MH Anshel, SJ Petruzzello SJ, EE Labbé (eds), APA handbooks in psychology series. APA handbook of sport and exercise psychology, Vol. 2. Exercise psychology. American Psychological Association, Washington.

Roos EM, Juhl CB 2012. Osteoarthritis 2012 year in review: rehabilitation and outcomes. Osteoarthritis and Cartilage 20, 1477–1483.

Rosenbaum S, Tiedemann A, Sherrington C et al 2014. Physical activity intervention for people with mental illness: a systematic review and meta-analysis. The Journal of Clinical Psychiatry 75(9), 964–974.

Rosenbaum S, Tiedemann A, Stanton R et al 2016. Implementing evidence-based physical activity interventions for people with mental illness: an Australian perspective. Australasian Psychiatry 24(1), 49–54.

Segal R, Zwaal C, Green E et al 2017. Exercise for people with cancer: a systematic review. Current Oncology 24(4), e290–2315.

Sherrington C, Michaleff ZA, Fairhall N et al 2017. Exercise to prevent falls in older adults: an updated systematic review and meta-analysis. British Journal of Sports Medicine 51, 1750–1758.

Tiedemann A, Sherrington C, Close JCT et al 2011. Exercise and Sports Science Australia position statement on exercise and falls prevention in older people. Journal of Science and Medicine in Sport 14(6), 489–495.

Yanai H, Adachi H, Masui Y et al 2018. Exercise therapy for patients with type 2 diabetes: a narrative review. Journal of Clinical Medicine Research 10(5), 365–369.

Zachariah G, Alex AG 2017. Exercise for prevention of cardiovascular disease, evidence-based recommendations. Journal of Clinical and Preventative Cardiology 6(3), 109–114.

NOTE

Exercise and Sports Science Australia (ESSA) is the self-regulating peak professional body for AEPs in Australia. All AEPs have to meet ESSA's standards, have recognised qualifications, and complete continuing education in order to be accredited and to practise as an AEP.

Role of the Medical Practitioner

Geoffrey Mitchell and Joel Rhee

The medical practitioner, along with the other health professionals, assists the patient to achieve their goals in self-care. Clearly, the role of medical practitioners is to identify medical and other problems and, in concert with the patient, devise strategies to manage them. Problems identified may require a medical intervention, such as a drug or an operation. However, many of the problems will require other assistance to manage them. This may involve health education, reassurance, allied health support, the arrangement of aids for daily living or attendance to psychological or spiritual issues. This is a very complex role (Stewart et al 2014) and often requires input from multiple professionals. Comprehensive care such as this necessitates the development of a clinical care plan. Such planning requires care coordination. Because of the longitudinal care that general practitioners (GPs) provide, such coordination is effectively their role. GPs, also known as family physicians or primary care physicians, are medical practitioners who have completed several years of specialist training for practice in primary care settings. In addition to GPs, medical practitioners of various specialties may be called upon to coordinate care in their particular sphere (e.g. oncologists in a cancer care team; a rehabilitation physician in a rehabilitation team).

However, this overarching role of the GP does depend on their role in the health system, which differs from country to country. In the United Kingdom, Canada, Australia, New Zealand, Singapore, the Netherlands and most Scandinavian countries, for example, the GPs function as 'gatekeepers' to the healthcare system, which means referrals to specialist care take place via them. In other countries, GPs do not have a 'gatekeeper' role. They are but one of many medical specialties to whom a patient can present directly. In these settings, the GP is very likely not to have longitudinal knowledge or continuity of care of their patients, so are often not involved in care coordination.

The care coordination role of GPs and the primary care sector leads to better outcomes. Starfield and colleagues have shown conclusively that the health of a nation's population is directly proportional to the degree to which the primary care sector is valued and resourced (1991, 1994; Macinko et al 2003), and more recent work (Basu et al 2019) still bears this out. One of the main reasons for this is that the absence of a central role for primary care may mean that no one coordinates care, with the result that some elements of care are duplicated and others are missed out on altogether. The patient and their family suffer as a result.

The funding of GP services can influence the conduct of multidisciplinary care. In Australia until 1999, GPs were funded by Medicare (Australia's universal public health insurance system) on a fee-for-service basis only, and no substitution of services by other health professionals on behalf of the GP was permitted. That is, the GP had to see the patient and deliver the service personally in order to attract government-supported payments. Practice staff could not render the service for them. This was in sharp contrast to the UK, which paid a per capita fee to each general practice to deliver primary care services to a defined group of patients, with additional incentive payments for meeting certain health targets (e.g. a percentage of patients immunised for influenza annually). Teamwork in this setting is clearly encouraged (Weller & Maynard 2004).

Since 1999, there has been a marked shift towards multidisciplinary care. Australian health planners recognised that comprehensive care cannot be delivered by GPs working in isolation, and funding models had to shift to accommodate this. Health outcomes are better when patients are cared for in teams, with purposive planning of the care. For example, in the care of chronic obstructive pulmonary disease (COPD), a Cochrane Systematic Review showed that patients have improved disease-specific quality of life and exercise capacity, and reduced hospital admissions, when they are treated by multidisciplinary teams (Kruis et al 2013). A systematic review of GP–specialist integration programs shows modest clinical gains, but higher patient satisfaction with integration of GPs and specialist teams (Mitchell, Burridge et al 2015).

The same systematic review identified six requirements for successful integration:
- interdisciplinary teamwork
- communication/information exchange
- shared care guidelines or pathways
- ongoing training/education
- accessible and acceptable to patients, and
- a viable funding model (Mitchell, Burridge et al 2015).

Such a system has evolved in Australia since 1999. GPs are funded by Medicare to take part in existing multidisciplinary care teams, such as those found in specialist palliative care services. Furthermore, any patient with chronic or complex health conditions can be provided with a care plan by their GP. Medicare funds the practice resources (GP and nurse time) taken to do this, as well as for communicating with health professionals from other disciplines while developing the plan (Trehearne et al 2014).

In addition, the funding scheme allows patients in certain vulnerable groups (people ≥75 years of age, people living in residential aged care homes, intellectually disabled people, refugees, certain children and adolescents, adults aged 45–49, people aged 40–49 years at a high risk of developing type 2 diabetes, Aboriginal and Torres Strait Islander patients) to undergo a comprehensive assessment to identify health problems that may not be readily detectable in a routine medical consultation (Australian Government Department of Health 2016). This allows appropriate multidisciplinary health interventions to be planned and delivered to prevent serious problems from arising at a later date. There is evidence that this approach works: the presence of a care plan in older diabetic patients reduces the rate of hospitalisations by 22% compared with no care plan (Caughey et al 2016).

Once a multidisciplinary management plan has been devised, the funding mechanism supports limited allied health interventions. While an ideal multidisciplinary team would have equal input from all team members, in this case the practicalities of general practice and community-based private allied health provider service patterns means that the allied health team members generally sign off on a GP generated plan. The GP has to allocate the small number of Medicare-supported allied health funding treatments (five per calendar year) among the providers, which creates dilemmas if effective treatment requires a different level of service (Foster et al 2009). A similar scheme has been developed for the care of mental health problems in the community, which facilitates access to clinical psychologists and other mental health professionals.

A final mechanism for promoting integrated care of chronically ill people is a case conference. Here the GP either arranges or participates in a conversation about complex patients with health professionals from at least two other disciplines. This differs from care plans which are generated by the GP, and communication occurs sequentially, one-on-one with the other health providers. Case conferences can be highly effective in developing a coordinated care plan, because the communication ensures all participants have a stake in the care plan development, and there is greater clarity in provider roles (e.g. Abernethy et al 2013; Mitchell, Zhang et al 2014).

Following are three examples of the way such programs can work. In Case Study 2.1 a multidisciplinary care program has been put in place within a rural general practice for diabetic patients. Under this model every diabetic patient is offered the service, and programmed recall is arranged every 3 months. The nurse works to a plan to review the patient, advising the GP

of findings to be reviewed. The GP then arranges for individualised, ongoing care (Ackermann & Mitchell 2006). In Case Study 2.2, uncontrolled diabetic patients are seen in a multidisciplinary clinic comprising a GP, specialist and a diabetic educator, based at a suburban general practice. Care plans are developed and the care is undertaken in the clinic until the patient is stabilised, at which point they are referred back to their GP with a care plan. This has resulted in significant reductions in HbA1c in an open label controlled trial (Russell et al 2013; Zhang et al 2015). In Case Study 2.3 (overleaf), case conferences take place between GPs, specialist heart or lung disease nurses and a palliative care physician to plan care for patients with end-stage heart or lung failure. A written care plan is generated and everyone is aware of their part in the plan. In a before-and-after designed study, dramatic reductions in hospital service utilisation result (Mitchell et al 2014).

CASE STUDY 2.1

EXAMPLE OF INTRA-PRACTICE MULTIDISCIPLINARY CARE

Setting: Regional Australian town: district population 25,000

Patients: All diabetic patients of the practice n = 700; 404 participated

Multidisciplinary team members: GP, practice nurse, visiting diabetic educator, visiting dietitian

Structure of multidisciplinary care: Patient reviewed by nurse, protocol of review developed by practice based on evidence-based best practice. GP reviews

patient, being alerted to features required to manage them. GP refers to other team members as required. Patient recalled for review every 3 months.

Outcomes: Population improvements in abdominal circumference, systolic and diastolic blood pressure, HDL and LDL cholesterol and 5-year risk of cardiovascular events, proportion of patients suffering severe hypoglycaemia in last 12 months, and proportion of foot lesions; proportion of patients at or below recommended blood pressure and cholesterol readings increased (all p < 0.05) over 2 years.

Ackermann & Mitchell 2006.

CASE STUDY 2.2

EXAMPLE OF INTRA-PRACTICE MULTIDISCIPLINARY CARE

Setting: Low socioeconomic suburb, Australia

Patients: Unstable diabetic patients at a tertiary hospital referred to a primary care integrated clinic, or to keep attending hospital specialist outpatients

Multidisciplinary team members: GP, practice nurse, visiting diabetic educator, visiting endocrinologist

Structure of multidisciplinary care: Comprehensive assessment by GP and diabetic educator. Case and

plan presented to attending endocrinologist, who refined the proposed management plan. Usual care – specialist endocrine outpatients in local tertiary hospital.

Outcomes: Percentage of patients achieving target HbA1c of 7% increased from 21% to 42% in integrated care, compared with a rise of 1% to 39% in control group; reduced unplanned hospitalisations by half.

Russell et al 2013; Zhang et al 2015.

CASE STUDY 2.3

EXAMPLE OF INTERDISCIPLINARY CARE PLANNING BETWEEN PRIMARY AND SECONDARY CARE: CASE CONFERENCES BETWEEN SPECIALISTS SERVICES AND GPs

Setting: Regional health service and surrounding community, Australia

Patients: Public hospital-based patients who have heart failure or lung disease approaching the end of life

Multidisciplinary team members: GP, palliative care specialist, heart failure or lung health nurse

Structure of multidisciplinary care: Case conference between health professionals, either at the GP surgery or by videoconference. An agreed written care plan is generated and each professional has tasks allocated. The care plan is reviewed by the patient and carers, amended if necessary, then enacted.

Outcomes: Before and after design. 23 case conferences. Annual rate of emergency department visits fell from 13.9 to 2.1 visits; annual rate of hospital admissions fell from 11.4 to 3.5 days, length of inpatient stay fell from 7.0 to 3.7 days.

Mitchell, Zhang, Burridge et al 2014.

CONCLUSION

Multidisciplinary care is well placed in primary care. Primary medical practitioners such as GPs have the opportunity to care for patients over many years, and thus develop a deep understanding of the person as an individual, as well as a knowledge of the family and microenvironment in which that person operates (Stewart et al 2014). This enables healthcare planning to take into account local factors, making the plans more attractive to the individual and thus more likely to be followed through. Newer models involving specialists working in conjunction with GPs are underway.

RECOMMENDED READING

Mitchell GK, Burridge L, Zhang J et al 2015. Systematic review of integrated models of health care delivered at the primary–secondary interface: how effective is it and what determines effectiveness? Australian Journal of Primary Health 21(4), 391–408.

Mitchell G, Senior H, Foster M et al 2011. The role of allied health in the management of complex conditions in primary care. Australian Primary Health Care Research Institute, Canberra.

REFERENCES

Abernethy APCD, Shelby-James T, Rowett D et al 2013. Delivery strategies to optimize resource utilization and performance status for patients with advanced life-limiting illness: results from the 'Palliative Care Trial'. Journal of Pain Symptom Management 45(3), 488–505.

Ackermann EW, Mitchell GK 2006. An audit of structured diabetes care in a rural general practice. The Medical Journal of Australia 185(2), 69–72.

Australian Government Department of Health 2016. Online. Available: www1.health.gov.au/internet/main/publishing.nsf/Content/mbsprimarycare-History

Basu S, Berkowitz SA, Phillips RL et al 2019. Association of primary care physician supply with population mortality in the United States, 2005–2015. JAMA Internal Medicine 179(4), 506–514.

Caughey GE, Vitry AI, Ramsay EN et al 2016. Effect of a general practitioner management plan on health outcomes and hospitalisations in older patients with diabetes. Internal Medicine Journal 46(12), 1430–1436.

Foster MM, Cornwell PL, Fleming JM et al 2009. Better than nothing? Restrictions and realities of enhanced primary care for allied health practitioners. Australian Journal of Primary Health 15(4), 326–334.

Kruis AL, Smidt N, Assendelft WJJ et al 2013. Integrated disease management interventions for patients with chronic obstructive pulmonary disease. Cochrane Database of Systematic Reviews 10, CD009437.

Macinko J, Starfield B, Shi L 2003. The contribution of primary care systems to health outcomes within Organization for Economic Cooperation and Development (OECD) countries, 1970–1998. Health Services Research 38(3), 831–865.

Mitchell GK, Burridge L, Zhang J et al 2015. Systematic review of integrated models of health care delivered at the primary–secondary interface: How effective is it and what determines effectiveness? Australian Journal of Primary Health 21(4), 391–408.

Mitchell G, Zhang J, Burridge L et al 2014. Case conferences between general practitioners and specialist teams to plan end of life care of people with end stage heart failure and lung disease: an exploratory pilot study. BMC Palliative Care 13, 24.

Russell AW, Baxter KA, Askew DA et al 2013. Model of care for the management of complex Type 2 diabetes managed in the community by primary care physicians with specialist support: an open controlled trial. Diabetes Medicine 30(9), 1112–1121.

Starfield B 1994. Is primary care essential? Lancet 344(8930), 1129–1133.

Starfield B 1991. Primary care and health. A cross-national comparison. The Journal of the American Medical Association 266(16), 2268–2271.

Stewart M, Brown JB, Weston WW et al 2014. Patient-centred medicine: transforming the clinical method, 3rd edn. Radcliffe Press, London.

Trehearne B, Fishman P, Lin EH 2014. Role of the nurse in chronic illness management: making the medical home more effective. Nursing Economics 32(4), 178–184.

Weller DP, Maynard A 2004. How general practice is funded in the United Kingdom. The Medical Journal of Australia 181(2), 109–110.

Zhang J, Donald M, Baxter KA et al 2015. Impact of an integrated model of care on potentially preventable hospitalizations for people with Type 2 diabetes mellitus. Diabetic Medicine 32(7), 872–880.

Role of the Occupational Therapist

Michelle Bissett and Lee Zakrzewski

Occupational therapists assert that daily life is comprised of participation and engagement in 'occupations' where occupations are the activities that people need or want to do. These occupations are typically classified as self-care (tasks people do to care for themselves, including showering and dressing), leisure (activities which are pleasurable, including playing sport or socialising) or productivity (activities that contribute to society, such as working or volunteering). Occupational therapists contend that occupational performance and engagement is the result of the interaction of three main factors: (1) the person and their particular skills and abilities; (2) the nature of the occupations in which they engage; and (3) the influence of various aspects of the environment. Engagement in occupations and people's abilities to self-select and perform meaningful tasks, are considered by occupational therapists to contribute to health, wellbeing and quality of life (Polatajko et al 2013).

Occupational performance and engagement can be reduced or eliminated when people experience illness or injury. Occupational decline is common in people with degenerative and progressive health conditions, and often correlates with deterioration of health status. Disability arising from chronic illness and disease can lead to a decline in occupational engagement, less diversity in occupations and a reduction in social relationships (Silvestri 2016). Occupational therapists work with these individuals to facilitate improvement or maintenance of their occupational performance and engagement (Lagueux et al 2018).

Occupational therapists are employed across the healthcare continuum, from acute care and rehabilitation to community care and health promotion. This provides many opportunities to work with people with chronic conditions. Nursing staff can refer any person who has occupational challenges for occupational therapy assessment and intervention. As occupational therapists consider both the physical and the psychological aspects of people, they are well placed to work with people who experience either chronic mental or physical health challenges.

In most scenarios, occupational therapists work with people to *improve* their occupational performance and engagement. This is done by determining the occupations that are important to an individual, assessing their occupational performance and prescribing therapeutic activities which address the issues impacting occupational engagement (Lagueux et al 2018; Leland et al 2017). The approach taken with people with chronic health conditions acknowledges that occupational performance will continue to decline as the health condition progresses. Therefore, occupational therapy with this group of people can aim to enhance performance but frequently focuses on *maintaining* current levels of occupational performance.

Occupational assessment of the person involves using a combination of both standardised and non-standardised assessments. A structured interview is typically used to understand the occupational profile of the person – that is, what are the occupations that make up the person's life? Additional assessments investigate how the person performs aspects of self-care, productivity and leisure and includes identification of individual assets and deficits. This process considers personal characteristics by assessing the areas of biomechanical, sensorimotor, cognitive, intrapersonal and interpersonal function. An environmental assessment is also included, as this considers the physical environment where individuals need to perform tasks and the social and cultural environments in which they perform their occupations.

Occupational therapists employ a person-centred practice philosophy (Townsend et al 2013). Therapists interact with individuals, carers and family members to establish goals and plans for therapy. As occupation selection is idiosyncratic, the person and family participate by identifying the occupational challenges that they would like to address. This varies between people and within practice settings. For example, a person on an acute medical ward may wish to be independent with showering, whereas a person living in the community, already independent in self-care tasks, may wish to be able to independently complete household shopping and meal preparation.

Occupational therapy intervention focuses on self-management strategies (Garvey et al 2015; Kos et al 2016; Pinxsterhuis et al 2015) to enable the person to achieve maximum occupational performance. While intervention focus is individualised, regularly used interventions are energy conservation, prescription of assistive devices and environmental modification.

Energy conservation is particularly important for people who experience decreased performance due to fatigue. Education about energy conservation is utilised to teach people to identify and adapt their daily activity patterns according to their fatigue (Garciá Jalón 2013; Kos et al 2016). Energy conservation includes educating and enabling behavioural changes to reduce energy expenditure (Asano et al 2015; Salomè et al 2019). The strategies implemented include planning ahead, delegation of tasks, balancing work and rest, using the body efficiently, modifying the task or the environment and using assistive technology (Martinsen et al 2016; Salomè et al 2019). These principles enable people to manage their energy use in order to have greater control and choice over activities in their day-to-day life. Similar strategies are also beneficial to people who experience pain due to their condition.

Assistive devices describe a variety of products that can be used to support engagement in daily occupations (Bondoc et al 2016; García et al 2019). Devices can be utilised to prevent further impairment, to compensate for loss of function such as decreased strength or movement, to promote safety and to manage pain (Bondoc et al 2016). Assistive devices can be used in a range of tasks, including dressing, feeding, grooming, communication, mobility and home management. The product prescribed can vary significantly depending on the functional problems being experienced by the individual. Products that are regularly prescribed include wheelchairs, modified cutlery, hand-held shower hoses, speaker phones, and easy-reachers. As part of therapy, individuals are able to trial assistive devices to determine the effectiveness and impact on their occupational performance.

Environmental modification is often required where individuals complete their occupations. This can include the home, work or social environment. Occupational therapists are trained to assess these different environments in order to identify barriers for occupational

performance and to recommend modifications that will enable ongoing participation (Aplin & Ainsworth 2018). This requires assessment of the environmental layout and the performance of the individual within that environment (Aplin & Ainsworth 2018). Modification of the home environment could include changing the design of taps for people with poor hand function or installation of external ramps for people who require wheelchair access into and around their home. Other examples of environmental modifications include workplace redesign and vehicle adaptation.

CONCLUSION

In summary, occupational therapists are concerned with people's ability to manage day-to-day activities, known as occupations. Occupational therapists assist people to maximise their occupational performance through individualised, person-centred treatment plans. Common strategies used with patients with chronic illness include education and application of energy conservation strategies, prescription of adaptive equipment and modification of their environments.

REFERENCES

Aplin T, Ainsworth E 2018. Clinical utility of the In-Home Occupational Performance Evaluation (I-HOPE) for major home modification practice in Australia. Australian Occupational Therapy Journal 65(5), 431–438.

Asano M, Berg E, Johnson K et al 2015. A scoping review of rehabilitation interventions that reduce fatigue among adults with multiple sclerosis. Disability and Rehabilitation 37(9), 729–738.

Bondoc S, Goodrich B, Gitlow L et al 2016. Assistive technology and occupational performance. American Journal of Occupational Therapy 70(Supplement 2), 1–9.

Garciá Jalón EG 2013. Energy conservation for fatigue management in multiple sclerosis: a pilot randomized controlled trial. Clinical Rehabilitation 27(1), 63–74.

García TP, Loureiro JP, González BG et al 2019. Assistive technology based on client-centred for occupational performance in neuromuscular conditions. Medicine 98(25).

Garvey J, Connolly D, Boland F et al 2015. OPTIMAL, an occupational therapy led self-management support programme for people with multimorbidity in primary care: a randomized controlled trial. BMC Family Practice 16, 59.

Kos D, Duportail M, Meirte J et al 2016. The effectiveness of a self-management occupational therapy intervention on activity performance in individuals with multiple sclerosis-related fatigue: a randomized-controlled trial. International Journal of Rehabilitation Research 39(3), 255–262.

Lagueux E, Dépelteau A, Masse J 2018. Occupational therapy's unique contribution to chronic pain management:

a scoping review. Pain Research and Management. Online. 5378451.

Leland NE, Fogelberg DJ, Halle AD et al 2017. Occupational therapy and management of multiple chronic conditions in the context of health care reform. American Journal of Occupational Therapy 71(1), 7101090010.

Martinsen U, Bentzen H, Holter MK et al 2016. The effect of occupational therapy in patients with chronic obstructive pulmonary disease: a randomized controlled trial. Scandinavian Journal of Occupational Therapy 24(2), 89–97.

Pinxsterhuis I, Sandvik L, Strand EB et al 2015. Effectiveness of a group-based self-management program for people with chronic fatigue syndrome: a randomized controlled trial. Clinical Rehabilitation 31(1), 93–103.

Polatajko H, Davis J, Stewart D et al 2013. Specifying the domain of concern: occupation as core. In: E Townsend, H Polatajko, Enabling occupation II: advancing an occupational therapy vision for health, well-being, and justice through occupation, 2nd edn. Canadian Association of Occupational Therapists, Ottawa.

Salomè A, Franchini G, Santilli V et al 2019. Occupational therapy in fatigue management in multiple sclerosis: an umbrella review. Multiple Sclerosis International.

Silvestri J 2016. Effects of chronic shoulder pain on quality of life and occupational engagement in the population with chronic spinal cord injury: preparing for the best outcomes with occupational therapy. Disability and Rehabilitation 39(1), 1–9.

Townsend EA, Beagan B, Kumas-Tan Z et al 2013. Enabling: occupational therapy's core competency. In: E Townsend, H Polatajko, Enabling occupation II: advancing an occupational therapy vision for health, well-being, and justice through occupation, 2nd edn. Canadian Association of Occupational Therapists, Ottawa.

Role of the Paramedic

Liam Langford and Graham Munro

Paramedics undertake a vital role in the interdisciplinary/multidisciplinary team through the delivery of care to patients with chronic illness and disabilities. Paramedics are autonomous registered healthcare professionals who predominantly deliver primary and emergency care in the out-of-hospital environment and are often the first point of healthcare access for patients. Paramedics provide care for a range of clinical and social presentations. These can vary from resuscitation to social welfare issues, from acute medical, traumatic and mental health conditions to the management of chronic illness in the community. This can occur in both public and private employment settings.

Patients with chronic illness and disabilities are likely to receive care from paramedics when their condition deteriorates suddenly, is exacerbated by an acute illness, and in cases of isolated injury or illness. Additionally, they can provide initial social support and navigation of the healthcare system for those affected by chronic illness and disabilities. Characteristic chronic illnesses encountered by paramedics include mental health presentations, commonly schizophrenia and depression; neurological conditions, including cerebrovascular accidents (CVAs); Parkinson's disease and dementia; diabetes; respiratory diseases, including asthma and chronic obstructive pulmonary disease (COPD); renal disease; heart failure and cancer. Furthermore, paramedics are often utilised to transport patients with chronic illness and disabilities between hospitals and health services, in both the routine management of the patient's condition or the requirement for the patient's care to be continued at a tertiary hospital.

Paramedics deliver clinical care through detailed patient assessments, including physical assessment, history-taking and vital signs assessments to assist in forming a diagnosis and associated patient management strategies. The provision and delivery of care can include a range of clinical, pharmacological and social interventions aimed at reducing morbidity and mortality, ensuring patient stabilisation and determining appropriate clinical referral pathways that may include transportation to hospital or other healthcare providers for further assessment and long-term management. Common therapeutic interventions include physiological monitoring, airway management, cardiovascular and respiratory support, immobilisation, haemorrhage control and pain management, along with emotional and psychological support. These clinical interventions are often provided in combination with pharmacological interventions, most commonly including bronchodilators, analgesia, antiemetics, thrombolytics, sedatives and a range of medications to assist the provision of care.

Robust emotional intelligence skills are an inherent requirement for paramedics, as they will encounter patients of various ages, ethnicity, culture, intellect and socioeconomic status that requires the ability to be adaptive in their communication approach, as well as ensure that the relevant information is shared between the paramedic, the patient and often their carers and/or family. This ability is of particular importance when treating patients with a chronic illness and disabilities, as the patient's health history is often extensive and complex. Comprehensive social and communication skills are also important when paramedics transfer the patient's care to a multidisciplinary healthcare team within the clinical setting.

The transfer of the information relating to the assessment and treatment provided in the out-of-hospital environment during handover is paramount in the ongoing treatment, safety and management of the patient. Paramedics routinely provide a verbal overview of the patient's background, history, medications given, assessments and treatments undertaken to nursing and medical health providers. The verbal report is then followed up with a formal written or electronic patient care record that provides the multidisciplinary team with detailed information of the patient care provided.

Paramedics utilise a range of critical thinking, prioritisation, time management and problem-solving skills to evaluate clinical findings and formulate a treatment plan to ensure that safe and effective care is delivered to each patient. Evidence-based practice and clinical practice guidelines (CPGs) are used to assist in the delivery of care and inform a paramedic's clinical decision-making and therapeutic plans. CPGs are developed by individual providers, but commonly include key information to aid with the assessment and provision of treatment, including medication dosing ranges, safety requirements, healthcare pathways and delineation of the scope of practice between paramedic skill levels. CPGs are often developed by the clinical advisory panel of a provider, comprised of a range of multidisciplinary health professionals who regularly evaluate the evidence base and update guidelines to help ensure the contemporary practice of paramedicine.

The scope of practice for paramedics is normally determined by the individual practitioner's education and experience in combination with the employer's clinical governance structures. Typically, several practice levels of paramedicine exist within the Australian setting, which includes the foundation level ambulance paramedic, and the more clinically and academically advanced intensive care paramedic, extended care paramedic and community paramedic (Paramedics Australasia 2012). Paramedics complete an undergraduate degree program in paramedicine and apply to become a Registered Paramedic (Paramedic Board of Australia 2020). It is then usual for them to undertake further clinical and professional experience through a graduate internship by an employer to transition into paramedic practice. A paramedic scope of practice is primarily geared around the recognition and management of a broad range of medical, mental health and trauma conditions that are commonly encountered in the delivery of out-of-hospital care.

Intensive care, extended care and community paramedics are further educated from the foundation paramedic role through additional internal training provided by the employer, in conjunction with postgraduate studies in paramedicine. This additional development, combined with extensive experience at the paramedic level provides the underpinning skills and knowledge to work within an extended scope of practice. This extended scope of practice often includes a better understanding of the healthcare system, more advanced clinical skills and additional medications that are utilised in the delivery of care to patients with complex out-of-hospital care needs.

Expanding models of care are also being developed in paramedicine to broaden the scope of practice for paramedics to provide a more holistic approach to care for people and reduce pressures on the healthcare system. Extended care paramedic roles have been used to reduce the number of patients transported to hospital emergency departments and to improve patient comfort. These paramedics operate under an extended scope of practice to provide advanced clinical services to patients within their own home or place of residence where some exacerbations of chronic illness can be treated by the paramedic, thus avoiding the need for emergency department attendance. The aim of this model is to avoid the need to transport patients to hospital by implementing care strategies with the patient, engaging multidisciplinary outpatient support such as community nurses, specialist outpatient nurses, GPs and community support workers. The extended care paramedic role appears to safely reduce hospital emergency department (ED) presentation rates where the service is in place, particularly with patients with chronic illnesses (Hoyle et al 2012; Swain et al 2010).

Paramedics also have a well-established role in responding to disasters, including floods, bushfires, earthquakes, cyclones and heat events, in which people with chronic illness are particularly vulnerable (Council of Ambulance Authorities [CAA] 2013). Paramedics can provide support outside the normal paramedic operational role in recovery settings, assistance in evacuations of hospitals and urban search and rescue. They can work autonomously within disaster health events or in multidisciplinary teams with other healthcare professionals. Formal response roles within disaster events, nationally and internationally, have been identified for paramedics. These events can include mass causalities, natural disasters (bushfire, storms and earthquakes), communicable disease outbreaks and chemical, biological, radiological, nuclear and explosive-related (CBRNE) events (Stevens 2010). There is also an identified role for paramedics to undertake the administration of vaccines in the general community or assist in the response to a communicable disease outbreak under temporary guidelines or protocols (Walz 2003). Paramedics are likely to provide clinical care, transport and support to patients with chronic illness and disabilities, who are often more vulnerable during disaster events due to the direct effect of the disaster, or the disruption to the normal care and treatment the disaster event has caused.

In Australia, there are over 100 employers of paramedics, ranging from the state ambulance services to private ambulance services; industrial employers, such as mines and oil rigs; hospitals and other healthcare institutions (National Rural Healthcare Alliance 2019). In addition, the role of paramedics will expand in the near future to include prescribing rights and the provision of primary healthcare in rural, regional and remote areas of Australia, which are severely underserviced, resulting in poorer health outcomes than urban residents.

CONCLUSION

Paramedics form an integral part of the interdisciplinary/multidisciplinary team that autonomously provides out-of-hospital assessment and treatment to patients. Paramedics are often the first healthcare professionals to provide care to patients with exacerbation or deterioration of chronic illness and disability. The paramedic's aim is to determine the initial severity of a condition, provide early medical treatment and reassurance before making a decision as to the disposition of the patient, which could include transporting the patient to hospital, where ongoing treatment and management are provided by a range of healthcare professionals that form the patient continuum of care. Paramedics are also likely to play a larger role in the interdisciplinary/multidisciplinary team into the future as more advanced roles are developed for paramedics to treat and support patients with the aim being for patients to remain in their own place of residence.

REFERENCES

Council of Ambulance Authorities 2013. Disaster and emergency management – the ambulance role. Council of Ambulance Authorities, Melbourne.

Hoyle S, Swain A, Fake P et al 2012. Introduction of an extended care paramedic model in New Zealand. Emergency Medicine Australasia: EMA 6, 652–656.

National Rural Healthcare Alliance (NRHA) 2019. The paramedic workforce in rural, regional and remote Australia. Fact sheet. Oct. 2019. NRHA, ACT.

Paramedic Board of Australia 2020. Regulating Australia's paramedics. Online. Available: www.paramedicineboard.gov.au/.

Paramedics Australasia 2012. Paramedic role descriptions. Online. Available: www.paramedics.org/content/2009/07/PRD_211212_WEBONLY.pdf.

Stevens G 2010. Determinants of paramedic response readiness for CBRNE threats. Biosecurity and Bioterrorism: Biodefense Strategy, Practice and Science 8(2), 193–202.

Swain A, Hoyle S, Long A 2010. The changing face of prehospital care in New Zealand: the role of extended care paramedics. New Zealand Medical Journal 1309, 11–14.

Walz B 2003. Vaccine administration by paramedics: a model for bioterrorism and disaster response preparation. Prehospital and Disaster Medicine 4, 321.

Role of the Pharmacist

Gisselle Gallego

Pharmacists are part of a multidisciplinary team, which includes doctors, nurses, other allied health professionals and consumers. Pharmacists can work in community pharmacies, hospitals or nursing homes, where they apply their clinical knowledge and skills to provide pharmaceutical care. They can educate patients about their chronic health conditions, as well as about the effects and possible side effects of their medications. They promote the judicious, appropriate, safe and efficacious use of medicines. Their role has evolved from medicine supply or dispensing to medicines management and adherence support, which are particularly important in chronic disease management (van Mil 2019).

Before a medication is dispensed, providing information on how side effects would be managed, should they occur in future, can be greatly reassuring to a patient who is worried about taking medication on a long-term basis (Marshall et al 2012). Services that a pharmacist can potentially offer to help patients effectively manage their chronic conditions include education and information, medication reviews and liaising with the person's GP and other healthcare providers as part of a care plan (Hwang et al 2017). Pharmacy services such as medication reviews may also reduce cardiovascular risk factors among adults with type 2 diabetes mellitus, hypertension or dyslipidaemia (Yuan et al 2019; Martínez-Mardones et al 2019).

'Adherence' implies choice, and that both patients and health providers have established both a medical regimen and a treatment goal (Ho et al 2009). Good and sustained adherence has been shown to improve signs and symptoms, prevent hospital admissions and reduce mortality (Touchette & Sharp 2019). Still, it is not uncommon for adherence to medication for chronic disease to temporarily decline, even when adherence-enhancing interventions are implemented (Nieuwlaat et al 2014). It is important to acknowledge that consumers play an important role, not only as self-managers but as shared managers of health and illness with healthcare providers (Rathbone et al 2017). Studies have described the link between non-adherence and lack of patient understanding of the disease and its treatment, resulting from inadequate education (Wilson et al 2020). Patients are more likely to be non-adherent with their medications if they do not understand their condition or the consequences of uncontrolled disease. Alongside other health professionals, pharmacists play a role in sustaining adherence by implementing interventions that target the changing needs of patients. This is particularly important for older adults, as their ability to adhere to complex medication regimens needed to treat numerous medical problems may also be challenged by cognitive changes (Hayes et al 2009). There are also age-associated changes in pharmacodynamics, pharmacokinetics and co-morbidity that may contribute to increased risk of adverse events (Fried et al 2014). Polypharmacy (the use of multiple medications) is more common among older adults (Rankin et al 2018), and it increases the risks of adverse drug reactions.

Pharmaceutical care may also need to adapt to address the medication-sensitive symptoms of people with a disability (Chrischilles et al 2014). In the case of people with hearing, sight or cognitive impairments, pharmacists need to be aware of how to tailor their advice. For example, if a person has a cognitive impairment, the communication style, information provided, skills and tools for self-management need to be tailored to the person (Sheerin et al 2019).

For people with an intellectual disability, pharmacists need to be able to assess the person's capacity to communicate and understand the information delivered to them (Sheerin et al 2019; Smith et al 2019). It is important that this process is collaborative, involving not only the person but other health professionals and, if appropriate, their carers. Davis and colleagues (2016) highlighted the importance of active listening to determine understanding of concepts and exercising care with language, to maximise adherence with inhaled asthma medications in people with intellectual disability. Pharmacists may also need to consider mobility needs (i.e. assistive aids for people with hand-dexterity weakness), swallowing difficulties and other circumstances that could have an impact on the person's medication use. For example, if the person has a visual impairment, an effort to understand the impairment should be made, tools for medication counselling should be used and detailed counselling should be provided (Lee & Lee 2019).

CONCLUSION

Pharmacists play an important role in empowering patients to be active and informed decision-makers. Including pharmacists as part of a well-integrated, multidisciplinary, patient-centred care medication management team helps optimise therapeutic outcomes by promoting the safe use of medicines and can lead to improved outcomes for different chronic conditions.

RECOMMENDED READING

National Heart Foundation of Australia 2011. Improving adherence in cardiovascular care. A toolkit for health professionals. Online. Available: Improving-adherence-in-cardiovascular-care-toolkit.pdf.

Vermeire E, Hearnshaw H, Van Royen P et al 2001. Patient adherence to treatment: three decades of research. A comprehensive review. Journal of Clinical Pharmacy and Therapeutics 26(5), 331–342.

REFERENCES

Chrischilles EA, Doucette W, Farris K et al 2014. Medication therapy management and complex patients with disability: a randomized controlled trial. Annals of Pharmacotherapy 48(2), 158–167.

Davis SR, Durvasula S, Merhi D et al 2016. Knowledge that people with intellectual disabilities have of their inhaled asthma medications: messages for pharmacists. International Journal of Clinical Pharmacy 38(1), 135–143.

Fried TR, O'Leary J, Towle V et al 2014. Health outcomes associated with polypharmacy in community-dwelling older adults: a systematic review. Journal of the American Geriatrics Society 62(12), 2261–2272.

Hayes TL, Larimer N, Adami A et al 2009. Medication adherence in healthy elders: small cognitive changes make a big difference. Journal of Aging and Health 21(4), 567–580.

Ho PM, Bryson CL, Rumsfeld JS 2009. Medication adherence: its importance in cardiovascular outcomes. Circulation 119(23), 3028–3035.

Hwang AY, Gums TH, Gums JG 2017. The benefits of physician–pharmacist collaboration. The Journal of Family Practice 66(12), E1–E8.

Lee BH, Lee YJ 2019. Evaluation of medication use and pharmacy services for visually impaired persons: perspectives from both visually impaired and community pharmacists. Disability and Health Journal 12(1), 79–86.

Marshall IJ, Wolfe CDA, McKevitt C 2012. Lay perspectives on hypertension and drug adherence: systematic review of qualitative research. British Medical Journal 345, e3953.

Martínez-Mardones F, Fernandez-Llimos F, Benrimoj SI et al 2019. Systematic review and meta-analysis of medication reviews conducted by pharmacists on cardiovascular diseases risk factors in ambulatory care. Journal of the American Heart Association 8(22), e013627.

Nieuwlaat R, Wilczynski N, Navarro T et al 2014. Interventions for enhancing medication adherence. The Cochrane Database of Systematic Reviews (11), CD000011.

Rankin A, Cadogan CA, Patterson SM et al 2018. Interventions to improve the appropriate use of polypharmacy for older people. Cochrane Database of Systematic Reviews (9).

Rathbone AP, Todd A, Jamie Ket al 2017. A systematic review and thematic synthesis of patients' experience of medicines adherence. Research in Social and Administrative Pharmacy 13(3), 403–439.

Sheerin F, Eustace-Cook J, Wuytack F et al 2019. Medication management in intellectual disability settings: a systematic review. Journal of Intellectual Disabilities 25(2), 242–276.

Smith MVA, Adams D, Carr C et al 2019. Do people with intellectual disabilities understand their prescription medication? A scoping review. Journal of Applied Research in Intellectual Disabilities 32(6), 1375–1388.

Touchette DR, Sharp LK 2019. Medication adherence: scope of the problem, ways to measure, ways to improve, and the role of the pharmacist. Journal of the American College of Clinical Pharmacy 2(1), 63–68.

van Mil JWF 2019. Definitions of pharmaceutical care and related concepts. In: F Alves da Costa, JWF van Mil, A Alvarez-Risco, The pharmacist guide to implementing pharmaceutical care. Springer International Publishing, Cham.

Wilson TE, Hennessy EA, Falzon L et al 2020. Effectiveness of interventions targeting self-regulation to improve adherence to chronic disease medications: a meta-review of meta-analyses. Health Psychology Review 14(1), 66–85.

Yuan C, Ding Y, Zhou K et al 2019. Clinical outcomes of community pharmacy services: a systematic review and meta-analysis. Health & Social Care in the Community 27(5), e567–e587.

Role of the Physiotherapist

Anthony Wright

Physiotherapy is a healthcare profession with a therapeutic focus on healthy movement, managing impairments, enhancing mobility and maintaining physical activity and quality of life. Physiotherapists are experts in exercise and physical activity, who assist people with movement-related problems and painful disorders, and help them to manage pain, improve and maintain movement, mobility and physical independence. They are key members of the interdisciplinary team in the management of a range of disabilities and chronic diseases, and work collaboratively with nurses, medical practitioners and a range of allied health practitioners.

Physiotherapists practise in a wide variety of settings, including hospitals, private practices, primary care facilities, schools and universities, aged care facilities, sports facilities, workplaces, mental health services and public health services. They also work with people across the entire lifespan, from premature babies in neonatal intensive care to the very elderly. Physiotherapists work closely with nurses in many different settings, including emergency departments (EDs), outpatient clinics, hospital wards and a range of community settings. Approximately half of all physiotherapists in Australia practise outside the public hospital system.

PHYSIOTHERAPY PROFESSION

Physiotherapists are primary contact practitioners whose services can be directly accessed by members of the public without medical referral. They are registered by the Physiotherapy Board of Australia (PBA) through the Australian Health Practitioners Regulation Agency (AHPRA). The Australian Physiotherapy Association (APA) is the national peak body representing the interests of Australian physiotherapists and their patients. The organisation is active in a wide range of advocacy roles on behalf of physiotherapists and their clients.

Physiotherapists are eligible for registration upon completion of an accredited educational program. This may be a 4-year Bachelor degree or a Masters degree (including an extended Masters degree) approved by the Australian Physiotherapy Council (APC). Many physiotherapists complete postgraduate studies in areas such as musculoskeletal disorders, sports physiotherapy, paediatrics and women's health. Physiotherapists also complete additional training to undertake extended scope of practice roles in areas such as EDs.

PHYSIOTHERAPY PRACTICE

The physiotherapy profession places a strong emphasis on the provision of care based on evidence-based practice linked to sound clinical reasoning and clinical expertise. The physiotherapist establishes a clinical diagnosis based on a detailed assessment of the client, including a clinical history and detailed clinical examination. Specific movement-related impairments will often be identified and goals of treatment will be established in consultation with the client. The physiotherapist will then develop an individualised treatment plan and a broad approach to assisting the client to manage their particular disorder. Physiotherapists utilise a wide range of non-drug-based therapies to achieve their therapeutic goals, and in most cases the treatment program will include an individualised exercise program and patient education related to prevention or management of the disorder. Commonly utilised treatments include manual therapies, specific movement re-education, therapeutic exercise, gait re-education, respiratory therapies, electro-physical agents, hydrotherapy, assistive devices, behavioural therapy and education. For most people with a disability or a chronic disease or condition, there is an emphasis on active interventions and empowering the individual and their carers to take an active role in self-management of their disorder and the promotion of health and activity.

CONDITIONS TREATED

Physiotherapists treat clients with a wide range of conditions, including musculoskeletal disorders, such as back pain, neck pain, headache and sports injuries (Jull et al 2015). This includes assisting patients to manage a wide range of chronic pain problems with an increasing emphasis on the use of a biopsychosocial model for chronic pain management (Briggs et al 2016). They are also actively involved in the management of patients who have various forms of arthritis by providing specific treatments, encouraging preventive strategies and providing postoperative management and rehabilitation for individuals who receive joint replacements. At a community level, physiotherapy places a strong emphasis on the importance of maintaining regular physical activity and exercise as a means of preventing or minimising the impact of arthritis (Skou & Roos 2019).

Physiotherapists are also active in the management of a range of chronic cardiopulmonary disorders such as asthma, COPD and cardiovascular disease (Denehy et al 2018). Interventions encourage exercise and physical activity, including specific exercises to retrain inspiratory muscle function and exercise programs to improve aerobic capacity (Denehy et al 2018). Physiotherapists have expertise in modifying exercise programs to ensure that they are safe for patients with significant pulmonary or cardiac pathology. The maintenance of optimal fitness is critical for many individuals living with significant pulmonary or cardiac disorders.

One of the most devastating outcomes of cardiovascular disease is stroke. Physiotherapists play a major role in the rehabilitation of patients after stroke. This includes movement re-education, re-education of gait and assisting patients to achieve the maximum possible level of functional independence. Physiotherapists often work closely with patients and their families for many months to ensure that they achieve the best possible outcomes and to assist them in adjusting to the major impact that stroke has on their lives (Pollock et al 2007).

Physiotherapy is also of benefit for patients with a variety of other neurological disorders, such as Parkinson's disease and multiple sclerosis (Lennon et al 2018). Physiotherapists work closely with clients to assist them in managing the impacts of these chronic diseases over time.

Physiotherapists are able to make an important contribution to the management of all chronic diseases for which exercise is known to be beneficial. This includes diseases such as diabetes mellitus and mental health problems such as depression (Hemmings & Soundy 2020; Ozdirenc et al 2004). Physiotherapists have expertise in designing exercise programs for at-risk populations and addressing particular problems that clients may experience, such as foot disorders and balance problems in patients with diabetes.

As indicated previously, physiotherapists work actively with clients across the entire lifespan. Paediatric physiotherapists work with families and children who experience a variety of conditions that may affect normal motor development (Campbell et al 2012). This includes conditions such as cerebral palsy. Paediatric physiotherapy places a strong emphasis on interdisciplinary practice and family-centred care. Physiotherapists work with parents to maintain and improve motor function in children with cerebral palsy and provide comprehensive rehabilitation programs after botulinum toxin injections and various surgical procedures (Yana et al 2019). There are a number of other paediatric conditions for which physiotherapy interventions are beneficial.

Many developed countries are experiencing a rapid ageing of the population with a significant increase in the number of people living with chronic diseases. Physiotherapists work with older individuals to assist them in managing their disorders and maintaining healthy physical activity within the confines imposed by multiple chronic conditions. They can also provide specific interventions to address the risk of falling and prevent the significant morbidity and mortality associated with falls (Hill 2018).

Physiotherapists also provide significant assistance for women with continence problems related to pelvic floor disorders following childbirth, including the use of ultrasound imaging to retrain pelvic muscle function (Whittaker et al 2007).

CONCLUSION

Physiotherapy plays an important role in the management of a broad range of disabilities and chronic conditions that affect people throughout the lifespan. Physiotherapists work closely with many other members of the healthcare team, including nurses, across a range of settings to assist patients in managing their conditions. Physiotherapists place significant emphasis on exercise and physical activity and are well equipped to tailor safe and effective exercise programs for people with a range of health conditions. Self-management and empowering and educating clients to take responsibility for the management of their own conditions are also important aspects of physiotherapy care. Other areas of emphasis include evidence-based interventions and primary and secondary prevention strategies.

REFERENCES

Briggs A, Chan MM, Slater H 2016. Models of care for musculoskeletal health: moving towards meaningful implementation and evaluation across conditions and care settings. Best Practice & Research: Clinical Rheumatology 30(3), 359–374.

Campbell S K, Palisano RJ, Orlin MN 2012. Physical therapy for children. Elsevier Saunders, St Louis, Missouri.

Denehy L, Granger CL, El-Ansary D et al 2018. Advances in cardiorespiratory physiotherapy and their clinical impact. Expert Review of Respiratory Medicine 12(3), 203–215.

Hemmings L, Soundy A 2020. Experiences of physiotherapy in mental health: an interpretative phenomenological analysis of barriers and facilitators to care. Physiotherapy 109, 94–101.

Hill AM 2018. Exercise interventions reduce the risk of injurious falls among older adults. Evidence Based Nursing 21(3), 75.

Jull G, Moore A, Falla D et al 2015. Grieve's modern musculoskeletal physiotherapy. Elsevier, Sydney.

Lennon S, Ramdharry G, Verheyden G 2018. Physical management for neurological conditions. Elsevier, Sydney.

Ozdirenc M, Kocak G, Guntekin R 2004. The acute effects of in-patient physiotherapy program on functional capacity in type II diabetes mellitus. Diabetes Research & Clinical Practice 64(3), 167–172.

Pollock A, Baer G, Pomeroy V et al 2007. Physiotherapy treatment approaches for the recovery of postural control and lower limb function following stroke. Cochrane Database Syst Rev(1), CD001920.

Skou ST, Roos EM 2019. Physical therapy for patients with knee and hip osteoarthritis: supervised, active treatment is current best practice. Clinical & Experimental Rheumatology 37 Suppl 120(5), 112–117.

Whittaker JL, Thompson JA, Teyhen DS et al 2007. Rehabilitative ultrasound imaging of pelvic floor muscle function. Journal of Orthopaedic & Sports Physical Therapy 37(8), 487–498.

Yana M, Tutuola F, Westwater-Wood S et al 2019. The efficacy of botulinum toxin A lower limb injections in addition to physiotherapy approaches in children with cerebral palsy: a systematic review. NeuroRehabilitation 44(2), 175–189.

Role of the Social Worker

Mark Hughes and Hilary Gallagher

Access to healthcare is a human right. The purpose of social work is to help people achieve optimal health and wellbeing within their own environment, which includes their family, community and society. In particular, social work is concerned with assisting those who are disadvantaged or marginalised by underlying social inequalities, such as discrimination on the basis of personal characteristics, identity, location, financial status or group affiliation according to ethnicity, gender, sexual identity, age, mental health, disability or addiction, to name a few. For example, access to Australian healthcare can vary, depending on whether people live rurally, remotely or in metropolitan environments; with school children living in rural areas experiencing poorer health outcomes (Maple et al 2019; Willis et al 2019). Thus, social work in the health arena promotes social justice and access to services for those experiencing disadvantage (Alston et al 2018).

In Australia, qualified social workers have undertaken either a 4-year undergraduate degree or a 2-year qualifying Masters degree, accredited by the Australian Association of Social Workers (AASW) in relation to a series of professional standards. While many social workers work in health, they are also employed in such areas as child protection, income security (Centrelink), housing, employment services, correctional facilities and schools. They could be working in government agencies or any number of community organisations ranging from large organisations, such as UnitingCare, to small agencies employing just a few staff, such as domestic violence shelters. Similarly, social work practice methods can be quite diverse – from individual case management and counselling to facilitating group interventions, to community development and social action, and policy writing.

HEALTH SETTINGS

In health settings, social workers are employed across a range of practice contexts; for example, Indigenous health, community mental health, alcohol and drug services, hospital emergency departments, palliative care, renal support, paediatrics and oncology. The role of a social worker in a health setting is to enhance social, emotional and practical outcomes by providing targeted interventions and referrals to other services and supports. The scope of practice of health social work may include bereavement, grief and loss, risk assessments, therapeutic interventions, socio-legal issues, discharge planning, family intervention and support, leadership, group facilitation, statutory reporting, advocacy, psychoeducation, crisis intervention, policy development, and research (AASW 2015a). Accredited mental health social workers, working in private practice, may also receive referrals from medical practitioners and be eligible for a Medicare Provider Number to provide focused psychological strategies for a person with a diagnosed mental health disorder. As with other allied health professions, increasingly social workers are providing services in an online environment (e.g. via online video conferencing, smartphone apps and instant messaging), which are particularly important for reaching people in remote parts of the country (Bryant et al 2018).

PSYCHOSOCIAL APPROACH

Social workers often draw on a psychosocial approach, which seeks to go beyond the traditional medical model to address the interplay between physical, psychological, environmental and social aspects of health and wellbeing. A key role for social workers in a multidisciplinary health team is carrying out psychosocial assessments which complement and inform the assessment/diagnostic tasks of other professionals. These use a person-in-environment approach that recognises the impact of the relationship between individual and social factors that influence health, wellbeing and recovery. When social workers undertake psychosocial assessments, they may explore challenges and strengths in social functioning, employment, financial and housing needs, family interactions and supports, significant relationships, social supports, and cultural and spiritual aspects, to name a few (AASW 2015b).

Critical to the effectiveness of the assessment process is forming an effective social work relationship with the client or patient. Social workers seek to 'start where the client is at', rather than impose predetermined assumptions. By building a meaningful relationship, people are enabled to disclose sensitive issues (such as previous experiences of abuse or trauma), which can have a significant impact on the person's wellbeing and recovery.

HEALTH INITIATIVES AND PRACTICE FRAMEWORKS

Government initiatives, such as Primary Health Networks and Preventative and Public Health Research, focus on strategies such as reducing hospitalisation by enabling integrated care in the community to people with chronic diseases and complex health needs. Social workers play a key role in assisting people to live independently in this way; for example, by mobilising available resources prior to a person returning home from hospital or by providing outreach or in-home support. They provide counselling to individuals, helping them adjust to and overcome limitations that might arise from their disability or illness. They work with partners, family members and friends and, in particular, provide support to caregivers and help strengthen caregiving networks. Social workers also advocate and lobby on behalf of clients' rights. For example, social workers may sometimes make a case for not discharging a patient home until appropriate community resources are put in place.

In the health and disability sectors, social workers often draw on a strengths-based approach, which aims to shift the focus away from a person's problems or deficits towards their capabilities or strengths (Chenoweth & McAuliffe 2017). It is argued that too much emphasis on a person's problems (such as their illness or disability) undermines their sense of competence and reduces their humanity to a label or diagnosis. While the approach does not ignore the challenges faced by the individual, it recognises their survival capacity and strengths in other areas of their life, and tries to emulate or build on these.

Like other professions, social work has also found much value in the social model of disability, which posits that disability arises not from the individual but from society's failure to accommodate the diversity of impairments that individuals experience (Oliver 2013). The focus is on society adjusting to individuals' incapacities rather than vice versa. Disability rights campaigns promote the social model of disability and call for disabled people to exercise more authority in the planning, delivery and evaluation of disability services.

This is especially important in the context of the implementation of the Australian National Disability Insurance Scheme (NDIS), which seeks to support people with a permanent and significant disability that impacts on their participation in everyday life. The full scheme has been progressively rolled out across all states and territories since July 2016. Agencies register to deliver supports or products to individual participants in the NDIS. Each participant has an individualised plan, outlining the outcomes they want and the supports they need. The rollout was completed in July 2020 with the aim that by 2025 an estimated 500,000 Australians would be able to access supports (NDIS 2020). It is hoped that the NDIS will provide opportunities for social workers and other professionals to work alongside clients to support them in gaining more control, not just over the services designated to respond to their needs, but also over other aspects of their lives.

CONCLUSION

Social work has long articulated a commitment to multidisciplinary practice. However, like other allied health professionals, social workers can experience challenges in team work, such as role overlap, differences in terminology and alternative ways of defining patient problems. There may also be power dynamics within teams – possibly reflecting wider social divisions (e.g. gendered labour patterns) – which impact on team members. Nonetheless, these sorts of difficulties are often overcome in everyday practice because optimal multidisciplinary healthcare relies on effective professional relationships that are focused on the needs of the client/patient.

RECOMMENDED READING

Australian Association of Social Workers (AASW) 2015. Scope of social work practice: social work in health. AASW, Melbourne.

REFERENCES

Alston M, McCurdy S, McKinnon J (eds) 2018. Social work: fields of practice. Oxford University Press, Melbourne.
Australian Association of Social Workers (AASW) 2015a. Scope of social work practice: social work in health. AASW, Melbourne.
Australian Association of Social Workers (AASW) 2015b. Scope of social work practice: psychosocial assessments. AASW, Melbourne.
Bryant L, Garnham B, Tedmanson D et al 2018. Tele-social work and mental health in rural and remote communities in Australia. International Social Work 61(1), 143–155.
Chenoweth L, McAuliffe D 2017. The road to social work and human service practice. Cengage, Melbourne.
Maple M, Pearce T, Gartshore S et al 2019. Social work in rural New South Wales school settings: addressing inequalities beyond the school gate. Australian Social Work 72(2), 219–232.
National Disability Insurance Scheme (NDIS) 2020. Online. Available: www.ndis.gov.au/
Oliver M 2013. The social model of disability: thirty years on. Disability & Society 28(7), 1024–1026.
Willis E, Reynolds L, Rudge T (eds) 2019. Understanding the Australian health care system. Elsevier Health Sciences, Sydney.

Role of the Speech Pathologist

Belinda Kenny

Speech pathologists are key members of an interdisciplinary team, who focus on enabling every individual to have optimal communication, swallowing and mealtime participation (Speech Pathology Australia 2016). Communication is a human right that is essential for an individual's participation in society, including interacting with others at home, in educational and vocational settings, and for taking an active role in healthcare decision-making. Speech pathologists enhance an individual's communication capabilities through spoken language, written language, sign language, augmentative and alternative communication and/or natural non-verbal communication.

Effective swallowing is essential for maintaining nutritional health and hydration, and quality mealtimes enable individuals to participate in social and cultural experiences with family and friends. Speech pathologists facilitate swallowing capabilities and mealtime experiences through saliva management and strategies to optimise swallowing function, eating and drinking.

Patients with diverse communication and swallowing needs may present to healthcare settings.

• People with lifelong disability may have complex communication needs and use forms of communication other than speech, referred to as augmentative and alternative communication (AAC) (Gormley & Light 2019). Speech pathologists can ensure patients have access to their communication aids or devices and educate others to communicate effectively with patients using AAC. Speech pathologists also support safe and enjoyable mealtime management practices during hospital admissions and community care.

- Patients who require a tracheostomy or artificial respiration during intensive care admission may experience temporary, sudden and significant changes in their communication abilities. Speech pathologists may educate patients preoperatively, and postoperatively provide communication aids to facilitate patients' expression of healthcare needs and concerns. Providing options for patients to communicate can prevent feelings of anger, frustration and disempowerment during acute stages of recovery (Freeman-Sanderson et al 2018). Speech pathologists also contribute to clinical management for patients with tracheostomies who experience difficulties swallowing saliva, food or fluids during intensive and high dependency care admissions.
- Patients may present with acquired communication and swallowing disorders resulting from cerebrovascular accident (CVA), laryngectomy and traumatic brain injury. These health conditions can significantly impact a patient's ability to understand, express verbal or written information, produce speech and/or use communication in a socially appropriate way. Acquired disabilities also include hearing loss and decline in cognitive functioning; frequently occurring concerns for people living in aged care facilities. Speech pathology intervention facilitates older adults' health and wellbeing by facilitating participation in communication activities and providing mealtime supports (Bennett et al 2015).
- Patients living with degenerative neurological conditions, including motor neurone disease, Parkinson's disease and multiple sclerosis, may report progressive changes in communication and swallowing skills. Speech pathologists work with these patients to maintain optimal communication. Swallowing issues frequently occur in life-limiting conditions, and speech pathologists are increasingly involved in supporting patients and their families to make informed decisions about safe and enjoyable mealtimes during palliative care (Kelly et al 2018).

Speech pathologists have an important role working with families and carers to establish and maintain communication as individuals' health and communication needs change across the lifespan. Communicating effectively provides patients with opportunities for connecting with carers, re-engaging with their community and coming to terms with major health changes (Brassel et al 2016). However, patients with communication impairment or complex communication needs may experience barriers in conveying messages about their health status, delaying responses for their care or

comfort needs (Beukelman & Nordness 2015), hence the importance of providing all patients with a means of effectively communicating with their healthcare team. Speech pathology intervention addresses patients' needs for accessible healthcare information and families' and healthcare professionals' needs for education to support communication interactions. This intervention may include reviewing how verbal or written information is presented in healthcare settings or educating nurses and other health professionals to apply supported communication strategies, so that individuals and families can participate in decision-making (Jensen et al 2015).

Speech pathology practice is guided by a professional framework that utilises the best available evidence and person, family and community-centred practice to meet the needs of individuals with communication and swallowing disorders. For example, during swallowing intervention, speech pathologists may conduct clinical bedside and instrumental evaluation (e.g. Videofluoroscopic Swallow Study), then implement evidence-based strategies to increase patients' strength, range and coordination of swallowing muscles or to compensate for loss of swallowing function. Speech pathologists' recommendations may include saliva management, managing the mealtime environment, non-oral nutritional measures or texture-modified diets and fluids. They work closely with patients and carers to address risks of aspiration and choking and maintain positive sociocultural aspects of eating. Respect and cultural responsiveness are core aspects of speech pathology practice in all health settings.

Nurses are constantly communicating with their patients and are highly aware of the impacts of communication disorders upon patient care. They may be the first member of the healthcare team to observe a patient experiencing difficulties in communicating with others. Nurses may also observe a patient and family members using communication strategies or AAC devices to successfully communicate. Nurses play a pivotal role in supervising patients and ensuring that swallowing needs are met, including oral hygiene, hydration and nutrition (Dondorf et al 2016). In acute settings, nurses are available on a 24-hour basis so they can observe patients experiencing difficulties at mealtimes, including coughing, choking, chewing solids or changes in respiratory status or temperature after meals. They may observe how families respond to mealtime issues. Nurses may also observe positive changes in patients' health status which may improve their ability to swallow. Hence, nurses can expedite referral to a speech pathologist and provide feedback based upon observations and interactions with family members.

Clearly, speech pathologists and nurses bring unique perspectives, skills and expertise to managing patients with communication and swallowing disorders. Interprofessional collaboration involves a partnership between health professionals and patients in a participatory, collaborative and coordinated approach that draws together their disciplinary expertise.

An important component of building collaborative partnerships is understanding each other's roles. Nurses cannot be expected to be knowledgeable about all types of communication and swallowing disability that may occur on a ward or all options to help make wards accessible communication environments. However, nursing observations and interactions are clearly important in supporting patients and families to participate in communication and mealtime activities.

In some healthcare settings, following training and consultation with speech pathologists, nurses may provide early identification for patients at risk of swallowing impairments. Nurses may also take an active role in feeding patients. To fulfil these roles, nurses must recognise risk signs, understand the dietary recommendations made by speech pathologists and be confident and competent in implementing safe swallowing strategies. Preparedness to listen and readiness to consider innovative problem-solving ideas are skills that both nurses and speech pathologists need to bring to such collaboration.

CONCLUSION

Communication is an essential component of effective collaborative practice (Kreps 2016). A challenge facing both nurses and speech pathologists is how best to maintain accurate and timely communication. Effective communication must navigate shifts and continuity of care across healthcare settings. Speech pathologists need to understand the ward structure and how to ensure that communication and swallowing strategies reach all nursing staff, whatever shift they are working on. Nurses need to seek opportunities to share observations with speech pathologists, who are frequently on the wards and consistently documenting changes in patients' communication and swallowing status. Willingness to identify barriers and suggest processes for streamlining verbal and written communication between nurses and speech pathologists will benefit the

team and ensure that patients and family members are informed and engaged in communication and mealtime management.

Communication and swallowing are essential for patients' health and wellbeing. Nurses and speech pathologists both have much to contribute to these health outcomes and, together with their patients, are the foundations of a strong collaborative team.

Acknowledgement

This chapter was revised from original contributions by Susan Balandin and Michelle Lincoln.

RECOMMENDED READING

Scope (Victoria) 2015. Communication access for all. Online. Available: www.scopeaust.org.au/wp-content/uploads/2014/12/A4-Communication-Access-for-All-Booklet-2015-web1.pdf

REFERENCES

Bennett MK, Ward EC, Scarinci NA et al 2015. Challenges to communication management in residential aged care. Journal of Clinical Practice in Speech–Language Pathology 17(2), 58–62.

Beukelman DR, Nordness A 2015. Patient–provider communication in rehabilitation settings. In: SW Blackstone, DR Beukelman, KM Yorkston (eds), Patient–provider communication: roles of speech-language pathologists and other health care providers. Plural, San Diego, CA.

Brassel S, Kenny B, Power E et al 2016. Conversational topics discussed by individuals with severe traumatic brain injury and their communication partners during sub-acute recovery. Brain Injury 30(11), 1329–1342.

Dondorf K, Fabus R, Ghassemi AE 2016. The interprofessional collaboration between nurses and speech-language pathologists working with patients diagnosed with dysphagia in skilled nursing facilities. Journal of Nursing Education and Practice 6(4), 17–20.

Freeman-Sanderson AL, Togher L, Elkins M et al 2018. Quality of life improves for tracheostomy patients with return of voice: a mixed methods evaluation of the patient experience across the care continuum. Intensive and Critical Care Nursing 46, 10.1016/j.iccn.2018.02.004.

Gormley J, Light J 2019. Providing services to individuals with complex communication needs in the rehabilitation setting: the experiences and perspectives of speech–language pathologists. American Journal of Speech–Language Pathology 28, 456–468.

Jensen LR, Løvholt AP, Sørensen IR et al 2015. Implementation of supported conversation for communication between nursing staff and in-hospital patients with aphasia. Aphasiology 29, 57–80.

Kelly K, Cumming S, Kenny B et al 2018. Getting comfortable with 'comfort feeding': an exploration of legal and ethical aspects of the Australian speech–language pathologist's role in palliative dysphagia care. International Journal of Speech–Language Pathology 20(3), 371–379.

Kreps GL 2016. Communication and effective interprofessional health care teams. International Archives of Nursing and Health Care 2, 51.

Speech Pathology Australia 2016. What is a speech pathologist? Online. Available: www.speechpathologyaustralia.org.au/SPAweb/Resources_for_the_Public/What_is_a_Speech_Pathologist/SPAweb/Resources_for_the_Public/What_is_a_Speech_Pathologist/What_is_a_Speech_Pathologist.aspx?hkey=7e5fb9f8-c226-4db6-934c-0c3987214d7a.

CHAPTER 3

Models of Care

VICKI DRURY

LEARNING OBJECTIVES

When you have completed this chapter you will be able to:

- critically examine existing models of management for long-term conditions
- describe and discuss the evidence base that has contributed to the self-management Model of Care
- describe the fundamental elements of the self-management Model of Care for people with long-term conditions
- identify opportunities and strategies for applying self-management approaches to the management of diverse long-term conditions
- apply a self-management approach in the delivery of care to people with long-term conditions.

KEY WORDS

models of care	Chronic Care Model
self-management	long-term conditions
chronic disease	

INTRODUCTION

Caring for populations who are living longer with chronic conditions is undoubtedly the current major global healthcare challenge (Hofmeijer 2020). The co-existence of co-morbid long-term conditions is increasing, with estimates that more than 80% of elderly people with a long-term condition have two or more co-morbid diseases (Harris 2019). Globally, almost 70% of all deaths are caused by chronic diseases (McGrady & Moss 2018). With the global population ageing, the impact of long-term conditions will place a significant burden both on the fiscal costs of healthcare as well as on the healthcare workforce (Atella et al 2019). Internationally, many countries have developed strategies to facilitate the development of clear, comprehensive, integrated approaches to the prevention, detection and management of long-term conditions (Hindi et al 2019; Holdsworth et al 2019; Thornicroft et al 2019). Producing long-term cost-effective public health policies is now the primary concern, and addressing lifestyle risks, such as physical inactivity and obesity, is a priority in the ongoing battle to halt widespread problems (Gill et al 2019; James et al 2019; Li et al 2018; Taylor et al 2017). However, the development and delivery of an effective strategy to assist people to alter their lifestyles and behaviour has been challenging. People at risk or living with long-term conditions need to develop and continue practising complex self-management strategies to allow them to live a healthier life (Cutler et al 2018). Current literature suggests that people with long-term conditions who effectively maintain self-management practices make better use of their health professionals' time, have better self-care and experience clearer clinical benefits (Cutler et al 2018; Hosseinzadeh & Shnaigat 2019; Nejhaddadgar et al 2019). Thus, there has been a growing popularity and emphasis on promoting formal self-management education programs across the developed world (World Health Organization 2015). Numerous models of care have arisen in the past decade in an attempt to manage the increasing burden of chronic disease. Common elements exist within all the models as governments adapt them to meet the needs of their populations.

MODELS OF CARE FOR PEOPLE WITH LONG-TERM CONDITIONS

The Chronic Care Model

Evidence suggests that the Chronic Care Model, developed by Wagner (1998) at the McColl Institute in the United States more than 20 years ago, is effective across a number of chronic conditions in improving both clinical and behavioural outcomes (Bauer et al 2019; Yeoh et al 2018). The key elements in this model that are viewed as being critical to effective management of patients with long-term conditions are community resources; the healthcare system; patient self-management; decision support; delivery system redesign; and clinical information systems (Carrier 2015; Davy et al 2015; González-Ortiz et al 2018). The key principles of the model include empowering people to manage their conditions, providing effective and responsible self-management support and organising community resources to meet the needs of people with long-term conditions (Carrier 2015). A revision of this model in 2003 led to the inclusion of cultural competency, patient safety, care coordination, case management and community policies (Carrier 2015). However, this model lacks a population health aspect and is therefore limited to impacting on those people with long-term conditions. It does not meet the need for a model that is inclusive of health promotion and health prevention

(Barr et al 2003). A recent randomised control trial of 5596 veterans found that implementing a collaborative Chronic Care Model improved patient outcomes in the general practice setting, especially for patients with complex mental health issues (Bauer et al 2019).

The Expanded Chronic Care Model

A Canadian team concluded that the Chronic Care Model did not meet the needs of health promotion or health prevention clinicians and integrated the Ottawa Charter for Health Promotion determinants with the key elements of the Chronic Care Model, enabling the inclusion of health prevention, social determinants of health and community participation in work concerning long-term conditions (Barr et al 2003; Coleman et al 2009) (see Fig. 3.1).

Innovative Care for Chronic Conditions Model

The World Health Organization (WHO), together with the McColl Institute, adapted the Chronic Care Model to develop a framework that expanded on the community and policy aspects and focused on improving care for people with long-term conditions at three levels: (1) the macro level (policy); (2) the meso level (healthcare organisations and community); and (3) the micro level (individual and family) (Carrier 2015). This

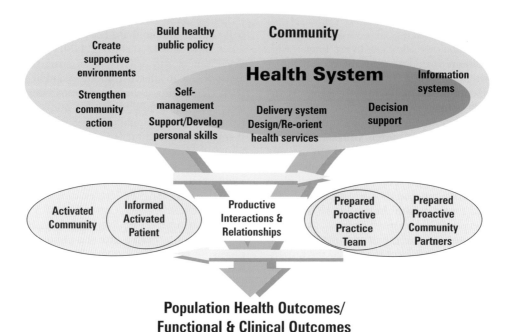

Population Health Outcomes/ Functional & Clinical Outcomes

FIG. 3.1 **The Expanded Chronic Care Model.** Barr et al 2003.

framework is relevant for both prevention and management of long-term conditions and provides an adaptable foundation on which to construct or redesign health systems within the local context (Carrier 2015).

The National Chronic Disease Strategy in Australia

The Australian Government developed the National Chronic Disease Strategy (NCDS) in acknowledgement that the existing system focused on acute short-term problems. This strategy aims to prevent or delay the onset of chronic diseases; reduce complications; reduce avoidable hospital admissions; and implement best practice in the prevention, assessment and management of chronic disease. Adopting a population health approach, the strategy contains four key areas (National Health Priority Action Council 2006):

1 Prevention across the continuum
2 Early detection and early treatment
3 Integration and continuity of prevention and care
4 Self-management.

This framework was superseded by the National Strategic Framework for Chronic Conditions in May 2017, which provides all states and territories within Australia with a uniform method of planning, implementing and evaluating policies and interventions that reduce the impact of chronic disease.

Nationally in Australia, the nine priority health areas for chronic disease are asthma, cancer, cardiovascular health, diabetes mellitus, mental health, injury prevention and control, obesity, dementia, and arthritis and musculoskeletal conditions. These diseases were highlighted as national priorities due to the excessive burden they place on Australian communities and the ability to minimise the effects of these diseases through lifestyle and behavioural changes and modifications within the environment by introducing policy and legislative changes (Australian Health Ministers' Advisory Council 2017). Fundamental to the Australian national strategy to reduce the burden of chronic disease and to improve the ability of individuals to effectively manage their conditions are the concepts of self-management and self-management support (Australian Health Ministers' Advisory Council 2017).

AN OVERVIEW OF THE HISTORICAL DEVELOPMENT OF SELF-MANAGEMENT PROGRAMS

The two approaches applied to self-management that are most evident in the literature are the Stanford approach, which uses peer leaders and is conducted in groups, and the Flinders Program, which is an individual, clinician-led approach underpinned by cognitive behaviour therapy principles (Grover & Joshi 2015). Both approaches have been credibly evaluated and are extensively used around the world (Convery 2019; Desborough et al 2019; McLaughlin 2019; Moreno et al 2019).

The first Chronic Disease Self-Management Program was developed by Kate Lorig and Stanford University in the 1970s. This program, designed specifically for people with arthritis, became a blueprint for subsequent programs (Lorig 1996). The Stanford Patient Education Research Center, under the leadership of Lorig, continues to develop, deliver and evaluate chronic disease self-management programs to patients and training for healthcare professionals and lay persons with chronic diseases. The Stanford program is a community-based group program led by pairs of trained lay people who have a chronic disease themselves (Carrier 2015; Martz 2017).

Despite global interest in the Stanford program, it was not until 1997 that both Australia and the United Kingdom developed similar programs. The Flinders Program in Australia (originally known as the Flinders Model) developed from the SA Health Plus coordinated care trial. The Flinders Program involves using designated tools that assist with assessment, goal setting and care planning. Unlike the Stanford program, the Flinders Program is an individual program that is initiated and supported by a health professional (Baird et al 2019). In the UK, the Living with Long Term Illness project was established in 1998. Findings from this project contributed to the Expert Patients Taskforce, established a year later. The aim of the taskforce was to combine both patient and clinical organisations to develop self-management programs (Carrier 2015). The current program is planned around three phases: case management; disease management; and self-management support. Recognising the need for integrated care for people with complex and/or comorbid chronic conditions, Wagner's Chronic Care Model and the Kaiser risk pyramid were later integrated into the UK model (Liddy et al 2016). The Chronic Disease Self-Management Program (CDSMP), the core Expert Patients Program, was introduced into the National Health Service (NHS) in 2002 (Silver 2018).

Although the aforementioned programs provide clinicians with specific guidelines and information, most long-term conditions are responsive to a generic approach to self-management (Silver 2018). Enabling people to accept responsibility for the self-management of their long-term condition is a complex issue that encompasses readiness for change, intrinsic motivation and high self-efficacy (Drury et al 2014; Tay et al 2014).

The Self-Management Framework

The self-management approach acknowledges that people must cope not only with the disease and the consequences of the disease, but also the impact that it has on their life.

Self-management is an approach to the management of a long-term condition that recognises the central role of the person in health promotion, disease prevention and successful management of the disease (Silver 2018). Self-management is the individual's ability to manage the disease process, the emotional consequences of living with the disease and the changes that occur to daily living as a consequence of the disease (Audulv et al 2019). With self-management, the person with the long-term condition is motivated to take responsibility for their health needs and is supported by health professionals and community services who work collaboratively to assist the individual to manage their chronic illness (Howell et al 2019).

Evidence shows that programs incorporating self-management skills can enhance health outcomes (Du et al 2017; Fortuna et al 2018; Vas et al 2017). Self-management is both a process, whereby education or training is provided to people with chronic illness, and an outcome, when people with long-term conditions achieve the skills and knowledge to manage the medical, emotional and role aspects of their illness.

The health professional works in partnership with the person, providing self-management support, and works with the person towards the achievement of common goals.

The literature identifies the following skills as being essential in facilitating self-management support for a person with a long-term condition (Barrecheguren & Bourbeau 2018; Dobkin 2016; Phillips et al 2018):

- assessing the person's readiness for change
- using motivational interviewing techniques
- assisting the person to set goals and develop a realistic and achievable action plan
- building self-efficacy.

Assessing readiness for change

It is essential that a person is assessed to determine whether they are motivated to make some changes in their life and also whether they want to take the lead role in managing their long-term condition. Understanding the readiness of a person in relation to changing behaviour affects the way you will communicate and respond to that person using motivational interviewing techniques.

Prochaska and DiClemente (1983) developed a model of behaviour change that provides an easy yet credible method of assessing an individual's readiness for change. In this model it is suggested that people go through a series of changes when altering their behaviour. It is acknowledged in the health promotion literature that people are often at different stages of change in relation to adopting self-management strategies (Vallis et al 2018). Furthermore, there is substantial evidence demonstrating that behaviour change is more effective when an individual's stage of change is considered in the development of goals and care planning (Vallis et al 2018). The Transtheoretical Model, also known as the Stages of Change, developed by Prochaska and DiClemente in the mid-1970s for use in smoking cessation, is commonly used to determine readiness for change (Jalilian et al 2019). In this model, 'stage' is a temporal construct that signifies when specific changes are likely to occur. Rather than behaviour change being viewed as an event, in this model change is viewed as occurring over time (this is the temporal aspect), with individuals moving through a series of five stages from pre-contemplation, when they have no intention to change, to a final stage of maintenance, where they have made changes and have implemented strategies to prevent relapse and sustain the behaviour change (DiClemente & Prochaska 1998).

The stages of change described in this model are summarised in Table 3.1.

Using motivational interviewing to facilitate behaviour change

In addition to assessing an individual's readiness for change, motivation, barriers to change, attitudes and self-efficacy also need to be assessed. Motivational interviewing has become an accepted communication strategy for working with individuals who do not appear to be ready to change behaviours that may be considered necessary by the healthcare professional (Binning et al 2019). Motivational interviewing is based on the premise that most people do not enter into consultation with a health professional ready and willing to make behaviour changes, thus the healthcare professional's role is to assist the individual to explore and resolve their ambivalence about behaviour change. Motivational interviewing differs from other forms of counselling as it is more focused and goal-directed. The motivation to change is intrinsic and elicited from the individual. Consequently, the gains for the individual are driven by internal needs

TABLE 3.1
Transtheoretical Model

Stage	Behaviour
Pre-contemplation	The person has no intention of making any changes in the next 6 months. While they may lack motivation, they may also lack the knowledge and skills that enable them to change behaviour.
Contemplation	In this stage the person is contemplating change within the next 6 months. Although aware of the benefits of changing behaviour, ambivalence occurs as the person focuses on the barriers and costs that will occur during the change period.
Preparation	Individuals in this stage are preparing to take action within the next month. They generally have a plan and may have already taken some action towards the change.
Action	The person has made modifications and action is observable and measurable. It is during this stage that ongoing support is essential as relapse is a high risk.
Maintenance	The changes have been made and the risk of relapse is decreasing. Individuals in this stage feel confident that they can continue the new behaviour.

DiClemente & Prochaska 1998; Prochaska & DiClemente 1983.

and goals. Individuals are encouraged and assisted to explore their feelings and concerns about the current behaviour and the potential new behaviour. This often results in ambivalence or mixed feelings, whereby the individual weighs up the costs and benefits of changing behaviours. Motivational interviewing is a continuous process of eliciting information from the individual, the provision of information by the healthcare professional and then eliciting information on the individual's understanding of the new information (D'Souza 2019). There are four fundamental phases in motivational interviewing: (1) engaging; (2) guiding; (3) evoking; and (4) planning (Miller & Rollnick 2012; Rollnick et al 2010) (see Table 3.2 and Fig. 3.2).

Goal setting and action planning

Goal setting and action planning are collaborative processes in which the clinician assists the individual to choose a behaviour change goal. Prior to setting goals the clinician has a responsibility to ensure that the individual has adequate information to make an informed choice. Once a goal has been agreed to, an action plan to assist with goal attainment is developed collaboratively (Moore et al 2019). The SMART

TABLE 3.2
Phases in Motivational Interviewing

Phase	Clinician's Role and Responsibilities	Communication Strategies
Engaging (express empathy)	Build a rapport with the person Use OARS: • Open-ended questions • Affirm • Reflective listening • Summarise Assess the individual's stage of change	How are things going? What do you want to do next? What are the good things about … and what are the less good things?
Guiding (develop discrepancy)	Explore the values and attitudes held by the individual Identify goals and break into small achievable and measurable steps Encourage the individual to identify the benefits and costs to changing behaviour Allow the individual to form their own argument concerning changing behaviour	How would you like things to be different? How do you think you could do that? How can I help you achieve that? Who is in your life that would support you making these changes?

Continued

TABLE 3.2
Phases in Motivational Interviewing – cont'd

Phase	Clinician's Role and Responsibilities	Communication Strategies
Evoking (role with resistance)	The individual has identified a goal aimed at changing behaviour and is motivated to make the change Use selective eliciting: elicit and selectively reinforce the individual's motivational statements, intention to change and ability to change • Do not argue • Use reflection • Summarise • Affirm the statements made	It sounds like this is really difficult for you … What is most important to you now? So what you are saying is …
Planning (support self-efficacy)	Identify and set goals using SMART criteria: • Specific • Measurable • Achievable • Realistic • Timely	How did you manage something like this in the past? How do you think you could do this?

Miller & Rollnick 2012; Rollnick et al 2010.

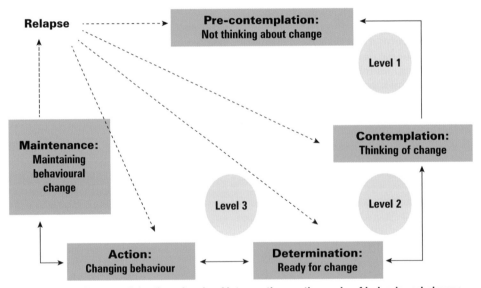

FIG. 3.2 **The impact of the three levels of intervention on the cycle of behavioural change.**

acronym can be applied to enable both the clinical staff and the individual to be able to measure whether goals have been attained (see Table 3.3).

A simple template for setting SMART goals contains the following:

• Goal
• When do I want to achieve it?
• How will I achieve it?
• How will I measure it?

Action planning results in a written commitment to action. Action plans are stated in measurable behavioural outcomes, so may be developed using SMART goals (Huffman et al 2019). When developing action plans from goals, assist the person to strive for a change

TABLE 3.3 Applying a SMART Goal	
Specific	Ensure the goal is specific to the problem. Get the person to start with 'my goal is to …'. This will make it specific. Ensure it is unambiguous. Describe goals in simple terms. What do they want to achieve? How will they achieve it? And when will they achieve it?
Measurable	The person needs to be able to determine if they have reached their goal. Write down how it will be measured if they reach their goal. You can also add in a starting point. If the goal is measurable, the person will be able to celebrate when they reach their milestone.
Achievable	The person needs to be able to think they CAN do this. Ask the following questions: What skills do you need to achieve this? What information and knowledge do you need? What help, assistance or collaboration do you need? What resources do you need? What barriers may block progress? Are you making any assumptions? Is there a better way of doing things? What steps do you need to accomplish your goal?
Realistic	The person must be able to expect to attain the goal. Don't allow them to set it too high to satisfy their friends or family or base their goals on someone else's aspirations. Write down 'I want to accomplish this goal because …'. Is this reasonable? This will keep them motivated.
Time Framed	The person must have a time frame within which to achieve their goal. This helps them stay focused and minimises procrastination. How long will it take to finish each step in the plan?

Bourbeau & Van der Palen 2009; Katch & Mead 2010.

that is behaviour-specific and always begin when a person has a confidence level of 7 or higher. You can determine the confidence level simply by asking the person on a scale of 0–10, with 10 being confident they can achieve the goal they have set, how confident they are that they will be successful (Speed 2019). A sample action plan is shown in Box 3.1.

Self-efficacy

Self-efficacy has been found to be essential in the development of self-management skills among people with long-term conditions (Milo 2017).

Bandura's Social Cognitive Theory posits that motivation and behaviour are moderated by cognitive, behavioural, personal and environmental factors

---

BOX 3.1
Goal-Behaviour Action Plan

Name: Natalie Doe **Date:** ………………….

Phone: …………..

The change I want to make is: Stop smoking.

My goal for the next 2 weeks is: To access information from the Quitline; gain support from family and friends; visit my family doctor for additional advice and support.

The steps I will take to achieve my goal are (what, when, where, how much, how often):

- I will identify reasons why I want to quit
- I will create a quit plan
- I will develop strategies to cope with cravings and stress.

The things that could make it difficult to achieve my goal include: Stressful events.

My plan for overcoming these difficulties includes:

- plan to quit at a time when no stressful life events are due to occur
- have a support person that I can seek advice and support from when I am facing challenges.

Support/resources I will need to achieve my goal include:

- friends and family
- family doctor
- Quitline (internet).

My confidence level (scale of 1–10, 10 being completely confident that you can achieve the entire plan): 8.

Review date: …………… (insert date for 2 weeks)

Review method: (phone, email, in person): In person with clinician.

(Schunk & Usher 2019). Bandura's seminal work in Social Cognitive Theory termed the interplay between these factors the Triadic Model of Reciprocal Causation and asserts that although each functions as an interacting element, they also influence each other bi-directionally (Bandura 2017). For example, a person's ability to self-manage their illness (behavioural factor) is influenced by how the person is affected (cognitive factors) by institutional policies and processes (environmental factors). Self-efficacy, an individual's belief that they have the ability to achieve in certain situations, lies at the heart of Bandura's Social Cognitive Theory. Basically self-efficacy is the 'I can' or 'I cannot' belief and reflects an individual's confidence in performing specific tasks. Bandura suggests that individual self-efficacy is acquired through four sources: (1) mastery experience; (2) vicarious experience; (3) social persuasion; and (4) physiological factors (Bandura 2017).

1. Mastery experience is performing a task successfully. Past experiences that show competence at mastering a similar skill or knowledge related to the skill contributes to a person's confidence in performing a task successfully. Success raises self-efficacy, failure lowers it!
2. Vicarious experience is when a person compares themselves to another person with similar abilities/disabilities and sees the person succeeding. This increases the person's self-efficacy; however, it needs to be noted that where they see the other person failing this will decrease their self-efficacy. In other words, the person thinks 'if they can do it, I can do it too'.
3. Social persuasions refers to either positive encouragement or negative comments. Positive encouragement increases a person's self-efficacy whereas negative persuasions decrease self-efficacy.
4. Physiological factors are our own emotional responses to situations. When a person is in a stressful situation physical symptoms may occur; for example, nausea and sweating. It is not the intensity of the symptoms; rather, it is how the person perceives and interprets them. Learning how to effectively manage stress and developing effective coping skills improves a person's self-efficacy.

In essence, self-efficacy involves helping people to set realistic goals, learn positive self-talk and learn the ability to visualise success. It is an intrinsic belief in your ability to perform a task successfully. Self-efficacy is an important component in self-management and it has been found that behaviour related to self-management is affected by individual self-efficacy (Wytrychiewicz et al 2019). Numerous research studies have demonstrated the importance of including self-efficacy in self-management programs across a number of chronic diseases; for example: cardiovascular disease (Irani et al 2019); chronic obstructive pulmonary disease (de Boer et al 2018); chronic kidney disease (Moktan et al 2019); diabetes (Lee et al 2019); ophthalmic disease (Drury et al 2017; Tey et al 2019); and arthritis (Zuidema et al 2019). Consequently, self-efficacy is usually incorporated into programs using a range of self-efficacy enhancing strategies, such as providing positive reinforcement, support in mastering new skills, modelling of new behaviours and building confidence (Nott et al 2019; Short 2019).

Self-Management Support

Key elements in self-management are the support and advocacy provided to people and their families to empower them to take a central role in managing their condition, set realistic and achievable goals, make informed decisions about their care and participate in healthy behaviours (Boucher et al 2019; Carey et al 2019; Lee et al 2019). Self-management support involves a partnership between the individual and the health professional where the health professional is the coach and the individual and their carers are the managers of daily care. In this model, the individual, family and carers and health professionals share information, understand the individual's goals and create an action plan that guides care at home as well as in the clinical setting (Howell et al 2019). The principles underpinning self-management support are to work collaboratively to:

- define the issues
- set goals and problem-solve
- provide active, sustained follow-up (Martz 2017).

The major difference between this model and the traditional medical model is that the patient is actively involved in their own care and works with the healthcare professional to manage the disease. The healthcare professional is the expert in the disease and the disease process while the patient is the expert about their life. The role of the healthcare professional is to provide support to the individual by assisting them to make informed choices, set their own goals and develop problem-solving skills (Boucher et al 2019).

The healthcare professional has a role of support when facilitating self-management with a person. Core knowledge and skills essential for healthcare professionals to provide self-management support can be centred around three platforms (Dineen-Griffin et al 2019):

1. Assessment skills, assessing:
   - readiness for change
   - risk factors
   - support systems
   - self-management ability.
2. Behaviour change skills:
   - effective use of motivational interviewing techniques
   - understanding theoretical models of behaviour change
   - able to assist the individual with goal setting, problem-solving and developing action plans.
3. Organisational strategies:
   - working in multidisciplinary teams
   - applying evidence to practice
   - sound knowledge of community resources.

The principles of self-management support, as discussed in the literature, include establishing a rapport and eliciting information from the individual about their progress, and the barriers and challenges they have confronted (Audulv et al 2019; Barrecheguren & Bourbeau 2018; Dineen-Griffin et al 2019; Martz 2017).

It is the role of the health professional to assess the individual's readiness for change and to help them understand and explore the consequences of current behaviours and any ambivalence towards change. These techniques require the health professional to have an understanding of the stages of change, as well as motivational interviewing techniques and Self-Efficacy Theory.

It is important to realise and accept that not all people will be ready to change. Pivotal to every self-management program is the development of an interpersonal relationship between the health professional and the individual. This relationship provides a safe environment for the health professional to help the individual to explore ambivalence and concerns, to provide education and help the individual understand their lifestyle and concerns.

INDIGENOUS AUSTRALIANS' HEALTH PROGRAMME AND CHRONIC DISEASE MANAGEMENT

In 2014 the Australian Government consolidated four extant funding streams, including the Aboriginal and Torres Strait Islander Chronic Disease Fund, into the Indigenous Australians' Health Programme. This program has a strong emphasis on the prevention, detection and management of chronic disease (Keleher 2019).

The Australian Government has contributed significant funding to facilitate the delivery of the Indigenous Chronic Disease package. This package has three major components:

1. Dealing with chronic disease risk factors
2. Improving chronic disease follow-up care and management
3. Expanding and supporting primary healthcare services (Gordon & Richards 2012).

The Chronic Care for Aboriginal People (Walgan Tilly) Clinical Services Redesign Project aimed to increase access to services and service utilisation and improve health outcomes for Aboriginal people in New South Wales. The application of this model requires health workers to possess certain skills that facilitate the building of trust with Aboriginal persons and communities. These skills are developed from meeting Aboriginal people and learning about their culture and values and being culturally sensitive (Pepler & Martell 2019).

Six statewide solutions were identified for NSW from the Walgan Tilly project. These are:

1. A Model of Care specifically for Aboriginal people
2. Greater cultural awareness and cultural sensitivity towards Aboriginal people
3. Integration of Aboriginal health and mainstream chronic disease services
4. Linkages with Justice Health
5. Improved access to primary healthcare services
6. Improved data quality (Scott 2011).

Previously the model was centred around vascular health; however, the Walgan Tilly project moved to a chronic disease approach focusing on four major diseases: cardiovascular disease, diabetes, chronic lung disease and kidney disease. The model may be used as a framework for the planning, monitoring and evaluation of service delivery initiatives and programs.

The Chronic Care for Aboriginal People Model of Care

After in-depth and extensive consultation, eight essential factors were identified as being vital to a Model of Care for working with chronic diseases in Indigenous Australian communities. These were: Identification, Trust, Screening and Assessment, Clinical Indicators, Treatment, Education, Referral and Follow-up (Gordon & Richards 2012).

The main factor that differs between this model and that of mainstream healthcare is the concept of trust. Indigenous Australians tend to mistrust mainstream healthcare services due to historical factors; trust and respect and the development of interpersonal relationships are integral to them participating in care (Lock 2018). The importance of communication – cups of tea and yarning – often viewed as time-consuming and unimportant in mainstream medicine, is inherent to the development of trust (Lin et al 2016).

PUTTING IT ALL TOGETHER

Theories such as the Transtheoretical Model, motivational interviewing and the Social Cognitive Theory have long provided a foundation for primary healthcare and health promotion strategies. However, many clinicians and healthcare students are perplexed by the different theories and have difficulties recognising the relationship between theories and how they can be integrated in clinical practice. Table 3.4 demonstrates the interrelationships between the Transtheoretical Model, motivational interviewing and Self-Efficacy Theory when facilitating self-management of long-term conditions.

In Case Study 3.1 we describe how the self-management framework, including Transtheoretical and Social Cognitive theories, were applied to a community-based project aimed at helping people with low vision regain optimal indepencence and remain safe within their own environments (Drury et al 2017; Tey et al 2019).

TABLE 3.4
Integrating Theoretical Concepts

Theories	Stage of Change (Transtheoretical Model)	Characteristics	Techniques	Health Professional's Role
Motivational interviewing Social Cognitive Theory – self-efficacy	Pre-contemplation	Not thinking about changing anything May be aware of problems, but lack the motivation to make any changes	Motivational interviewing (Rollnick et al 2010) Mastery experience (Bandura 2005) Vicarious experience (Bandura 2005)	Raise doubt about perceived risks and problems associated with current issue and with changing behaviours • Ask the client if they want to change this area of their life • Encourage the client to consider whether changes could improve their lifestyle. At this stage you are encouraging the client to reflect rather than act • Does the client need further education or resources?
	Contemplation	Not sure whether they want to change or not – ambivalent		Suggest reasons to change and risks to not changing Increase the client's self-efficacy for change • Ask the client if they want to change this area of their life • Explore changing the behaviour with the client: What effect would changes have on them? their family and friends? What are the pros and cons? • Can you identify some positive outcomes for them to consider?

TABLE 3.4
Integrating Theoretical Concepts – cont'd

Theories	Stage of Change (Transtheoretical Model)	Characteristics	Techniques	Health Professional's Role
Motivational interviewing Social Cognitive Theory – self-efficacy	Preparation	Have been trying to change or are planning to act	Motivational interviewing (Rollnick et al 2010) Mastery experience (Bandura 2005) Vicarious experience (Bandura 2005) Social persuasions (Bandura 2005) Psychological symptoms (Bandura 2005)	Help the client decide on the best course of action to take to … • Help your client to problem-solve • Identify social support and resources available • Verify that they have the skills and knowledge to change • Help them set small goals so that they have a sense of achievement
Motivational interviewing Social Cognitive Theory – self-efficacy Write – action planning	Action	Practising new behaviour for 3–6 months	Motivational interviewing (Rollnick et al 2010) Action planning (Scobbie et al 2011) Mastery experience (Bandura 2005) Vicarious experience (Bandura 2005) Social persuasions (Bandura 2005) Psychological symptoms (Bandura 2005)	Support the client to set goals and initiate the change • Focus on restructuring cues and social support • Bolster self-efficacy for dealing with obstacles • Combat feelings of loss and reiterate long-term benefits
	Maintenance	Continued commitment to sustaining new behaviour Post-6 months to 5 years		• Provide ongoing support and follow-up • Give positive reinforcement • Discuss coping with relapse
	Relapse	Go back to previous behaviour		Don't let the client get hindered by relapse; rather, assist them to rekindle their motivation for change • Help client determine the trigger for relapse • Re-evaluate motivational readiness and barriers to getting back on track • Plan coping strategies with your client to deal with triggers and barriers

Brody et al 2005; Curtin et al 2008; Johnston-Brooks et al 2002.

CASE STUDY 3.1

DESCRIPTION OF INTERVENTION

The Singapore Low Vision Self-Management Program is an innovative health promotion intervention implemented at primary health level via invitation to participate from tertiary hospital clinics and the Singapore Association for the Visually Handicapped (SAVH) (Tey et al 2019). It is led by medical social workers trained in self-management and psycho-social interventions, who are assisted by registered nurses also trained in self-management strategies. It targets people with low vision due to chronic eye diseases such as macular degeneration. The program is run over 4 weeks and is designed to address universal challenges faced by people with low vision. Learning activities included self-care, the use of visual aids, coping strategies, problem-solving and information related to chronic eye conditions.

APPLICATION OF THE TRANSTHEORETICAL MODEL AND SOCIAL COGNITIVE THEORY

Two conceptual approaches form the basis of the program: the Transtheoretical Model and Social Cognitive Theory (SCT). The Transtheoretical Model, as previously discussed, assesses individual readiness to change behaviour, while SCT promotes self-efficacy behaviours and beliefs.

ASSESSING READINESS FOR CHANGE USING THE TRANSTHEORETICAL MODEL

The Transtheoretical Model (Prochaska & DiClemente 1986) posits that people have varying levels of motivation or readiness to change. Accordingly, by using strategies effective for each stage, the program assists participants to move through the different stages of change. Initially, potential participants are assessed by a member of the team, who asks a number of questions to assess readiness for change. For example, potential participants are asked if they have tried anything to assist themselves with managing their low vision in activities of daily living. If the response is negative then the interviewer probes deeper to determine whether the person is ready for change or unwilling to change.

The first session of the program highlighted the advantages of changing health behaviours, particularly for those people in the pre-contemplation phase where individuals may have been resistant to change or unaware of the need to change. Setting goals each week and sharing reflections of the activity with program members facilitated individuals to move from a stage of contemplation, where they were aware and open to change, to the preparation phase, where they were ready to change. The weekly sessions helped individuals identify barriers, plan action for change and set realistic and achievable goals, while also providing positive affirmation and building self-efficacy.

ENHANCING SELF-EFFICACY

An important aspect of SCT (Bandura 2017) is enhancing self-efficacy, the confidence in one's ability to solve difficulties related to behaviour change and in increasing self-regulatory skills, including setting goals, solving problems and monitoring and rewarding oneself.

A number of factors were incorporated into the program to enhance self-efficacy behaviours and beliefs.

1. Individuals were encouraged to share successes and challenges. Therefore, self-efficacy was built through vicarious experience; that is, individuals were able to view the success of others and believe that they could also achieve the same result.

2. Positive feedback was provided by both staff and program members promoting positive encouragement among individuals, as well as emotional feelings of achievement and pride.

Weekly program sessions adopted motivational interviewing techniques. As part of this technique, participants were encouraged to talk as much as, or more than, the group leaders. Group leaders relied primarily on reflective listening and positive affirmations rather than direct questioning, persuasion or giving advice.

OUTCOMES OF THE PROGRAM

Narratives from patients were positive with individuals asserting that they gained independence and new and useful skills from the program. Intrinsic motivation has been found to be an important factor in ensuring positive outcomes in low vision self-management programs (Perlmutter & Hussey 2017; Yue'e et al 2016). The program has been revised and adopted across a number of organisations in Singapore. A Caregiver's program has also been developed and is being delivered to caregivers of people with low vision.

IMPLICATIONS FOR PRACTICE

This case demonstrates how a relatively simple intervention can be adapted within a group setting in the community. By training peers as leaders it is cost effective, while at the same time self-efficacy is enhanced as the peer leaders transmit values, behaviours and attitudes to others who model their behaviours accordingly.

These concepts can be adapted and implemented into practice individually, as well as in a group setting. When any patient with a chronic disease or disability presents to a health professional there is an opportunity to assess readiness to change behaviours, and use motivational interviewing to encourage people to identify and decrease feelings of ambivalence, leading to a motivation to change behaviour. The fundamental constructs to build self-efficacy can be utilised to increase individual confidence that changes can be made and sustained successfully.

CONCLUSION

The traditional medical model is not a sustainable model for people with long-term conditions. Managing a chronic disease is complex, multi-faceted and time-consuming. The person with the chronic disease has to manage the disease and live with the consequences of the disease daily, so it makes sense that they should be provided with the resources and skills to do this. The role of the health professional is to offer support, advice and facilitate access to resources. Self-management programs aim to change patient behaviour by increasing self-efficacy, encouraging the patient to gain new knowledge and skills and empowering patients to take control of their health. Changes in behaviour lead to better health outcomes, reduced utilisation of health services and fewer hospital admissions. Embedding these principles into the healthcare system requires clinicians and patients to embrace working as partners in care.

Reflective Questions

1 With the current move towards self-management for all long-term conditions and disabilities and the evidence supporting this model, why are some health professionals reluctant to move away from the traditional medical model and what can be done at a systems level to facilitate change?

2 With the dispersion of population in Australia and limited access to professional development for many clinicians, what tools could be developed that would facilitate patient engagement with self-management practices and clinician expertise in providing self-management support?

3 If working collaboratively as partners in care is an underlying principle of self-management, what strategies are needed to facilitate patient and clinician behaviour changes and embed this into practice?

RECOMMENDED READING

Hu J, Basit T, Nelson A, Crawford E et al 2019. Does attending Work It Out – a Chronic Disease Self-Management Program – affect the use of other health services by urban Aboriginal and Torres Strait Islander people with or at risk of chronic disease? A comparison between program participants and non-participants. Australian Journal of Primary Health 25(5), 464–470.

Prochaska JO, DiClemente C 1986. Toward a comprehensive model of change. Springer, Boston.

Tey CS, Man REK, Fenwick EK et al 2019. Effectiveness of the 'living successfully with low vision' self-management program: Results from a randomized controlled trial in Singaporeans with low vision. Patient Education and Counseling 102(6), 1150–1156.

Wang LH, Zhao Y, Chen LY et al 2020. The effect of a nurse-led self-management program on outcomes of patients with chronic obstructive pulmonary disease. The Clinical Respiratory Journal 14(2), 148–157.

REFERENCES

Atella V, Piano Mortari A, Kopinska J et al 2019. Trends in age-related disease burden and healthcare utilization. Aging Cell 18(1), e12861.

Auduly Å, Ghahari S, Kephart G et al 2019. The Taxonomy of Everyday Self-management Strategies (TEDSS): a framework derived from the literature and refined using empirical data. Patient Education and Counseling 102(2), 367–375.

Australian Health Ministers' Advisory Council 2017. National Strategic Framework for Chronic Conditions. Australian Government, Canberra.

Baird M, Bristow S, Moses A 2019. Self-management and empowerment chronic care nursing: a framework for practice. Cambridge University Press, Cambridge.

Bandura A (ed.) 2017. Psychological modeling: conflicting theories. Transaction Publishers, New Brunswick.

Bandura A 2005. The primacy of self-regulation in health promotion. Applied Psychology 54(2), 245–254.

Barr VJ, Robinson S, Marin-Link B et al 2003. The expanded Chronic Care Model: an integration of concepts and strategies from population health promotion and the Chronic Care Model. Hospital Quarterly 7(1), 73–82.

Barrecheguren M, Bourbeau J 2018. Self-management strategies in chronic obstructive pulmonary disease: a first step toward personalized medicine. Current Opinion in Pulmonary Medicine 24(2), 191–198.

Bauer MS, Miller CJ, Kim B et al 2019. Effectiveness of implementing a collaborative chronic care model for clinician teams on patient outcomes and health status in mental health: a randomized clinical trial. JAMA Network Open 2(3), e190230–e190230.

Binning J, Woodburn J, Bus SA et al 2019. Motivational interviewing to improve adherence behaviours for the prevention of diabetic foot ulceration. Diabetes/Metabolism Research and Reviews 35(2), e3105.

Bourbeau J, Van Der Palen J 2009. Promoting effective self-management programmes to improve COPD. European Respiratory Journal 33(3), 461–463.

Boucher LM, O'Brien KK, Baxter LN et al 2019. Healthy aging with HIV: the role of self-management support. Patient Education and Counseling 102(8), 1565–1569.

Brody BL, Roch-Levecq A, Thomas RG et al 2005. Self-management of age-related macular degeneration at the 6-month follow-up: a randomized controlled trial. Archives of Ophthalmology 123(1), 46–53.

Carey M, Agarwal S, Horne R et al 2019. Exploring organizational support for the provision of structured self-management education for people with Type 2 diabetes: findings from a qualitative study. Diabetic Medicine 36(6), 761–770.

Carrier J 2015. Managing long-term conditions and chronic illness in primary care: a guide to good practice: Routledge, London.

Coleman K, Austin BT, Brach C et al 2009. Evidence on the chronic care model in the new millennium. Health Affairs 28(1), 75–85.

Convery EA 2019. Hearing loss self-management in older adults. PhD thesis, University of Queensland, School of Health and Rehabilitation Sciences.

Curtin RB, Walters BAJ, Schatell D et al 2008. Self-efficacy and self-management behaviors in patients with chronic kidney disease. Advances in Chronic Kidney Disease 15(2), 191–205.

Cutler S, Crawford P, Engleking R 2018. Effectiveness of group self-management interventions for persons with chronic conditions: a systematic review. Medical–Surgical Nursing 27(6), 359.

D'Souza A 2019. Motivational interviewing: the RULES, PACE, and OARS. Current Psychiatry 18(1), 27–28.

Davy C, Bleasel J, Liu H et al 2015. Effectiveness of chronic care models: opportunities for improving healthcare practice and health outcomes: a systematic review. BMC Health Services Research 15(1), 194.

de Boer GM, Mennema TH, van Noort E et al 2018. Intrinsic factors influence self-management participation in COPD: effects on self-efficacy. ERJ Open Research 42(2), 00011–02018.

Desborough J, Parkinson A, Korda R et al 2019. The practical use of the Patient Enablement and Satisfaction Model in nurse-led outpatient cardiac clinics. Collegian 26(4), 415–421.

DiClemente CC, Prochaska JO 1998. Toward a comprehensive, Transtheoretical Model of change: stages of change and addictive behaviors. In: WR Miller, N Heather (eds), Treating addictive behaviors, 2nd edn. Plenum, New York.

Dineen-Griffin S, Garcia-Cardenas V, Williams K et al 2019. Helping patients help themselves: a systematic review of self-management support strategies in primary health care practice. PloS one, 14(8).

Dobkin BH 2016. Behavioral self-management strategies for practice and exercise should be included in neurologic rehabilitation trials and care. Current Opinion in Neurology 29(6), 693.

Drury VB, Aw AT, Shiow PLH 2017. Self-management of vision impairments. In E Martz (ed.), Promoting self-management of chronic health conditions: theories and practice. Oxford Press, New York.

Drury V, Chiang PP, Tey CS et al 2014. Assessing the willingness to change: optimising behaviour change in the management of chronic eye conditions. International Journal of Ophthalmic Practice 5(5), 182–188.

Du S, Hu L, Dong J et al 2017. Self-management program for chronic low back pain: a systematic review and meta-analysis. Patient Education and Counseling 100(1), 37–49.

Fortuna KL, DiMilia PR, Lohman MC et al 2018. Feasibility, acceptability, and preliminary effectiveness of a peer-delivered and technology supported self-management intervention for older adults with serious mental illness. Psychiatric Quarterly 89(2), 293–305.

Gill D, Blunt W, Silva NBS et al 2019. The HealtheSteps™ lifestyle prescription program to improve physical activity and modifiable risk factors for chronic disease: a pragmatic randomized controlled trial. BMC Public Health 19(1), 841.

González-Ortiz LG, Calciolari S, Goodwin N et al 2018. The core dimensions of integrated care: a literature review to support the development of a comprehensive framework for implementing integrated care. International Journal of Integrated Care 18(3).

Gordon R, Richards N 2012. The Chronic Care for Aboriginal People program in NSW. NSW Public Health Bulletin 23(4), 77–80.

Grover A, Joshi A 2015. An overview of chronic disease models: a systematic literature review. Global Journal of Health Science 7(2), 210.

Harris RE 2019. Epidemiology of chronic disease: global perspectives. Jones & Bartlett Learning, Burlington, MA.

Hindi AM, Schafheutle EI, Jacobs S 2019. Community pharmacy integration within the primary care pathway for people with long-term conditions: a focus group study of patients', pharmacists' and GPs' experiences and expectations. BMC Family Practice 20(1), 26.

Hofmeijer I 2020. Global risks report 2020. Online. Available: www3.weforum.org/docs/WEF_Global_Risk_Report_2020.pdf.

Holdsworth S, Corscadden L, Levesque JF et al 2019. Factors associated with successful chronic disease treatment plans for older Australians: implications for rural and Indigenous Australians. Australian Journal of Rural Health 27(4), 290–297.

Hosseinzadeh H, Shnaigat M 2019. Effectiveness of chronic obstructive pulmonary disease self-management interventions in primary care settings: a systematic review. Australian Journal of Primary Health 25(3), 195–204.

Howell D, Richardson A, May C et al 2019. Implementation of self-management support in cancer care and normalization into routine practice: a systematic scoping literature review protocol. Systematic Reviews 8(1), 37.

Huffman JC, Feig EH, Millstein RA et al 2019. Usefulness of a positive psychology–motivational interviewing intervention to promote positive affect and physical activity after an acute coronary syndrome. The American Journal of Cardiology 123(12), 1906–1914.

Irani E, Moore SE, Hickman RL et al 2019. The contribution of living arrangements, social support, and self-efficacy to self-management behaviors among individuals with heart failure: a path analysis. Journal of Cardiovascular Nursing 34(4), 319–326.

Jalilian H, Pezeshki MZ, Janati A et al 2019. Readiness for diet change and its association with diet knowledge and skills, diet decision making and diet barriers in type 2 diabetic patients. Diabetes & Metabolic Syndrome: Clinical Research & Reviews 13(5), 2933–2938.

James S, Halcomb E, Desborough J et al 2019. Lifestyle risk communication by general practice nurses: an integrative literature review. Collegian 26(1), 183–193.

Johnston-Brooks CH, Lewis MA, Garg S 2002. Self-efficacy impacts self-care and HbA1c in young adults with type 1 diabetes. Psychosomatic Medicine 64(1), 43–51.

Katch H, Mead H 2010. The role of self-efficacy in cardiovascular disease self-management: a review of effective programs. Patient Intelligence 2, 33–44.

Keleher H 2019. Primary health care in Australia. In: E Willis, L Reynolds, T Rudge (eds), Understanding the Australian health care system. Elsevier, Sydney.

Lee AA, Piette JD, Heisler M et al 2019. Diabetes self-management and glycemic control: the role of autonomy support from informal health supporters. Health Psychology 38(2), 122.

Li Y, Pan A, Wang DD et al 2018. Impact of healthy lifestyle factors on life expectancies in the US population. Circulation 138(4), 345–355.

Liddy C, Johnston S, Nash K et al 2016. Implementation and evolution of a regional Chronic Disease Self-Management Program. Canadian Journal of Public Health 107(2), e194–e201.

Lin I, Green C, Bessarab D 2016. 'Yarn with me': applying clinical yarning to improve clinician–patient communication in Aboriginal health care. Australian Journal of Primary Health 22(5), 377–382.

Lock M 2018. Australian healthcare governance and the cultural safety and security of Australia's first peoples: an annual critique. No. 1: Focussing on knowledge governance. Committix, Newcastle.

Lorig K 1996. Chronic disease self-management: a model for tertiary prevention. American Behavioral Scientist 39(6), 676–683.

Martz E 2017. Promoting self-management of chronic health conditions: theories and practice: Oxford University Press, New York.

McGrady A, Moss D 2018. Chronic illness, global burden, and the pathways approach: integrative pathways. Springer, New York.

McLaughlin R 2019. The effects of a self-management programme (Stanford model) on adults in County Donegal with long term health conditions. International Journal of Integrated Care, 19.

Miller WR, Rollnick S 2012. Motivational interviewing: helping people change. Guilford Press, New York.

Milo RB 2017. Patient knowledge, perceived self-efficacy, and self-management among patients with type II diabetes mellitus. Doctor of Nursing. University of San Diego, San Diego.

Moktan S, Leelacharas S, Prapaipanich W 2019. Knowledge, self-efficacy, self-management behavior of the patients with predialysis chronic kidney disease. Ramathibodi Medical Journal 42(2), 38–48.

Moore A, Esquibel KA, Hilliard TC et al 2019. Improving health through motivational interviewing. Nursing Made Incredibly Easy 17(5), 18–25.

Moreno EG, Mateo-Abad M, de Retana García LO et al 2019. Efficacy of a self-management education programme on patients with type 2 diabetes in primary care: a randomised controlled trial. Primary Care Diabetes 13(2), 122–133.

National Health Priority Action Council 2006. National Chronic Disease Strategy. Australian Government, Canberra.

Nejhaddadgar N, Darabi F, Rohban A et al 2019. The effectiveness of self-management program for people with type 2 diabetes mellitus based on PRECEDE-PROCEDE model. Diabetes & Metabolic Syndrome: Clinical Research & Reviews 13(1), 440–443.

Nott M, Wiseman L, Seymour T et al 2019. Stroke self-management and the role of self-efficacy. Disability and Rehabilitation 1–10.

Pepler E, Martell RC 2019. Indigenous model of care to health and social care workforce planning. Healthcare Management Forum 32(1), 32–39.

Perlmutter M, Hussey G 2017. Living life with vision loss: a community-based self-management program for people with low vision. OT Practice 2017, 24–26.

Phillips R, Hogden A, Greenfield D 2018. Motivational interviewing to promote self-management. In: E Martz (ed.), Promoting self-management of chronic health conditions: theories and practice. Oxford University Press, Melbourne.

Prochaska JO, DiClemente CC 1986. Toward a comprehensive model of change. In: WR Miller, N Heather (eds), Treating addictive behaviors. Springer, Boston, MA.

Prochaska JO, DiClemente CC 1983. Stages and processes of self-change of smoking: toward an integrative model of change. Journal of Consulting and Clinical Psychology 51(3), 390.

Rollnick S, Butler CC, Kinnersley P et al 2010. Competent novice: motivational interviewing. BMJ: British Medical Journal 340(7758), 1242–1245.

Schunk DH, Usher EL 2019. Social Cognitive Theory and motivation. The Oxford handbook of human motivation. In: R Ryan (ed.), The Oxford handbook of human motivation. Oxford University Press, Oxford.

Scobbie L, Dixon D, Wyke S 2011. Goal setting and action planning in the rehabilitation setting: development of a theoretically informed practice framework. Clinical Rehabilitation 25(5), 468–482.

Scott M 2011. Evaluation of Walgan Tilly Project. NSW Health Chronic Care For Aboriginal People Program. NSW Health, Sydney.

Short AL 2019. Enhancing migraine self-efficacy and reducing disability through a self-management program. Journal of the American Association of Nurse Practitioners 33(1), 20–28.

Silver I 2018. Bridging the gap: person centred, place-based self-management support. Future Healthcare Journal 5 (3), 188.

Speed S 2019. The use of motivational interviewing to determine smoking cessation readiness: literature review. (DNP), South Dakota State University. Online. Available: https://openprairie.sdstate.edu/con_dnp/124.

Tay KCP, Drury VB, Mackey S 2014. The role of intrinsic motivation in a group of low vision patients participating in a self-management programme to enhance self-efficacy and quality of life. International Journal of Nursing Practice 20(1), 17–24.

Taylor D, Binns E, Signal N 2017. Upping the ante: working harder to address physical inactivity in older adults. Current Opinion in Psychiatry 30(5), 352–357.

Tey CS, Man REK, Fenwick EK et al 2019. Effectiveness of the 'living successfully with low vision' self-management program: results from a randomized controlled trial in Singaporeans with low vision. Patient Education and Counseling 102(6), 1150–1156.

Thornicroft G, Ahuja S, Barber S et al 2019. Integrated care for people with long-term mental and physical health conditions in low-income and middle-income countries. The Lancet Psychiatry 6(2), 174–186.

Vallis M, Lee-Baggley D, Sampalli T et al 2018. Equipping providers with principles, knowledge and skills to successfully integrate behaviour change counselling into practice: a primary healthcare framework. Public Health 154, 70–78.

Vas A, Devi ES, Vidyasagar S et al 2017. Effectiveness of self-management programmes in diabetes management: a systematic review. International Journal of Nursing Practice 23(5), e12571.

Wagner EH 1998. Chronic disease management: what will it take to improve care for chronic illness? Effective Clinical Practice: ECP 1(1), 2.

World Health Organization (WHO) 2015. World report on ageing and health [Internet]. 2015. WHO, Geneva. Online. Available: https://apps.who.int/iris/bitstream/handle/10665/186463/9789240694811_eng.pdf;jsessionid=566BF1D4CDC22EAD1EE416F51C7031DC?sequence=1.

Wytrychiewicz K, Pankowski D, Bargiel-Matusiewicz K et al 2019. The role of psychological and medical variables in the process of adaptation to life with chronic illness in a group of COPD outpatients. Psychology, Health & Medicine 24(10), 1243–1254.

Yeoh E, Wong MC, Wong EL et al 2018. Benefits and limitations of implementing Chronic Care Model (CCM) in primary care programs: a systematic review. International Journal of Cardiology 258, 279–288.

Yue'e Y, Lingzhi N, Wang A 2016. The effect of intrinsic motivation on self-efficacy and quality of life for low vision patients. Chinese Journal of Practical Nursing 32(1), 45–49.

Zuidema R, van Dulmen S, Nijhuis-van der Sanden R et al 2019. Efficacy of an online self-management enhancing program for patients with rheumatoid arthritis: explorative randomized controlled trial. In: R Zuidema (ed.), Participatory development and evaluation of an online self-management enhancing program for patients with rheumatoid arthritis. PhD thesis. Radboud University, The Netherlands.

CHAPTER 4

Spirituality

JOHN XAVIER ROLLEY • ESTHER CHANG • AMANDA JOHNSON

LEARNING OBJECTIVES

When you have completed this chapter you will be able to:

- understand spirituality as a key concept of nursing practice
- appreciate the central role spirituality plays in human living and dying
- appreciate the diversity of spiritual expression people and their families bring to experiences of suffering and illness
- appreciate and recognise the role of the nurse in providing spiritual care for people with chronic illness and/or disability
- reflect on your own spirituality and the influence this has on the delivery of nursing care.

KEY WORDS

hope	spirituality
self-awareness	suffering
spiritual care	

INTRODUCTION

Spirituality is an essential and dynamic human phenomenon. It influences your life and the lives of those you interact with, whether you are aware of it or not. Spirituality is a human experience which is profoundly subjective and mysterious. As a nurse working with people with chronic and complex needs, you will encounter spirituality flowing through people's lives and experiences of illness, suffering and wellbeing.

As evidenced throughout this book, practice is best founded on principles rather than tasks. In order to assist you to negotiate the concepts of this chapter, some guiding principles for practice are given below and integrated into the discussion.

There is a need for nurses to be:

- aware of how spirituality is expressed in their lives and living
- informed of the current best practice in spiritual care, and
- sensitive to diverse spiritual needs and expressions.

DEFINING SPIRITUALITY

Defining spirituality is problematic and iterative in nature (Lalani 2020). Spirituality is a multifactorial, interconnected, universal human meta-concept (Lasair 2020). Factors include culture, religious background, socioeconomic status, educational level, gender and sexuality. For example, atheists may express spirituality in terms that exclude religion or religious process, while secular humanists may deny the existence of spirituality as a valid element of human expression. Whatever the perspective, defining spirituality is a complex and subjective process.

The essence of spirituality appears to be deeply integrated with how people derive and live out meaning in and of life (Lasair 2020). It includes how the individual defines their 'world view'; that is, information gathered from the world around them through multiple 'filters' such as familial, social, cultural, religious and personal experiences. It is difficult to simply describe what is a dynamic and multifactorial process. As this chapter will discuss, spirituality is a common human experience that sits above and behind personal religious belief and practice.

An important note of caution is required. Whenever reading, reflecting on and discussing spirituality, it is important to consider the contexts of all involved. The influence of those filters cannot be underestimated.

Spirituality as Connection

Spirituality incorporates both the internal and personal experiences, as well as what is experienced through connection with others (Sadat Hoseini et al 2019). Essentially, spirituality is a relational concept. The dimension beyond the self involves connection with an 'other', which is the purpose and process of spiritual experience and expression. It includes the big questions people ask about life and its meaning, as well as how their relationships impact on the self (Lasair 2020). These relationships involve the connections of family, support networks, including friends, groups and the community, and, in some cases, the divine, in whichever way that is perceived and defined.

According to Holopainen and colleagues (2017), caring is experienced in the encounter between the nurse and the person they are caring with. It is in the experience of reaching and touching that relationships are established; a core process to human relating and caring. Connection and, importantly for the nurse, the intention of the connection, allow relationships to develop. Both the nurse and the person move from the experience of 'otherness' as the space between them is bridged through mutual connection.

Families, Friends and Human Connection

Relationships help bring meaning to life. They provide a context, space or place for growth and expression. As social beings, humans need to relate, share, tell stories, hear and be heard, express emotion, love, loss and grieve. It is in the nexus of relationships that people come to learn who they are and develop meaning. Isolate an infant, for example, and they run the risk of 'failure to thrive' due to deprivation of interaction, touch and intimacy (Arel 2019). Indeed, it is intimacy between a person, their family, friends and life partner that is essential to survival.

As stated above, spirituality is a relational concept: relationship with the self and with an 'other' or 'others'. Hawkins (1987, cited in Burkhardt & Nagai-Jacobson 2002, p. 266) said this about the spirituality of relationships:

> When we attempt to lead our spiritual lives apart from the nurture, support and accountability of others, we end up distorting our spiritual growth. The presence of fellow travellers is essential for our growth. We need companionship and communion with others.

Nowhere is this more vital than in illness. Chronic illness, in particular, brings added strain to the person experiencing the illness, let alone the relationships that form their social fabric. Yet, it is these relationships that are essential to the healing of the person. The role of nurses, then, is to support and role-model these healing relationships. The nurse becomes one who comes alongside the person and their family; not to replace but to enhance (see Case Study 4.1).

CASE STUDY 4.1

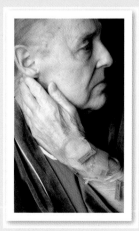

iStockphoto/Instants.

Two weeks ago Mr Darren Marcs, a 54-year-old man, was diagnosed with end-stage prostate cancer with spread to his regional lymph nodes and metastatic disease to his spine and liver (Grading: T4 N1 M1). He first detected a problem after noting worsening back pain which was not relieved with analgesia. Darren had not had any routine prostate screening, despite being over the age of 45.

Darren was raised a Roman Catholic, yet has not adhered to any religious observance for over the past 25 years, and has, since that time, avowed atheism. Darren was divorced 6 years ago in difficult circumstances and of his three children, only one, Michael (aged 22), the eldest, has maintained any contact. Darren has requested that his former wife and two remaining children are not to be told of his diagnosis or prognosis. Darren is in considerable pain, which staff are struggling to treat effectively, and he is showing signs of depression. When he is with his son, Michael, Darren is often teary and clearly distressed.

CASE STUDY 4.1 – cont'd

Other members of the healthcare team have reported Darren to be 'difficult' and 'prickly' to engage with.

Michael approaches you and confides that he is worried about his father's depression. He says his father is deeply afraid of death. Michael, the only member of the family to identify with his father's religious convictions, states that he is at a loss as to how to console his father.

CASE STUDY QUESTIONS

1. Spend some time reflecting on the effects of the disease process on Darren's sense of self, relationships and spirituality.

2. What are some important things to consider when approaching spiritual care for people who identify as being atheist?

3. Is there such a thing as an atheistic spirituality?

4. Reflect on the effect of suffering on Darren's life. What impact is this having on his health?

5. What approaches could you, as the nurse, take to engage Michael in Darren's care?

6. Hold a debate: does atheism automatically preclude a person from identifying as a spiritual person?

Religion, Human Ritual and Spirituality

At one time, being religious and being spiritual were synonymous, as evidenced by the lack of an equivalent term for 'spirituality' in the Judeo–Christian religious tradition. However, it could be argued that if a person needed to be religious in order to be authentically spiritual, the experiences of many people, including scientists, healthcare professionals, artists, poets, musicians and philosophers, would mean little. Social changes after World War II, together with the challenge to the authority of religion, have given rise to secularism in the West. When the influx of Eastern spiritual traditions into the West is considered, the once clearly held ideas of traditional religious belief no longer hold prominence. In Australia, the most recent Census revealed that 30% of the population reported 'no religion' (ABS 2017).

As discussed above, spirituality involves the 'stuff' of life. This does not mean religion does not or cannot play an important role in the process of life, nor does it mean that the person is required to engage in religious practice or belief. Rather, religion may provide a structure for spiritual expression where beliefs may assist the individual in constructing a view of the world and thereby derive meaning for living their lives. People living with chronic conditions have reported benefit from religious involvement (Krause et al 2019). Yet, the opposite is equally true, where people can find religious structures and talk distressing (Broom 2016). As the responses to religious practice are diverse, the nurse must be sensitive to the person's unique spiritual and religious perspective (see Table 4.1).

Some religions are theistic, meaning they hold a central belief in the existence of a god or gods. Others, such as Buddhism, do not believe in a god as such, but rather in the process of evolution of each soul towards enlightenment and the release of the need for Karma or purification through reincarnation.

Most religions include complex constructions of the world, how it came about and the place of people in relation to the world. They often prescribe the behaviour of their members regarding these world views, moral values, practice and worship. The Judeo–Christian tradition has a long yet varied history representing two of three major theistic branches of monotheism. The other monotheistic religion, Islam, holds similar beliefs about the value of life and the need for caring for the sick as an extension of belief in God (Heydari et al 2016). Furthermore, many of the advances in medicine, science and mathematics prior to the Western European Renaissance were due to the work of Islamic scholars. Regardless of the religious paradigm, it is important to realise that spirituality flows beyond religious structures.

Atheism, on the other hand, never describes itself as a religion, but has similar, albeit opposite, beliefs to theism. More recently, there has been an emerging debate about the place of spirituality among those who identify as atheist. Two philosophers have tackled this in the popular press: Alain de Botton and André Comte-Sponville. Both argue for an atheism that engages the 'best' of religious traditions, in terms of universal values of love, community, aesthetics, kindness or compassion and ritual (Comte-Sponville 2006; de Botton 2012). In their discussion, the notion of spirituality avoids the supernatural and superstitious. Their approach is not without criticism from within atheist circles, and serves to remind nurses of the complexity and subjective nature of spirituality. Furthermore, it underscores the need for nurses to avoid categorising people.

TABLE 4.1
Religious Diversity – Key Points

Belief	Type of religion	Core beliefs	Core practices
Atheism	Atheistic	• The existence of God cannot be demonstrated • All of existence can be explained through rational means • What is yet unexplainable will one day be explainable using rational methods • There is no life beyond death	• Various • Usually humanistic approaches to personal reflection
Baha'i	Theistic	• God is one • The various religions of the world are manifestations of the One God • Baha U'llah, born Mizra Husayn-Ali Nuri, is considered the prophetic fulfilment by Baha'i of Islamic, Christian and other religious traditions • There is life beyond death	• Daily prayer • Pilgrimage • Reading of holy scriptures
Buddhism	Atheistic	• Life is a cycle of birth, death and rebirth • The soul progresses towards enlightenment and the end of the need to suffer • Nirvana is the ultimate form of being and is essentially absolute unity, or Buddha-hood, with all things • Various sects have differing approaches to Buddhism with varying beliefs about the existence of deities and the place of ritual	• Meditation • Good deeds • Reading of sacred texts
Christianity	Theistic	• God is one yet a union of three 'persons': Father, Son and Holy Spirit • God as creator who is above and beyond the created order • Jesus as Son of God and Saviour to those who believe • The word of God is found in the Holy Bible • The 'Church' is the body of Christ on earth • One becomes a Christian through baptism • There is life beyond death • Many sects have varying beliefs about these core beliefs and practices	• Daily prayer • Reading of the Bible • Attendance at church services • The Holy Communion, Eucharist or Mass as the central act of worship for most Christians
Hinduism	Polytheistic	• Oldest 'living' religion • All life is sacred • God is expressed in many ways and forms • Life is a cycle of birth, death and rebirth • Karma is an infinite force for teaching and purifying the soul on its many reincarnations • People are born into various casts which orders society and is determined by Karma • There are several sects with devotees focused on the deities associated with them, for example, Shivism (Shiva), Krishna Consciousness (Krishna or Vishnu) and Brahmanism (Brahma)	• Meditation • Attendance at temple for important feasts and milestones • The importance of the dharma or teachings found in the many texts such as Vedas, Sutras or sacred writings • The importance of social conventions regarding caste and family obligations

TABLE 4.1
Religious Diversity – Key Points – cont'd

Belief	Type of religion	Core beliefs	Core practices
Islam	Theistic	• God is one • God created all things and is above and beyond the created order • Muhammad is the last and greatest prophet • The word of God is found in the Quran • There is life beyond death	• Daily prayer • Reading the holy scriptures • Attending corporate prayer • Fasting at certain times, including the great fast of Ramadan
Judaism	Theistic	• God is one • God created all things and is above and beyond the created order • There is life beyond death	• Daily prayer • Recitation of the scriptures with emphasis on the Torah or Law
Shinto	Animistic; Polytheistic	• Japanese Indigenous spirituality • There is life beyond death • There are several sects	• Daily reverence of the 'kami' or spirits of the ancestors • Attendance at special shrine observances
Sikh	Theistic	• God is one • God created all things and is above and beyond the created order • The word of God is found in Guru Granth Sahib or holy scriptures • Baptism is the way a person becomes a Sikh • There is life beyond death	• Daily prayer • Attendance at festivals and temple events • Reading of the holy scriptures

THE ROLE OF RITUAL IN SPIRITUALITY

Human beings are essentially ritualistic. While the term 'ritual' may imply religious practice, it is an essential human phenomenon beyond religion alone. Including religious observances, such as going to a sacred space, human ritual extends to every part of human existence. Rites of passage in life (birthday celebrations, coming of age and celebrating successes), rituals of connecting with another person (the bow, handshake, hug or kiss), and the marking of changes in intimate relationships (such as the first date, engagement or betrothal, marriage and death), all express the milestones of life. Other more mundane examples, such as how people choose their clothes, bathe and eat, as well as how they celebrate 'special' occasions such as birthdays and anniversaries, and mark grief and loss, speak of the ritual existence humans are living. They connect with some sense of meaning and use ritual to express that meaning. As such, ritual plays an important role in the lives of those living with chronic illness and/or disabilities, and such experiences can bring significant challenges to their sense of self and world view.

Those who identify with religion may use ritual as a source of connection with a higher reality or being. Prayer, meditation, corporate forms of worship, spiritual reading and contemplation form the core of most religious expression. While debate rages as to the empirically measurable benefits of these activities, many report a deep satisfaction and increased sense of wellbeing through engaging in ritual practice. As such, it continues to be a vital aspect of how human beings gain meaning in life and overcome barriers.

In summary, the concepts of spirituality, religion and ritual can inform and flow into each other. Spirituality is the broader context for both religion and ritual, both of which form expressions of spirituality. This is illustrated in Fig. 4.1.

WHY SPIRITUALITY IS IMPORTANT TO NURSING

Nursing is a healthcare profession focused on more than just disease and injury. The World Health Organization (WHO), in its fundamental definition of health, recognises that health concerns people's wellbeing

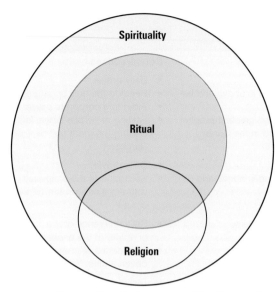

FIG. 4.1 **The relationship between spirituality, religion and ritual.**

rather than the absence of disease (WHO 1948). What this means for nurses regarding spirituality is complex.

As discussed earlier, spirituality is a human process of finding meaning in life and life's experiences. The individual moves beyond the objective biological determinants of life to the metaphysical (a term that literally means 'beyond or above the physical'). The challenge nurses face when clients, often in distress, ask 'Why is this happening to me?', cannot be answered by citing test results or biological measures alone. Other approaches are necessary.

The imperative of competent spiritual care at the core of nursing does not lie in any sacred or divine calling placed on nurses. Rather, it is the patterns of care, where nurses provide extensive, extended and often intimate support, that lie at the heart of this challenge.

Nursing the Whole Being

Nursing theorists have championed the adoption of other models and frameworks for viewing and responding to the human condition. Taking a humanistic approach, these theories often incorporate the need to approach the person as a complete, connected entity: body, mind and spirit. This integration is referred to as 'holism'. As a term, it has been classically defined simply as 'the whole is greater than the sum of its parts', and has often been considered synonymous with nursing (Kinchen 2015). From a health viewpoint, it includes biological, psychological,

sociological and spiritual dimensions. The indivisible nature of the union is essential to understanding holism. It will not do to define holism as a deconstruction of a whole, that is, biological 'bits', psychological 'bits', social 'bits' and spiritual 'bits'.

Several nursing theorists engage in integrative notions where the environment, health, the person and nursing converge. The most significant aspect of these notions are the relationships formed between the client and the nurse. Easley (2007) describes this in terms of harmony, where the coming together of a conducive environment, engaging of the client and the nurse, and time, are integral in building the relationship.

Spirituality and Suffering

Suffering is a recurrent theme in spirituality and health. It is considered one of the most profound of human experiences and one that the individual negotiates alone. Cassell (2004, p. 32), writing what has become a seminal work on the topic, defined suffering as '… the severe distress associated with events that threaten the intactness of the person'. Importantly, this notion of threat to 'intactness' or integrity of a person is not solely reliant on an event, but rather the perception of what that event means for the individual (Vance 2019). Ellis and colleagues (2015), reporting on a qualitative study that investigated the perceptions of suffering experienced by people with advanced cancer, found suffering to be a complex and context-dependent experience. Suffering is a shared human physical and emotional experience that encompasses loss, yet, interestingly for the participants, led to an experience of transformation (Ellis et al 2015). It was in that transformational space that the notions of spirituality were expressed. For nurses, the uniqueness of the person's experience is paramount and suffering has the power to alter the individual's perception of meaning (Cassell 2004; Ellis et al 2015). Given a significant enough confrontation, through an event or perceived consequence of an event, the constructed meaning of the individual's worldview can crumble. It is through the crumbling process that the person experiences suffering.

Suffering is a deeply personal experience, which may engender feelings of isolation and vulnerability leading to hopelessness. Hopelessness, experienced as despair or the belief that they are without hope, is a significant experience of those who suffer. Through these experiences, it is important to note that the extent to which people experience hopelessness varies with the individual, and the circumstances, such as those encountered in chronic illness, where the feeling may be transitory (Leite et al 2019).

The idea of 'transition' as a psychological process, where the person seeks new meaning, is critical to how people navigate chronic illness and disability health journeys (Munck et al 2018). Yet, in the context of this chapter, it is equally important to see transition as essentially spiritual, as it speaks to the process of human meaning-making. The process of transition entails progression towards new perceptions, not the return to an older perception. The experience renders the notion of 'return' to a previous state impossible, as the person has had to engage in the consequences of the stimulus to their suffering (Munck et al 2018).

Holding Hope

Traversing suffering requires resilience that is born of another human trait: the holding of hope. The focus is on a future that is grounded in a perceived reality that is essentially subjective, yet vital to life and wellness (Clarke 2003). Without hope, the individual soon loses their emotional connection to life, and death may follow (Clarke 2003). Suffering is so confronting due to its effect on the perceived reality of things that to 'lose hope' is to let go of the desire to survive the experience. Losing hope or despairing is the opposite of hope, which, as Fitzgerald Miller (2007, p. 14) states, '… saves persons from the agony of despair'. An Australian philosopher, Zournazi (2002, p. 22), wrote this about hope:

What does hope involve in everyday life and experience? Imagine you have a friend who is sick or a loved one who is dying: there is a trust that situations or events, even in adversity, have an element that could sustain our belief in the world. This hope has no logical or clear definition to it. It may be the hope that things could be different or the cherishing of life, where courage marks the strength to continue, and where aspects of grief, mourning and death become part of life, and the movement is one away from despair. If we can understand hope as composing life as it emerges, there is the possibility of joy and a hopeful vision for the world.

Hope is not the denial of reality presented by suffering. Rather, it is the incorporation of it into the person's experience. Hope has been connected with the feeling of power or empowerment in the midst of suffering (Olsman et al 2016). As such, it implies relationship. It is in that relational space created through suffering and hope that the nurse provides care. Olsman and colleagues (2016) describe the process of caring or solicitude as:

… the power of hope and empowerment, which are supported by mutually dependent relationships. On the other hand, solicitude includes compassion, which is the shared recognition of fragility and suffering, in which the difference between giving and receiving is transcended.

THE NURSE AS A SPIRITUAL BEING

How often do nurses ask themselves who they are or what causes them to think and act a certain way? While uncovering answers to such questions takes a lifetime, it is a quest every nurse is encouraged to take. Self-awareness is a critical aspect of a nurse's professional development and impacts on their capacity to engage others appropriately in spiritual care. The heart of this quest is in understanding the motivators for values, beliefs and resulting actions. It is a journey of discovery about what it is to be a human being. Reflection is essential for professional and personal development.

Several tools can be used to assist nurses with the reflective process, and include, yet are not limited to: reflective journalling, artwork, meditation, dream analysis, physical movement and ritual. Choosing the best approach is an individual process.

Tools for Reflective Practice

Journalling is a common approach to self-discovery. Confidentiality is important if this method is to be used, and so the journal should be kept in a safe place. Writing for most people causes anxiety. The following is a guide to aid the reader, adapted from Bolton (2001):

1. Find a space that is quiet and where you will not be distracted for 30–40 minutes.
2. Write for about 6 minutes without stopping – try not to think about the process, just write whatever comes into your head. This is to help get the 'juices' flowing.
3. Pause, reread but do not judge what you have written.
4. Sit quietly again, and focus on what you feel you need to reflect on.
5. Start writing and keep doing so for about 20–40 minutes.
6. Spend some time rereading and reflecting on what you have written. Keep the following in mind:
   i. Do not worry about grammar, punctuation or spelling
   ii. Allow reaction and emotion to flow unhindered
   iii. Remember that what you are writing is your perspective
   iv. Refrain from judgement.

Writing for reflection takes time. What is more, there will be times when reflective writing will play a larger part in life than other times. The important thing is to engage in the process.

People may also prefer a visual approach using one of many artwork genres. It may be drawing, painting, sculpture or craft work, such as the use of textiles, wood or metal. Instead of words, colour, pictures or symbols are used for reflection.

Using a similar approach to writing described above, allow yourself to settle in a quiet space free from distraction. Choose a medium (e.g. painting, drawing, clay or collage) that suits you best. Focus on what it is you want to reflect on and allow it to flow, ensuring to refrain from judgement.

Clinical Supervision

Having someone to talk with about your spiritual needs is essential. This is especially true for nurses who work with patients and families experiencing grief and loss repeatedly during the trajectory of chronic illness and death (Ryan & Seymour 2016). The following are examples of personal spirituality questions to promote reflection for nurses (see Case Study 4.2):

- What do I believe in?
- What do I value in my life?
- What gives my life meaning?
- What do I hope for?
- How do I cope with adversity?
- Who do I love and who loves me?
- How am I with others?

CASE STUDY 4.2

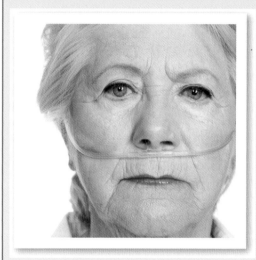

iStockphoto/STEEX.

Janet is a registered nurse with 3 years experience in intensive care and a total of 5 years experience since she graduated from university. She is caring for Phyllis, aged 68, who has a long history of chronic respiratory and cardiac illness. Phyllis was brought into hospital by her daughter, Elaine, following deterioration from a bout of influenza. Phyllis has been admitted several times in the past 3 months due to either exacerbation of chronic respiratory disease or pulmonary oedema secondary to congestive heart failure.

The most recent admission resulted in Phyllis being admitted to the intensive care unit (ICU) and intubated, requiring full ventilation support. Her admission was characterised by sepsis and multi-organ failure. All attempts at weaning her off ventilation have failed. Her deterioration has been so profound that medical staff feel Phyllis will not survive an extubation. Janet has been appointed as the primary nurse managing Phyllis's care and has been working extensively with the family. Janet understands that the prognosis is not good and has been subtly preparing the family for Phyllis's possible death.

A family conference is called. Elaine, who has been providing the majority of care for Phyllis, and her two other siblings and their partners, are in attendance. The healthcare team present include the ICU doctor in charge of Phyllis's medical care, Janet as the primary nurse caring for Phyllis, the respiratory doctor and a social worker. The ICU doctor spells out Phyllis's medical condition, current treatment, challenges to making any improvement and prognosis. When he suggests that the only option left is to extubate, provide medication to keep her comfortable and allow 'nature to take its course', Elaine becomes deeply distressed and lashes out. Elaine refuses to accept that her mother will not recover and 'walk out of this horrid place'. Janet is surprised at Elaine's reaction. She feels she has failed Elaine and her family by not preparing them more adequately for Phyllis's death.

CASE STUDY QUESTIONS

1. What is your initial reaction to Phyllis's situation?
2. Reflect on your own values and beliefs regarding the end of life. You may choose to use techniques discussed earlier in this chapter.
3. Reflect on the two perspectives: Janet, the nurse, and Elaine, the daughter and carer.
4. How can a person be 'prepared' for the death of a loved one?
5. What do you feel is an appropriate response for Janet?
6. What is the nurse's role in supporting people's struggle with end-of-life issues?
7. What does this say about the spiritual processes of Janet, Elaine and her family?

SPIRITUAL CARE IN NURSING PRACTICE

Considering the value of life and its meaning will help to enhance your spirituality, as well as sustain you in supporting the spiritual needs of your patients and their families. The nurse needs to have the knowledge and skills in order to conduct a systematic approach in spiritual care when dealing with patients who are suffering from chronic illness and/or disability. Spiritual care involves the need for assessment and the implementation of a range of interventions. Interventions may include, but are not limited to, supporting the patient and their family in engaging their religious practice, reading inspirational texts, reminiscing and providing music, therapeutic use of self, symptom management and healing presence (Ghorbani et al 2020).

Assessing Spiritual Needs

A thorough assessment depends on being aware of the spiritual experiences of a patient. Methods of assessment consist of three broad approaches: spirituality screening, patient qualitative histories and in-depth comprehensive interviews with care planning (Balboni et al 2017). The majority of nurses would use a patient history approach through the ongoing interaction between nurse, patient and family. As such, listening is one of the most important aspects of a nurse's role in assessing and supporting spiritual care. When nurses are active listeners they offer support to patients who are seeking meaning of their illness experience. A good listener needs to listen with their heart along with their ears. To be an effective listener it is crucial to give full attention to the person, engaging how they express themselves in terms of verbal and non-verbal cues. Nurses need to be aware that their patients may be uncomfortable in disclosing the innermost aspects of self. Fostering disclosure is based on building a trusting and caring relationship between nurse and patient. As such, it is vital for the nurse to provide an environment characterised by respect and openness where the individual is supported to discuss spiritual matters. The ability of the nurse to influence the health and wellbeing of their patients in a positive manner depends on the nurse's capacity to build a caring relationship with the patient.

Several tools have been developed to assist healthcare professionals in assessing spiritual care needs (see Table 4.2 for a list of tools and scales). They are often designed with specific populations of patients in mind; for example, people living with chronic and life-limiting illness. Given the subjective nature of spirituality, many of the items are open-ended rather than using numerical rating scales. As such, the intention is for the

TABLE 4.2 Selected Spiritual Healthcare Assessment Tools				
Authors	**Year**	**Title**	**No. of Items**	**Intended Use**
Paloutzian & Ellison	1982	Spiritual Well-being Scale	20 in two sub-scales	Scale to measure spiritual and existential wellbeing
Reed	1987	Spiritual Perspective Scale	20	For administration to patients in general clinical settings
Maugans	1996	SPIRITual: S (Spiritual belief system); P (Personal spirituality); I (Integration with a spiritual community); R (Ritualised practices); I (Implications for medical practice); T (Terminal events planning)	22	Primary care setting-focus. Open-ended questionnaire to be used by healthcare professionals while taking a medical history
Puchalski & Romer	2000	FICA: F (Faith, belief and meaning); I (Importance and influence); C (Community); A (Address)	11	Primary care setting-focus. Open-ended questionnaire to be used by healthcare professionals while taking a medical history
Anandarajah & Hight	2001	HOPE: H (Sources of hope, comfort, strength, peace, love and connection); O (Organised religion); P (Personal spirituality & practice); E (Effects on medical care and end-of-life issues)	20	Teaching tool for healthcare professionals

continued

TABLE 4.2				
Selected Spiritual Healthcare Assessment Tools – cont'd				
Authors	**Year**	**Title**	**No. of Items**	**Intended Use**
Peterman, Fitchett, Brady et al	2002	FACIT-Sp-12: Functional Assessment of Chronic Illness Therapy – Spirituality - 12	12	Spirituality sub-scale for use with people with chronic illness
Delaney	2003	The Spirituality Scale	23 in three sub-scales	
Neely & Minford	2009	FAITH: F (Faith/spiritual beliefs); A (Application); I (Influence, importance of faith in life, this illness and healthcare decisions); T (Talk / terminal events planning); H (Help)	18	Primary and acute care setting-focus Open-ended questionnaire to be used by healthcare professionals while taking a medical history
Dhar, Chaturvedi & Nandan	2011	Spiritual Health Scale 2011	114	Self-administered inventory of spiritual health
LaRocca-Pitts	2015	Four FACTs Spirituality Assessment Tool		Chaplains in clinical settings

Note: see references for full citations.

tool to guide comprehensive assessment rather than determining a 'score'.

The use of spirituality assessment tools in clinical practice has been criticised in the literature. Several tools contain biases towards cultural and religious experiences; for example, the use of certain terms consistent with one religion over another. In particular, the earlier assessment tools were developed in North America and have a decidedly Christian focus (Blaber et al 2015). There is also a lack of empirical testing to validate these tools so that the practitioner can use them with enough certainty that the tool is measuring what it says it will measure. For example, the lack of a definitive definition of spirituality and spiritual practice is a perpetual flaw of most of these tools.

Interventions to Support Spiritual Wellbeing

In order to deliver spiritual care with commitment and competence, the nurse needs to reflect on what this means in practice and how it can be attained. Without meaningful actions and provision of relevant resources, the spiritual dimension becomes simply an empty gesture. Attentive presence brought by the nurse to the patient interaction, with respect for the individual's uniqueness upheld, is essential to effective spiritual care. Open-ended questions within the context of the nurse–patient–family relationship can be used to begin a conversation about spiritual matters. Besides listening and giving consideration to the spiritual needs, it

may be necessary for the patient to be referred to a chaplain or appropriate minister; or in the case of a person who avows no religion, a support person they trust to assist them in their experience. The nurse should offer to call an appropriate chaplain or the church, temple, mosque or synagogue, for all patients who identify with a specific faith. Spiritual care should not be provided by any one person in isolation; rather, it should be provided with the support of a multidisciplinary team that includes a strong spiritual counsellor or chaplain (Koper et al 2019). The most important consideration is the need for the nurse to respect the individual spiritual perspectives of their patients without imposing the nurse's own personal spiritual views. An example of intervention that poses potential problems for the nurse–patient relationship is prayer (Taylor et al 2014). Caution is needed when choosing to pray with patients and family. Without proper understanding of the person's individual spiritual views, disruption of the therapeutic relationship may create a barrier to the delivery of safe and quality care (Taylor et al 2014).

Barriers to spiritual care have been well documented and include the perception that nurses have not made adequate preparation and have insufficient time to meet spiritual needs (Ramezani et al 2014). Increasing opportunities for nurses to learn about the role that spirituality plays in the lives of themselves and others, together with greater knowledge of effective interventions, will go a

Box 4.1
Highlighting Research

Oh and Kim evaluated 15 research papers reporting results of studies into spiritual interventions with people with cancer. A combined total of 889 patients from all the studies were included in the final analysis. Interventions included individual or group spirituality-focused psychotherapy sessions, spiritual counselling as an adjunct to weight-loss counselling, and purpose-developed nursing interventions. Nurses represented the largest group of health professionals delivering the interventions. Other health professionals included clinical psychologists, an oncologist and a dietitian.

While the studies had considerable variation in their methodological quality, three key points emerged:

- Spiritual interventions with patients with cancer have beneficial effects, particularly related to spiritual wellbeing, meaning of life and depression.
- Nursing interventions conducted over time with a minimum of eight sessions were found effective.
- The evidence remains weak due to the limitations of the included studies.

In concluding their work, Oh and Kim emphasise the need for further research using controlled trials to more accurately measure the effects of spiritual interventions with people with cancer.

Oh & Kim 2014.

long way towards meeting the needs of people with chronic and complex needs.

There is a growing body of research supporting the use of a range of alternative therapies to support people's spiritual wellbeing. The use of expressive modalities, including music (Moss 2019), art therapy (Wiswell et al 2019), and storytelling (Enzman et al 2015), form valuable avenues for exploring the experience of illness and suffering. Developing knowledge about these modalities will enhance practice, particularly when nurses are caring for people with chronic and complex conditions (see Box. 4.1).

CONCLUSION

Nurses often do not take much time to care for their own spirituality. For nurses to provide optimal spiritual care to their patients they need to examine their own life experiences and what meaning this has for them. Suffering and the spirituality experience are unique to the individual and nurses need to understand the influence of various cultures, belief systems and philosophies that affect a person's view of the meaning and value of life. The nurse needs to be accountable and responsible for the sensitive and safe practice of spiritual care for their patients' welfare. Finally, spirituality is more than a domain of health; it resides within the centre of the person's experience of life. For nurses, it forms the glue that holds the healing process together.

Reflective Questions

1. In what diverse ways is spirituality expressed in those living with chronic illness and/or disability?
2. When reflecting on the ways spirituality has been expressed in your life, how has it influenced the ways you think and feel about health, illness and wellbeing?
3. What are among the key principles underpinning spiritually sensitive and safe care that nurses must consider when supporting people living with chronic illness and/or disability?

RECOMMENDED READING

Ghorbani M, Mohammadi E, Aghabozorgi R et al 2020. Spiritual care interventions in nursing: an integrative literature review. Supportive Care in Cancer, 1–17.

Holopainen G, Nyström L, Kasén A 2017. The caring encounter in nursing. Nursing Ethics 26(1) 7–16.

Sadat Hoseini AS, Razaghi N, Khosro Panah AH et al 2019. A concept analysis of spiritual health. Journal of Religion and Health 58(4), 1025–1046.

REFERENCES

Anandarajah G, Hight E 2001. Spirituality and medical practice: using the HOPE Questions as a practical tool for spiritual assessment. American Family Physician 63, 81–89.

Arel SN 2019. Disgust, shame, and trauma: the visceral and visual impact of touch. In: R Ganzevoort, S Sremac (eds), Trauma and lived religion. Palgrave studies in lived religion and societal challenges. Palgrave Macmillan, Cham.

Australian Bureau of Statistics (ABS) 2017. Religion in Australia 2016: Census of Population and Housing: reflecting Australia – stories from the Census 2016, cat no. 2071.0 ABS, Canberra. Online. Available: www.abs.gov.au/ausstats/abs@.nsf/Lookup/by+Subject/2071.0~2016~Main+Features~Religion+Data+Summary~70.

Balboni TA, Fitchett G, Handzo GF et al 2017. State of the science of spirituality and palliative care research. Part II: screening, assessment, and interventions. Journal of Pain and Symptom Management 54(3), 441–453.

Blaber M, Jones J, Wilis D 2015. Spiritual care: which is the best assessment tool for palliative settings? International Journal of Palliative Nursing 21(9), 430–438.

Bolton G 2001. Reflective practice: writing and professional development. Paul Chapman Publishing, London.

Broom A 2016. Dying: a social perspective on the end of life. Taylor Francis, Sydney.

Burkhardt MA, Nagai-Jacobson MG 2002. Spirituality: living our connectedness. Delmar, Albany.

Cassell EJ 2004. The nature of suffering and the goals of medicine, 2nd edn. Oxford University Press, New York.

Clarke D 2003. Faith and hope. Australasian Psychiatry 11(2), 164–168.

Comte-Sponville A 2006. The little book of atheist spirituality. Penguin, London.

de Botton A 2012. Religion for atheists. Hamish Hamilton, London.

Delaney C 2003. The spirituality scale: development, refinement and psychometric testing of an instrument to assess the human spiritual dimension. PhD Thesis. The University of Connecticut.

Dhar N, Chaturvedi SK, Nandan D 2011. Spiritual health scale 2011: defining and measuring 4th dimension of health. Indian Journal of Community Medicine 36(4), 275.

Easley R 2007. Harmony: a concept analysis. Journal of Advanced Nursing 59(5), 551–556.

Ellis J, Cobb M, O'Connor T et al 2015. The meaning of suffering in patients with advanced progressive cancer. Chronic Illness 11(3), 198–209.

Enzman Hines M, Wardell DW, Engebretson J et al 2015. Holistic nurses' stories of healing of another. Journal of Holistic Nursing 33(1), 27–45.

Fitzgerald Miller J 2007. Hope: a construct central to nursing. Nursing Forum 42(1), 12–19.

Ghorbani M, Mohammadi E, Aghabozorgi R et al 2020. Spiritual care interventions in nursing: an integrative literature review. Supportive Care in Cancer, 1–17.

Heydari A, Khorashadizadeh F, Nabavi FH et al 2016. Spiritual health in nursing from the viewpoint of Islam. Iranian Red Crescent Medical Journal 18(6), e24288.

Holopainen G, Nyström L, Kasén A 2017. The caring encounter in nursing. Nursing Ethics 26(1), 7–16.

Kinchen E 2015. Development of a quantitative measure of holistic nursing care. Journal of Holistic Nursing 33, 238–246.

Koper I, Pasman HRW, Schweitzer BPM et al 2019. Spiritual care at the end of life in the primary care setting: experiences from spiritual caregivers – a mixed methods study. BMC Palliative Care 18(1), 98.

Krause N, Pargament KI, Hill PC et al 2019. Exploring religious and/or spiritual identities: part 1 – assessing relationships with health. Mental Health, Religion & Culture 22(9), 877–891.

Lalani N 2020. Meanings and interpretations of spirituality in nursing and health. Religions 11(9), 428.

LaRocca-Pitts M 2015. Four FACTs spiritual assessment tool. Journal of Health Care Chaplaincy 21(2), 51–59.

Lasair S 2020. A narrative approach to spirituality and spiritual care in health care. Journal of Religion & Health 59(3), 1524–1540.

Leite ACAB, Garcia-Vivar C, Neris RR et al 2019. The experience of hope in families of children and adolescents living with chronic illness: a thematic synthesis of qualitative studies. Journal of Advanced Nursing 75(12), 3246–3262.

Maugans TA 1996. The spiritual history. Archives of Family Medicine 5(1), 11–16.

Moss H 2019. Music therapy, spirituality and transcendence. Nordic Journal of Music Therapy 28(3), 212–223.

Munck B, Björklund A, Jansson I et al 2018. Adulthood transitions in health and welfare: a literature review. Nursing Open 5(3), 254–260.

Neely D, Minford E 2009. FAITH: spiritual history-taking made easy. The Clinical Teacher 6(3), 181–185.

Oh P, Kim SH 2014. The effects of spiritual interventions in patients with cancer: a meta-analysis. Oncology Nursing Forum 41(5), E290–301.

Olsman E, Willems D, Leget C 2016. Solicitude: balancing compassion and empowerment in a relational ethics of hope – an empirical–ethical study in palliative care. Medicine, Health Care, and Philosophy 19(1), 11–20.

Paloutzian RF, Ellison C 1982. Loneliness, spiritual well-being, and quality of life. In: LA Peplau, D Perlman (eds), Loneliness: a sourcebook of current theory, research and therapy. Wiley, New York.

Peterman AH, Fitchett G, Brady MJ et al 2002. Measuring spiritual wellbeing in people with cancer: the Functional Assessment of Chronic Illness Therapy–Spiritual Wellbeing Scale (FACIT–Sp). Annals of Behavioral Medicine 24, 49–58.

Puchalski CM, Romer AL 2000. Taking a spiritual history allows clinicians to understand patients more fully. Journal of Palliative Medicine 3, 129–137.

Ramezani M, Ahmadi F, Mohammadi E et al 2014. Spiritual care in nursing: a concept analysis. International Nursing Review 61(2), 211–219.

Reed PG 1987. Spirituality and well-being in terminally ill hospitalized adults. Research in Nursing and Health 10(5), 335–344.

Ryan L, Seymour J 2016. Death and dying in intensive care: emotional labour of nurses. End of Life Journal 3(2), 1–9.

Sadat Hoseini AS, Razaghi N, Khosro Panah AH et al 2019. A concept analysis of spiritual health. Journal of Religion and Health 58(4), 1025–1046.

Taylor EJ, Park CG, Pfeiffer JB 2014. Nurse religiosity and spiritual care. Journal of Advanced Nursing 70(11), 2612–2621.

Vance MC 2019. Recognizing trauma in the healer. Health Affairs 38(5), 868–871.

Wiswell S, Bell JG, McHale J et al 2019. The effect of art therapy on the quality of life in patients with a gynecologic cancer receiving chemotherapy. Gynecologic Oncology 152(2), 334–338.

World Health Organization (WHO) 1948. Constitution of the World Health Organization. Online. Available: http://apps.who.int/gb/bd/PDF/bd47/EN/constitution-en.pdf?ua=1.

Zournazi M 2002. Hope: new philosophies for change. Pluto Press, Sydney.

CHAPTER 5

Psychosocial Care

KAREN STRICKLAND

LEARNING OBJECTIVES

When you have completed this chapter you will be able to:

- recognise the complex factors that influence a person's experience of chronic illness or disability
- describe the features that affect the quality of life for people with chronic illnesses or disabilities
- explore how diversity across individuals and population groups impacts on the way in which health services are delivered to people with chronic illnesses or disabilities
- consider how nurses can empower the person with a chronic illness or disability to live a full and contributing life
- identify opportunities and strategies for enabling families and carers to support a person with a chronic illness or disability.

KEY WORDS

carers	diversity
chronic illness	empowerment
disability	psychosocial

INTRODUCTION

This chapter discusses the psychosocial considerations for a person living with a chronic illness or disability – that is, the range of factors that contribute to that person's psychological and social wellbeing. All people have their own unique and complex lives; the experience of a chronic illness or disability adds to that complexity. For a person to live their life to the full, symptoms of the chronic illness or disability must be managed in the context of the person's life, including their psychosocial needs. This is best achieved with the acknowledgement that no one knows the life of a person better than the person who is living that life. This chapter considers how nurses can help the person with a chronic illness or disability to make decisions about the management of their illness or disability, including their psychosocial needs, to fit with the particular set of circumstances of their life.

Central to helping the person address their psychosocial needs is the recognition by nurses that people are

diverse. As discussed in later sections of this chapter, differences between people are a consequence of their psychosocial characteristics – that is, their personal (including emotional, cognitive and behavioural) attributes, family influences, age, gender, sexuality, cultural background, level of education, socioeconomic and employment status, social networks, spiritual and political beliefs, as well as the community and physical environment in which they live. Addressing the psychosocial needs of people with chronic illnesses or disabilities is just as important as addressing their medical needs. This is because it is the psychosocial aspects of the person's life that frame their quality of life. Supporting functions of the body, prescribing medicines, implementing therapies and other health-related interventions will have only limited outcomes – the lived experience of a chronic illness or disability is much bigger than a diagnosis and treatment intervention.

For this reason it is important that nurses are aware of the various ways in which they can work in partnership with the person who has a chronic illness or disability. This includes being aware of how to employ the principles of person-centredness and collaborative decision-making, and thereby empower the person and their families or carers to make the best decisions for their situation. Ultimately, the aim of these psychosocial approaches is to support the person with a chronic illness or disability to improve their quality of life, and live a full and contributing life, notwithstanding the symptoms they may be experiencing.

CHRONIC ILLNESS VERSUS ACUTE ILLNESS

Useful illustrations to explain the differences between chronic and acute illnesses can be drawn from sport. For example, if chronic illness were a sport it might be a test cricket match, while an acute illness might be a 100-metre sprint. These two events have much in common: they are both sports, involve physical competition, include spectators and competitors, have a beginning and an end, and have defined rules. But as sporting events they are also very different. A cricket match can last for five days (and still be a draw), whereas a sprint can be over in 10 seconds.

This analogy works for chronic and acute illnesses in several important ways. For example, one way is that a small error or a tactical decision in the sprint can have immediate and permanent consequences on the outcomes of the event. In contrast, in a five-day test cricket match there are many twists and turns; it is difficult to say that any one error is directly responsible for the outcome, and tactics followed by the players may be changed many times, in response to how the match is played. In chronic illness, as in cricket, there is time to make decisions, review them and try different approaches without immediate or permanent consequences.

LIVED EXPERIENCE VERSUS HEALTH CONDITION

Other people may tell you that cricket is more than a sport. They say that it is also about the sound of leather on willow, white flannel on green fields surrounded by picket fences, good sporting conduct and courtesy to others. Of course, it is debatable whether these aspects of the game of cricket are the defining features of what it means to play cricket, but it is true to say that there is more to cricket than the game itself. In other words, for cricket lovers, the lived experience of cricket involves more than just the game.

Likewise, the lived experience of people with a chronic illness or disability involves more than just a diagnosis or recommended treatment interventions. Previous models of care relied upon biomedical approaches that focused on the structure and function of parts of the body, and the pathophysiology of a particular disease process or health condition (Alonso 2004). In contrast, holistic and person-centred models of care take into account the complex interplay between the illness experience, as well as the psychological, social and cultural needs of the individual to promote healing (Jasemi et al 2017). Holistic and person-centred models of care acknowledge the lived experience of an illness or disability encompasses a much wider – and, as such, far more complex – approach to all of the aspects of what it means to have an illness or disability (Jasemi et al 2017; McCance & McCormack 2017; Watson 2015). The experience of chronic illness includes not only the symptoms that result from the effects of the condition on the body's systems, but also the wide-ranging economic, functional, occupational, psychological, sexual, social and spiritual effects of the illness. In addition, the experience of chronic illness includes the responses to the effects of chronic illness or disability, of the person's family, carer(s), and the community in which the person lives (Nelson et al 2016).

At this point it is important to note that biomedical approaches to healthcare place a strong emphasis on the 'curing' of a disease or illness and, as such, do not necessarily fit with the lived experience of people with illnesses or disabilities, nor do they offer person-centred or holistic approaches to the assessment of the individual (Kogan et al 2016). For example, a cure is usually not possible for a chronic illness or disability; consequently, attempts to find a cure may work against the person moving on to adapt to a chronic health condition or disability and live a full and contributing life. There is another parallel here to the game of cricket. In some test cricket matches, the aim is not always to win the match, but rather to avoid a loss and, consequently, effect a draw!

Caring for someone with a chronic illness or disability is also different from caring for someone with acute health needs. People with an acute illness require nursing care for a short period of time, after which they are likely to resume their previous lifestyle. For example, in acute episodes, treatment decisions are often made by members of the multidisciplinary team, with the need for decisive action great and the potential consequences of delay profound. There may be little opportunity for the person who is acutely unwell to participate in decision-making under these circumstances – for this reason, in acute situations the 'patient' adopts a 'sick' or passive role and follows the advice of health professionals to overcome the illness, injury or disease (Hamann et al 2015; Kon et al 2016).

In contrast, for people with chronic illnesses, the aims of the interventions employed are to minimise the impact of the health condition; to adapt to the changes that result from the health condition (economic, functional, physical, psychological, sexual, social and so on); and live a full and satisfying life. This process occurs through ongoing collaborative partnerships between the person with the chronic illness or disability and all members of the multidisciplinary team, including nurses; with the person taking an active role in setting goals and carrying out the collaborative decisions negotiated (Friesen-Storms et al 2015). While there may be a need to revisit and revise these decisions on an ongoing basis, dependent upon changing circumstances, it is the person, not the health professional, who is 'captain of the team', making the calls that best suit their lived experience of the chronic illness or disability.

PSYCHOSOCIAL CONSIDERATIONS

Before considering how best to give psychosocial support to people with chronic illnesses or disabilities, there is a need to define the term 'psychosocial care'. The overall psychosocial context within which a person lives is complex, and includes (without being limited to) their individual or personal characteristics (including emotional, cognitive and behavioural), family influences, age, gender, sexuality, cultural background, level of education, socioeconomic and employment status, social networks, spiritual and political beliefs, as well as the community and physical environment in which they live. Psychosocial care, then, is complex, involving many different aspects of the person's life.

For this reason, it is important that nurses are aware of the various ways in which they can develop a therapeutic relationship, conveying empathy for the individual and their lived experience and taking account of the wide-ranging factors that affect the lived experience of the person with a chronic illness or disability – not just the biological or medical factors. To provide truly holistic and person-centred care requires more than knowledge and understanding of biology, pathophysiology and medical interventions; psychosocial care also requires knowledge and understanding of people, their health needs, experiences, preferences – and aspirations

and the ability to convey empathy (Siyun Chen et al 2017).

For example, each person has unique personal characteristics and circumstances that may inform their response to illness. The personal characteristics that may make one person's response to a chronic illness very different from the next person's include life skills, values and world view, levels of resilience, as well as capacity to be creative and adapt to change (Ambrosio et al 2015). Likewise, among the circumstances that influence the broad range of social factors that affect a person's response to chronic illness are the economic aspects of the person's life, with low socioeconomic status and unemployment having a significant impact on a person's level of physical and mental health. Again, a person's cultural background affects their perceptions of health, illness and disability. This is because our cultural background influences our beliefs and values; it also determines, in large part, our behaviours. As such, awareness of cultural diversity and the delivery of culturally appropriate care is an essential part of providing psychosocial care (Browne et al 2016; López-Sierra & Rodríguez-Sánchez 2015).

No less significant are the social roles of people. Significantly, a person with a chronic illness or disability will have many roles in life that are essential to describing them as a person. For example, a person with chronic back pain is not only a person with a chronic illness; they may also be a spouse or partner, a parent, a leader or manager, a carer. The way in which the chronic illness or disability affects the person's roles will be dependent on a range of factors, including the physical, psychological and mental health changes experienced by that person. These changes may alter a person's self-perceptions, including the way in which they fulfil their roles in light of their chronic illness or disability. The changes experienced by a person with a chronic illness or disability may also alter the perceptions of others on the capability of the person to fulfil the roles they had in the past. Exploring the different ways in which roles can be fulfilled can take time for all those involved, but provides an important means by which the person with the chronic illness or disability can live a satisfying life.

Diversity

The concept of diversity is useful when thinking about and caring for people with a chronic illness or disability because it recognises that people are different from one another and have unique needs, preferences and aspirations. As already noted, a person is a composite of a range of factors, including those related to the individual, family, age, gender, sexuality, culture, level of education, socioeconomic and employment status, social networks, spiritual and political beliefs, the community, and surrounding physical environment. By acknowledging diversity, nurses are demonstrating awareness of the many different factors that influence the ways in which people live their lives. This awareness is important, as the healthcare systems within which nurses practise often do not cater for difference, but instead take a 'one size fits all' approach to delivering services (Allen 2019; Ancheta et al 2015; Cloitre 2015).

One of the clearest examples of diversity is found in cultural diversity, which has already been mentioned as a major psychosocial consideration when supporting people with chronic illness or disability. Contemporary Western societies are almost always multicultural societies – that is, they comprise people and population groups from countries such as Africa, the Americas, Asia-Pacific, Europe, the Middle East and others. The delivery of culturally appropriate care involves an acknowledgement of this cultural diversity – and the need to respond appropriately to people from diverse cultures. For example, mainstream healthcare systems are based on Western scientific and philosophical ways of thinking, which may not necessarily be reflected in the beliefs and values of Aboriginal or Torres Strait Islander people or of other ethnic groups living within the community (Battersby et al 2018; Fung & Linn 2015; Kilcullen et al 2018; van der Greef et al 2015). In addition, a person's cultural background influences the meaning they give to notions of health and ill-health. For example, some groups of people may believe that ill-health or disability is a form of punishment. This creates challenges for nurses helping people who belong to these cultures, to consider ways of living a full and satisfying life despite illness or diversity. Cultural background also influences the way in which some people view health professionals – for example, some people expect to receive paternalistic advice or directions from nurses, and view it as disrespectful to question people 'in authority'. The person may therefore be unfamiliar with approaches that focus on collaborative partnerships to develop strategies and goals.

Culturally appropriate approaches by nurses do not necessitate an understanding of each and every culture that may be encountered in health settings; however, being sensitive to the cultural needs and experiences of people from culturally diverse backgrounds is essential for providing culturally safe care (Battersby et al 2018; Brooks et al 2019). Culturally

appropriate care is delivered when the nurse takes the following three steps.

1. Firstly, nurses must understand their own beliefs and values, including the ways in which these beliefs and values influence notions of how people 'should' respond to a particular set of circumstances. When nurses develop this understanding they are more able to listen to and acknowledge cultural viewpoints that are different to their own. No one culture is better than another culture – rather, diversity shows the richness of humankind. Understanding of their own beliefs and values, and how these beliefs and values are culturally constructed, enables nurses to approach cultural diversity with greater levels of acceptance, including a recognition of how much a person's cultural background can shape them as a person.

2. The second step involves the nurse acknowledging that there is no 'one size fits all' approach to delivering health services. Western health settings have been established on Western values, with many of the services delivered having been developed on the presumption that most people will conform to these values. For this reason, nurses may have to pave the way for people from diverse cultures to access a service, adapting the way in which the services are delivered according to the person's needs.

3. The third step in the process involves nurses exploring how best they can work collaboratively with the person from another culture to consider which interventions or services best fit with their particular view of the world (Filmer & Herbig 2020). This may involve carers and/or families, and even the communities with which the person lives. It may also involve ensuring that the person has access to translators. For example, cultural diversity often means linguistic diversity – and some people may have limited or no ability to speak, read or write in the dominant language (e.g. English) used in Western health settings, and so be unable to ask for help or information. Others again may have unresolved issues related to past experiences and trauma (Cleary & Hungerford 2015) – for example, refugees may be experiencing symptoms of post-traumatic stress disorder (PTSD), but be unable to express what is happening to them. These many considerations add to the complexities involved in supporting people with psychosocial care.

Quality of Life

We have established that the emphasis when helping people with chronic illness or disability is not on seeking a cure, but rather on supporting the person to live a full and contributing life and/or experience a satisfying quality of life (Lassen 2015). It is important, then, to consider what it means to live life to the full or to experience a satisfying quality of life.

Psychosocial factors that contribute to quality of life include good physical and mental health, financial stability, positive family dynamics and cohesiveness, strong social support networks, maintenance of an optimal level of cognitive functioning and personal control (de Jong et al 2015; Park et al 2015; Sánchez et al 2016). Nurses must consider these factors, as they are closely connected to the way in which they approach the delivery of psychosocial care to a person. For example, questions the nurse could ask a person to consider when developing goals may be: What is the financial situation of the person? How well does the person relate to family members and friends? Has the person been assessed for depression? What steps could be taken to help empower the person?

In a public health context, quality of life measures, such as 'burden of disease', aim to quantify the experience of chronic illness. These measures make use of the notions of years of life lost and/or years of healthy life lost due to disability, to calculate 'disability-adjusted life years'. 'Disability-adjusted life years' (DALY) represents one year of healthy life lost from living with an illness or disability ('years lived with disability' or YLD) (Australian Institute for Health & Wellbeing [AIHW] 2019). While this approach is useful for governments and large health service organisations to support strategic planning, it is also important to recognise the significance of the lived experience of people with chronic illnesses. For example, the public health approach is one of deficit rather than a strength-based approach, considering only what has been lost rather than what has been added to a person's life as a result of the chronic illness or disability.

Other researchers have made use of qualitative approaches to consider the quality of life of people with a chronic illness or disability. This includes personal interviews, focus group discussions and questionnaires that explore a range of factors affecting people with the lived experience of the illness or disability.

Together, both quantitative and qualitative approaches consider the notion of quality of life from a variety of stances – illustrating the complexity of what it means to live a full and contributing life. What is perhaps most important is to recognise that different people have different values, and so they will place different emphases on different parts of their life. Consequently, nurses must ask the person with a chronic illness or disability what it is that they value most in their life; and ascertain the person's preferences in relation to the support they receive to address their psychosocial needs and live life to the full.

Grief, Loss and Uncertainty

Diagnosis of a chronic illness or disability will often give rise to feelings of grief and loss for a person, and also family members and carers. Even in the early stages of some conditions, when a person may feel relatively well, there can be strong feelings of loss (Strickland et al 2017). Some factors that influence the length and intensity of grief include the level of social support available, the nature and significance of other stressors in life, and the perception of lost opportunities due to the illness for the person and family members or carers (Holland et al 2015).

Another major challenge for people living with a chronic illness is uncertainty (Cypress 2016; Hoth et al 2015; Strickland et al 2017). There is uncertainty before and at the time of diagnosis, uncertainty about how the illness will progress, and about the potentially unpredictable nature of the illness. Other common psychosocial features that may emerge related to this are anxiety, depression, stress and feelings of powerlessness.

Such responses suggest the need for nurses to help the person to reflect on their feelings, and how they are coping with and/or adapting to their new or ongoing circumstances. If the person seems to need additional or specialist help, it is essential that the nurse refers the person to the most appropriate health professional for further assessment. Grief, loss and uncertainty are responses that require psychosocial care first and foremost, rather than medical interventions. It is the nurse's role to support the person to receive that care.

Stigma

Stigma, and experiences of discrimination, are factors that will influence a person's quality of life (Knaak et al 2017). Stigma occurs when a condition or way of being is perceived in a negative way (Ditchman et al 2016; Hungerford et al 2015). Stigma has the effect of discriminating between those who are accepted as 'normal' or 'acceptable' and those who are not, and can lead to social marginalisation (Ditchman et al 2016; Jackson et al 2016). Stigma is a particular problem for people who experience chronic illnesses or disabilities that other people can see or will notice.

For example, some chronic illnesses or disabilities such as paraplegia are visible; other chronic health conditions, such as diabetes, are not so visible. People with a chronic illness or disability may be subjected to unfair treatment from others on the basis of their illness or disability, whether it is visible or not. However, the more visible the illness or disability, the more likely it is that the person will experience stigma (Roberts et al 2017). Therefore, in many cases, people may not disclose and may even actively conceal their health conditions, for fear of being discriminated against. A part of providing healthcare to people with a chronic illness or disability, then, is to explore if and how the person and their family or carers are experiencing stigma or discrimination, and work with those involved to address the issues.

MODELS

We have already considered how people are different, including the wide range of factors that influence the different needs and preferences of people. It is also important to note that there is a wide range of chronic illnesses and disabilities – moreover, the lived experience of a chronic illness or disability is very different for each person. For example, a person with a chronic illness will go through many changes throughout the course of their illness, which may include adaptation, deterioration and/or rehabilitation.

Chronic illness models or frameworks, like all models of care, provide an important means of understanding the processes at play and guiding the practice of the nurse (Crowe & Deane 2018). With regard to chronic illness, models of care enable deeper insight into the adaptation, deterioration and/or rehabilitation phases, and illustrate the many factors involved, including a

person's past experiences of health and ill-health, capacity to cope, cognitive ability, as well as the person's social networks, availability of resources to support them, and environment (Livneh & Parker 2005). These models also show that, in the process of adaptation, most people move towards renewed personal growth and capacity to function (Livneh & Parker 2005). In the following sections, two models are explained: the Corbin and Strauss Illness Trajectory Model and Paterson's Shifting Perspectives Model.

The Corbin and Strauss Illness Trajectory Model

The Illness Trajectory Model is a seminal work developed by Corbin and Strauss (1991), which suggests that the goals of the person with a chronic illness, together with the health professional(s), are best viewed in the context of a long journey (Corbin 2001). The journey is shown in different phases of the chronic illness experience for the person with the chronic illness. At different times along the trajectory, different elements of care will come to the fore.

Most often, the trajectory is non-linear and people may skip phases or return to previous phases more than once. The Illness Trajectory Model describes the goals of treatment according to each phase (Corbin 2001). For example, in the stable phase the goal of care is to maintain stability and the usual activities of life, while in the crisis phase the goal is to avert the specific threat to the person's life. Table 5.1 and Case Study 5.1 illustrate the phases and goals of care.

TABLE 5.1
Trajectory Phases

Phase	Definition	Goal of Management
Pre-trajectory	Genetic factors or lifestyle behaviours that place an individual or community at risk for the development of a chronic condition	Prevent onset of chronic illness
Trajectory onset	Appearance of noticeable symptoms; includes a period of diagnostic work-up and announcement by biographical limbo as person begins to discover and cope with implications of diagnosis	Form appropriate trajectory projection and scheme
Stable	Illness course and symptoms are under control. Biography and everyday life activities are being managed within limitations of illness. Illness management is centred in the home	Maintain stability of illness, biography and everyday life activities
Unstable	Period of inability to keep symptoms under control or reactivation of illness. Biographical disruption and difficulty in carrying out everyday life activities. Adjustments being made in regimen with care usually taking place at home	Return to stable

TABLE 5.1 Trajectory Phases – cont'd		
Phase	**Definition**	**Goal of Management**
Acute	Severe and unrelieved symptoms or the development of illness complications necessitating hospitalisation or bed rest to bring illness course under control. Biography and everyday life activities temporarily placed on hold or drastically cut back	Bring illness under control and resume normal biography and everyday life activities
Crisis	Critical or life-threatening situation requiring emergency treatment or care. Biography and everyday life activities suspended until crisis passes	Remove life threat
Downward	Illness course characterised by rapid or gradual physical decline, accompanied by increasing disability or difficulty in controlling symptoms. Requires biographical adjustment and alterations in everyday life activity with each major downward step	To adapt to increasing disability with each major downward turn
Dying	Final days or weeks before death. Characterised by gradual or rapid shutting down of body processes, biographical disengagement and closure and relinquishment of everyday life interests and activities	To bring closure, let go and die peacefully

Corbin 2001.

CASE STUDY 5.1

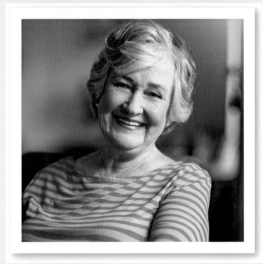

iStockphoto/PeopleImages.

PART 1

Gwen is a 69-year-old woman. She was born in Wales and moved to Australia with her parents and three siblings – an older and younger brother and young sister – when she was 10 years old. Her family moved to Australia for what her father termed 'a better life'. He was a manual labourer who was attracted by perceptions of the Australian people, the climate and the promise of work on big new infrastructure projects. He was a very reserved man, who, although he loved his children, found it difficult to express this. As a result, his children saw him as stern and unapproachable. Gwen's mother deferred to her husband. She was a loving, stay-at-home mother who was always 'there' for her children.

Gwen experienced asthma, particularly in spring, but despite this was an active child who was involved in a range of team sporting activities; she played hockey in winter, women's cricket in summer, and netball all year round. She was also an avid follower of the local football team.

When Gwen was 16 her mother died suddenly. Gwen remembers this as a very difficult time – she saw her father cry for the first time and become a shadow of his former self overnight. Gwen left school and took on many of her mother's roles, running the household, caring for her father and older brother, and raising her younger siblings. Soon after her mother died, Gwen's father, a heavy smoker, was diagnosed with Chronic Obstructive Pulmonary Disease (COPD). This meant that Gwen also became a nurse of sorts, tending to her father's deteriorating health needs, until one day he died suddenly from a massive cardiac arrest.

continued

CASE STUDY 5.1 – cont'd

Throughout this time, Gwen continued to follow her interest in sport. In her mid-twenties Gwen met Tony, who was also involved in the local football club, and they fell in love and married. Tony worked at the local bank. Gwen and Tony soon had five children – three boys and two girls – and Gwen kept busy being a mother and home-maker.

Tony was offered a promotion, which required the family to move to the city. The family moved and set up their home in the new, much bigger and busier environment. The family was happy in their new home, particularly Gwen, who became involved in supporting the children's sporting interests and also joining the local sporting club.

The children soon grew up, and grandchildren arrived. Gwen became a very involved grandmother and looked forward to the day Tony would retire. She was devastated when, like her father, he died of a sudden heart attack, but she soon realised there was no changing events and it was best just to manage things as best she could and get on with her life. She was still active, able to continue living in the family home, helping out with her grandchildren and being involved with her sporting interests.

As time went by, Gwen noticed that her legs were a bit swollen at times and that the skin had become darker. Her legs were not really sore, but it felt good when she sat in her recliner chair and put them up for a while.

Recently Gwen bumped her leg just above her ankle and tore the skin. The small wound did not heal and actually seemed to be getting bigger. Gwen decided she needed to put her leg in the sun at least once daily to help dry it out. She also told herself that if it persisted another week, she would see her general practitioner about it. She had developed a good relationship with her GP over the years while raising her children and now helping out with her grandchildren.

CASE STUDY QUESTIONS

1. What are the main factors in Gwen's life, past and present, that may influence how she maintains her health and wellbeing?

2. In light of these factors, how do you think she would respond to having a chronic illness?

One of the ways in which the Illness Trajectory Model is useful in clinical practice is that it helps the person with the chronic illness and the nurse to discuss the person's needs and goals at different times in the illness journey (Frost et al 2017). Every person will experience their illness trajectory in different ways; this model provides opportunities for conversations between the person and the nurse about the illness which, in turn, may lead to a shared understanding of a person's unique trajectory through the illness.

Paterson's Shifting Perspectives Model

The Shifting Perspectives Model (Paterson 2001) recognises that at times the person with a chronic illness will see themselves as well, with the illness in the background, while at other times they will see themselves as unwell, with the illness in the foreground. The shift from the perspective that the person is well may be precipitated by, for example, an exacerbation of symptoms. This shift in perspective will revert once symptoms are well managed and the illness is no longer to the fore. The Shifting Perspectives Model suggests that a person's perceptions of their chronic illness will change according to their needs and circumstances, in a pendular fashion; consequently, the person's perception of themselves as well or unwell will change accordingly (Livneh & Parker 2005).

The shifting perspective conceptualisation of illness or disability serves a useful function for two reasons. Firstly, when a person sees themselves as well, their behaviour is more likely to include activity that increases participation in the activities of life and promotes interaction and self-esteem. Secondly, when a person sees themselves as unwell, they are more likely to engage in behaviours that decrease the effects of ill-health or re-establishes the healthy frame (Paterson 2001). These activities include working towards the goals developed to enable improved quality of life or to living full and contributing lives.

PRINCIPLES OF CARE

As already noted, each person's lived experience of a chronic illness or disability is different. This is because the person is a product of their personal (including emotional, cognitive and behavioural) characteristics, family influences, age, gender, cultural background, level of education, socioeconomic and employment status, social networks, spiritual and political beliefs, as well as the community and physical environment in which they live. To ensure that the care and support that nurses give to a person is appropriate – that is, it encompasses the psychosocial considerations as well as the biological or medical needs – it is important that a person-centred approach is taken.

CASE STUDY 5.1

PART 2

Gwen's leg wound did not change for the better, despite her sunning it regularly. When she visited her GP, he decided it was most likely a venous leg ulcer caused by problems with the venous circulation to the legs. He advised Gwen on some lifestyle changes that she could make, including keeping her leg up on a stool when she was sitting down and perhaps taking a zinc supplement. He also asked her not to put the leg out in the sun, explaining that current research suggests that this is not the best thing. He also gave her a referral to the community nursing service to assess and dress the wound. Many of his patients were visited by the community nurses and he had come to know the strengths of what they could provide and how the professions of nursing and medicine could complement one another. He also knew that the community nurses have a particular expertise in wound management and are able to access a wide range of dressing products that may be helpful.

Prior to visiting the doctor, Gwen had been dressing the wound herself. She had purchased some gauze from the chemist and had cut a crepe bandage into smaller sections to hold the gauze squares in place. The wound was quite moist and she believed she had to change the dressing several times a day to ensure it was clean. She was happy to do this as it meant that she could still maintain her active lifestyle. It also meant the bandages looked clean, so people wouldn't think that she couldn't take care of herself.

CASE STUDY QUESTIONS

3. Consider the Shifting Perspectives Model. Do you think that Gwen sees herself with a leg ulcer as well or unwell?

4. How does Gwen's view of herself influence the way in which she approaches her wound management?

Person-centredness

A person-centred approach focuses on the person and their lived experience, rather than the health condition and how medical science can achieve a cure. When any member of the multidisciplinary team is positioned as the holder of knowledge, an unequal power base is established, including the presumption that the person will follow the advice of the health professional. In contrast, when the focus of care is on the person and their needs and preferences, the outcomes achieved become more meaningful for the person with the chronic illness or disability (Battersby et al 2018; Eaton et al 2015).

A person-centred approach includes giving due acknowledgement to the range of factors that may influence the decisions made by the person with the health condition. Rather than providing solutions that may lack relevance or applicability for the person in their particular situation, the nurse works alongside or with the person. This more equal partnership enables the person to explore the range of options or interventions available, and decide for themselves the best possible solutions for their particular set of circumstances.

Partnership

In the early stages of an illness, the person with the chronic illness may rely on the professional knowledge provided by the nurse. Over time, however, it is the person with the health condition who becomes the expert as they learn about the condition and what it is like to live with the illness. While the person may not be able to communicate this knowledge using the medical terminology that nurses are more likely to use, the person's knowledge is authentic. The lived experience also provides fertile ground for the nurse and the person to work together, in partnership, towards common goals.

For example, the person with a lived experience of a chronic illness will know how it feels to experience that illness, what circumstances and events make them feel better or worse, what time of day is the most difficult for them and what strategies they use to help them to cope with these more difficult times. This information is vital for managing symptoms and identifying goals of the psychosocial care being delivered.

Consequently, nurses must demonstrate an understanding or common sense of humanity – even humility – when working with the person with a chronic illness (Foronda 2020; Manookian et al 2016). This would include the nurse considering how to demonstrate respect and acceptance of the person's knowledge, together with the capacity to engage with the person to establish and develop their role as partners in care. Through the very 'ordinariness' of these kinds of interactions, nurses will find that they are able to connect meaningfully with the people they help, while at the same time using their knowledge and skills to build a collaborative working partnership that addresses psychosocial needs (Manookian et al 2016).

CASE STUDY 5.1

PART 3

The community nurse, Sharon, visited Gwen at home. She conducted a thorough health history, meticulously completing the admission form. Sharon then assessed the wound. In her eyes it had all the clinical signs of a venous ulcer. It was moist, had irregular edges and there was brown staining of the skin around the wound edges and lower leg. Sharon performed a Doppler ultrasound to see if there is evidence of arterial involvement. She knew that her treatment decisions depended on being very sure of Gwen's peripheral vascular status. Sharon also decided to phone the GP and suggest he make a referral to the vascular specialist for more thorough investigations. In the meantime Sharon dressed the wound conservatively, keeping Gwen's comfort in mind.

Over the next few weeks Sharon visited regularly to dress the wound. Gwen was happy with the arrangement and quite liked Sharon's visits.

Before too long, Gwen visited the vascular specialist: venous insufficiency was confirmed and arterial disease ruled out. Sharon was very pleased with this diagnosis as it meant that she could feel comfortable about applying compression therapy, which she knew would help heal the wound.

A four-layer bandaging system was commenced and Sharon announced to Gwen that she wouldn't need to come to see her quite as often any more as this type of dressing could be left in place for a week. Gwen, however, was sceptical about leaving a dressing for that long. She was accustomed to changing it several times a day. Also, she felt that the dressing was too tight, too bulky-looking, and too hot with the warm weather. Sharon responded by carefully explaining the reasons for compression therapy and how it worked. She assessed Gwen's understanding by giving her opportunities to ask questions and express her understanding in her own words. Sharon was confident that the education she provided to Gwen was thorough and adequate.

As time went by, however, Gwen continued to express concern about the tightness, bulk and discomfort of the dressing when she was out and about. Sharon therefore suggested to Gwen that she limit her activity for the time being, especially during the summer months. In her view, this would help expedite the healing and Gwen could then resume her activities. Sharon reiterated that it is only by working together that the wound would heal.

There are, however, a variety of reasons why a person may not talk openly about their illness or disclose how their illness affects their life. Reasons may include inadequate trust and fear of hospitalisation or other treatments (Hungerford et al 2015). Alternatively, the person may not want to be seen as complaining or they may be concerned that an intervention they have found useful is about to be withdrawn (O'Dowd 2015).

Another reason a person may not talk openly to the nurse about their lived experience is a lack of confidence in the person's knowledge base. Nurses bring with them knowledge, clinical evidence, and a comprehensive understanding of the conditions and treatments. This information is vital in developing a plan of care – but may have the effect of undermining a person's confidence. Also, nurses must be careful not to make assumptions about the lived experience of the person with the chronic illness. The nurse's experience and knowledge may suggest that a particular approach or strategy is acceptable because it has worked in the past, but they might find it is not acceptable to the person they are supporting. In this case, the nurse's experience can, in a way, present a barrier to care rather than a useful addition to the relationship. Even so, sometimes nurses must 'unknow' the things they have learned and take care with assumptions when supporting the person (Munhall 1992). 'Unknowing' means looking at each person's experience as new and unique – and responding accordingly.

CASE STUDY 5.1

PART 4

Gwen intensely disliked the compression bandaging. She couldn't get over the fact that it was too tight, too bulky and too hot. She understood Sharon's explanation of why it was necessary, but she was not happy about it because it reduced her outside activities, including her involvement with her grandchildren and sport. She had also found it necessary to change the way she dressed, wearing tracksuit trousers instead of her usual dresses. This makes her feel 'low class' and embarrassed about her appearance.

By combining the expertise from both the person and the nurse into a collaborative partnership, it is likely that the quality of life for that person will be enhanced. This collaborative partnership will rely on reflective listening and the validation of the emotions of the person with a chronic illness (Karazivan et al 2015; Pomey et al 2015; Smith et al 2015). From this, information may be given, myths or misunderstandings addressed, and a plan of care negotiated. This cannot be achieved, however, without recognising the broader social context of the life of the person with a chronic illness.

Values and beliefs are unique to each person and will affect the decisions and choices that a person makes in their life. It is important, then, that nurses are aware of their own personal values and beliefs; that they do not force onto the person their own values and beliefs, particularly in relation to the way in which things 'should' be done (Mannix et al 2015; Orvik et al 2015).

Finally, good collaborative partnerships will take time to build. Likewise, realistic goals will take time to achieve. Consequently, there is a need to avoid unrealistic expectations in relation to a 'normal' time frame to achieve goals. Rather, each person must be allowed to progress in their own way, in their own time.

CASE STUDY 5.1

PART 5
Over the next 2 months, Sharon visited Gwen every week and applied the dressing. They had arranged a weekly Wednesday morning routine where Gwen removed the bandaging layers, placed them in a bag and cleaned her wound in the shower. After the shower, she would cover the wound with a clean pad and wait for Sharon to arrive. When Sharon arrived, she would look at the old dressings and apply new ones.

While the routine was clearly working, Sharon was alarmed that the wound itself was not healing and, in fact, seemed to be getting worse. Sharon was concerned as the evidence suggested that Gwen was having the correct treatment for her condition. Gwen, in turn, was becoming frustrated and impatient with the treatment – and Sharon.

Sharon began to ask questions of Gwen, to try and work out what was going on. After some time, Gwen reluctantly admitted that a couple of hours after Sharon left the house, she had taken to adjusting the dressing so that she could wear her shoes. Sharon felt frustrated and annoyed that Gwen was not complying with the treatment.

Carers

The presence of family members or carers who can provide support to the person with a chronic illness is another factor that influences that person's lived experience (Sav et al 2015). For example, the caring role is very demanding, with high levels of stress that can impact adversely on the carers' psychosocial needs (Mansfield et al 2016; Sav et al 2015; Strickland et al 2015). Carers have quite specific needs, including ongoing emotional support, as well as engaging with health professionals to exchange information; and to be recognised by health professionals for the crucial role they play in caring for consumers (Strickland et al 2015). Carers also express some confusion when negotiating the complex and confusing health-related services and systems. This confusion can contribute to 'carer burden', which comprises the psychosocial stressors experienced by carers and also serves to hinder the inclusion of carers in the process of decision-making with the person with a chronic illness or disability. It is of concern, then, that the majority of carers report high levels of stress and low levels of support from health professionals (Strickland et al 2015).

For this reason, careful consideration must be given by nurses to the level of support and care that can be given, over time, by families or carers of people with a chronic illness or disability. This is particularly important if carers are older people with chronic illnesses of their own. The questions must be asked, how long will the older person be able to care for their spouse or family member? Alternatively, the person with the chronic illness or disability may have adult children. But how accessible are these adult children? Do they live some distance away? Are they in full-time employment? Do they have children of their own to care for or other responsibilities that will inhibit their capacity to give support to their family member? Answers to these questions must be factored into any plans that are made with or for the person with a chronic illness or disability.

While family members and carers provide ongoing support to people with chronic illnesses, it is essential that nurses consider the psychosocial needs of carers and refer them to appropriate health services for assessment and support as required (Langbecker & Yates 2015; Long et al 2015). Without support, carers or family members will be unable to care for the person, leaving the person less likely to achieve a satisfying quality of life.

CASE STUDY 5.1

PART 6

Sharon felt troubled by Gwen's admission that she was adjusting the dressing, and couldn't understand why Gwen wouldn't adhere to the recommended treatment. In Sharon's view, if Gwen would just persist with the treatment for a couple of months, she most likely would not need a dressing at all. Sharon also wondered how Gwen had been dressing her leg herself for so long without Sharon knowing about it. It was then that Sharon realised that perhaps she had been doing a lot of talking at Gwen, rather than listening.

Sharon wondered if perhaps she had missed out on developing a good therapeutic relationship with Gwen, and instead focused on the best treatment for the leg ulcer. She also acknowledged to herself that Gwen had to live with the leg ulcer and so was in the best position to understand the way it impacted on her life. Sharon resolved that at the next visit she would backtrack and spend some time talking with Gwen about her life, her goals, and how they could truly work in partnership together.

Collaborative Decision-Making

An important step in caring for the person with a chronic illness or disability is to agree on the goals for managing the symptoms of the illness or the disability. These goals, and the interventions they comprise, must be acceptable to the person. For example, a nurse may believe that compression bandaging is likely to heal a leg ulcer within a relatively short period of time, but this may mean that the person cannot wear their bowling shoes because the feeling of tightness causes discomfort. If the nurse cannot negotiate interventions that are acceptable to all those concerned, it is unlikely the intervention will work.

Goals may be the healing of a wound, better management of symptoms, or the regaining of a level of functioning that allows that person to engage in a particular activity (Bernoth et al 2016). Once the goal is established, the nurse and the person with the chronic illness or disability must determine, together, the most acceptable way of attaining the goal. By using the nurse's experience and knowledge of options and interventions, combined with the person's understanding of their own life, strategies can be decided upon and implemented together (Fonseca et al 2015).

CASE STUDY 5.1

PART 7

At the next visit, Sharon asked Gwen if it would be okay to spend a bit more time talking about her situation. Fortunately, Gwen didn't have any pressing engagements or appointments and agreed. Sharon expressed her appreciation at being given the opportunity and then acknowledged that Gwen clearly knew what was important in her life and also what she was capable of doing. Sharon congratulated Gwen on her perseverance, including the changes in diet and lifestyle that she had undertaken. Sharon went on to say that she had cared for many different people with leg ulcers and, while everyone was different, she had a good understanding of some of the challenges and possibilities that Gwen might have come across.

Sharon suggested that in their therapeutic relationship from this point forwards she would like the emphasis to be on what she could do to better support Gwen. Sharon promised to listen to what Gwen had to say; and to work with Gwen to help her to meet her needs.

Sharon went on to ask, 'How have things been for you since you developed this leg ulcer?'

Gwen answered, 'I hate it. I feel unclean all the time and I worry that people will think I can't look after myself.'

'Why didn't you tell me how you felt?' asked Sharon.

'Well, since we're being honest here – you were very bossy and in fact I did tell you, but you weren't really interested.'

Sharon was somewhat taken aback by Gwen's words, but could see how her actions may have been interpreted. She acknowledged Gwen's feelings and explained that she really did want to help. 'While I am not an expert when it comes to your life, I would like to try to work together a bit more and I'll try not to come across as too bossy.'

Sharon went on to ask about the dressing and why Gwen took it off. 'I know you told me the dressing was bulky, hot and tight. Was this why you took it off? There isn't much we can do about those things, but if it's too much, would you like to try something else?'

Gwen recognised Sharon's genuine interest in working together.

'No, I can handle those things really; it's just that I can't fit my shoes on. I take it off on Wednesdays so that I can wear my shoes for bowls. I'm careful though, I cover the wound and look after it and I put the bandages back on when I get home.'

Sharon didn't realise the extent of Gwen's interaction with the wound and was very surprised that the dressing was totally removed less than 2 hours after it was applied. However, by listening more, Sharon heard that Gwen was

CASE STUDY 5.1 – cont'd

captain of her lawn bowling team and that they were currently winning the regional championship. Gwen loved bowling, loved the competitive nature of the sport, and had many good friends in and around the bowling club. For Gwen, wearing her bowling shoes was a higher priority than wearing her bandages.

Gwen explained that she didn't tell Sharon about it as she was worried she would 'be in trouble'.

Both Gwen and Sharon felt that this frank conversation allowed them to start working together. They were able to develop goals that drew on Sharon's expert knowledge of wound management and also on Gwen's expert knowledge of her life, resources and capacities.

In the end, managing the issues was a simple matter of rearranging the timing of the visits. Gwen still took the bandage off prior to going to lawn bowls, put on a temporary dressing which Sharon prepared and taught her how to apply. Gwen then went bowling. In the afternoon, after Gwen returned home, Sharon would visit and apply the full four-layer compression bandage system. This way, the dressing was able to stay on for almost a whole week. Both Sharon and Gwen acknowledged that while the system was not perfect, they also both felt that it was a good middle ground. Gwen's wound did begin to heal and they both found this very reassuring.

Compliance Versus Adherence

The term 'compliance' is often used in the context of the goals and strategies of health interventions and implies a power relationship between the health professional and the person with the illness (Fox & Reeves 2015); for example, for health professionals, the 'non-compliant' person is generally 'not doing what I told them to do'. The concept of non-compliance fails to acknowledge the range of factors that may influence decisions made by different people at different points in time. If agreed-upon goals are negotiated as acceptable to both the person with the health condition and the nurse, and the person is given the support and resources to work towards those goals, 'non-compliance' is less likely (Zhang et al 2015).

Given the increasing awareness of the negative implications of the term 'compliance', alternative terms such as 'adherence' or more recently 'concordance' have gained popularity (Bush et al 2015; Fox & Reeves 2015; Randall & Neubeck 2016; Wilson et al 2020). This terminology readjusts the implications slightly by using less power-laden language; however, even these terms suggest that people should 'stick' to doing what is asked of them, regardless of the factors influencing their life (Wilson et al 2020). Thinking about approaches to caring for people in terms of giving personalised information and agreed-upon goals is useful, regardless of whether we are talking about compliance or adherence (Randall & Neubeck 2016; Wilson et al 2020).

For example, the person with diabetes who eats whatever they want and does not give themselves injections is non-compliant with their diet and medications. Even so, in Western countries, there is no law against people making decisions that impact adversely on their health. This is sometimes very difficult for nurses to accept. Even so, rather than applying the label of 'non-compliant' to a person with a chronic illness or disability, it is more helpful to consider ways of developing an effective partnership between the nurse and the person. This would involve exploring the patterns of behaviour with the person, including factors that discourage the person from making health choices.

On the other hand, where a person is cognitively unable to make a reasoned, informed decision about their healthcare, as may be the case for people with, for example, dementia or some mental illnesses, ensuring compliance may be exactly the approach called for. Occasionally, it may be reasonable – even necessary – for a health professional to make unilateral decisions relating to a person's treatment, occasionally by placing a community treatment order, which allows for the provision of treatment without consent for individuals with severe mental health problems (Weich et al 2020). Great care must be taken with this approach, however, to ensure that the rights of the person and their family members or carers are respected; and clear and transparent communication is upheld between all people.

Empowerment

One of the roles of the nurse is to empower the person they are helping so that the person can manage their own care. This may include addressing some structural barriers to self-care or providing information or education to the person and also their carers (Grisot et al 2018). Empowerment does not refer to a division of labour; nor does it describe what the nurse will and will not do, and what the person with the chronic illness should or should not do. Instead, empowerment is about supporting people to make their own choices or decisions, to 'self-determine' (McCallum et al 2019; Zoffmann et al 2016).

What happens when a nurse believes a person should assume responsibility for some aspect of care, but the person believes the nurse should do it? One common example is in the self-administration of subcutaneous injections. In a biomedically influenced world, it is a common perception that the administration of medications via this route must be performed by a medically focused health professional. This can be quite a challenge to a person with a new diagnosis of, for example, diabetes. How are these conflicts resolved?

When the nurse and person have developed a good collaborative partnership, which includes trust and good communication skills, the result will most often include the resolution of conflicting expectations. Discussing and accepting a person's fears and uncertainties will help nurses to consider ways they can address these fears and uncertainties and, in the process, achieve outcomes that are acceptable to the person with a chronic illness or disability.

Another aspect of empowerment relates to engagement. For example, sometimes it is a part of the nurse's role to facilitate engagement with the multidisciplinary team. This could involve advocacy – that is, speaking on behalf of or representing the needs and wishes of the person with a chronic illness (Chapman 2015; PinChoi 2015). A more significant and lasting contribution is the one that is made when the person has the knowledge, resources and self-belief to speak for themselves. Questions the nurse could ask the person or family member may include: What is stopping you from speaking up? What are your fears? What would help you to speak up? Working towards addressing such questions with the person with a chronic illness or disability is an important way of empowering the person.

Storytelling

Some people like to talk about their experiences of illness. This type of storytelling provides a crucial means by which people (and health professionals) can potentially make meaning of an illness and their lives (Frank 2015; Morales-Asencio et al 2015; Strickland et al 2017). By listening to a person's stories and finding out what is important to them, nurses can facilitate a shared understanding of the needs of the person. Giving time to the person, together with giving the person permission to ask questions and seek answers, may enhance the partnership between the person and nurse. Such activities will also help the person to incorporate the experience of the illness into their life and attach meaning to their illness, which, in turn, may improve their coping and adaptation in positive ways (Egnew 2018; Metersky & Schwind 2015; Riegel et al 2019).

It is interesting to note that along with suffering comes adaptation and resilience, giving up old versions of self and establishing a new identity. Sometimes living with a chronic illness or disability can be seen as a very positive thing in someone's life. Many people say that their life is richer for the new perspectives they have attained; or that they have learned things about themselves they did not know prior to their illness. Examples may be appreciating things that they have previously taken for granted, such as the beauty of a sunrise or time spent with children, or recognising one's own strength through completing some very difficult rehabilitation. These things may also be true for nurses who work with people with a chronic illness.

Self-Management

One of the most powerful and practical approaches to the management of chronic illness is self-management. Self-management is a dynamic process and involves the person with the chronic illness actively taking responsibility for the management of their condition in their daily life (Riegel et al 2019). The role of the nurse is to support self-management; the role of the person with a chronic illness or disability is to 'do' the self-management. This means the person takes on a new role – of a consumer of healthcare. The person actively seeks information to understand the illness or disability and to learn new skills. The person becomes an active and informed participant in the relationship with healthcare providers and makes decisions based on best available evidence, personal preferences and availability of resources. The person then actively integrates self-management into their lives (Randall & Neubeck 2016; Riegel et al 2019). Self-management may give the person a sense of control and may be the process that brings order back into their life (Riegel et al 2019).

CASE STUDY 5.1

PART 8

Four months later, Sharon visited Gwen for the last time until a new need arose. Gwen gave her a card and a box of chocolates to share with the health team. They had worked together to arrive at a place where Gwen felt safe and comfortable with her care. Gwen was applying moisturiser to her leg and had bought stockings with a degree of compression.

Sharon learned something very valuable about herself as a registered nurse and how she might at times be perceived. She also learned about the success that can be had through working towards shared goals. Finally, she had to acknowledge that she had learned a lot about lawn bowls!

CONCLUSION

People lead complex lives that are influenced by personal (including emotional, cognitive and behavioural) characteristics, family influences, age, gender, sexuality, cultural background, level of education, socioeconomic and employment status, social networks, spiritual and political beliefs, as well as the community and physical environment in which they live. No one knows the life of a person better than the person who is living it. The psychosocial care that is delivered to the person with a chronic illness or disability will depend on the knowledge, skills and attitudes of the nurse in recognising the value of the experience of the person, including what the person knows about themselves and their life; and working alongside the person to achieve relevant, shared goals. Collaborative partnerships provide a foundation for delivering psychosocial care, and involve the nurse and the person with a chronic illness working together to maximise the person's capacity to live life to the full, despite the illness; and minimising the adverse impacts of their illness. Recognising diversity, supporting self-management and empowering people to engage with healthcare systems and other aspects of life are important person-centred strategies that are applied within the collaborative partnership to bring about better health outcomes, improved quality in life, and lives that are lived to the full.

Reflective Questions

1. Think about your own culture. How does your culture influence your perception of health and ill-health?

2. Consider a person with a chronic illness that you know or have supported. How has the person's perception of their chronic illness changed over time, according to their needs and situation? Likewise, how has the care they have received changed over time?

3. What are the main psychosocial needs of the carer of the person with a chronic illness or disability? How could the nurse best support those needs?

RECOMMENDED READING

Allen D 2019. Care trajectory management: a conceptual framework for formalizing emergent organisation in nursing practice. Journal of Nursing Management 27(1), 4–9.

Ambrosio L, Senosiain García JM, Riverol Fernández M et al 2015. Living with chronic illness in adults: a concept analysis. Journal of Clinical Nursing 24(17–18), 2357–2367.

Australian Institute for Health & Wellbeing (AIHW) 2019. Australian burden of disease study: impact and causes of illness and death in Australia 2015. Online. Available: www.aihw.gov.au/reports/burden-of-disease/burden-disease-study-illness-death-2015/summary

Friesen-Storms JH, Bours GJ, van der Weijden T et al 2015. Shared decision making in chronic care in the context of evidence based practice in nursing. International Journal of Nursing Studies 52 (1), 393–402.

McCormack B, McCance T 2017. Person-centred practice in nursing and health care. Theory and practice, 2nd edn. Wiley Blackwell, Chichester.

REFERENCES

Allen D 2019. Care trajectory management: a conceptual framework for formalizing emergent organisation in nursing practice. Journal of Nursing Management 27(1), 4–9.

Alonso Y 2004. The biopsychosocial model in medical research: the evolution of the health concept over the last two decades. Patient Education and Counseling 53(2), 239–244.

Ambrosio L, Senosiain García JM, Riverol Fernández M et al 2015. Living with chronic illness in adults: a concept analysis. Journal of Clinical Nursing 24(17–18), 2357–2367.

Ancheta IB, Carlson JM, Battie CA et al 2015. One size does not fit all: cardiovascular health disparities as a function of ethnicity in Asian-American women. Applied Nursing Research 28(2), 99–105.

Australian Institute of Health and Welfare (AIHW) 2019. Australian burden of disease study: impact and causes of illness and death in Australia 2015. Australian Burden of Disease series no. 19. Cat. no. BOD 22. AIHW, Canberra.

Battersby M, Lawn S, Kowanko I et al 2018. Chronic condition self-management support for Aboriginal people: adapting tools and training. Australian Journal of Rural Health 26(4), 232–237.

Bernoth M, Burmeister OK, Morrison M et al 2016. The impact of a participatory care model on work satisfaction of care workers and the functionality, connectedness, and mental health of community-dwelling older people. Issues in Mental Health Nursing 37(6), 429–435.

Brooks LA, Manias E, Bloomer MJ 2019. Culturally sensitive communication in healthcare: a concept analysis. Collegian 26(3), 383–391.

Browne CV, Ka'opua LS, Jervis LL et al 2016. United States Indigenous populations and dementia: is there a case for culture-based psychosocial interventions? The Gerontologist 4(1), 1–9.

Bush R, Brown K, Latz C 2015. Compression therapies for chronic venous leg ulcers: interventions and adherence. Chronic Wound Care Management and Research 2, 11–21.

Chapman S 2015. Reflections on a 38-year career in public health advocacy: 10 pieces of advice to early career researchers and advocates. Public Health Research & Practice 25(2), e2521514.

Cleary M, Hungerford C 2015. Trauma-informed care and the research literature: how can the mental health nurse take the lead to support women who have survived sexual assault? Issues in Mental Health Nursing 36(5), 370–378.

Cloitre M 2015. The 'one size fits all' approach to trauma treatment: should we be satisfied? European Journal of Psychotraumatology 6, doi: 10.3402/ejpt.v6.27344.

Corbin J 2001. Introduction and overview: chronic illness and nursing. In: R Hyman, J Corbin (eds), Chronic illness: research and theory for nursing practice. Springer, New York. © Ruth Hyman.

Corbin JM, Strauss A 1991. A nursing model for chronic illness management based upon the trajectory framework. Scholarly Inquiry for Nursing Practice 5(3), 155–174.

Crowe S, Deane F 2018. Characteristics of mental health recovery model implementation and managers' and clinicians' risk aversion. Journal of Mental Health Training, Education & Practice 13(1), 22–33.

Cypress BS 2016. Understanding uncertainty among critically ill patients in the intensive care unit using Mishel's Theory of Uncertainty of Illness. Dimensions of Critical Care Nursing 35(1), 42–49.

de Jong M, de Boer AG, Tamminga SJ et al 2015. Quality of working life issues of employees with a chronic physical disease: a systematic review. Journal of Occupational Rehabilitation 25(1), 182–196.

Ditchman N, Kosyluk K, Lee EJ et al 2016. How stigma affects the lives of people with intellectual disabilities: an overview. In: K Scior, S Werner (eds), Intellectual disability and stigma. Palgrave Macmillan, London.

Eaton S, Roberts S, Turner B 2015. Delivering person centred care in long term conditions. British Medical Journal (Clinical Research Ed.) 350, h181.

Egnew TR 2018. A narrative approach to healing chronic illness. The Annals of Family Medicine 16(2), 160–165.

Filmer T, Herbig B 2020. A training intervention for home care nurses in cross-cultural communication: an evaluation study of changes in attitudes, knowledge and behaviour. Journal of Advanced Nursing 76(1), 147–162.

Fonseca C, Lopes M, Ramos A et al 2015. Nursing interventions in prevention and healing of leg ulcers: systematic review of the literature. Journal of Palliative Care & Medicine 5, 238, DOI: 10.4172/2165-7386.1000238.

Foronda C 2020. A theory of cultural humility. Journal of Transcultural Nursing 31(1), 7–12.

Fox A, Reeves S 2015. Interprofessional collaborative patient-centred care: a critical exploration of two related discourses. Journal of Interprofessional Care 29(2), 113–118.

Frank AW 2015. Asking the right question about pain: narrative and phronesis. British Journal of Pain 9(1), 209–225.

Friesen-Storms JH, Bours GJ, van der Weijden T et al 2015. Shared decision making in chronic care in the context of evidence based practice in nursing. International Journal of Nursing Studies 52(1), 393–402.

Frost J, Foster K, Ranse K 2017. Unfolding case study and Mask-Ed™ high fidelity simulation for chronic illness education: a case study. Collegian 24(5), 433–439.

Fung FY, Linn YC 2015. Developing traditional Chinese medicine in the era of evidence-based medicine: current evidences and challenges. Evidence-based Complementary and Alternative Medicine 2015, Article ID 425037.

Grisot M, Moltubakk AK, Hagen L et al 2018. Supporting patient self-care: examining nurses' practices in a remote care setting. Studies in Health Technology and Informatics 247, 601–605.

Hamann J, Mendel R, Cohen R et al 2015. Psychiatrists' use of shared decision making in the treatment of schizophrenia: patient characteristics and decision topics. Psychiatric Services 60(8), 1107–1112.

Holland JM, Graves S, Klingspon KL et al 2015. Prolonged grief symptoms related to loss of physical functioning: examining unique associations with medical service utilization. Disability and Rehabilitation 1–6.

Hoth KF, Wamboldt FS, Ford DW et al 2015. The social environment and illness uncertainty in chronic obstructive pulmonary disease. International Journal of Behavioral Medicine 22(2), 223–232.

Hungerford C, Dowling M, Doyle K 2015. Recovery outcome measures: is there a place for culture, attitudes, and faith? Perspectives in Psychiatric Care 51(3), 171–179.

Jackson JW, Williams DR, VanderWeele TJ 2016. Disparities at the intersection of marginalized groups. Social Psychiatry and Psychiatric Epidemiology 51(10), 1349–1359.

Jasemi M, Valizadeh L, Zamanzadeh V et al 2017. A concept analysis of holistic care by hybrid model. Indian Journal of Palliative Care 23(1), 71–80.

Karazivan P, Dumez V, Flora L et al 2015. The patient-as-partner approach in health care: a conceptual framework for a necessary transition. Academic Medicine: Journal of the Association of American Medical Colleges 90(4), 437–441.

Kidd S, Kenny A, McKinstry C 2015. The meaning of recovery in a regional mental health service: an action research study. Journal of Advanced Nursing 71(1), 181–192.

Kilcullen M, Swinbourne A, Cadet JY 2018. Aboriginal and Torres Strait Islander health and wellbeing: social emotional wellbeing and strengths-based psychology. Clinical Psychologist 22(1), 16–26.

Knaak S, Mantler E, Szeto A 2017. Mental illness-related stigma in healthcare: barriers to access and care and evidence-based solutions. Healthcare Management Forum 30(2), 111–116.

Kogan AC, Wilber K, Mosqueda L 2016. Person-centered care for older adults with chronic conditions and functional impairment: a systematic literature review. Journal of the American Geriatrics Society 64(1), e1–e7.

Kon AA, Davidson JE, Morrison W et al 2016. Shared decision making in ICUs: an American College of Critical Care Medicine and American Thoracic Society policy statement. Critical Care Medicine 44(1), 188–201.

Langbecker D, Yates P 2015. Primary brain tumor patients' supportive care needs and multidisciplinary rehabilitation, community and psychosocial support services: awareness, referral and utilization. Journal of Neuro-Oncology 1–12.

Lassen AJ 2015. Keeping disease at arm's length – how older Danish people distance disease through active ageing. Ageing and Society 35(7), 1364–1383.

Livneh H, Parker RM 2005. Psychological adaptation to disability perspectives from chaos and complexity theory. Rehabilitation Counseling Bulletin 49(1), 17–28.

Long A, Halkett GK, Lobb EA et al 2015. Carers of patients with high-grade glioma report high levels of distress, unmet needs, and psychological morbidity during patient chemoradiotherapy. Neuro-Oncology Practice 3(2), 105–112.

López-Sierra HE, Rodríguez-Sánchez J 2015. The supportive roles of religion and spirituality in end-of-life and palliative care of patients with cancer in a culturally diverse context: a literature review. Current Opinion in Supportive and Palliative Care 9(1), 87–95.

Mannix J, Wilkes L, Daly J 2015. 'Good ethics and moral standing': a qualitative study of aesthetic leadership in clinical nursing practice. Journal of Clinical Nursing 24 (11–12), 1603–1610.

Manookian A, Chereghi MA, Nasrabadi AN 2016. Ontology of human dignity in nursing. International Journal of Advanced and Applied Sciences 3(2), 74–77.

Mansfield E, Bryant J, Regan T et al 2016. Burden and unmet needs of caregivers of chronic obstructive pulmonary disease patients: a systematic review of the volume and focus of research output. COPD: Journal of Chronic Obstructive Pulmonary Disease 1–6.

McCallum M, Gray CM, Hanlon P et al 2019. Exploring the utility of self-determination theory in complex interventions in multimorbidity: a qualitative analysis of patient experiences of the CARE Plus intervention. Chronic Illness, DOI: 10.1177/1742395319884106.

McCance T, McCormack B 2017. The person-centred practice framework. In: B McCormack, T McCance (eds), Person-centred practice in nursing and health care. Theory and practice, 2nd edn. Wiley-Blackwell, Oxford.

Metersky K, Schwind JK 2015. Interprofessional care: patient experience stories. International Journal of Person Centered Medicine 5(2), 78–87.

Morales-Asencio JM, Martin-Santos FJ, Kaknani S et al 2015. Living with chronicity and complexity: lessons for redesigning case management from patients' life stories: a qualitative study. Journal of Evaluation in Clinical Practice 22(1), 122–132.

Munhall PL 1992. 'Unknowing': toward another pattern of knowing in nursing. Nursing Outlook 41 (3), 125–128.

Nelson G, Macnaughton E, Curwood SE et al 2016. Collaboration and involvement of persons with lived experience in planning Canada's At Home/Chez Soi project. Health & Social Care in the Community 24(2), 184–193.

O'Dowd A 2015. Older people are afraid to complain, says ombudsman. BMJ: British Medical Journal (Online), 351, h7012.

Orvik A, Vågen SR, Axelsson SB et al 2015. Quality, efficiency and integrity: value squeezes in management of hospital wards. Journal of Nursing Management 23(1), 65–74.

Park LG, Howie-Esquivel J, Whooley MA et al 2015. Psychosocial factors and medication adherence among patients with coronary heart disease: a text messaging intervention. European Journal of Cardiovascular Nursing 14(3), 264–273.

Paterson BL 2001. The shifting perspectives model of chronic illness. Journal of Nursing Scholarship 33(1), 21–26.

PinChoi P 2015. Patient advocacy: the role of the nurse. Nursing Standard 29(41), 52–58.

Pomey M-P, Ghadiri DP, Karazivan P et al 2015. Patients as partners: a qualitative study of patients' engagement in their health care. PLoS ONE 10(4), e0122499.

Randall S, Neubeck L 2016. What's in a name? Concordance is better than adherence for promoting partnership and self-management of chronic disease. Australian Journal of Primary Health 22(3), 181–184.

Riegel B, Jaarsma T, Lee CS et al 2019. Integrating symptoms into the middle-range theory of self-care of chronic illness. ANS. Advances in Nursing Science 42(3), 206.

Roberts RM, Neate GM, Gierasch A 2017. Implicit attitudes towards people with visible difference: findings from an Implicit Association Test. Psychology, Health and Medicine 22(3), 352–358.

Sánchez J, Rosenthal DA, Tansey TN et al 2016. Predicting quality of life in adults with severe mental illness: extending the International Classification of Functioning, Disability and Health. Rehabilitation Psychology 61(1), 19.

Sav A, King MA, Whitty JA et al 2015. Burden of treatment for chronic illness: a concept analysis and review of the literature. Health Expectations 18(3), 312–324.

Siyun Chen C, Wai-Chi Chan S, Fai Chan M et al 2017. Journal of Nursing Research 25(6), 411–418.

Smith J, Swallow V, Coyne I 2015. Involving parents in managing their child's long-term condition – a concept synthesis of family-centered care and partnership-in-care. Journal of Pediatric Nursing 30(1), 143–159.

Strickland K, Worth A, Kennedy CM 2017. The liminal self in people with multiple sclerosis: an interpretative phenomenological exploration of being diagnosed. Journal of Clinical Nursing 26(11–12), 1714–1724.

Strickland K, Worth A, Kennedy CM 2015. The experiences of support persons of people newly diagnosed with multiple sclerosis: an interpretative phenomenological study. Journal of Advanced Nursing 71, 2811–2821.

van der Greef J, van Wietmarschen H, Schroën Y et al 2015. Systematic approaches to evaluation and integration of Eastern and Western medical practices. Medical Acupuncture 27(5), 384–395.

Watson M 2015. Listening to the wherewho: a lived experience of schizophrenia. Schizophrenia Bulletin 41(1), 6–8.

Weich S, Duncan C, Twigg L et al 2020. Use of community treatment orders and their outcomes: an observational study. Health Services and Delivery Research 8.9. NIHR Journals Library, Southampton.

Wilson TE, Hennessy EA, Falzon L et al 2020. Effectiveness of interventions targeting self-regulation to improve adherence to chronic disease medications: a meta-review of meta-analyses. Health Psychology Review 14(1), 66–85.

Zhang KM, Dindoff K, Arnold JMO et al 2015. What matters to patients with heart failure? The influence of non-health-related goals on patient adherence to self-care management. Patient Education and Counseling 98(8), 927–934.

Zoffmann V, Hörnsten Å, Storbækken S et al 2016. Translating person-centered care into practice: a comparative analysis of motivational interviewing, illness-integration support, and guided self-determination. Patient Education and Counseling 99(3), 400–407.

CHAPTER 6

Stigmatisation of People Living with a Chronic Illness or Disability

DIANNE E. ROY • LYNNE S. GIDDINGS

LEARNING OBJECTIVES

When you have completed this chapter you will be able to:

- identify and name examples of stigmatising processes that could lead to stereotyping, labelling and 'othering' of people who live with chronic illness and/or impairment
- use self-reflexive questioning to assist in deconstructing situations that may marginalise and discriminate against people who live with chronic illness and/or impairment
- develop strategies to identify, name and challenge stigmatising processes experienced by people who live with chronic illness and/or impairment
- apply specific principles of nursing practice to avoid stigmatising people who live with chronic illness and/or impairment
- become 'part of the solution' to prevent the marginalisation and discrimination of people who live with chronic illness and/or impairment.

KEY WORDS

discrimination
health disparities
marginalisation

stereotyping
stigma

INTRODUCTION

This chapter focuses on the concept of stigma and related processes, such as stereotyping, labelling and othering, and their effects on people who live with chronic illness and/or impairment. Such processes not only affect individuals, families and their communities, but also contribute to disparities in healthcare. For the purposes of this chapter we focus our discussion on how nurses can challenge these stigmatising processes in the context of working with people with chronic illness and/or impairment. We acknowledge that the 'isms', such as racism, sexism, heterosexism and classism, also intersect within the healthcare context. It is also important to acknowledge the distinction between chronic illness, impairment and disability. Illness is caused by disease (and may or may not involve impairment), whereas disability is created within societal

structures (Oliver 2009, 2013; World Health Organization [WHO] 2018). As outlined in the United Nations Convention on the Rights of People with Disability, disability is an evolving concept that results from the interaction between people living with an impairment and attitudinal and environmental barriers that hinder their full and effective participation in society on an equal basis with others (United Nations 2006). When these terms are used synonymously it is difficult to challenge the stigmatising processes that make invisible the different needs of people living with an impairment who experience disability. We next explore issues relating to nurses and the processes of stigma and the value of using the social model of disability to guide self-reflexive practice. 'Self-reflexive' in the context of this chapter refers to a process of critical self-reflection on such things as one's preferences, prejudices, biases and actions (Schwandt 2007). Finally, we will discuss various principles of nursing care using fictitious case study scenarios derived from our clinical experience.

NURSES AND STIGMA

Stigma, defining people as abnormal if they do not meet an expected norm, is related to being different; it pervades all levels of society and crosses all cultures. We are all affected by it, we are all part of the problem, but we can also make ourselves part of the solution. Nurses who care for people who live with chronic illness and/or impairment are well positioned to challenge the everyday processes of stigmatisation. Through the naming of the processes and their effects, possibilities for conscious action are opened up at the personal, professional and socio-political levels. One of the first principles to be aware of as healthcare providers is to 'know ourselves' in relation to who we are in the world so that we are able to deconstruct (identify and name) the stigmatising processes that lead to marginalisation and discrimination of others.

Knowing Ourselves

Many nurses believe that they treat everyone the same and/or they are not privileged or oppressed in any way. We challenge this position as we believe that all of us contribute to disparities within society and the healthcare system. If we start with the premise that we all use stigmatising processes and are all affected by them, we can get somewhere with challenging them. We offer here some self-reflexive questions that can assist nurses to care effectively for people who are different from themselves, such as those who live with chronic illness and/or impairment. These questions have been informed by the work of Porter (1996), Maeve (1998), Smith (1999) and Giddings (2005a).

1. Am I acknowledging my position of power and privilege in relation to the people with chronic illness and/or impairment whom I work alongside or care for?
2. Am I actively trying to understand and accept the validity of each individual's experience?
3. Am I recognising the expertise/developing expertise of people in living with their illness and/or impairment?
4. Am I working with and supporting the personally developed strategies for self-management of people living with chronic illness and/or impairment?

Self-reflexive approaches to nursing practice are grounded in respect and regard for people. They help position nurses as potential advocates and social activists

by making visible stigmatising processes such as stereotyping, labelling and othering, and their outcome: social isolation, powerlessness and health disparities (see Table 6.1). These processes and outcomes are complex and interlink to produce a society in which some people and groups within certain contexts are privileged while others are marginalised and discriminated against. Of course, how one views these processes depends on where one is standing. Those people who are privileged by belonging to a dominant cultural/social group, such as being male, white, heterosexual, middle-class and able, may not be able to 'see' that just belonging to a mainstream group can advantage them in relation to others. Conversely, those people who are identified as belonging to a group that is marginalised within society may effectively internalise the dominant cultural attitudes and so believe them to be true (Giddings 2005a; Hickey 2015; Johnson 2006); they have an acquired social consciousness or false consciousness, so they self-fulfil or act out the stereotypical behaviour (Giddings 2005b). For example, a person who is living with diabetes may self-label as 'a diabetic' or may accept a 'sick role' of unnecessary dependency (Luyckx et al 2016), while a person with HIV/AIDS may decide to conceal their condition in situations when revealing the truth opens them to stigmatisation (Bruce et al 2019). All groups within society, including the disabled community, marginalise and discriminate from within. For example, a person who is able to

---

TABLE 6.1
Definitions of Stigmatising Processes

Stigmatising Process	Definition
Stereotyping	Involves categorising and prejudging (prejudice) individuals based on an over-simplified set of beliefs about the nature and characteristics of particular groups
Labelling	The application of negative stereotypes by naming individuals and their identified group as problematic
Othering	The social construction of people with certain characteristics into named groups that are viewed as 'different' in some way from what is widely believed in society to be 'normal'

articulate their experiences and needs (able–disabled) may privilege themselves to speak for those who live with both intellectual and physical impairment and are less able to speak for themselves (disabled–disabled). Such discriminatory processes can inadvertently be supported by otherwise sound and beneficial policies, such as the New Zealand Disability Strategy (Ministry of Health NZ 2001; 2016) and the Australian National Disability Strategy (Department of Social Services 2011), by creating an assumption that 'one size fits all'.

In the broadest terms, we are arguing that people coming into the healthcare system, no matter what their difference, need to be culturally safe; that is, receive effective and safe healthcare (Curtis et al 2019; Mackean et al 2019; Nursing Council of New Zealand 2011; Papps 2015; Ramsden 2002). Nurses need to not only be aware and sensitive to the effects of stigmatising processes within society and the healthcare system, but also have a social consciousness that enables action by developing strategies for implementing change: working with, not against (Francis et al 2019; Giddings et al 2007; Hickey 2015; Roy & Giddings 2012), naming not blaming; and deconstructing power relations rather than passively accepting the status quo (Giddings 2005b; Johnson 2006).

Deconstructing (Identifying, Naming and Challenging) Societal Stigmatising Processes

Even today it is not uncommon to hear stigmatising or othering terms used to describe people who live with chronic illness and/or impairment. For example, people are sometimes described as being 'handicapped', 'crippled', 'retarded', 'suffering from', 'mongoloid' or 'wheelchair-bound'. They may also be labelled by their condition, for example, 'an arthritic', 'a diabetic', 'a lunatic', 'an asthmatic', 'a spastic', 'a quadriplegic' or 'an epileptic'. Identifying such labelling is one of the first steps in challenging the processes of stigmatisation. It can assist in making stereotypes and related health disparities visible and open to critique. Nurses need to be aware, however, that many people living with chronic illness and/or impairment may wish to conceal and keep their condition secret in an attempt to pass as 'normal'. These attempts, although a protective response to the marginalising and discriminatory practices within society, feed into their hidden nature and make them difficult to challenge. It is important to challenge stigmatising processes as they not only have negative effects for the individual living with chronic illness and/or impairment, but also for their family, friends and community, and can even extend to those

who care for them. Within nursing itself, for example, there are processes that marginalise and discriminate (Neal-Boylan 2019a, 2019b; Zlotnick & Shpigelman 2018). Nursing educational programs often exclude people with disabilities (Marks & McCulloh 2016; Neal-Boylan & Smith 2016), and nurses living with chronic illness and/or impairment often report difficulties with maintaining employment and/or achieving promotion (Giddings 1997; Hickey 2015; Neal-Boylan 2019a, 2019b).

Self-reflexive practice that identifies, names and challenges stigmatising processes can be guided by the social model of disability first described by Oliver (1983, 1996, 2009, 2013). It was developed in the 1980s and 'has demonstrated success for disabled people in society, challenging discrimination and marginalisation, linking civil rights and political activism and enabling disabled people to claim their rightful place in society' (Owens 2015, p. 385). The model has been extensively reviewed, critiqued and used to inform research, policy and practice (see, for example, Goering 2015; Levitt 2017; Ministry of Health NZ 2001; Mitra 2006; Office for Disability Issues 2016; Oliver 2009, 2013; Owens 2015; Retief & Letšosa 2018; Shakespeare 2008). Within this model it is argued that people, as individuals, live with impairments. Concomitantly (Oliver 1996, p. 33):

> Disability is all the things that impose restrictions on disabled people; ranging from individual prejudice to institutional discrimination, from inaccessible public buildings to unusable transport systems, from segregated education to excluding work arrangements, and so on. Further, the consequences of this failure do not simply and randomly fall on individuals but systematically upon disabled people as a group who experience this failure as discrimination institutionalised through society.

The social model of disability moves the problem of disability away from the individual to society. The onus is on society, therefore, to adapt and cater for the needs of individuals and families who live with chronic illness and/or impairment. An ongoing case in New Zealand highlights institutional discrimination against families who provide specific disability-related care for their 'adult disabled children' (Human Rights Commission 2016). Although the adult-aged children, all living with significant impairments, were assessed by the Ministry of Health as requiring this care, policy prior to 2013 stated that only non-family members could be paid (Human Rights Commission n.d.). Families providing disability-related care successfully challenged this policy by employing human rights legislation. A Human Rights Review Tribunal concluded in

2010 that the policy was discriminatory under the *Human Rights Act 1993* as discrimination on the basis of family status is prohibited (Human Rights Commission n.d.). The Ministry appealed the decision through the High Court and the Court of Appeal. Both courts, however, upheld the decision, with the High Court noting that the Ministry's policy was at odds with the New Zealand Disability Strategy (Ministry of Health NZ 2001) and the Convention on the Rights of Persons with Disabilities (United Nations 2006). In response to the court decisions, the government passed the *New Zealand Public Health and Disability Amendment Act (No. 2) 2000/2013*, which prohibits payment to family members, except in accordance with Funded Family Care policy developed by the Ministry of Health (NZ) (2016). The policy permits payments to some family members (but not partners and at a lesser rate than non-family members) in some narrow circumstances. The legislation (Part 4A) also prevents any future claims being taken to the Human Rights Commission, the Human Rights Review Tribunal or the courts (Human Rights Commission 2016). Since implementation of Funded Family Care, the legislation and policies have remained a concern to the Commission and many other groups, including disabled people and their whānau (families). In January 2020, the New Zealand Government announced significant changes that took effect from September 2020. This included removing the discriminatory elements of the *Public Health and*

Disability Amendment Act (No. 2) 2000/2013 through a repeal of Part 4A that prevented disabled people and their whānau making a complaint on the grounds of discrimination (Ardern & Genter 2020; Ministry of Health 2020). Among other changes announced, eligibility criteria now enables access to the scheme not only by disabled people with high or very high support needs, but also those with needs related to long-term health conditions, mental health and addiction, and aged care. Partners/spouses and children aged 16 years and over are now eligible to receive payments (Ministry of Health NZ 2020).

Similarly, evidence of institutional discrimination has been reported in Australia in relation to the National Disability Insurance Scheme (NDIS) (Department of Social Services 2011), which began a full rollout nationally in 2016. Early reviews of the scheme have shown, for example, that health inequalities can be further entrenched (Malbon et al 2019), some groups (such as those living with intellectual impairment) are marginalised (Perry et al 2019), and it is not responsive to the needs of many people, particularly Aboriginal and Torres Strait Islander people (Avery 2018; Gordon et al 2019).

Presented in Case Study 6.1 are common scenarios that can help you explore the principles of nursing care that can guide your self-reflexive practice in relation to identifying, naming and challenging stigmatising processes while caring for and working with people who live with chronic illness and/or impairment.

CASE STUDY 6.1

PART 1

Serena (32 years) and her partner Nigel (30 years) have been living with Serena's parents, Muriel and Keith, in their large suburban home for the last 2 years. They are in the process of moving into a place of their own in the inner city. Serena works full-time as a case manager for a family carer support organisation and Nigel is an architect for the city council. Serena was born with spina bifida, has paralysis of her lower body and uses a wheelchair; Nigel has lived with diabetes (type 1) since he was 16 years old. Adding to the complexity of the family situation, Muriel has lived with multiple sclerosis for nearly 20 years.

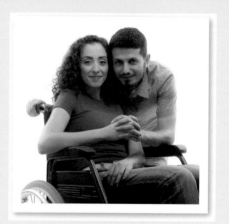

iStockphoto/ozgurdonmaz.

CASE STUDY 6.1 – cont'd

Serena and Nigel frequently go to the movies, often enjoying a coffee or meal before the show. Although the local theatre is accessible for wheelchairs, the cafés and restaurants in the area have narrow doorways and often steps. Once she has made it into a café, Serena then has to negotiate her wheelchair to a table, often a difficult task. Recently, on Nigel's birthday when they were ordering a coffee, the person behind the counter looked down at Serena, then turned to Nigel and asked, 'What type of coffee does she want?'

Nigel replied, 'You can ask her.'

The young woman leaned over the counter and talking slowly and loudly asked, 'What—type—of—coffee—do—you—want?'

Serena replied, 'I do not have a hearing impairment and I would like a trim latte with two sugars, please. My partner will have a double shot, long black, no sugar. And while we are at it, we will have two pieces of that delicious-looking apple cake, thanks.'

While they were consuming the coffee and cake, Serena chuckled and said, 'What if the practice nurse catches you eating *that*, Nigel?'

Nigel laughed and replied, 'She would be shocked, I'm sure. She just doesn't seem to understand that sometimes on a special occasion you just have to have it.'

Serena needed to go to the toilet. The café's toilet facilities were outside, down some steps and near the storeroom. Such inaccessibility necessitated that she wait until they reached the movie theatre. Although the theatre has two wheelchair-accessible toilets, they are both situated in the women's and men's toilet areas respectively. As Serena requires assistance with toileting, no matter which they choose they often receive disapproving looks from other patrons. Nigel reflects on the irony posed by such situations given his work as an architect.

PART 2

Nigel injured his leg while playing club rugby. He was transported to the emergency department (ED) by ambulance with a suspected fracture of the tibia. With the focus on his acute injury, his belongings, including his medication and blood glucose meter, were left behind in the changing rooms. He alerted the ambulance staff to the fact he has type 1 diabetes. They immediately tested his blood glucose level (BGL), which was found to be within normal range at 5.2 mmol/L. On arrival at the ED, Nigel was triaged and sent to the acute area for further assessment. Soon after, he began to feel strange and experienced a tingling sensation around his mouth; symptoms he recognised as signalling the beginning of a hypoglycaemic episode. He pressed the call bell, which was eventually answered by a nurse. Nigel told the nurse he was experiencing a 'hypo' and requested some food or glucose tablets. He explained that his 'gear' had not come with him so he could not self-test. The nurse checked his chart. She said that as his BGL was 5.2 mmol/L only half an hour earlier, treatment was not necessary. Nigel explained that he had been playing rugby and because of his accident had not had his planned snack at half-time. He knew his BGL had dropped and that he must have some glucose or food immediately. The nurse replied that he was not allowed anything to eat because of his injury, but she would do a repeat BGL to see if it was low. The nurse left the room. Ten minutes later another nurse escorting Serena to Nigel's bedside found him semi-conscious, sweating profusely and tachycardic. She immediately called for emergency assistance.

PART 3

In anticipation of their move, Serena changed her primary care provider from the health centre she had attended since childhood to an inner-city practice belonging to the same primary health organisation. Prior to the move, she checked out the accessibility of the building and the clinic, and arranged for her health records to be transferred. In due course, Serena made an appointment for a routine cervical smear. On arrival she was informed by the nurse that the clinic's height adjustable examination table was broken and she was unsure when it would be fixed. As Serena was unable to transfer to a regular height examination table, the nurse offered to arrange a home visit so Serena could have the smear taken on her own bed. Serena accepted the offer. Two weeks later she was surprised to receive an invoice for $120. She immediately phoned the practice. On asking why it was so high, she was told by the practice manager that 'This is the standard charge for a home visit'. Serena explained what had happened, but the practice manager said there was nothing she could do about it. Serena asked to speak to the nurse. On asking, 'What is the standard cost for a smear?', the nurse replied, '$20'. Serena pointed out that the home visit resulted from the fact that the equipment was malfunctioning and asked why she should pay more than other women for this preventative health service. The nurse paused, then replied, 'Oh, I see your point. I'm sorry; I have never thought of it that way before. I agree, you shouldn't be asked to pay more than other women. I will take this case to the practice management team meeting tomorrow morning.'

Next morning at the meeting, members of the practice management team initially expressed surprise when the issue was raised, as surely it only required the equipment to be repaired. The nurse argued that the issue was broader and similar situations may arise when the practice

continued

CASE STUDY 6.1 – cont'd

is not able to provide equitable services for people living with impairment. Following robust discussion, the team came to agreement that the charge was discriminatory and would be changed and that a policy review was required. The nurse offered to draft a document that could be circulated to extend the discussion to include other practices in their primary health organisation.

PART 4

Serena's mother, Muriel, had elective surgery for a hysterectomy. She was admitted to a four-bed room in a surgical unit. The morning following surgery when the nurse finished checking her wound, he stressed to Muriel the importance of walking soon after surgery and instructed her to walk to the end of the ward and back. Some time later the nurse returned and asked Muriel if she had been for her walk. Muriel shook her head, but before she could explain, the nurse loudly remarked, 'I don't know why some people can't help themselves', and left the room.

Sally in the neighbouring bed chortled, 'Well, that was a good telling-off.'

Muriel responded, 'Actually, I live with multiple sclerosis and would have been lucky to make it to the door prior to my surgery, let alone now!'

Silence hung between them.

PART 5

For a number of years Muriel has been on the committee of a local community action group. Six months previously, the committee were notified that their meeting room, which had been made available at no cost, was to be demolished. Finding a new no-cost or low-cost venue proved difficult. Eventually one was found, but access was via two flights of stairs. With Muriel's increasing level of physical impairment, access was prohibitive to her attending meetings. Still keen to be actively involved on the committee, she put her name forward for the position of treasurer. The position had been notoriously hard to fill and Muriel knew that she had the skills and could do the work from home, thanks to computer and internet technology. Being treasurer, she reasoned, meant she could continue her contribution to the group without attending the meetings in person. She withdrew her nomination, however, when it became clear that this was not acceptable to all members of the committee.

At the recent annual general meeting no nominations were received for treasurer. On the incoming committee, however, was a nurse who, on hearing of Muriel's earlier self-nomination, challenged the processes that excluded her from the position. The nurse successfully argued that there were options, including the treasurer's work being done electronically and communicated via emails as Muriel had suggested or, in the longer term, applying for funding so the committee could pay for a venue that would be accessible to everyone.

PART 6

Serena received a call at work from Kerry, a woman who cares for her adult-aged son, who lives with severe physical and intellectual impairments resulting from a rare congenital condition. Kerry was seeking advice on what day-service options might be available for her son, Malcolm. He had recently been made redundant following the closure of the facility where he had worked for 5 years in a supported environment. The chances of him finding another job within his capability were limited. Kerry expressed concern that since Malcolm had not been going to work each day, he had lost contact with his friends and colleagues. She struggles to get him out of the house. Kerry said:

Going to work meant so much more to him than the money; it was his life. It gave structure to his day and the opportunity to be with his friends. And even though he couldn't focus on a task for more than a few minutes at a time, when he completed one of his jobs he had a real sense of pride. The money didn't really matter to him. And then, of course, there is the impact on my life. I am just so tired and life is so much more of a juggle than before. I used to be able to have a bit of a break when he was at work and get some things done. Like now I can only go to the supermarket at night when my daughter can come and be with her brother because he can't be left alone. And if I take him, then we have to endure people staring when his behaviour becomes socially unacceptable – which is quite often. Honestly, Malcolm going to work is what got me through the week; sort of recharged my batteries.

PRINCIPLES OF NURSING CARE WHEN WORKING WITH PEOPLE LIVING WITH CHRONIC ILLNESS AND/OR IMPAIRMENT
Working with People in Context

The stories of people who live with chronic illness and/or impairment may have some similarities, but each person's journey is unique (Giddings et al 2007; Guerin et al 2017; Heid et al 2018; Sheridan et al 2019; Vijayasingham 2018). Rather than generalising experiences with the risk of stereotyping, such as 'the difficult arthritic in cubicle three', nurses need to work within the context of the person's everyday life

(Digby et al 2016; Giddings et al 2007; Roy & Giddings 2012; Sheridan et al 2019).

Working with the person in context means getting to know them and their families and how they live with, or are learning to live with, their chronic illness and/or impairment. It means supporting the person to develop their capacity and capability to self-manage. Nursing decisions can then be guided by what the person needs and perceives as working uniquely for them (Francis et al 2019; Heid et al 2018; Roy & Giddings 2012; Sheridan et al 2019). The nurse needs to be ready to step in and help by offering suggestions, strategies and support, and at times taking over care. They also need to be ready to step back when not required (Giddings et al 2007).

Historically, nursing practice has been underpinned by a biomedical approach to care with a focus on the individual, pathophysiology and cure. This model, although successful in treating acute diseases and acute events within chronic illnesses, is limited for general use in the overall management of chronic illness and/or impairments (Conroy et al 2017; Francis et al 2019; Hogan 2019). As well as having a sound knowledge of pathophysiology and protocols of care informed by contemporary chronic care approaches, nurses need to be self-reflexive so they are constantly alert to when they are 'taking over', labelling or using generalised norms and beliefs about how someone should behave or act.

Nursing care based on a social model of disability and chronic care approaches can complement the biomedical model in such a way that the expertise and resourcefulness of people living with chronic illness and/or impairment are more easily recognised and valued. This involves nurses working consciously in partnership with their clients and supporting self-management, rather than always taking control and prescribing strategies (Franklin et al 2019; Giddings et al 2007; Sheridan et al 2019; Wilkinson et al 2016). Nurses need to recognise that 'Each day, [people] decide what they are going to eat, whether they will exercise and to what extent they will consume prescribed medicines' (Bodenheimer et al 2002, p. 2470). The question is not whether people self-manage their chronic illness and/or impairment, but how? The focus should be on supporting a person's right to self-determination in self-management decisions (Francis et al 2019; Peters & Cotton 2015; Roy et al 2011). This serves to empower them to act rather than accept the status quo of health disparities and discrimination. This was evident when Serena challenged the charge for the home visit that enabled her to have a cervical smear (Case Study 6.1, part 3). Although

maybe unintentional, this form of institutional discrimination, embedded in policy, could have created a barrier to Serena accessing appropriate health services.

If nurses use self-reflexive questioning while working with a client, they will remain alert to when they are making stereotypical assumptions that could stand in the way of their giving contextualised care. It is also more likely that they will be able to see and name such assumptions when played out in society. Take, for example, the barista who assumed that because Serena used a wheelchair, that she had hearing and cognitive impairments (Case Study 6.1, part 1). Each time such incidences are named and challenged within the healthcare system and society generally, the world becomes a safer place for those who are different in some way from the mainstream.

Working effectively with the person in context involves developing therapeutic relationships to enable communication processes and comprehensive assessments that are appropriate to the person's situation. Most people living with chronic illness and/or impairment receive healthcare within their community. Hospitalisation only occurs if they are receiving treatment for an acute exacerbation or a co-morbid condition. Knowledge of a person's situation and of the possibility of co-morbidity is essential for comprehensive assessment and delivery of effective care of the person in context, whether in the community or in hospital (Green et al 2013; Heid et al 2018; O'Brien et al 2011; Roy & Giddings 2012). Co-morbidity adds further complexity to the lives of people living with chronic illness and/or impairment and has been shown to increase the risk of stigmatisation (Francis et al 2019). The nurse caring for Muriel following her hysterectomy, for example, did not contextualise his care (Case Study 6.1, part 4). By insisting Muriel walk to the end of the ward and back, he based his care on expected norms, perhaps the prescribed clinical pathway, and was not mindful of her diagnosis of multiple sclerosis. In a 2017 review of 22 studies of the experiences of patients with co-morbidity (van der Aa et al 2017), the key overarching theme across the studies was the experience of a lack of holistic care. This was compounded by a range of system- and professional-related issues with healthcare delivery that showed little regard paid to a person's co-morbidities. In Muriel's case, good assessment skills and an understanding of her unique context would have enabled the nurse to recognise her co-morbidities. Muriel could have then been encouraged to mobilise in a way that prevented postoperative complications and promoted recovery but that was within her ability. Instead, the care that was offered marginalised Muriel, labelling her 'non-compliant' and not wanting to 'help herself' in her recovery.

Nurses need to adapt to the ever-changing client context. Client care cannot be prescribed by strict clinical protocols that ignore the ever-changing nature of a person's experience. Nurses need to be flexible and open to being guided by the self-knowledge of their clients while being vigilant to signs of tension or change. Many chronic illnesses, such as multiple sclerosis and rheumatoid arthritis, are characterised by periods of remission and periods of exacerbation of disease activity, when there may be a need for hands-on nursing care. Age and life stage, along with the ebb and flow of relationships and family life, also impact on the experience (Avieli et al 2019; Heid et al 2018; Roy & Giddings 2012). The impact on Kerry's life, for example, when Malcolm was made redundant (Case Study 6.1, part 6) demonstrates the complexity and ripple effects within the family that is living with chronic illness, and/or impairment that goes beyond the pathophysiological.

There may not always be the need for direct nursing care when working with people living with chronic illness and/or impairment, but nurses must remain aware of and work with the ever-changing client context. They need to continually challenge stigmatising processes that get in the way of contextualising care.

Recognise and Value Expertise and Resourcefulness

Nurses need to recognise and work with the expertise/developing expertise of their clients. This is essential for effective care (Francis et al 2019; Giddings et al 2007; Reeve & Cooper 2016; Roy & Giddings 2012). Over time, people and their families who live with the daily reality of chronic illness and/or impairment develop self-knowing as well as effective strategies for self-management and care. These strategies are not only informed through the person–health professional relationship, but also through social and media sources, such as family, friends, magazines and the internet. Nigel demonstrated expertise when he recognised the beginning of a hypoglycaemic episode (Case Study 6.1, part 2). He based this on his self-knowledge developed through having experienced similar episodes over the past 14 years. Had the nurse recognised and valued his expertise and self-knowing, the subsequent emergency situation may have been avoided.

Recognising and valuing the unique expertise of the person is empowering to both parties in the person–health professional relationship. There is a fine balance between stepping in and holding back in offering care that requires nurses to know their clients in context. This balance can only be achieved by establishing processes of negotiation, with two-way communication within an ongoing therapeutic relationship that is mutually respectful of each other's expertise (Koch et al 2004; Sheridan et al 2019). Such a relationship, which enhances the person's highly tuned knowledge of themselves, can make the difference between effective and ineffective care and self-management (Franklin et al 2019; Giddings et al 2007; Roy & Giddings 2012; Roy et al 2011). At a societal level, it is essential that people living with chronic illness and/or impairment are included in decision-making processes and that their expertise is valued, listened to and acted upon when plans are made for provision of services, design of buildings and so forth (Hertel et al 2019; Jackson 2018). Nurses, too, need to take responsibility, not only in advocating for this client group, but also in becoming politically active. The nurse (Case Study 6.1, part 3) advocated for Serena when she took the issue of the charge for the home visit to the practice management team meeting. She demonstrated political action when she broadened the issue to one of equity for all people living with an impairment.

Support Rights to Self-Determination

Nurses play an important role in providing education and care that is not only appropriate and timely, but also presented in a way that respects a person's right to self-determination. For example, nurses, along with other health professionals, are often required to prescribe and reinforce what a person should or should not do in living with a chronic illness and/or impairment, such as giving guidance about appropriate dietary modifications to people with diabetes. The techniques and strategies suggested may at times, however, be at odds with the person's everyday reality. There are always tensions between what people 'should do', 'can do' or 'choose to do' (Francis et al 2019; Roy 2001; Roy et al 2011). Rather than setting rigid protocols, nurses need to respect their client's self-determination by acknowledging and working with such tensions. They can talk with the person about how they might realistically and individually incorporate dietary modification (for example) into their everyday lives, establishing a pathway for success, not failure. Such strategies would incorporate 'what matters most' and enable them to live positively with the inevitable tensions. For example, when Serena and Nigel were at the café (Case Study 6.1, part 1), Nigel chose to have a piece of cake, in spite of the dictatorial voice of the practice nurse ringing in his ears. On this occasion 'what mattered most' was Serena and Nigel's celebration, not his dietary adherence. Nigel knew this was a special occasion and that the consequence would be close monitoring of his blood glucose levels and possible increase of his next insulin dose. He also probably knew it was not something he would do every day if he wished to avoid long-term complications.

Be Aware of the Potential for Social Isolation

Nurses need to remain vigilant in relation to their clients' overall wellbeing. Numerous studies have shown that people living with chronic illness and/or impairment experience depression, loneliness and social isolation (e.g. see Brunes et al 2019; Schafer 2018; Warner et al 2019; Waterworth et al 2015). They are less likely to socialise with friends outside the home or to be involved in religious, recreational or any other groups or activities (Neille & Penn 2015; Wilson et al 2017). Brunes and colleagues (2019) found in their study of 736 adults with low vision that loneliness was associated with younger age, blindness, having other impairments, unemployment, and a history of bullying or abuse. They also experienced higher levels of social isolation and lower levels of life satisfaction than the general population.

Social isolation and loneliness in many instances results from the disabling effects of discrimination and marginalisation that limit opportunities for such things as travel, socialising and employment. These situations continue to exist despite the ratification of the United Nations Convention on the Rights of Persons with Disabilities (2006) in New Zealand and Australia in 2008 and legislation, such as the Australian *Disability Discrimination Act 1992* and the New Zealand *Human Rights Act 1993*, aimed at 'abolishing discrimination against people living with disabilities and to encourage equal opportunities for people in all areas' (Varnham 2004, p. 48). With the loss of employment, Malcolm experienced increased social isolation and loneliness (Case Study 6.1, part 6). When he was made redundant, he lost not only his salary but also the structure to his day, contact with his friends and doing work that reinforced his sense of self-worth.

Societal attitudes that do not value contributions made in different ways by people who are differently abled can contribute to the social isolation. Similarly, many people living with chronic illness and/or impairment are unable to find paid employment, often due to the inflexibility of workplace practices and the attitudes of employers (McDonnall & Crudden 2018; Murfitt et al 2018). Labour force statistics show significantly lower employment rates for people living with chronic illness and/or impairment than the general population (Australian Bureau of Statistics 2019; Shandra 2018; Statistics New Zealand 2019). This is significant given that unemployment has been shown to have a strong association with ill-health and depression (Dixit 2019; Robertson et al 2019).

Nurses need to work with individuals and families in strategising ways to offset the possibility of social isolation. They also need to be aware of the increased potential for depression in people who live with chronic illness and/or impairment. Referral to other providers may be necessary for the individual and other family members. Being mindful of possible barriers to inclusion, challenging these and seeking new or different ways of doing things are actions nurses can take within their work situations or within the broader community. The nurse elected to the community action group committee (Case Study 6.1, part 5) demonstrated such action in suggesting short- and long-term solutions to overcome the barriers that were excluding Muriel from participation on the committee, concomitantly reducing the risk of social isolation.

CONCLUSION

Nurses who work with people living with chronic illness and/or impairment can act to maintain the status quo of marginalisation and discrimination (do nothing) or challenge it (do something). Nurses who use the social model of disability and incorporate self-reflexive practice in their approach to care can challenge their own positions of privilege and take actions that uncover the often hidden processes of stigmatisation of their clients. They need to continually challenge stigmatising processes within the clinical setting, their communities, in the media and within their own social milieu. Actions can be at:

- a personal level: being alert to stigmatising processes such as stereotyping, labelling and othering
- a professional level: working with people in context; recognising and valuing their expertise and resourcefulness; supporting their rights to self-determination and remaining mindful of the risks of social isolation
- a socio-political level: making visible and challenging stigmatising practices that marginalise and discriminate against people with chronic illnesses and/or impairments.

Reflective Questions

1. How can self-reflexive questioning assist you in reviewing your positions of power and privilege in relation to people living with chronic illness and/or impairment?

2. How can you become more aware of actions that unintentionally marginalise and discriminate against people in your work and social contexts?

3. How can you challenge everyday situations in nursing practice where people who live with chronic illness and/or impairment are marginalised and discriminated against?

RECOMMENDED READING

Oliver M 2013. The social model of disability: thirty years on. Disability and Society 28(7), 1024–1026.

Shandra CL 2018. Disability as inequality: social disparities, health disparities, and participation in daily activities. Social Forces 97(1), 157–192.

Wilson NJ, Jaques H, Johnson A et al 2017. From social exclusion to supported inclusion: adults with intellectual disability discuss their lived experiences of a structured social group. Journal of Applied Research in Intellectual Disabilities 30(5), 847–858.

REFERENCES

Ardern J, Genter JA 2020. Government restores fairness for family carers. New Zealand Government, Wellington.

Australian Bureau of Statistics (ABS) 2019. Disability, ageing and carers, Australia: summary of findings, 2018. Online. Available: www.abs.gov.au/ausstats/abs@.nsf/0/C258C88A7AA5A87ECA2568A9001393E8?Opendocument.

Avery S 2018. Indigenous peolple with disability have a double disadvantage and the NDIS can't handle that. Online. Available: https://theconversation.com/indigenous-people-with-disability-have-a-double-disadvantage-and-the-ndis-cant-handle-that-102648.

Avieli H, Band-Winterstein T, Araten Bergman T 2019. Sibling relationships over the life course: growing up with a disability. Qualitative Health Research 29(12), 1739–1750.

Bodenheimer T, Lorig K, Holman H et al 2002. Patient self-management of chronic disease in primary care. JAMA: The Journal of the American Medical Association 288(19), 2469–2475.

Bruce A, Beuthin R, Sheilds L et al 2019. Holding secrets while living with life-threatening illness: normalizing patients' decisions to reveal or conceal. Qualitative Health Research 0(0), 1–19.

Brunes AB, Hansen M, Heir T 2019. Loneliness among adults with visual impairment: prevalence, associated factors, and relationship to life satisfaction. Health & Quality of Life Outcomes 17(1), 1–7.

Conroy T, Feo R, Alderman J et al 2017. Building nursing practice: the fundamentals of care framework. In: J Crisp, C Douglas, G Rebeiro et al (eds), Potter & Perry's fundamentals of nursing: Australian Version, 5th edn. Elsevier Australia, Chatswood, NSW.

Curtis E, Jones R, Tipene-Leach D et al 2019. Why cultural safety rather than cultural competency is required to achieve health equity: a literature review and recommended definition. International Journal for Equity in Health 18(1), 174.

Department of Social Services 2011. National Disability Strategy 2010–2020. Commonwealth of Australia. Online. Available: www.dss.gov.au/our-responsibilities/disability-and-carers/publications-articles/policy-research/national-disability-strategy-2010-2020.

Digby R, Lee S, Williams A 2016. The experience of people with dementia and nurses in hospital: an integrative review. Journal of Clinical Nursing 29(9–10), 1152–1171.

Disability Discrimination Act 1992. Statutes of Australia. Online. Available: www.legislation.gov.au/Details/C2016C00763

Dixit S 2019. Employment status depression and desire for social freedom. International Journal of Social Sciences Review 7(4), 772–774.

Francis H, Carryer J, Wilkinson J 2019. Patient expertise: contested territory in the realm of long-term condition care. Chronic Illness 15(3), 197–209.

Franklin M, Lewis S, Willis K et al 2019. Controlled, constrained, or flexible? How self-management goals are shaped by patient–provider interactions. Qualitative Health Research 29(4), 557–567.

Giddings LS 2005a. Health disparities, social injustice, and the culture of nursing. Nursing Research 54(5), 304–312.

Giddings LS 2005b. A theoretical model of social consciousness. Advances in Nursing Science 28(3), 224–239.

Giddings LS 1997. In/visibility in nursing: stories from the margins. Doctoral thesis, University of Colorado, Denver.

Giddings LS, Roy DE, Predeger E 2007. Women's experience of ageing with a chronic condition. Journal of Advanced Nursing 58(6), 557–565.

Goering S 2015. Rethinking disability: the social model of disability and chronic disease. Current Reviews in Musculoskeletal Medicine 8(2), 134–138.

Gordon T, Dew A, Dowse L 2019. Listen, learn, build, deliver? Aboriginal and Torres Strait Islander policy in the National Disability Insurance Scheme. Australian Journal of Social Issues 54(3), 224–244.

Green J, Jester R, McKinley R et al 2013. Nurse–patient consultations in primary care: do patients disclose their concerns? Journal of Wound Care 22(10), 534–539.

Guerin BM, Payne DA, Roy DE et al 2017. 'It's just so bloody hard': recommendations for improving health interventions and maternity support services for disabled women. Disability and Rehabilitation 39(23), 2395–2403.

Heid AR, Gerber AR, Kim DS et al 2018. Timing of onset and self-management of multiple chronic conditions: a qualitative examination taking a lifespan perspective. Chronic Illness 0(0), 1–17.

Hertel E, Cheadle A, Matthys J et al 2019. Engaging patients in primary care design: an evaluation of a novel approach to codesigning care. Health Expectations 22(4), 609–616.

Hickey H 2015. Nursing and working with disability. In: D Wepa (ed.), Cultural safety in Aotearoa New Zealand, 2nd edn. Cambridge University Press, Melbourne.

Hogan AJ 2019. Social and medical models of disability and mental health: evolution and renewal. CMAJ: Canadian Medical Association Journal 191(1), E16–E18.

Human Rights Act 1993. Statutes of New Zealand. Online. Available: www.legislation.govt.nz/act/public/1993/0082/latest/DLM304212.html.

Human Rights Commission 2016. Payments for providing care for disabled adult family members. HRC, Wellington.

Jackson M 2018. Models of disability and human rights: informing the improvement of built environment accessibility for people with disability at neighborhood scale? Laws 7(1), 10.

Johnson AG 2006. Privilege, power and difference. McGraw-Hill, New York.

Koch T, Jenkin P, Kralik D 2004. Chronic illness self-management: locating the 'self'. Journal of Advanced Nursing 48(5), 484–492.

Levitt JM 2017. Exploring how the social model of disability can be re-invigorated: in response to Mike Oliver. Disability & Society 32(4), 589–594.

Luyckx K, Rassart J, Aujoulat I et al 2016. Self-esteem and illness self-concept in emerging adults with Type 1 diabetes: long-term associations with problem areas in diabetes. Journal of Health Psychology 21(4), 540–549.

Mackean T, Fisher M, Friel S et al 2019. A framework to assess cultural safety in Australian public policy. Health Promotion International. DOI: https://doi.org/10.1093/heapro/daz011

Maeve MK 1998. A critical analysis of physician research into nursing practice. Nursing Outlook 46(1), 24–28.

Malbon E, Carey G, Meltzer A 2019. Personalisation schemes in social care: are they growing social and health inequalities? BMC Public Health 19(1), 805.

Marks B, McCulloh K 2016. Success for students and nurses with disabilities: a call to action for nurse educators. Nurse Educator 41(1), 9–12.

McDonnall MC, Crudden A 2018. Predictors of employer attitudes toward blind employees, revisited. Journal of Vocational Rehabilitation 48(2), 221–231.

Ministry of Health NZ 2020. Funded family care 2020. Online. Available: www.health.govt.nz/funded-family-care-2020.

Ministry of Health NZ 2016. Funded family care. Ministry of Health, Wellington.

Ministry of Health NZ 2001. The New Zealand Disability Strategy: making a world of difference. Whakanui Oranga, Wellington. Online. Available: www.odi.govt.nz/nz-disability-strategy/about-the-strategy/new-zealand-disability-strategy-2001/2001-strategy-read-online/.

Mitra S 2006. The capability approach and disability. Journal of Disability Policy Studies 16(4), 236–247.

Murfitt K, Crosbie J, Zammit J et al 2018. Employer engagement in disability employment: a missing link for small to medium organizations – a review of the literature. Journal of Vocational Rehabilitation 48(3), 417–431.

Neal-Boylan LJ 2019a. Having a disability may make you a better nurse. Workplace Health & Safety 67(11), 567–568.

Neal-Boylan LJ 2019b. The nurse with a profound disability: a case study. Workplace Health & Safety 67(9), 445–451.

Neal-Boylan LJ, Smith D 2016. Nursing students with physical disabilities: dispelling myths and correcting misconceptions. Nurse Educator 41(1), 13–18.

Neille J, Penn C 2015. Beyond physical access: a qualitative analysis into the barriers to policy implementation and service provision experienced by persons with disabilities living in a rural context. Rural and Remote Health 15(3), 1–15.

New Zealand Public Health and Disability Amendment Act (No. 2) 2000/2013. Statutes of New Zealand. Online. Available: www.legislation.govt.nz/act/public/2013/0022/latest/whole.html.

Nursing Council of New Zealand 2011. Guidelines for cultural safety, the Treaty of Waitangi and Māori health in nursing education and practice (rev. ed). Online. Available: www.nursingcouncil.org.nz/Public/Nursing/Standards_and_guidelines/NCNZ/nursing-section/Standards_and_guidelines_for_nurses.aspx?hkey=9fc06ae7-a853-4d10-b5fe-992cd44ba3de.

O'Brien R, Wyke S, Guthrie B et al 2011. An 'endless struggle': a qualitative study of general practitioners' and practice nurses' experiences of managing multimorbidity in socio-economically deprived areas of Scotland. Chronic Illness 7(1), 45–59.

Office for Disability Issues 2016. New Zealand Disability Strategy 2016–2026. Wellington, NZ. Ministry of Social Development. Online. Available: www.odi.govt.nz/nz-disability-strategy/.

Oliver M 2013. The social model of disability: thirty years on. Disability and Society 28(7), 1024–1026.

Oliver M 2009. Understanding disability: from theory to practice, 2nd edn. Palgrave Macmillan, Basingstoke.

Oliver M 1996. Understanding disability: from theory to practice. St Martin's Press, New York.

Oliver M 1983. Social work with disabled people. Macmillan, Basingstoke.

Owens J 2015. Exploring the critiques of the social model of disability: the transformative possibility of Arendt's notion of power. Sociology of Health and Illness 37(3), 385–403.

Papps E 2015. Cultural safety: daring to be different. In: D Wepa (ed.), Cultural safety in Aotearoa New Zealand, 2nd edn. Cambridge University Press, Melbourne.

Perry E, Waters R, Buchanan A. 2019. Experiences of National Disability Insurance Scheme planning from the perspective of adults with intellectual disability. Australian Journal of Social Issues 54(3), 210–223.

Peters K, Cotton A 2015. Barriers to breast cancer screening in Australia: experiences of women with physical disabilities. Journal of Clinical Nursing 24(3–4), 563–572.

Porter S 1996. Men researching women working. Nursing Outlook 44(1), 22–26.

Ramsden IM 2002. Cultural safety and nursing education in Aotearoa and Te Waipounamu. PhD in Nursing, Victoria University of Wellington. Online. Available: https://croakey.org/wp-content/uploads/2017/08/RAMSDEN-I-Cultural-Safety_Full.pdf.

Reeve J, Cooper L 2016. Rethinking how we understand individual healthcare needs for people living with long-term conditions: a qualitative study. Health and Social Care in the Community 24(1), 27–38.

Retief M, Letšosa R 2018. Models of disability: a brief overview. HTS Teologiese Studies/Theological Studies 74(1), 1–8.

Robertson J, Beyer S, Emerson E et al 2019. The association between employment and the health of people with intellectual disabilities: a systematic review. Journal of Applied Research in Intellectual Disabilities 32(6), 1335–1348.

Roy DE 2001. The everyday always-thereness of living with rheumatoid arthritis. PhD thesis, Massey University, Auckland.

Roy DE, Giddings LS 2012. The experiences of women (65–74 years) living with a long-term condition in the shadow of ageing. Journal of Advanced Nursing 68(1), 181–190.

Roy DE, Mahony FM, Horsburgh MP et al 2011. Partnering in primary care in New Zealand: clients' and nurses' experience of the Flinders Program™ in the management of long-term conditions. Journal of Nursing and Healthcare of Chronic Illness 3(2), 140–149.

Schafer MH 2018. (Where) is functional decline isolating? Disordered environments and the onset of disability. Journal of Health & Social Behavior 59(1), 38–55.

Schwandt TA 2007. Reflexivity. In: TA Schwandt (ed.), The SAGE dictionary of qualitative inquiry, 3rd edn. Sage, Thousand Oaks, CA.

Shakespeare T 2008. Debating disability. Journal of Medical Ethics 34(1), 11–14.

Shandra CL 2018. Disability as inequality: social disparities, health disparities, and participation in daily activities. Social Forces 97(1), 157–192.

Sheridan NF, Kenealy TW, Fitzgerald AC et al 2019. How does it feel to be a problem? Patients' experiences of self-management support in New Zealand and Canada. Health Expectations 22(1), 34–45.

Smith LT 1999. Decolonizing methodologies: research and Indigenous peoples. Zed Books/University of Otago Press, London/Dunedin.

Statistics New Zealand 2019. Labour market statistics (disability): June 2019 quarter. Online. Available: www.stats.govt.nz/information-releases/labour-market-statistics-disability-june-2019-quarter.

United Nations 2006. Convention on the rights of persons with disabilities and optional protocol. United Nations, Online. New York. Available: www.un.org/disabilities/documents/convention/convoptprot-e.pdf.

van der Aa MJ, van den Broeke JR, Stronks K et al 2017. Patients with multimorbidity and their experiences with the healthcare process: a scoping review. Journal of Comorbidity 7(1), 11–21.

Varnham S 2004. Current developments in Australia. Education and the Law 16(1), 47–59.

Vijayasingham L 2018. Work right to right work: an automythology of chronic illness and work. Chronic Illness 14(1), 42.

Warner CB, Roberts AR, Jeanblanc AB et al 2019. Coping resources, loneliness, and depressive symptoms of older women with chronic illness. Journal of Applied Gerontology 38(3), 295–322.

Waterworth S, Arroll B, Raphael D et al 2015. A qualitative study of nurses' clinical experience in recognising low mood and depression in older patients with multiple long-term conditions. Journal of Clinical Nursing 24(17/18), 2562–2570.

Wilkinson M, Whitehead L, Crowe M 2016. Nurses, perspectives on long-term condition self-management: a qualitative study. Journal of Clinical Nursing 25(1–2), 240–246.

Wilson NJ, Jaques H, Johnson A et al 2017. From social exclusion to supported inclusion: adults with intellectual disability discuss their lived experiences of a structured social group. Journal of Applied Research in Intellectual Disabilities 30(5), 847–858.

World Health Organization (WHO) 2018. Disability and health. Online. Available: www.who.int/en/news-room/fact-sheets/detail/disability-and-health.

Zlotnick C, Shpigelman CN 2018. A 5-step framework to promote nursing community inclusivity: the example of nurses with disabilities. Journal of Clinical Nursing 27(19–20), 3787–3796.

CHAPTER 7

Sexuality

TINASHE M. DUNE

LEARNING OBJECTIVES

When you have completed this chapter you will be able to:

- comprehend the multifactorial issues of the topic
- relate to the way people may experience changes to their sexuality due to chronic illness and/or disability
- explore the resources available
- articulate clinical scenarios where intervention is necessitated
- comprehend alterations to quality of life for this group of people.

KEY WORDS

chronic illness	sexual health
disability	sexual wellbeing
sexuality	

INTRODUCTION

The purpose of this chapter is to explore how adults may experience changes to their sexuality when living with chronic illness and/or disability. The topic is vast because sex and sexuality are complex areas of human experience across the lifespan. Issues of sexuality for children or adolescents with chronic illness and/or disability are not explored in this chapter. To structure our exploration of the topic, we draw on research data to understand the biological, psychological and social impact on sex and sexuality when people are living with chronic illness and/or disability. We also discuss promotion of sexual health and wellbeing, as well as identify the implications and strategies for nursing practice.

Sexual expression is a part of life, and of course sex is important because it means that the human species can propagate! Satisfaction with sexual relationships is important to quality of life (Deans et al 2015). Even though sex and sexual expression are fundamental parts of life, it may be a taboo topic of conversation for many people. This may be even more so for adults with chronic conditions and/or disability, because sex is

often associated with beauty and physical fitness; therefore, people with a visible disability or illness may be perceived by others to be non-sexual (Dune et al 2015). People with disability or illness, however, are sexual beings and often have to overcome uninformed judgements and attitudes in addition to personal and physiological barriers to sex and sexuality (Andrews & Lund 2016). For example, disability and illness may result in many physical and psychological changes to movement, bodily sensations, abilities to communicate, continence, behaviour, relationships and sexual functioning. These changes may affect sexuality, body image and the feelings that people have about themselves (Nguyen et al 2016). In addition, symptoms such as pain and fatigue, and prescribed treatments and medicines, may also affect sexual desire and sexual function (Nguyen et al 2016). For people with chronic illness and/or disability, sex can be a source of comfort, intimacy and pleasure when illness has changed so many aspects of life (Andrews & Lund 2016). People with chronic illness and disability can experience problems with arousal, lubrication, fear, position, exacerbating pain, low confidence, performance worries and relationship problems and also difficulties when initiating new relationships (Kattari & Turner 2017). Although the physical demands of sexual activity can be high, few chronic illnesses require restriction of sexual activity, but rather may require rethinking, trialling and adapting to changed approaches (Loeser et al 2018). The range of problems and people's preferences for help suggest that multidisciplinary intervention is required (Dune & Mpofu 2017).

Effective nursing care has as its foundation the health worker understanding the whole body, yet the topic of sexual health for people with illness and/or disability may be a neglected element within the scope of holistic nursing care (Lee et al 2015; Rowniak & Selix 2015). Certainly, training in sexual health is limited (Lee et al 2015). Sexuality and sexual functioning are a nursing concern because they are important aspects of a person's sense of wellbeing and quality of life (Lee et al 2015). While health workers may not be able to affect the progression or physiological impact of chronic illness, they may be able to make a difference to people by affirming and validating the issues people experience and providing supportive advice and navigation towards resources (Dune & Mpofu 2017). Health workers may need to work with people to access information or participate in conversations about sexuality with people who are learning to live with an altered body as a consequence of illness or disability (Rowniak & Selix 2015). It is important, however, that health workers who may need to counsel people on this topic are comfortable with talking about sex and sexuality (Uslu et al 2016).

BACKGROUND

The dialogue quoted in this chapter has come from a research program that compiles the findings of multiple inquiries with people learning to live with chronic illness and/or disability. Much of the dialogue has been extracted from a study that aimed to understand how people living with cerebral palsy make sense of their sexuality and sexual lives. A series of interviews between the author and nine people (six men and three women) living with various forms and severity of cerebral palsy took place during a 2-year period (2009–11). They shared their lives and stories through a series of in-depth interviews and rapid ethnography.

The use of a series of in-depth interviews allowed the author to engage with the participants' lived experiences across a period of time and across a range of events within the participants' lives (e.g. the beginning and end of intimate relationships, experiences of dating and navigating their sexual wellbeing needs with

health practitioners). This method of using interviews is corroborated by Dune and Mpofu (2017), who explained that multiple interviews provoke a reflective or analytical perspective from the participant, while preliminary interviews focus on presenting and clarifying experiences. The decision to engage in rapid ethnographic encounters allowed the author to better understand what a day in the life of a person with cerebral palsy was like and the relationship their daily routine may have on their sexual lives. Isaacs (2012) explains that rapid ethnography is a quicker method than those used in traditional anthropology to more swiftly come to understandings. This method to engage with participants' experiences of their daily and sexual lives was dually beneficial as it gave a means to maintain the involvement of the ethnographer as a core element in the process of learning about other people's lives and experiences (Isaacs 2012).

The result of these methodologies revealed multi-layered experiences with a major focus on how people with cerebral palsy perceive sexual health and wellbeing, with experiences with others (interactional) being the most significant factor in their understanding of their sexuality. Public influences (e.g. media representations of chronic illness and disability) was the second most important factor for the participants' understanding of their sexual health and wellbeing. Finally, private factors (e.g. the ways in which participants thought about themselves) were the least influential factor in their experiences and understandings.

This research also supports understanding these interactional, private and public factors in the context of transitions over the life course for people living with chronic illness and disability. Transition encompasses people's responses during a passage of change. Life and living involve transitional processes (Dune 2016). A transitions approach to disruptive life events such as chronic illness creates a focus on what is changing, how we experience those changes and how we can respond. It is not a focus on the illness or disease. Times of transition can be very difficult periods in people's lives. People experience transition when one chapter of their life is over and another begins (e.g. the end or beginning of a relationship or acquired disability and rehabilitation). They look for ways to move through the turmoil to create some order in their lives by reorienting themselves to new situations (Silverberg & Kaufman 2016). Transition may also provide people with the opportunity to review their life, get rid of some old baggage and find new ways of living. Transition can involve testing new ways through trial and error living, doing and being (Dune 2016).

The impact of changed ability on sexuality was therefore a central topic of conversation for participants in their explorations of navigating changes in their lives, relationships and sexuality. It was evident that chronic illness and/or disability can have a profound impact on the individual and partner, and the effects can be multifactorial (Loeser et al 2018).

DEFINING THE TERMS

There have been many definitions of the terms 'sex', 'sexuality', 'sexual health' and 'sexual wellbeing'. Some writers suggest there have been no adequate definitions that can be broadly utilised in healthcare (Dune 2016). Sex has been defined as sexual activity, such as sexual intercourse, and sexuality as a person's self-concept which is shaped by their personality and societal up-bringing (Dune 2016). The term sexuality is a broad concept that has many meanings. In this chapter:

> Sexuality is a fundamental part of human wellbeing and health. It is made up and informed by emotional, physical and sociological factors. It includes nurturing and protecting the sexual and reproductive health of both you and your partner as well as getting the most from your sexual life while also feeling happy and confident about yourself.

As indicated in this definition, a key aspect of (sexual) wellbeing and health is feeling confident and good about oneself, a key concept which the participants in the research highlighted in their experiences and understandings of sexual health, sexuality and sexual wellbeing. In addition to this definition, there are many variations, inclusions, uses and meanings of the term. For example, sexual wellbeing and sexual health are often used interchangeably, especially with regards to the psychosocial aspects of sexual health (e.g. body image, sexual self-esteem, sense of desirability, sexual satisfaction) (Ebrahim 2019). As such, there are many ways to understand constructions of sexual health, sexuality and sexual wellbeing.

Furthermore, some sexuality educators use a model called the circles of sexuality. This model includes five interconnected circles that represent five broad areas of sexuality: sensuality, intimacy, sexual identity, sexual health, and reproduction and sexualisation. In this model, sexuality is represented as much more than sexual arousal, intercourse and orgasm. This way of thinking about sexuality highlights the importance of all the feelings, thoughts and behaviours associated with being a certain gender, being attracted to someone or being in a loving or intimate relationship (Loeser et al 2018). According to this model and the above

definition, sexuality – and its many elements – is a fundamental and natural part of being human for people of all ages. So, while defining sexuality can be difficult, it is nevertheless present throughout the lifespan. Notably, Peta and colleagues (2017) assert that sexuality is the expression of an age-blind desire for meaningful intimacy and connection with others.

As mentioned, a key aspect of sexuality is sexual health. Although the term sexual health is also expansive and complicated, definitions are generally in agreement with one another. For the purposes of this chapter, sexual health, as defined by the World Health Organization (2016), is:

> … a state of physical, emotional, mental and social well-being in relation to sexuality; it is not merely the absence of disease, dysfunction or infirmity. Sexual health requires a positive and respectful approach to sexuality and sexual relationships, as well as the possibility of having pleasurable and safe sexual experiences, free of coercion, discrimination and violence. For sexual health to be attained and maintained, the sexual rights of all persons must be respected, protected and fulfilled.

In order to maintain sexual health, healthcare providers and institutions must play an important role. However, if older people (who represent a majority of people living with chronic illness and disability) are not acknowledged as sexual or having sexuality, programs designed to address the sexual health needs of such people will not be successful – to the detriment of their overall sexual wellbeing (Fileborn et al 2015).

Given that sex, sexuality and sexual health are complementary concepts, how does sexual wellbeing factor in and what does it mean? Similar to the term 'sexual health', sexual wellbeing is the healthy and satisfactory experience of one's sexuality (Dune & Mpofu 2017). The meanings of the terms 'sex' and 'sexuality' are closely linked, and by citing these definitions we do not suggest that it is the same for all people. On the contrary, sex and sexuality experiences, meanings, wellbeing and understandings change throughout the lifespan and as a result of different experiences.

Sexual activity continues across the lifespan yet older people may be perceived as being incapable of a sexual relationship and therefore not requiring support, advice or education in this area (Kattari & Turner 2017). Sexual health needs are often a delicate balance of emotional and physical issues, and those seeking advice may be worried and concerned about misconceptions. For example, upbringing, belief imprinted in the formative years and societal values are deterrents to older people requesting advice, as it is not necessarily the 'done thing', and this negative stereotype is supported in the media, where ageing and sexuality are not positively portrayed (Fileborn et al 2015).

Sexual development and sexual identity evolve throughout the lifespan. However, many factors shape the sexual attitudes and needs of individuals, which may alter at times throughout the lifespan in response to given circumstances (Kattari & Turner 2017). For example, people who have a past history of sexual abuse or assault may interpret sexuality differently (Terrein-Roccatti 2017). When chronic illness or disability becomes a part of people's lives, surgical intervention and medical treatments may result in their appearance being altered and symptoms such as pain, stiffness, fatigue and depression may change the way they feel about their sexual selves, especially in relation to their experiences of sexuality (Dune & Mpofu 2017). In order to better understand these impacts, the researcher asked people living with chronic illness and disability what sexuality meant to them. Trevor, who has severe spastic quadriplegic cerebral palsy, thoroughly explained how his perception of sexual experiences with others has influenced his perspectives on sexuality.

Trevor: There are three key sexual transitions in my life. The first was entering into my first romantic relationship as a teenager. Getting to actually go on dates, and to call someone my girlfriend, was a very liberating experience at the time. The second was my first physical sexual experience and the loss of my virginity. This was key, because I'd been waiting for it for so long, and when it happened, a large part of me regretted it. It was not, looking back, an enjoyable experience. The final transition occurred very recently, when I finally had a physical sexual experience that was purely enjoyable. I had become sexually aroused prior to this, but never fully enjoyed the act.

The best sexual experience I ever had was with my current girlfriend, and only occurred a month or so ago. It was the best because she took the time to physically explore my body, and not simply accept that what is supposed to feel good, should feel good. The experience was accompanied by a very open and honest dialogue between the two of us, and allowed me to grow in sexual confidence. I was able to fully embrace the limitations, but more importantly the abilities, of my body and use them to full effect. It was also the first time that I was able to let go of my need to pleasure my partner, and allow myself to be pleasured without feeling obligated to reciprocate immediately.

Ultimately, sexuality, to me, is all about sexual exploration. It is all about a physical dialogue between the partners, where we find out what works for each other and for us as a couple. It is about not accepting that something feels good, because that is the way that it is typically done, but about creating your own version of typical. My desire

to push the boundaries of my disability, and finding a partner who is willing to go on that journey with me is the hallmark of a positive and good sexual experience. The biggest detriment to sex for me is when we are just 'going through the motions'. Good sex is about pure and unrestricted physical expression.

Trevor highlights that each of the major sexual transitions in his life (all interactional) allowed personal and sexual growth: 'The first was entering into my first romantic relationship as a teenager … The second was my first physical sexual experience and the loss of my virginity … The final transition occurred very recently, when I finally had a physical sexual experience that was purely enjoyable.' Trevor's illustration of the best sexual encounter he had experienced included the several factors discussed earlier in the chapter. For example, good sexual experiences included several factors: 1) peer acceptance of impairment and atypical sexual experiences: 'My desire to push the boundaries of my disability, and finding a partner who is willing to go on that journey with me is the hallmark of a positive and good sexual experience'; 2) the reconstruction of sexual expectations: 'It is about not accepting that something feels good, because that is the way that it is typically done, but about creating your own version of typical'; 3) exploring one's sexuality: 'Ultimately, good sex, to me, is all about sexual exploration'; 4) accepting oneself: 'I was able to fully embrace the limitations, but more importantly the abilities, of my body and use them to full effect'; 5) feeling worthy of sexual experiences with others: 'It was also the first time that I was able to let go of my need to pleasure my partner, and allow myself to be pleasured without feeling obligated to reciprocate immediately'; 6) communication and validation: 'The experience was accompanied by a very open and honest dialogue between the two of us, and allowed me to grow in sexual confidence'; 7) feeling sexually liberated: 'Good sex is about pure and unrestricted physical expression'. Trevor's description of his sexuality emphasises the salience of positive interactional experiences with others in order to circumvent detrimental public sexual expectations and consolidate positive internal dialogue.

THE IMPACT OF CHRONIC ILLNESS AND/ OR DISABILITY ON SEXUALITY AND SEXUAL HEALTH

The effects of chronic illness and/or disability on sexuality and sexual health can be classified as biological, psychological and social (Dune 2016). Biological or physical factors that affect sexuality and sexual health are those associated with the illness, disability or treatments. Examples may be reduced cardiovascular or pulmonary function, fatigue and pain. Surgical procedures and treatments may result in altered function and/or appearance. Psychological factors relate to changed relationships, depression, anxiety and grief associated with loss and change associated with chronic illness and/or disability. Social factors relate to challenges such as stigma and how others perceive people with illness and disability (Ebrahim 2019). While these factors will be discussed separately, they are entwined in the realities of everyday life for people with chronic illness. We will now discuss these factors in more detail.

Biological Impact

Sexual dysfunction is caused by different conditions, with even more differences occurring between men and women. The desire and capacity to engage in sexual activity can be affected by illness and disability in multiple ways through neurological, vascular and endocrine systems and, as a consequence, symptoms such as pain and fatigue may be prioritised in people's lives (Silverberg & Kaufman 2016). In addition, the effects of medications and treatments and surgical intervention can also affect an individual's capacity and desire to engage in sexual activity (Silverberg & Kaufman 2016).

There is a lot of importance placed on a sexually functioning body and the popular ideal is for people to be thin, fit and healthy (Kattari & Turner 2017). The reality, however, is that people have an assortment of body shapes, and illness and/or disability can further reshape the human body, which can significantly affect a person's sexuality, as Leah explains:

> I often wonder what it would be like to be a guy with CP (cerebral palsy), because as a girl who is meant to be dainty and delicate and, you know, somewhat helpless for men, there's some ability for people to reconcile that with your physical weakness because you're a girl anyway. Whereas I wonder what it's like for guys when they're physically weak and how that affects their concept of their masculinity and their sexual confidence and what a relevant issue it is.

The biological or physical impact of illness and disability can cause significant change in a person's life, as Alex and Trevor revealed:

> Alex: My level of mobility also influences my sexuality because I can't perform all of the same functions as an able-bodied person, so I often feel inadequate. I think the fact that I have had mostly one-night stands also influences how I experience sexuality, because I feel like I won't find anything long term due to my disability.

> Trevor: As I grew older, sexual thoughts developed from 'playing house' into [being] more sexual, or sexually charged, in nature. But, due to my physical limitations, I was not able to fully explore those feelings as early as some people might.

When illness or treatments made visible changes it was evident that those changes dominated the illness experience. People perceive that a beautiful, sexual body is a body without illness. John explained:

> I mean the issue really is if you really claim that you really love someone and that you want to spend your life with them under what terms is that mediated. I mean … the standard marriage vows go 'in sickness and in health' and that's fine. But it doesn't go 'in sickness and in constant disease and in constant doctor's appointments and in constant co-morbidities'.

Leah described how her changed body altered the meaning of sexual activity because illness forced changes to both sexual activity and sexual satisfaction:

> I mean we still try to do the normal stuff. But if my leg goes spastic I just go 'hip, hip' whichever one it is. 'Move it, move it, move it, no I can't go there!' It's not always painful; sometimes it is, but sometimes that helps, so you just stay with the pain because you get a pay-out. There are a few positions we tried because they're meant to be easy on your hips but you don't get a lot from them.

As with other life activities, the person who is learning to live with chronic illness and/or disability may have to make adaptations in their life. For example, sexual activity may be less spontaneous and require planning in order to prepare for issues such as fatigue, pain, breathlessness, and bowel and bladder evacuation, as the nerves servicing the reproductive organs can be impaired, leading to changes in sexual functioning (Liddiard & Slater 2018). Slowed arousal time, reduced libido or desire and altered orgasmic response are not uncommon experiences. Fatigue also dampens sexual desire (Ekström et al 2018). Men with illness or disability may experience erectile dysfunction (a common problem that can have serious physical and psychological effects – also known as impotence) or difficulty due to physiological factors or medication that may respond to further investigations (Smith et al 2015). Some people with illness and disability may need to learn to incorporate prosthesis or another permanent intervention, such as an indwelling urinary catheter into their lives and sexual activity (Logan 2020). Adaptations to be made may include trying different positions during sex activity, expanding their sexual repertoire or a partner playing a more active role (Kattari & Turner 2017). Masturbation may enable experimentation with changing bodily sensations

(Loeser et al 2018). It can be important for people with an illness or disability that impairs the neurological system to identify areas of the body that allow sensation and to use those areas to augment sexual expression (Silverberg & Kaufman 2016). Other forms of sexual expression may also be used. This may call for experimentation and alternative methods of pleasuring. Assistive devices may be useful for some people (Silverberg & Kaufman 2016) – these can be purchased discreetly via the internet.

Psychological Impact

Media images portray traditional images of stereotypical male and female roles and what may define the gender role. For example, men are often represented as aggressive, physically strong, being in powerful positions. Alternatively, women are represented as sexualised, fashion-conscious and nurturers. Further, sexuality is attributed to youth and a pastime for those who are physically attractive and socially desirable. For many people these messages are internalised and create pressure to act in the same ways as those represented in the media – standards which are impossible for the average person to meet. These images, therefore, reflect a very commercialised and narrow representation of humanity and ignore not only human diversity but also sexual diversity, possibly leaving many people feeling inadequate and abnormal (Dune 2016). Alex, a gay man, described how public depictions of romance reinforced his sense of being different:

> I guess my idea [of romance] comes from media depictions and what I see played out at bars, but I have no real life experience to draw from. I honestly feel that romance is only in the movies and that because I am 'different', I will not find it conventionally or long term.

Leah felt that exclusionary messages about sexuality implied that she was socially and/or sexually inadequate.

> And then when you've got someone who … the messages they are getting is that you're not sexually attractive, you're not going to get anyone to do that [have sex with you]. You're not going to have someone who is going to love you outside of your family. Because I think that's what a lot of people get because then it's going to affect your social development.

Chronic illness and disability impact on the dynamics of relationships (Wilson et al 2019). Trevor reflected on both the impact of disability on his sexuality and the relationship dynamics required to accommodate for these changes.

> My care needs do influence my sexuality. I think this is a result of how much physical assistance I require. It tends to make my sexual partners very apprehensive and unsure of

> how to handle the situation. I need help with all of my daily functioning, and it is not often that I found someone who is truly comfortable with my level of disability. So, yes, my disability does influence my sexuality.

Changes to sexuality for some people because of illness and disability may mean managing their partner's sexual needs at a time when illness results in restrictions (Wilson et al 2019). Alex's experiences with relationships led to his view of an ideal partner for someone living with an illness or a disability.

> My ideal partner would be extremely open-minded. It would be helpful if they have had some experience with the disabled community, but I realise how rare that is. I tend to think that I would date someone older, only because they have more life experience. My lack of physical ability means that I am relying on my partner to accept that they need to facilitate much of the movement.

Pre-existing relationship issues may be exacerbated by the challenges of illness. For some people their lover may become their carer. Some people may prioritise aspects of illness or disability or for other reasons may not feel like being sexually active and may avoid being sexual with their partner. Research also indicates that changes in sexual desires may negatively affect relationships (Friedman 2019). Loss of sexual desires and the inability to meet their partner's sexual needs can therefore create friction within the relationship and become a barrier to effective communication about changing sexual needs and desires (Friedman 2019). Participants' narratives were imbued with limitations to self-esteem as a result of living with a disability in the context of a society which did not seem to accept atypical functioning or physical forms. Alex explains:

> Most of the time I don't feel desirable in this manner. This may also be a result of social ostracism due to my disability – and the projection of attitudes surrounding disability back on to me.

Within many relationships where a partner experiences illness or disability, the creation of a common dialogue around sexuality is integral. Participants noted that this was sometimes difficult and may reflect the broader societal attitudes to sexuality, which foster discomfort in talking about the topic. This can be very difficult if dialogue between partners around sex and sexuality has not previously existed – such as in new relationships. Ian indicated what might be included in such communications:

> I also try to prepare my partners for how a sexual encounter with me would be different than with an able-bodied individual … It just means that a partner has to communicate and reconstruct what sex can be when they are with me.

Communication is not only integral to intimate relationships in the context of chronic illness and disability, but is an important component in all relationships (Dune & Mpofu 2017). When a disability or illness exists, it becomes important that partners and individuals are given the opportunity to discuss thoughts, feelings, needs, wants and how they can mutually satisfy each other. How do people begin to talk about sex and sexuality if they have not done so before? Health workers may assist by initiating discussion in a matter-of-fact but sensitive way, and letting people know that sexuality is considered to be an important aspect of their health (Linton & Rueda 2015).

Social Impact

Sometimes our ideals and values about sexuality and disabilities have to do with unwritten rules (Dune 2016). In our society, we judge harshly those who break rules about sexuality and sexual behaviour (Dune & Mpofu 2017). Unfortunately, most of the rules are not formally taught, but are learned incidentally and vary according to the age, situation and culture. Take culture, for example. While a general definition of sexuality was presented earlier in the chapter, both sexuality and disability are constructed and therefore understood in varying ways in various cultures (Dune et al 2015). Further, cultures are consistently evolving and intermingling, meaning that constructions of sexuality and disability have changed and do change over time and across cultures. As such, cultural competency, in addition to the acknowledgement of sexuality, is integral to understanding and supporting healthy sexuality for people living with chronic illness and/or disability from various cultural, ethnic, religious or language groups (Mpofu et al 2018).

As such, people living with chronic illness or disability may need to incorporate many changes into their lives and identities (Dune 2016). In line with social and cultural factors, some changes may include traditional gender roles that were previously valued and are a defining factor for a person's identity (Simon & Gagnon 1986, 1987, 2003, 2011). Illness or disability may affect a person's ability to continue to perform those roles in a way that they value (Dune 2016). Certain types of movement, playing a sport, wearing certain clothing or participating in paid work may no longer be possible. Further, fatigue or pain can affect energy levels and limit activities. These effects can lead people to feel that they are not leading a valued life. Chronic illness and disability can provide an opportunity for individuals to redefine what is important to them, as Trevor revealed in the following story about how he felt before and after a major surgery:

I have never really seen my body as sexy, but I've recently begun to explore that side of my sexuality more. I am not there yet, but I'm definitely starting to change my view.

Gender (being a man, woman or gender diverse) is closely linked to roles and not being able to fulfil certain familiar roles can feel threatening. Reliance on a traditionally more dominant partner may be intimidating and frightening, causing tension, anxiety and distress. Brian considered how disability affects perceptions of masculinity and gendered roles, especially with respect to initiating relationships.

Males are competitive, so I mean if I'm after one female and there are three other able-bodied males, where is she going to go? I was talking to this girl and there were other guys who walked in and they didn't say 'hello' or anything, but they could stand and face her. I was in the room, but I might as well not have been there.

The judgement of others can have a significant impact on how people perceive themselves and people with chronic illness and/or disability often need to develop ways to protect themselves from those judgements, as Leah explained.

I think it's a social thing. Because if you went around saying to everyone 'of course I'm sexy, why wouldn't I be?' I think some of it is that you would get some negative feedback, so if part of me thinks I'm sexy, it's the part of me I'm going to keep to myself because you don't let people see everything that feeds your soul.

Sometimes, in the face of negative reactions, people with chronic illness and/or disability learn ways to protect themselves. Evident in their responses is that they developed certain principles to maintain self-worth. Mary indicated:

Well that's actually advice that my German friend gave me. 'You need to walk around naked more.' So, okay, I started to do that and I felt, 'this feels strange,' but you know, if you don't actually look at your body enough, you're going to be more uncomfortable with it or showing it to anybody else.

People with illness and/or disability may become socially withdrawn if they think they are judged by others. People who are gay or lesbian and living with disability and/or chronic illness may be reluctant to disclose and discuss issues regarding their sexuality. For example, Alex describes the contention in managing multiple identities and their impact on others' perceptions.

> *Obviously my coming out of the closet was a very important transition in my life. However, I also think that I had to come out twice: as gay and disabled. That happened when I starting meeting sexual partners. It was at that point that I truly understood the impact of my disability.*

Research has reported that lesbian women and gay men are reluctant to seek care when they have health concerns because of past negative experiences with the health sector (Mpofu et al 2018). It can also be difficult for people whose illness or disability is not visible or whose condition may be treated with suspicion or has social stigma attached to it, such as people living with chronic pain or HIV (Silverberg & Kaufman 2016).

IMPLICATIONS FOR HEALTH PRACTICE

If sex and sexuality are often taboo subjects, why should health workers raise this issue with people? The assumption that people with chronic illness or disability are non-sexual can present a barrier to people gaining information and having open discussion about a major aspect of their life (Dune 2017). Health workers have a significant role to play in addressing barriers to sexual fulfilment that are a result of disability, chronic illness and treatments.

For example, the constant contact that health workers have with clients provides them with the opportunity to facilitate communications about sexuality and to ensure that sexuality is accorded the same priority as other health issues (Mpofu et al 2018). In doing so, a foundation of acceptance and respect for the whole person is established, which provides people with permission to ask questions or seek assistance with sex and sexuality issues (Peta et al 2017). However, McCabe and Holmes (2014) found that when interviewed on this topic nurses cited competing priorities as principal reasons why they did not discuss sexual health issues with their clients. A nurse from their study explained (p. 82):

> *Quite honestly, it [sexual health] is not something that I think of upfront, because we are dealing with such bigger issues. Are they going to get a cold this winter? How will they manage their secretions? … those kinds of things are so much more a part of their ongoing life and their priorities.*

The research by McCabe and Holmes (2014) also showed that although nurses were keen to have discussions about sexuality with their clients, institutional or systemic issues restricted such discussions. Jenna shared her perspective:

> *It's not that they only don't have actual physical time to ask those questions. But the whole concept of having a discussion on sexuality usually takes more time and there's a comfort level when you are asking that type of question … I don't think that the system is designed to allow for that.*

The acknowledgment of the sexual aspect of a person by a health worker and the willingness to assist in this area is extremely affirming for people who are coming to terms with the effects of disability and/or chronic illness. Examples of interventions are provided in Case Studies 7.1 and 7.2. Sexuality is a sensitive and

---

CASE STUDY 7.1

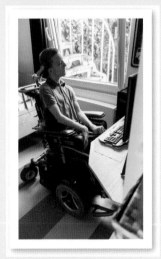

iStockphoto/funky-data.

BACKGROUND

My name is Amin and I am 22 years old. Following a complicated birth in which I was without oxygen for some time, I acquired severe spastic quadriplegic cerebral palsy in the minutes following my birth. This was diagnosed when I was 2 and has meant that I have always needed to live with a carer as I have high-level care needs. As a child and teenager I lived with my mother and stepfather, then in a fully accessible residential building at the university where I completed my undergraduate studies in law. At university I was provided with living support from nurses and nurse trainees within the university's attendant care program for students with disabilities. After university, my mother (who was my primary carer when I lived at home) passed away and I now live in an aged care facility as it is the only place equipped to meet my health and daily needs within my community. I require daily assistance with all activities of daily living, including eating, bathing, getting dressed, getting out of bed and getting into bed. On Facebook I often see that my peers from university are dating, travelling, trialling employment options and even having children. On the other hand, I am the youngest resident in the aged care facility and have little opportunity for interaction with anyone my age or people outside the facility.

I have a good relationship with the nursing staff at the aged care facility and have told them that I am feeling quite negatively about myself, my prospects and how frustrating it is that I cannot be around my peers or have the chance to participate in intimate relationships. At least when I was at university there were opportunities to be supported outside of the residential colleges as it was supported by the university and my fees. Now it is too expensive to have someone assist me outside of the aged care facility.

Without a job I can hardly do anything. Even then I do not feel like I belong anywhere. I sometimes think that there is no use for me except for being a good doorstop – perhaps I and the world would be better off without me.

I thought maybe I should have a chat with my stepfather, who pays for my stay at the aged care facility, about all the issues I am having and how I don't have any friends or opportunities for intimate relationships. He told me that it was up to me to make it happen. He said that living with a severe disability moves a player from the field and onto the bench – I don't like when he uses sporting analogies for someone like me who is in a wheelchair most of the time.

value-laden area, and individuals range in both their attitudes and their comfort levels with regard to sexuality. It is important that health workers develop an awareness of their own values about sex and sexuality

in order to facilitate open communications (Logan 2020). Creating a comfortable environment and using lay sexual terms are effective ways of communicating about sexuality (Kattari & Turner 2017).

BOX 7.1
Amin's Experience

Issues identified by the nurse in collaboration with Amin and his stepfather:

- tight muscles and joints
- difficulty communicating – speech impairment
- diminished sense of self
- diminished sense of purpose
- diminished sense of belonging
- lack of sexual and relationship intimacy.
  Collaborative assessment between the nurse, Amin and his stepfather led to:
- a physical assessment which identified acute muscle and joint tightness, resulting in scoliosis and discomfort
- medication review (GP/local pharmacist) to relieve limb spasticity and encourage mobility
- weekly physiotherapy session to relieve limb spasticity and encourage mobility
- review of the communication/interaction between healthcare providers and Amin and his stepfather
- allowing Amin access to the aged care facility accessible vehicle, which can be scheduled ahead of time if Amin would like to attend events with his peers outside of the facility
- connecting Amin and his stepfather with a disability support liaison officer to seek additional funding for him to engage in regular youth-focused events and

activities away from the aged care facility several times a week
- allowing Amin a more relaxed care provision schedule if he would like to participate in activities with peers or have a guest visit him at the aged care facility.
  Amin was keen to be allowed these privileges, but was warned that he also had to make an effort to connect with his peers online and in person in order to avoid feeling helpless and socially withdrawn.
  Amin's collaborative plan of care:
- Meet with aged care facility counsellor to discuss weekly events, feelings and accomplishments
- Take daily medication to relax the muscles
- Referral to physiotherapy for pool exercises to increase mobility and flexibility
- Referral to occupational therapy to assess for adaptive device modifications or other equipment.
  At the next appointment the plan of care was reviewed:
- Amin felt he had improved his social skills by talking with the counsellor weekly
- muscle tension was reduced
- weekly pool exercises reduced pain and mobility and limb flexibility increased
- Amin used the accessible vehicle once a month to visit friends he had made while at university.

continued

BOX 7.1
Amin's Experience – cont'd

AMIN'S OUTCOMES

I am so glad that I have had the chance to speak with a healthcare provider from the aged care facility, who understands and recognises the issues I have been having and who worked with my family to help me out – things were getting really dire and frustrating. The nurse brought together a whole team of people who I could actually talk to about my feelings and needs, so that everyone understood what I was going through and what I wanted to achieve. I am beginning to feel less annoyed about life and like I am good for nothing or that no one will ever see me as anything but a flawed mass of flesh. I still feel irritated and influenced by what others say and do with regards to my disability, but at least I am getting more of a chance to meet people and have a chance – before this new plan I didn't even have that. It is hard to start conversation or know how to use the best pick-up lines, especially because I am out of practice since leaving university, so I might need some help to build up my confidence and self-esteem a bit more so that I can be less preoccupied with

what others are thinking. It seems things have changed with my stepdad as well. He has started to invite me to his monthly football club outings at the local ex-servicemen's club. Even though I am not really into sports, I am happy to be invited and have the opportunity to connect with my stepdad and other people at the club. It's nice to just be out and doing what other people do with friends. Since I started going to the footie club with my stepdad I also notice that his friends and their families and children are not as distanced as they were before. It's like being out and about has made them less fearful and reduced the stigma of disability in the group. The nurse and counsellor at the aged care facility have also made some contacts for me with The Cerebral Palsy Foundation, who ran some camps when I was a kid. It was great to be reunited with people I hadn't seen for a while and have another opportunity to meet others with and without disabilities to interact with and learn from. These changes have helped me see that perhaps I'm not just good as a doorstop.

CASE STUDY 7.2

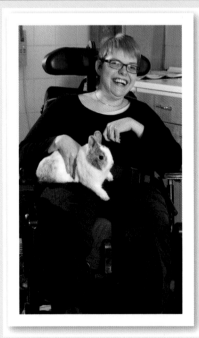

iStockphoto/Horsche.

BACKGROUND

Hi, my name is Sienna and when I was 30 years old I was involved in a motor vehicle accident. I have been told that the car in which I was a passenger was travelling at a speed of 160 km per hour at the time of the accident. Apparently, I was thrown from the car and suffered a partial spinal cord injury (L2–4). I still have partial sensation in my thighs and groin, but I no longer have bladder and bowel control.

At the time of my accident I was engaged to Billy (he was not involved in the accident). After the accident Billy spontaneously ended the relationship – I was devastated. A year later, and after I had started to get a handle on pressing health issues, I started seeing Morgan, who I have been with for the past couple of years. Things have gotten quite serious between us and Morgan is interested in having children. Morgan has asked me if I wanted to try for a baby. I haven't given my answer as I am unsure about whether or not I can conceive, or carry a child to term or parent. No one ever discussed things with me since my injury 3 years ago – I wish someone had.

Now that most of my health needs are stabilising I am hoping to get assistance continence management. Although I have performed clean self-intermittent catheterisation (CSIC) twice–daily, urinary incontinence is still a major concern for me. Although Morgan is really supportive and tells me he doesn't mind my toileting issues,

CASE STUDY 7.2 – cont'd

I sometimes feel that having limited continence is simply not sexy. I was keen to talk to someone about this at the rehabilitation centre, but given my past experience where no one bothered to discuss this with me I doubted that I would get the outcomes I was looking for.

When I went to the first few visits the nurse seemed receptive, but I wasn't sure if this would last and how much I needed to say about my personal and/or sexual life. It's not every day that you have these types of conversations with someone you don't know, so it was a bit weird and confronting for me to say this stuff out loud. The nurse was actually really attentive and gave me time to speak and listened to my concerns. This was reassuring because the nurse did not dismiss my concerns or ideas, but was instead really supportive of my sexual and reproductive needs. I began to trust and build rapport with the nurse and began discussing some of my deeper thoughts and feelings about whether or not I was a 'real' woman, considering that I may have fertility issues and whether I could be a parent. For instance, I was particularly concerned that being in a wheelchair meant that I was not the best partner for Morgan and would not be a good parent to potential children.

I have always wanted children and my own family, but since my injury I feel that such a dream is now out of the question. I assume this to be the case because if I had a chance at these life goals someone would have already discussed this with me. Perhaps the health workers didn't mention it because they didn't want to disappoint me. I have been trying to find resources online but am left very confused by the positive as well as negative anecdotal experiences from parents with spinal cord injury. I long to talk to someone knowledgeable before I decide on what I will tell Morgan.

BOX 7.2
Sienna's Experience

ISSUES IDENTIFIED BY SIENNA AND THE NURSE

Sienna was devastated because:

- her first partner had left her without explanation
- she is unsure of her womanhood
- she is worried that she will be a bad parent
- she does not want to disappoint Morgan.

Collaborative assessment between the nurse, Sienna and Morgan led to:

- the recognition that Sienna's experiences and expectations of womanhood may have changed since the injury, but that this should not mean she is no longer a sexual being with sexual and reproductive desires. The nurse acknowledged that sexuality and sexual wellbeing are important aspects of everyone's life and relationships, and that injury and disability require the support from all health and social support workers to develop strategies for Sienna to express and experience her sexuality.

- the nurse being able to engage Sienna and Morgan in discussions about their sexual and reproductive needs by providing sensitive strategies. This permitted Sienna and Morgan to review and reflect on information and a variety of strategies (e.g. via pamphlets and videos of other families in similar circumstances) in order to facilitate discussions with the health team.

- exploration of Sienna and Morgan's sexual and reproductive concerns through opportunities for both the healthcare team and the clients to learn more about disability and pregnancy and parenthood. The health team has organised monthly online workshops and focus groups led by parents in similar circumstances to discuss and share their stories which Sienna and Morgan are keen to attend.

- addressing issues within the team's expertise and boundaries. The nurse has noted that some of the issues which are important to Sienna and Morgan are best addressed by other health workers, such as an obstetric/gynaecologist and maternal physiotherapist. The addition of these practitioners to the team will help to support all aspects of the pre- and post-maternal experience.

- referral and advocacy. Sienna will need continued follow-up with respect to her psychosexual concerns about womanhood and parenting. The nurse has referred Sienna and Morgan to a sexual therapist who works with women with disabilities and their families to support her in this ongoing journey.

Collaborative plan of care developed with Morgan:

- review oral fluid intake (mainly soft drink or coffee)
- implement routine bowel management – Movicol daily
- continue CSIC
- consent to a medication review
- weekly online discussions with a midwifery trainee, sexual health nurse, obstetric/gynaecologist and maternal physiotherapist who have been trained in supporting pregnancy for women with disability and their partners and who have a range of experience with parents with disability

continued

BOX 7.2
Sienna's Experience – cont'd

- monthly online focus group with other families in similar circumstances
- regular visits with the sexual therapist.

OUTCOMES
Sienna's Viewpoint
After 1 month of my collaborative plan I have become more comfortable with the idea of parenting with a disability. I have decided that I do want to try to have a child with my partner on the condition that Morgan helps me organise a group for parents with disabilities in our local community. The online group hosted by the health workers is great, so it would be wonderful to have parents in our community who we could visit and spend time with too. After having a few meetings with the online health team and learning some strategies to work with my reproductive system and to build strength and comfort where I could, I discovered I was pregnant! I was so glad to tell the online and community group – everyone was so supportive and celebrated this wonderful life event. I was then excited to tell my parents and siblings. I was disappointed and a bit surprised by their concern and trepidation. Instead of showering me with congratulations they started to ask many questions about how I was going to deal with a baby who was incontinent when I continued to have continence issues. Sometimes I am quite worried about how society would welcome this news. Even so, given the help and support I have from the online health team, online focus groups and community group, I try not to worry so much about what others think about my ability to be a pregnant woman with a disability or to be a parent.

During the first trimester of my pregnancy Morgan and I continued running our local parents with disabilities group and invited expert members of the online health team to come and provide accurate information and advice about parenting, relationships, sexuality and health. I also invited my parents and siblings to sit in at the meetings. They were doubtful about the information which would be provided, but became clearer on the benefits and challenges to someone in my situation. Overall, I feel more capable as a partner and parent than when I started this process. Through the support and assistance I have received, my knowledge, skills and perspectives have been validated by a range of people who I consider important in my life. I have realised this through continued sessions with my sexual therapist, who reinforces at every visit that I am valuable, that I am worthy of a partner and a family, and that I can be a great parent.

Nursing Reflections
Some nurses may struggle with being comfortable or knowing what to say and how to address patient concerns. This is often the result of limited opportunities for professional development and education about sexuality and the range of ways people can experience a healthy sexual life. It is therefore important for nurses to be provided, and to engage with, education and training opportunities to improve their ability to support healthy sexuality for patients with chronic illness and disability (Blockmans 2019). Notably, training must include how to address sexual concerns, provide information and treatment interventions, as well as deal with comfort issues and attitudes about sexuality, illness and disability (Dune 2017). However, in order for nurses and other health professionals to be competent in this area of healthcare, organisations need to commit to the provision of sexual education, counselling and support when patients are receiving treatment or care. The timing of this acknowledgement and integration of sexuality into patient care in relation to the onset of the illness or injury can be crucial to future psychosexual wellbeing (Dune 2016). Although several tools, such as the PLISSIT, Kaplan, ALLOW and Sexual Counselling Framework models (discussed further below), have been indicated for the provision of sexual counselling in rehabilitative care, their use by staff may be infrequent due to unfamiliarity with how to approach sexual issues with their clients.

In consideration of an increasingly interprofessional and interdisciplinary approach to the management of chronic illness and disability, educational and interactive processes are necessary to effectively support patient goals. For instance, the Recognition Model (as described by Andrews & Lund 2016) reinforces both the importance and impact of engaging in discussions about sexuality with clients. Within this model, recognition supports sensitive skills of acknowledgement, normalisation, affirmation and validation. These can be used even when a practitioner does not wish, or is unable, to facilitate exploration of sexuality. Further, recognition also helps to facilitate a positive response to the unsought sexual disclosure. Practitioners who dismiss or ignore unsought inquiries are contributing, albeit unwittingly, to the asexualisation of the disabled person. In order for nurses to be better prepared for such conversations and engagement, a review of relevant models is required.

MULTIDISCIPLINARY APPROACHES TO ADDRESSING SEXUAL HEALTH AND WELLBEING NEEDS

Given that there is still a need for the integration of sexuality counselling in the provision of healthcare, much has changed to support clients in their sexual wellbeing journeys. These changes address the differences that people with disability and chronic illness may face regarding their sexuality, but also acknowledge the normalcy of their sexual wellbeing needs. While clients may attempt to engage with healthcare providers on the topic of sexuality, providers need to be both ready and competent in addressing these topics. In doing so, it is important that clients are not left to fumble with subtle hints or questions about sexual concerns or having to resort to making jokes in attempts to manage their sexual concerns, organised sexual counselling sessions and referrals to sexual health professionals. To provide a more competent framework of sexuality support (see Table 7.1), a multidisciplinary approach can

TABLE 7.1
Multidisciplinary Approach to Sexuality Counselling Summary

Approach	Key Features	Issues to Consider
PLISSIT	PLISSIT stands for Permission to discuss sexuality, provision of Limited Information regarding sexuality, Specific Suggestions regarding the person's sexual issues, and Intensive Therapy with an expert when needed	Giving permission may reinforce a doctor/patient hierarchy Limiting information may undermine a client's right to informative/comprehensive sexual health Intensive therapy may pathologise and problematise variations in human sexual experience and expectations
Kaplan model	The Kaplan model focuses on the chief complaint, sexual status, psychiatric status, family and psychosocial history, relationship assessment, summary and the provision of recommendations	Focusing on a chief complaint may pathologise and problematise variations in human sexual experience and expectations Referral systems which do not include continuity of care may send clients on an expensive, time-consuming and redundant healthcare journey
ALLOW	ALLOW stands for Ask the patient about sexual activity and function, Legitimise the patient's concerns by acknowledging them as relevant within their rehabilitative program, addressing Limitations presented by lack of knowledge and comfort, Open discussions about sexual issues for assessment and the provision of referrals to a specialist, and Work collectively in or to develop a treatment plan	The term and ideology of a treatment plan may pathologise and problematise variations in human sexual experience and expectations
Sexual Counselling Framework	A sexual counselling program using three dimensions of sexuality: person-related pre-existing factors, disease-specific factors and the patient's and partner's response. The three dimensions address patient sexual functioning and dysfunction, the impact and influence of illness or disability on the patient's sexual experiences and finally the psychosexual and sociosexual state of both the patient and their partner	The onus remains on individual healthcare practitioners or healthcare institutions to integrate the model into their rehabilitative programs Implementation and administration may be time-consuming and resource-intensive Practitioners may need to take time to learn about or receive instruction about the model, as well as take time to administer it to all clients
The Recognition Model	Recognises the sexuality of people living with a disability, their needs and desires. Includes five stages for health teams to engage with: 1) the recognition of the service user as a sexual being; 2) permission to discuss their sexual concerns; 3) exploration; 4) addressing issues within the team's expertise and boundaries; and 5) referral on and advocacy	Effectiveness of this approach rests on a team that is keen not only to work together, but also to work together on the topic of sexuality The result of several practitioners' lack of willingness or capacity to engage in such counselling may leave one (or none) of the team members to support the sexual needs of the client

Dune 2018.

help practitioners discuss sexual issues, as well as provide treatment or interventions where necessary (i.e. PLISSIT, Kaplan, ALLOW, the Sexual Counselling Framework and the Recognition Model).

As can be seen in Table 7.1, there is a range of frameworks to support client sexuality. However, given changes to context of healthcare practice, a more in-depth focus on interdisciplinary and interprofessional service deliver is important. Take, for example, the Recognition Model. This model is a shift from one that is problem focused, and the role of individual health practitioners can be seen in this model, which was developed following extensive research into the practice of multidisciplinary teams (e.g. occupational therapists,

nurses, physiotherapists, speech and language therapists and psychologists) working in the area of physical disability (Andrews & Lund 2016). This model seeks to 'recognise' the sexuality of people living with a disability and that their needs and desires are like those of their typical counterparts. The model includes five stages (see Fig. 7.1) for health teams to engage in: 1) the recognition of the service user as a sexual being; 2) permission to discuss their sexual concerns; 3) exploration; 4) addressing issues within the team's expertise and boundaries; and 5) referral on and advocacy.

The Recognition Model responds to findings from research which indicate that health practitioners felt that sex was not on the health and social care agenda,

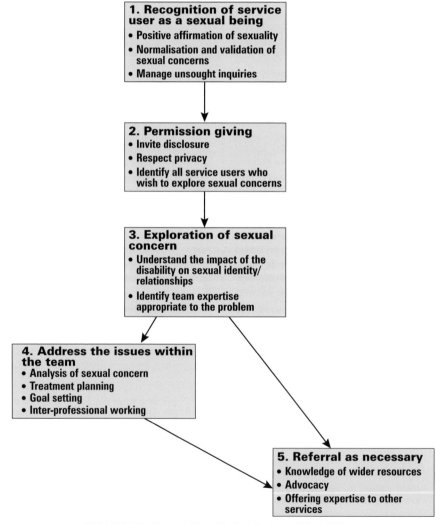

FIG. 7.1 **The Recognition Model.** Andrews & Lund 2016.

with asexualising attitudes in society permeating into healthcare (Andrews & Lund 2016). As such, an important feature of this model, unlike the others, is the recognition of the multitude of practitioners engaged in rehabilitation and disability support. Thus, the model supports a team approach to sexual counselling and acknowledges that not every individual in the team may be willing, or able, to work at all stages. It therefore becomes the role of the team, and not the individual health worker, to ensure that all five stages of the model are included in services provision. This approach further supports the sexuality of people with disabilities by reinforcing a truly holistic approach to sexual counselling and support.

While this model presents a holistic and team framework for sexual counselling, the effectiveness of this approach rests on a team that is keen not only to work together, but also to work together on the topic of sexuality. Although this is mentioned in the model's description, the result of several practitioners' lack of willingness or capacity to engage in such counselling may leave one (or none) of the team members to support the sexual needs of the client. As such, while the model clearly indicates how team-based sexual counselling can be employed, this can only be achieved if health workers are aware of and support the social model of disability, understand and counteract myths of asexuality and disability as part of their daily practice and actively seek to learn more about the sexual lives and experiences of people with chronic illness and disability (e.g. through training, engagement and experience).

CONCLUSION

This chapter has revealed that the ways in which people respond to illness, disability and sexuality are diverse but central to their wellbeing. Despite this, only a minority of people receive help for sexual concerns. As noted by Rohleder and colleagues (2019) and Zivani and colleagues (2004), limitations on receiving support from health workers about illness or disability and sexuality can result from practitioners waiting for clients to initiate such conversations. People who participated in the inquiries reported in this chapter would have benefited from health professionals who were prepared to confront and explore sexuality issues and their relationship to other aspects of their lives. This confirms the findings of other authors (Dune 2016) which indicate that clients would welcome health workers initiating discussion about the impact of illness on sexuality.

Rohleder and colleagues (2019) suggest that health workers may assist clients to communicate about the way sexual feelings are affected by illness by developing confidence in their own ability to listen and respond. Conversations can begin with the promotion of sexual health. Health promotion may include talking about acting within one's own value system to prevent unplanned pregnancies, seeking early prenatal care, or avoiding contracting or transmitting sexually transmitted diseases. Health-promoting behaviours, such as self-examination for breast and testicular cancer and regular check-ups, are responsible ways to identify potential problems. With knowledge of resources and services in the sexuality health area people can be facilitated towards expanded opportunities for appropriate assistance and support. A health worker might say during a conversation with a client, 'Many people with your condition find they have some sexual concerns … is this area a concern for you?' The client may have been wanting the topic of sex and sexuality to be raised. Of course, the health worker should also be prepared if the person does not respond. It may be, however, that the door has been opened for conversation to occur at a later time.

Although ageing (even in healthy individuals) may contribute to changes in the sexual dynamics of a relationship, a number of treatment modalities are available, both psychological and medical (Ekström et al 2018). Doctors and other healthcare providers are expected to be able to manage the sexual health issues of their patients. Even those who are not trained experts in sexual health can provide help simply by minimally expanding what they are already trained to do: first, assess and evaluate; second, treat and/or refer. Simply initiating a discussion of sexual concerns is often the most valuable component of treatment for couples. By asking about sexuality, the healthcare provider informs the patient that it is appropriate to discuss sexual problems in that setting and validates a patient's self-perception as a sexual being (Dune 2016). It is hard to provide an effective intervention, regardless of the type of treatment, if there is no mention of a problem (Valvano et al 2018).

Despite the increasing acknowledgement and acceptance of sexuality as a fundamental aspect of wellbeing, many people hold onto fairly restrictive and conservative views of what is 'appropriate' and 'normal' (Dune 2016). Therefore, appropriate intervention may involve helping people to redefine 'normal' sexual activity. Change does not have to be extreme for couples to notice significant improvement in sexual fulfilment. It may be something as simple (but often not considered) as suggesting that couples engage in sexual activity in the morning when pain and fatigue are less of an issue, rather than late in the evening when there is a greater likelihood of fatigue. Options can also include using different positions and using pillows as needed. It can be important to talk with people about establishing ways of communicating about sexual need and desire. This is important in the case of progressive illness where some adjustment or change may be constant. Communication itself can be seductive, enticing and sexual. Effective communication in everyday life is also important for the quality of the overall relationship, which is also critical to the sexual lives of couples.

This chapter has only 'touched' on the broad topic of sexuality. However, in every clinical contact people living with illness and/or disability need to feel that their concerns and experiences are affirmed. Openly addressing issues of sex and sexuality can be complex, so health workers should create space and time for such conversations with clients. Sexuality is such an intrinsic part of people's lives and is integral to holistic health and wellbeing. When illness changes how people experience their lives, changes to their experience of sexuality are to be expected. Although physical concerns may have a great impact on the ways they engage with their sexuality, people who live with chronic illness or disability continue to emphasise the importance of remaining connected to their sexuality and sexual identity. It is therefore paramount that health workers avoid assumptions that sexuality is no longer a concern for clients because of illness or disability. Acknowledging that most clients embrace opportunities to talk about sexuality reinforces that they are a sexual being and affirms them as a whole person.

Reflective Questions

1. What are the differences between sexuality, sexual health and sexual wellbeing?
2. What are the prevalent barriers people with chronic illness and/or disability experience in regard to sexual health and wellbeing?
3. How can health workers help to promote and facilitate sexual health and wellbeing for people with chronic illness and/or disability?

Acknowledgement: The author would like to thank Debbie Kralik and Norah Bostock for their contribution to this chapter.

RECOMMENDED READING

Dune TM 2016. 'You just don't see us': the influence of public schema on constructions of sexuality by people with cerebral palsy. Development and the Politics of Human Rights, 223–248.

Dune TM, Mpofu E 2017. Understanding sexuality and disability: using interpretive hermeneutic phenomenological approaches. Handbook of Research Methods in Health Social Sciences, 1–21.

Friedman C 2019. Intimate relationships of people with disabilities. Inclusion 7(1), 41–56.

Silverberg C, Kaufman M 2016. The ultimate guide to sex and disability: for all of us who live with disabilities, chronic pain, and illness. Cleis Press.

REFERENCES

Andrews EE, Lund EM 2016. Silenced no more: a review of supporting disabled people with their sexual lives. Sexuality and Disability 34(2), 227–233.

Blockmans IG 2019. Encounters with the white coat: confessions of a sexuality and disability researcher in a wheelchair in becoming. Qualitative Inquiry 25(2), 170–179.

Deans R, Liao LM, Wood D et al 2015. Sexual function and health-related quality of life in women with classic bladder exstrophy. BJU International 115(4), 633–638.

Dune TM 2018. Sexuality. In: E Chang, A Johnson (eds), Living with chronic illness and disability: principles for nursing practice, 3rd edn. Elsevier, Sydney.

Dune TM 2016. 'You just don't see us': the influence of public schema on constructions of sexuality by people with cerebral palsy. In: SN Romaniuk, M Marlin (eds), Development and the politics of human rights. CRC Press, US.

Dune T, Mapedzahama V, Hawkes G et al 2015. African migrant women's understanding and construction of sexuality in Australia. Advances in Social Sciences Research Journal 2(2).

Dune TM, Mpofu E 2017. Understanding sexuality and disability: using interpretive hermeneutic phenomenological approaches. Handbook of Research Methods in Health Social Sciences, 1–21.

Ebrahim S 2019. Disability porn: the fetishisation and liberation of disabled sex. In: P Chappell, M de Beer (eds), Diverse voices of disabled sexualities in the global south. Palgrave Macmillan, Cham.

Ekström M, Johnson MJ, Taylor B et al 2018. Breathlessness and sexual activity in older adults: the Australian Longitudinal Study of Ageing. NPJ Primary Care Respiratory Medicine 28(1), 1–6.

Fileborn B, Thorpe R, Hawkes G et al 2015. Sex, desire and pleasure: considering the experiences of older Australian women. Sexual and Relationship Therapy 30 (1), 117–130.

Friedman C 2019. Intimate relationships of people with disabilities. Inclusion 7(1), 41–56.

Isaacs E 2012. The value of rapid ethnography. In: B Jordan (ed.), Advancing ethnography in corporate environments. Routledge, London.

Kattari SK, Turner G 2017. Examining more inclusive approaches to social work, physical disability, and sexuality. Journal of Social Work in Disability & Rehabilitation 16(1), 38–53.

Lee K, Devine A, Marco MJ et al 2015. Sexual and reproductive health services for women with disability: a qualitative study with service providers in the Philippines. BMC Women's Health 15(1), 87.

Liddiard K, Slater J 2018. 'Like, pissing yourself is not a particularly attractive quality, let's be honest': learning to contain through youth, adulthood, disability and sexuality. Sexualities 21(3), 319–333.

Linton KF, Rueda HA 2015. Dating and sexuality among minority adolescents with disabilities: an application of sociocultural theory. Journal of Human Behavior in the Social Environment 25(2), 77–89.

Loeser C, Pini B, Crowley V 2018. Disability and sexuality: desires and pleasures. Sexualities 21(3), 255–270.

Logan K 2020. An exploration of men's experiences of learning intermittent self-catheterisation with a silicone catheter. British Journal of Nursing 29(2), 84–90.

McCabe J, Holmes D 2014. Nursing, sexual health and youth with disabilities: a critical ethnography. Journal of Advanced Nursing 70(1), 77–86.

Mpofu E, Athanasou JA, Harley D et al 2018. Integration of culture in teaching about disability. In: K Keith (ed.), Culture across the curriculum: a psychology teacher's handbook. Cambridge University Press, Cambridge.

Nguyen TTA, Liamputtong P, Monfries M 2016. Reproductive and sexual health of people with physical disabilities: a metasynthesis. Sexuality and Disability 34, 3–26.

Peta C, McKenzie J, Kathard H et al 2017. We are not asexual beings: disabled women in Zimbabwe talk about their active sexuality. Sexuality Research and Social Policy 14(4), 410–424.

Rohleder P, Braathen SH, Carew MT et al 2019. Disability and sexual health: a critical exploration of key issues. Routledge.

Rowniak S, Selix N 2015. Preparing nurse practitioners for competence in providing sexual health care. Journal of the Association of Nurses in AIDS Care 27(3), 1–7.

Silverberg C, Kaufman M 2016. The ultimate guide to sex and disability: for all of us who live with disabilities, chronic pain and illness. Cleis Press, San Francisco.

Simon W, Gagnon JH 2011. Sexual conduct: the social sources of human sexuality. Transaction Publishers, New Jersey.

Simon W, Gagnon JH 2003. Sexual scripts: origins, influences and changes. Qualitative Sociology 26(4), 491–497.

Simon W, Gagnon JH 1987. Sexual theory: a sexual scripts approach. In: J Greer, W O'Donoghue (eds), Theories and paradigms of human sexuality. Plenum Press, New York.

Simon W, Gagnon JH 1986. Sexual scripts: permanence and change. Archives of Sexual Behavior 15 (2), 97–120.

Smith AE, Molton IR, McMullen K et al 2015. Brief report: sexual function, satisfaction, and use of aids for sexual activity in middle-aged adults with long-term physical disability. Topics in Spinal Cord Injury Rehabilitation 21(3), 227–232.

Terrein-Roccatti N 2017. PL-25 Emotional and psychological expressions of the elements included in sexuality. The Journal of Sexual Medicine 14(5), e218.

Uslu E, İnfal S, Ulusoy MN 2016. Effect of PLISSIT Model on solution of sexual problems. Psikiyatride Guncel Yaklasimlar – Current Approaches in Psychiatry 8(1), 52–63.

Valvano AK, Rollock MJ, Hudson WH et al 2018. Sexual communication, sexual satisfaction, and relationship quality in people with multiple sclerosis. Rehabilitation Psychology, 63(2), 267.

Wilson NJ, Frawley P, Schaafsma D et al 2019. Issues of sexuality and relationships. In: JL Matson (ed.), Handbook of intellectual disabilities: integrating theory, research and practice. Springer, Cham.

World Health Organization (WHO) 2016. Sexual and reproductive health: defining sexual health. Online. Available: www.who.int/reproductivehealth/topics/sexual_health/sh_definitions/en/

Ziviani J, Lennox N, Allison H et al 2004. Meeting in the middle: improving communication in primary health care consultations with people with an intellectual disability. Journal of Intellectual and Developmental Disability 29(3), 211–235.

CHAPTER 8

Health Disparities and People with Intellectual and Developmental Disability

NATHAN J. WILSON • DAVID CHARNOCK

LEARNING OBJECTIVES

When you have completed this chapter you will be able to:

- define intellectual and developmental disability
- explain the causes of intellectual and developmental disability
- understand contemporary frameworks for conceptualising intellectual and developmental disability and health
- identify the specific health issues faced by people with intellectual and developmental disability and describe how these can be minimised
- describe the current and future roles for nurses who support people with intellectual and developmental disability and their families.

KEY WORDS

health promotion	intellectual and developmental disability
inclusion	participation
individualised supports	

INTRODUCTION

People with intellectual and developmental disability share more in common with their fellow citizens than they have differences. Notwithstanding these common-alities, however, people with intellectual and developmental disability often need care and support with some aspects of, or at certain times in, their lives. Despite the closure of many segregated settings (e.g. residential institutions), even in a modern and wealthy nation such as Australia people with all types of disabilities, and particularly intellectual and developmental disability, still experience significant disadvantage compared with their non-disabled peers (Emerson et al 2013). For people with intellectual and developmental disability, this disadvantage is particularly stark when it concerns their health and wellbeing. Hence, health

professionals, such as nurses, can play a pivotal role in countering lifelong disadvantage and promoting health and wellbeing.

The specialist area of intellectual and developmental disability has always been and remains a multidisci-plinary field where the role of the nurse has been central historically and should remain so into the future. Grounded in Article 25 of the principles of the United Nations Convention of the Rights of Persons with Dis-abilities (2006), this chapter introduces readers to this area of practice with a focus on the specific health issues faced by people with intellectual and developmental dis-ability. In addition, it provides a summary of contempo-rary issues on health promotion, health screening and the role of the healthcare professional in the lives of people with intellectual and developmental disability.

The UN Convention, which promotes human rights and freedoms for all in relation to health promotion and the prevention of illness, states:

> *Provide persons with disabilities with the same range, quality and standard of free or affordable health care and programmes as provided to other persons … provide those health services needed by persons with disabilities specifically because of their disabilities, including early identification and intervention as appropriate … provide these health services as close as possible to people's own communities, including in rural areas … require health professionals to provide care of the same quality to persons with disabilities as to others (p. 18).*

DEFINING INTELLECTUAL AND DEVELOPMENTAL DISABILITY

Intellectual and developmental disability is an umbrella term encompassing a range of different lifelong developmental problems that are united by their effect on the individual during childhood that limits their function and/or independent participation in activities such as communication, mobility, self-care and learning (National Center on Birth Defects and Developmental Disabilities 2016). Examples of developmental disabilities include, but are not limited to, intellectual disability, autism spectrum disorders (ASD), Down syndrome, cerebral palsy, ADHD (in the United States) and fetal alcohol syndrome. It is important to note that although someone may have a developmental disability, such as an ASD, this does not automatically infer that they have an intellectual disability, yet a person with intellectual disability does have a developmental disability. The reason that we use the umbrella term is related to the reality that most health professionals and specialists work with both as intellectual and developmental disability often co-occur.

The classification of intellectual and developmental disability is not as straightforward as it might appear and this has historically been the case where once accepted classifications are superseded by new classifications. Over time, the acquisition of new knowledge and changing social norms have seen terms like *idiot* and *handicapped* evolve into the more common internationally accepted term *intellectual and developmental disability*. Nehring (2010) provided a concise historical overview and explained how terms like idiot and its sub-classifications (e.g. genetous idiocy, epileptic idiocy and traumatic idiocy) originally had a scientific basis despite, with the benefit of hindsight, their demeaning interpretation in more contemporary times. That is, our specialist forebears such as Ireland, Kerlin,

Down, Goddard and Doll were working towards improving the classification of individuals in order to promote better treatment, support and outcomes. It was only recently, however, in the United States that the term *mental retardation* was replaced by *intellectual disability* (ID) as it better reflected the person–environment interaction inherent in modern constructs of disability, as well as being less offensive and more internationally consistent (Schalock et al 2007). The American Association on Intellectual and Developmental Disabilities defines intellectual disability as being characterised by significant limitations in both intellectual functioning and in adaptive behaviour, and that occurs before the age of 18 (Schalock et al 2010). Intellectual functioning is usually determined via IQ tests and adaptive behaviour refers to the conceptual (e.g. money, time, self-direction), social (e.g. interpersonal skills, self-esteem, naiveté, ability to follow social rules), and practical (e.g. activities of daily living (ADLs), travel, safety) skills needed to function in the community. By contrast, in the United Kingdom the term *learning disability* is used and is defined as a reduced ability to learn about and understand new skills and complex information and the reduced ability to independently cope, which starts during the developmental years and has a lasting effect on development (Department of Health 2001). How long it takes for the term intellectual and/or learning disability to be superseded by something more reflective of the times and less offensive to a new generation remains open to conjecture, but the point remains that a classification system is necessary and confers benefits to the individual and their family as it opens access to a range of supports that would otherwise not be accessible.

PREVALENCE OF INTELLECTUAL AND DEVELOPMENTAL DISABILITY

Prevalence is a public health term concerned with reporting the number of old and new cases of a given disease or disorder within a population over a nominated period of time. This is in contrast to the term incidence, which is the number of new cases within a population arising at a stated point in time (Fryers 1993). Accurate estimates of the prevalence and incidence of intellectual and developmental disability, in particular across global contexts, is difficult in part due to the differing definitions (e.g. ADHD is included in the United States, but not elsewhere), and also due to the multitude of variable social contexts in which the person with intellectual and developmental disability lives. For example, a person with a mild intellectual disability living in a small rural village in India where subsistence farming dominates their life, faces a very different disabling experience and requires very different adaptive behaviour skills when compared with a person with a mild intellectual disability living in a major Western city where technology, mobility and communication are vital to full and meaningful participation.

Notwithstanding these challenges based on definitions, terms and constructs, and therefore the reliability of the data, there are some noteworthy data to report. Looking solely at the prevalence of intellectual disability, Maulik and colleagues (2011) conducted a meta-analysis of population-based studies and reported a prevalence of approximately 1%. By contrast, the Australian Institute of Health and Welfare (AIHW) (2008) reported a 3% prevalence across Australia. Nevertheless, if we then consider US data for developmental disability in children, which by definition includes ADHD and other learning disorders (e.g. dyslexia), then the prevalence of developmental disability heads towards 14% of the population (Boyle et al 2011). As these data suggest, the problems of not having a standardised disability identifier, not using population data, and the reality that much of the data are collected by proxy rather than by direct individual assessment,

means that accurately estimating prevalence continues to be fraught with difficulty (Davis et al 2014). Yet, there are some clear trends that are worth mentioning: more males than females have intellectual and developmental disability (approximately 60% for males compared to 40% for females), there are greater reported prevalence rates in children than in older people, low income countries tend to have a higher prevalence, data from household surveys rather than disability service administrative data report a greater prevalence, and studies that use a broad screening tool rather than disability-specific criteria also report a greater prevalence (Emerson & Hatton 2014).

CAUSES OF INTELLECTUAL AND DEVELOPMENTAL DISABILITY

Although for most people with intellectual and developmental disability the cause remains unclear, advances in genetic screening, molecular and neuro-imaging techniques mean that more will be known in the years ahead. There are, however, several known causes which, based primarily on comprehensive description and discussion by Hellings and colleagues (2010), are summarised in Table 8.1. In addition to the causes listed in the table, there are other less

TABLE 8.1
Main Causes of Intellectual and Developmental Disability

Cause	Description	Common Health Problems
Down syndrome	Chromosomal disorder; Trisomy 21. Most common cause of intellectual and developmental disability, affecting 1 in 700–1000 births. Significantly reduced total brain volume with under-developed temporal lobes	Congenital heart defects, endocrine disorders, eye and vision problems, poor muscle tone, atlantoaxial instability, prone to obesity, risk of early-onset Alzheimer's disease
Fragile X syndrome	X-chromosome disorder twice as common in males. Autistic behavioural tendencies. Caudate nucleus (part of basal ganglia) abnormality	Connective tissue laxity, strabismus, scoliosis
Prader-Willi syndrome	Paternal deletion of the 15q11–q13 chromosome region	Hyperphagia, hypogonadism, OCD, prone to obesity, risk of type 2 diabetes
Angelman syndrome	Maternal deletion of the 15q11–q13 chromosome region	Epilepsy, sleep disturbance, dysphagia
Velo-cardio-facial syndrome	22q11.2 deletion syndrome affecting in 1 in 5000 births. Cleft palate, cardiac malformation. Autistic behavioural tendencies are common	Dysphagia, heart problems, mental health problems, renal abnormalities, scoliosis, low muscle tone
Rett syndrome	Mainly occurs in females; about 1 in 9000 female births. Autistic behavioural tendencies and classic 'hand wringing' movements	Ataxia

Continued

TABLE 8.1

Main Causes of Intellectual and Developmental Disability – cont'd

Cause	Description	Common Health Problems
Fetal Alcohol Syndrome (FAS)	Estimates vary between 0–10.7 per 1000 births in the United States; more common in socially deprived areas such as in Indigenous Australia and parts of South Africa	Renal and cardiac defects, vision and hearing problems
Autism Spectrum Disorders (ASD)	Approximately 1 in 100 people have ASD with males affected at 4 times the rate of females. No known single cause	Sensory problems, seizures
Cerebral palsy	Results from an insult to the developing brain of the fetus or infant causing CNS damage and motor impairment	Dysphagia, epilepsy, hearing and vision impairment, prone to being underweight, hypo- or hyper-tonic muscles, scoliosis

Hellings et al 2010; Wilson-Jones & Morgan 2010.

common ones, including metabolism disorders (e.g. phenylketonuria), fetal infections (e.g. cytomegalovirus, toxoplasmosis and congenital syphilis), exposure to heavy metals (e.g. lead and mercury), maternal iodine deficiency and CNS abnormalities (e.g. Dandy–Walker cyst). Further, some noteworthy environmental causes of intellectual and developmental disability during the childhood years include lifelong cognitive impairments from trauma, poisoning, drowning and assault.

HEALTH ISSUES FOR PEOPLE WITH INTELLECTUAL AND DEVELOPMENTAL DISABILITY

It is an undisputed reality that people with intellectual and developmental disability have more health problems, do not receive the same level of healthcare, and have mortality rates that are far greater than in the general population (Davis et al 2014). They are one of the most marginalised sub-groups in society as they experience direct and indirect inequality and face multiple numbers of the social determinants of poor health (Emerson & Hatton 2014). Moreover, recent studies also point to the greater likelihood that people with intellectual and developmental disability will die from potentially avoidable causes (Trollor et al 2017). Despite it being decades since the end of deinstitutionalisation and the widespread implementation of policies aimed at promoting self-determination, people with intellectual and developmental disability still have fewer choices about and less control over their health than the general population (Wullink et al 2009). Furthermore, the prevalence of health problems is likely to

be underestimated as most studies of health problems rely on proxy data rather than from direct assessment of individuals by skilled nurses or physicians.

Although people with intellectual and developmental disability are vulnerable to a myriad of problems, only the key issues will be focused on within this chapter.

Mortality as an Indicator of Health Problems

Although there has been a trend in the gradual reduction of mortality for people with intellectual and developmental disability over time, they still have a shorter life expectancy than the general population across all age ranges (Emerson & Hatton 2014). For example, in 1929 people with Down syndrome had a life expectancy of 9 years, whereas by 1997 this had increased to 49 years (Yang et al 2002). Although this is a remarkable change that reflects advances in science and medicine and improvements to health and social care, disparities in life expectancy remain. The first known population-based study in Australia was carried out on data collected from a defined population in North Sydney during 1989–1990 and showed that standardised mortality rates (SMR – ratio of observed by expected number of deaths where a ratio greater than 1.0 is considered excess deaths) for people with intellectual disability was 4.9, with the death rates highest at each end of the age range (Durvasula et al 2002). Using a much larger sample of NSW population data from 2005–2011, Florio and Trollor (2015) reported an SMR of 2.48 for people with intellectual disability across all ages. In the UK, using population data from 2002 to 2014, Glover and colleagues (2016) reported an SMR of

3.18 across all age ranges with a life expectancy at birth 19.7 years lower than in people without intellectual disability.

Although international data have reported that mortality rates are decreasing, there remains a significant disparity between people with and people without intellectual and developmental disability, which should be of major concern to all health professionals. A major cause for concern has been the link between mortality rates and preventable or premature deaths in people with intellectual and developmental disability. For example, in the UK, MENCAP has been at the centre of a national campaign to highlight the number of preventable deaths of people with intellectual and developmental disability through the failings of mainstream health services. In Wales (UK), the Paul Ridd Foundation has spearheaded a campaign to improve health outcomes for people with intellectual and developmental disability using a range of strategies such as training champions within acute care services. An example of the health inequalities faced by people with intellectual and developmental disability, through

factors such as diagnostic overshadowing, is presented in Case Study 8.1.

Diabetes

Diabetes is a long-term condition which occurs when either the pancreas fails to produce insulin or the body has difficulty processing the insulin produced (International Diabetes Federation 2020). There are two types of diabetes requiring different treatment regimens. Type 1 diabetes (T1D) develops when cells in the body responsible for the production of insulin are destroyed. Patients with this type require treatment with doses of insulin on a daily basis. Type 2 diabetes (T2D), on the other hand, is caused when the cells responsible for insulin production are not productive enough or the insulin simply fails to work properly. The patient with this type of diabetes often requires medication and needs to make changes to their diet and lifestyle.

According to the World Health Organization (WHO 2020), the number of people diagnosed with diabetes has more than doubled since the 1980s, resulting in a global prevalence rate of 8.5%, identifying it as the

---

CASE STUDY 8.1

A PREVENTABLE DEATH

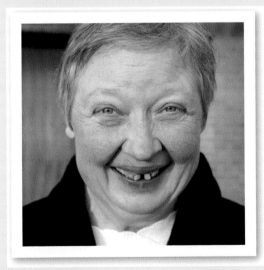

iStockphoto/SilviaJansen.

Carole Foster died on 2 October 2006 after Pennine Acute Hospital Trust and Pennine Care NHS Foundation Trust failed to treat her for gallstones. Instead, staff interpreted the change in her behaviour as symptomatic of her learning disability and mental ill-health.

Carole's family complained to the hospital. In September 2007 they wrote to the Chief Executive of the Trust to express their concerns that, one year on, no satisfactory explanation had been given as to why Carole had died.

The case was referred to the ombudsman in December 2007, but the final report was not published until November 2011, just over 5 years after Carole died. The ombudsman's investigation identified *a catalogue of service failures and concluded that Carole's death could have been avoided.**

CASE STUDY QUESTIONS

1. How does diagnostic overshadowing potentially lead to such poor outcomes?
2. What can health professionals do to avoid reaching disablist conclusions about the presentation of people with intellectual and developmental disability in acute care settings?
3. What type of disability-specific training do healthcare professionals need to provide better care to people with intellectual and developmental disability?

*Emphasis added
MENCAP 2012, p. 18.

seventh leading cause of death worldwide. Despite differences in the intellectual and development disability literature with regard to diabetes, there is general consensus that the prevalence is higher when compared to the general population (Flygare et al 2018; McVilly et al 2014; Taggart et al 2013). In a study conducted in Stockholm, Sweden, Flygare and colleagues (2018) reported a prevalence rate higher than the general population between the ages of 19 and 84. The only group where prevalence was significantly lower when compared to the general population was among those with Down syndrome aged 50 to 64. This in part supports results reported by Taggart and colleagues (2013), of higher prevalence for both T1D and T2D for people with intellectual and developmental disability, although the authors acknowledge that for T2D the figure is not consistent across studies, possibly as a result of problems with definition and access to primary healthcare. Although difference and uncertainty remain, the evidence does suggest that focus on this health condition is essential for those working with people who have intellectual and developmental disability.

Risk factors associated with T2D and people with intellectual and developmental disability, including obesity, poor diet and sedentary lifestyles, should be of particular concern to care workers (Taggart et al 2013; Bryant et al 2018; Tyler et al 2020). Bryant and colleagues (2018) raise specific concerns regarding higher morbidity from diabetes directly related to obesity and physical activity among people with intellectual and developmental disability compared to the general population. The authors recommend a focus on the management of weight and sedentary lifestyles. It is critical that care workers are mindful of these risk factors and provide the right support to establish strategies that acknowledge complex needs and lifestyle choices (Tyler et al 2020). Other factors which appear to significantly increase the risks associated with intellectual and developmental disability and diabetes are social and economic deprivation and health inequalities (Phillips 2016). Again this suggests a greater emphasis on the health needs of people with intellectual and developmental disability, which focuses on the delivery of personalised healthcare plans.

It is important to encourage people with intellectual and developmental disability to work towards the self-management of their diabetes where this is possible (Rouse & Finley 2016; Whitehead et al 2016; Maine, Dickson et al 2017). How self-management is encouraged and maintained will be significant if people with intellectual and developmental disability are to develop the necessary autonomy. In a study conducted by Rouse and Finley (2016), they point to the success of developing supportive narratives to help empower individuals. Similarly, in work by Whitehead and colleagues (2016) and Maine, Brown and colleagues (2018), the negotiation of autonomy and the maintenance of it was identified as critical to successful self-management. All three studies note the importance of support to this process in order to promote good and safe care. However, Maine, Dickson and colleagues (2017) advise caution that the support and well-intentioned persuasion offered does not result in compliance, which may endanger autonomy. In addition, these authors point to the lack of vicarious experiences in diabetes management for people with intellectual and development disability. This type of experiential learning may be significant in helping people to self-manage their diabetes. Assumptions can be made regarding a person's ability to develop the necessary knowledge to self-manage based purely on their intellectual and developmental disability. However, in a study by Hale and colleagues (2011), the researchers found that people with intellectual and developmental disability with T2D often had some useful knowledge about their condition. It is therefore essential that healthcare workers establish the patient's knowledge base and assist the individual to develop and improve this through active support and education or, in the case of those with more severe intellectual and developmental disability, ensure that the correct strategies are in place to establish consistent control of diabetic symptoms. In a more recent study, Trip and colleagues (2016) noted that a concentration on lifestyle, education and collaborative working by those supporting people with intellectual and developmental disability is central to the success of diabetes care.

Evaluative research has been conducted to identify the essential components of adapted mainstream educational programs for people with intellectual and developmental disability (Maine, Brown et al 2017). In addition, specific projects have been conducted for the development of specifically designed programs for this group of people (see Maine, Brown et al 2017, 'Walking Away from Diabetes Programme'; Dunkley et al 2017, 'STOP Diabetes Programme'). There is a need for further testing of these programs, but this demonstrates that these interventions are needed to help people with intellectual and developmental disability manage diabetes more effectively.

Obesity and Underweight

Obesity is a major issue for the whole population, but for people with intellectual and developmental disability the issue of being underweight is also problematic. Obesity is simply defined as excess body fat as a result of too much energy input (e.g. food) and too little energy output (Bray 1987). Although excess body fat may not be a critical issue in the short term, longer term it has significant implications for one's health and wellbeing. This includes being at greater risk of cardiac and circulatory problems, respiratory problems, musculoskeletal problems, gastric problems and endocrine disorders such as T2D. Research about people with intellectual and developmental disability reports that they are significantly more likely to be obese than the general population, with a diagnosis of ASD, spina bifida or Down syndrome a significant added causative factor (Slevin & Northway 2014). National Core Indicators data from the United States, however, did not show a significant difference in obesity between the general population and people with intellectual and developmental disability, but of those who were obese, risk factors included being female, having Down syndrome, having a milder intellectual disability and living in more independent community settings (Stancliffe et al 2011). This suggests that greater staff support when living in residential services is potentially associated with greater scrutiny over food choices, preparation and consumption. Importantly, being underweight is more common among people with intellectual and developmental disability, in particular more so for males who are substantially more likely to be underweight than the general male population (Bhaumik et al 2008). These findings have significant implications for health and wellbeing in addition to suggestions for a research focus on how these findings relate to body image and masculinity for men and boys with intellectual and developmental disability (Wilson et al 2012).

Nutritional interventions aimed at promoting an appropriate intake of the right kinds of foods and to better understand portion sizes are needed, yet there is a paucity of research about nutrition and intellectual and developmental disability (Humphries et al 2009). This leaves the onus on health professionals to provide understandable, accessible and adaptable nutrition education support programs. The pictorial examples illustrated in Fig. 8.1 from the US Department of Agriculture (2016) provide an excellent concrete communication starting point that can be used as part of an overall nutrition plan.

Oral Health

Oral health is a major issue for people with intellectual and developmental disability, with problems including a greater rate of unhealthy teeth and gums and more

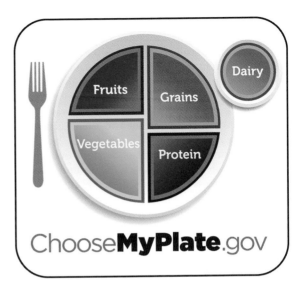

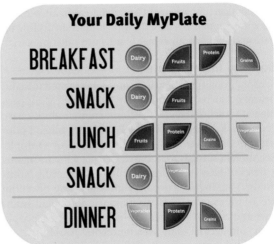

FIG. 8.1 Pictorial example for nutrition plans. © US Department of Agriculture (2016). Choose My Plate. Retrieved from www.choosemyplate.gov/.

dental decay than in the general population (Emerson & Hatton 2014). For example, in a population health study conducted in Northern Sydney, dental disease was found to be the most frequent health problem, occurring in 86% of the entire sample of people with intellectual and developmental disability (Beange et al 1995). Recent literature reviews have identified that people with intellectual and developmental disability have poorer oral hygiene and a higher prevalence and greater severity of periodontal disease than in the general population (Anders & Davis 2010; Wilson, Lin,

Villarosa & George 2019). A discussion about how to counter these problems concluded that a 'one size fits all approach' likely will not succeed as the unique needs of people with intellectual and developmental disability and their caregivers will differ significantly (Wilson, Lin, Villarosa, Phillip et al 2019). These issues are really vital as there is a clear link between poor oral health and respiratory problems, related to silent aspiration and dysphagia. For healthcare professionals, key practice issues include the need to not overlook oral health in comprehensive health assessments, to find ways to counter poor access to mainstream oral health services, provide access to oral health education for caregivers, and initiate individualised oral health support for people with intellectual and developmental disability. Although there are some practice-based interventions reported in the literature – for example, an oral health intervention where dental specialists trained disability support staff (Mac Giolla et al 2013) – that show a post-intervention improvement in oral health knowledge, they are limited by their lack of long-term follow-up data and significantly better oral health outcomes.

Sensory Impairments

Sensory impairments include problems related to sight, hearing, touch, taste and spatial awareness. More people with intellectual and developmental disability have co-morbid sensory impairments than the general population (Bosch & Bass-Ringdahl 2010). For example, SeeAbility (2016) is a UK-based website which contains a series of facts (see references; note UK-specific terminology) stating that people with a learning disability are 10 times more likely to have a serious sight problem and 6 out of 10 require glasses. Further, people with intellectual and developmental disability are more likely to have an unnecessary vision impairment as a result of not having their near or long sightedness corrected by glasses (Woodhouse 2010). A review of the literature indicated that people with intellectual disability have somewhere between 40 and 100 times the rate of hearing impairments than the general population, with having Down syndrome a significant risk factor (Radhakrishnan 2010). Given the major senses are our usual way of interacting with and participating within our environment, these are important areas of support that need innovative and timely interventions from health professionals.

Case Study 8.2 offers an insight into the impact that a sensory impairment can have on a person's mobility and participation around the home. Healthcare professionals need to know about interventions to help promote participation in people with intellectual and

developmental disability and co-morbid sensory impairments, such as creating an even lighting environment within a home, minimising contrasting floor coverings and colours, and eliminating trip hazards for people with a vision impairment. It is also vital for healthcare professionals to provide support and education in how to clean, care for and store aids such as glasses and hearing aids. Anecdotal evidence noted by the authors suggests that the number of people with intellectual and developmental disability who have sensory impairments but are never supported by staff to wear an appropriate aid is very high!

Sexual Health

Sexual health is integral to quality of life, integrating the physical, cognitive, social and emotional aspects of our sexuality, but is often negatively affected by having intellectual and developmental disability (UN 2006). Having a healthy sexuality is not just about avoiding undesirable outcomes, such as contracting a sexually transmitted infection (STI) or the news of an unintended pregnancy; rather, it is about having the skills, understanding, education and sexual behaviours to be sexually healthy throughout one's life. Yet, research about the sexual lives of people with intellectual and developmental disability highlights a particularly adverse picture of negative sexual experiences, high rates of sexual abuse, sexual health problems, unplanned pregnancies, and high rates of testicular cancer (McCarthy et al 2016; Wilson et al 2010). People with intellectual and developmental disability also encounter opposition to sexual activity and those who support them struggle to wade through the myriad of complex and ethical issues (Eastgate & Moyle 2014).

Recent Australian research highlighted that young adults with intellectual and developmental disability experience their sexual lives through a pathological and fear-based paradigm: men fear doing the wrong thing; women fear being vulnerable (Frawley & Wilson 2016; Wilson & Frawley 2016). This research also showed that current models of sex education are not working for young people with intellectual and developmental disability. Further, when and how people with intellectual and developmental disability access mainstream sexual health services is largely unknown as many mainstream services do not collect data using a standardised disability identifier. Major research gaps include testicular examination, screening for prostate cancer, prevalence of STIs and effective sexual health education programs. There are limited international data about how people with intellectual and developmental disability understand, educate themselves or

CASE STUDY 8.2

THE IMPACT OF SENSORY IMPAIRMENT

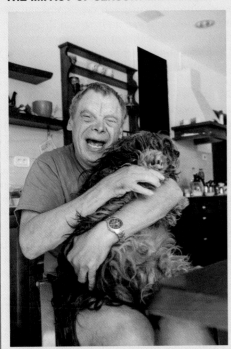

iStockphoto/CasarsaGuru

Bob Evans was an older man with Down syndrome and early stage Alzheimer's disease, living in a community group home that had been his home for 20 years. Bob had limited verbal communication and started having falls around the home, which his support staff put down to his old age and Alzheimer's disease as Bob couldn't tell staff why he kept falling over. The staff initiated a range of strategies to reduce falls, which included restricting his movement around his home at times of low staff-to-client support ratios.

During a routine health screening assessment at a specialised developmental disability clinic, the doctor noted that Bob had a misty appearance to his eyes and referred him to an ophthalmologist. Bob had cataracts, which would have significantly impaired his vision. Upon getting the cataracts removed, Bob started to mobilise more freely around his home and no longer experienced the same number of falls.

CASE STUDY QUESTIONS

1. What would have been a better support for Bob rather than an assumption that his behaviour change was down to early-stage Alzheimer's disease?
2. What interventions could staff have implemented around the home to reduce the risk of falls rather than restricting his movements?
3. If the cataracts had not been diagnosed, what would the likely long-term outcome be from restricting Bob's movement around his home?

make informed decisions about their sexual health, including their experience of accessing sexual health services. Future research needs to focus on accessible sexuality and relationship education; potential areas for innovative practice include peer mentoring approaches that are starting to be used in Australia (Frawley et al 2011).

HEALTH PROMOTION FOR PEOPLE WITH INTELLECTUAL AND DEVELOPMENTAL DISABILITY

Community-based health promotion is seen as a cost-effective and viable public health approach to preventing chronic disease that extends beyond clinical settings and takes a multifaceted approach (Marks & Sisirak 2014). Examples include programs that utilise multiple interventions (e.g. advertisements, screening, contests, self-help programs and environmental interventions) to reduce the rates of cardiovascular disease,

to change attitudes towards and rates of smoking, and HIV prevention programs (Merzel & D'Afflitti 2003). Yet, many of these programs directly or indirectly exclude people with intellectual and developmental disability by not being accessible or by not using adapted content such as plain English advertising booklets. For example, a study of barriers to breast screening in Australia included the need for a direct invitation to attend, unhelpful stereotypes of the perceived need for screening in women with intellectual and developmental disability, and co-morbid physical disability making the procedure far too complex for many women due to the machine being unable to accommodate physical differences (Sullivan et al 2004). Typical strategies to promote breast screening to women from the general population might include mail via listed addresses on the electoral roll, yet how many women with intellectual and developmental disability are enrolled to vote? Therefore, our knowledge about the effect of health promotion interventions on people with intellectual and developmental disability is largely unknown, apart from some exemplars that are described below. The inclusion of people with intellectual and developmental disability in community health promotion programs will reduce some of the known health disparities they face. In addition, they foster opportunities for social inclusion and the creation of valued social roles as active and healthy citizens (Hallawell et al 2013).

Healthy Ageing – an Example of an Inclusive Intervention to Promote Active Ageing

Health problems are one of the major causes of involuntary retirement – and hence social and economic exclusion – for people with disabilities (Brotherton et al 2020; Denton et al 2013) and so finding ways to promote active ageing are needed. The Transition to Retirement (TTR) project (Stancliffe et al 2013), although not directly labelled as a health promotion intervention, was a project that promoted the principles of active ageing. Active ageing is about enhancing quality of life by optimising the health, participation and security of individuals and populations (WHO 2002). The TTR project was probably the first controlled intervention study to support older people with intellectual and developmental disability reduce their days at sheltered workshops by participating in meaningful activities with the general aged population. Each individual was supported to drop a day at work and either join a community or a volunteer group that older people without a disability might join. Examples from the TTR Workbook (Stancliffe et al 2013) included Joanne, who joined a local walking and knitting group; Jeff, who joined a Men's Shed; and Ken, who joined the volunteers at the aviation museum. That is, all participants increased their physical activity, their community participation, made new friends and experienced a significantly greater sense of social satisfaction (Stancliffe et al 2015).

Using a program logic method, the TTR project had a multifaceted health promotion approach based on the individual's needs, actively encouraging family input, promoting change at disability services, and by increasing community capacity to be able to support people with intellectual and developmental disability (Bigby et al 2014). As the flowchart in Fig. 8.2 describes, the health promotion outcomes were not just from working with an individual, but were about supporting the individual through a deliberate and targeted approach that included underpinning *all* aspects of their life. Using this approach, the health and social care professional is acting as a case manager who is promoting change for individuals, services and communities to create better health and wellbeing

outcomes for an individual now while providing exemplars, or 'champions', that will help promote better health and wellbeing for other individuals. That is, other people with intellectual and developmental disability start to think, if he can do it, so can I! Community groups start to realise that providing support is not that hard and including other people with a disability in the future will not appear so daunting.

Health Matters – an Example of a Health Promotion Program from the United States

Health Matters is one of the few evidence-based health promotion interventions designed for and tested on people with intellectual and developmental disability (Marks et al 2010). Key outcomes from preliminary studies illustrate the power of utilising a multifaceted approach where staff support and organisational commitment are just as important as individualised support to people with intellectual and developmental disability. Using exercise classes and integrated health education classes, the goals of Health Matters were to:

- improve flexibility, aerobic capacity, balance and strength
- increase knowledge about healthy lifestyles
- teach staff and caregivers how to support participants to achieve these goals (Marks et al 2010, p. 80).

Using a controlled intervention research design, a staff 'train-the-trainer' Health Matters program demonstrated significant positive differences in psychosocial health status, perceived pain and self-efficacy when the intervention group was compared with a matched group who did not participate in the program. Furthermore, staff also reported better health and wellbeing outcomes following their participation as trainers. These are worthy outcomes and the workbook by Marks and colleagues (2010) provides anyone wishing to create and implement such a program with a 'how to' guide covering how to embed principles of universal design and plain English into the program.

One of the possible downsides of the approach taken by Marks and colleagues (2010) is the disability-specific group nature of the program and the reliance on staff, rather than a more targeted and individualised approach that uses pre-existing community resources. One major barrier, however, to using existing community resources such as the local gym, is the monthly cost that may be prohibitive for many people with intellectual and developmental disability. An alternative to group-based exercise currently being analysed in Australia is an approach aimed at embedding physical activity in the everyday life of people with intellectual and developmental disability (Lante et al 2014). For

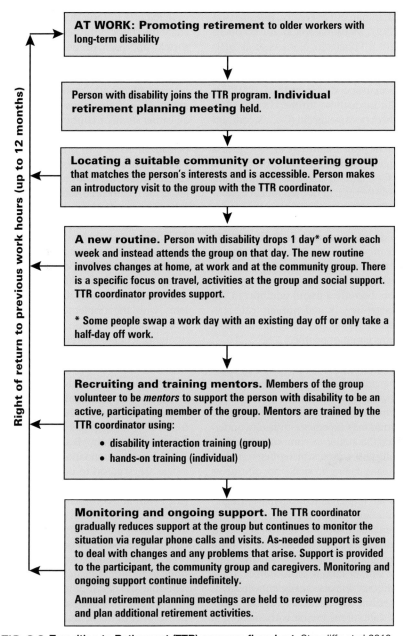

Right of return to previous work hours (up to 12 months)

AT WORK: Promoting retirement to older workers with long-term disability

Person with disability joins the TTR program. **Individual retirement planning meeting** held.

Locating a suitable community or volunteering group that matches the person's interests and is accessible. Person makes an introductory visit to the group with the TTR coordinator.

A new routine. Person with disability drops 1 day* of work each week and instead attends the group on that day. The new routine involves changes at home, at work and at the community group. There is a specific focus on travel, activities at the group and social support. TTR coordinator provides support.

* Some people swap a work day with an existing day off or only take a half-day off work.

Recruiting and training mentors. Members of the group volunteer to be *mentors* to support the person with disability to be an active, participating member of the group. Mentors are trained by the TTR coordinator using:
- disability interaction training (group)
- hands-on training (individual)

Monitoring and ongoing support. The TTR coordinator gradually reduces support at the group but continues to monitor the situation via regular phone calls and visits. As-needed support is given to deal with changes and any problems that arise. Support is provided to the participant, the community group and caregivers. Monitoring and ongoing support continue indefinitely.

Annual retirement planning meetings are held to review progress and plan additional retirement activities.

FIG. 8.2 **Transition to Retirement (TTR) program flowchart.** Stancliffe et al 2013.

example, walking to the corner store to buy milk rather than driving to the supermarket, or doing pre-taught exercises during each ad-break of a favourite TV program. Preliminary findings demonstrate that an individualised approach resulted in significantly better exercise self-efficacy when compared to a group-based approach (Stancliffe et al 2014).

HEALTH CHECKS FOR PEOPLE WITH INTELLECTUAL AND DEVELOPMENTAL DISABILITY

Poor health and the issue of mortality in populations of people with intellectual and developmental disability in the developed world, highlighted earlier in this chapter, is again presented in the literature in support of health checks (Chapman 2012; Lennox & Robertson 2014; Martin et al 1997; Macdonald et al 2018; Robertson, Hatton et al 2014; Robertson, Roberts et al 2011; Slowie & Martin 2014; Walmsley 2011; Ware & Lennox 2016). Concern is raised regarding preventable death in people with intellectual and developmental disability resulting from health inequalities. In the UK the effectiveness of health checks was being cited as a significant factor in physical health gain at a time when deinstitutionalisation was at its peak (Martin et al 1997). It is clear that this is a significant factor in the promotion of effective healthcare for this group and that health professionals should include this as part of their practice (Robertson et al 2014). With the exception of the UK and the Republic of Ireland, specialist practitioners for people with intellectual and developmental disability are no longer part of service provision. This raises a challenge to the health status of this group and, as a consequence, it is essential that health check tools, such as those suggested in this section, become a useful addition to the assessments undertaken by GPs and primary care specialists, who may not have the knowledge to promote optimal health for this group of people.

Health checks are recognised as offering a proactive method for improving the health of people with intellectual and developmental disability (Lennox & Robertson 2014; Robertson, Hatton et al 2014; Robertson, Roberts et al 2011; Macdonald et al 2018). They are particularly important as this group may experience difficulty understanding or may lack the ability to communicate effectively when something goes wrong, which often results in the person or their carer failing to make appointments with their GP. Lennox and Robertson (2014) indicate that when health checks are implemented they have the potential to improve the knowledge of people with intellectual and developmental disability. As a consequence, they may become increasingly aware of their own health and be able to communicate symptoms when attending future appointments with healthcare professionals. There may also be an additional impact on the knowledge of carers as they may become more able to recognise symptoms related to the health of the person with intellectual and developmental disability. An added benefit may be that support workers are less likely to misinterpret behaviours, as in the case of diagnostic overshadowing highlighted in Case Study 8.1 earlier in this chapter.

Implementation of health checks and the identification of indicators of success can be complex as they are normally conducted in primary care by staff with little education or experience of the needs of people with intellectual and developmental disability. Macdonald and colleagues (2018), in their RCT of practice nurse-led health checks, concluded that the nurses in their study were happier to carry out the check if they were able to adapt the check to the person. Although this may appear a useful approach, the authors argue that in doing so the nurses failed to use the breadth of the health check, which may have had an impact on the potential benefits for the person with intellectual and developmental disability. This adaptation is also reflected in the findings of an earlier study by Durbin and colleagues (2016), but in this case adaptation was to the environment and not the person. In essence, in order to conduct the check some aspects had to be adapted as a result of the practice focus. Related to the community covered by the practice or a specific health need staff had particular knowledge of, aspects of the check were approached in different ways. Unsurprisingly, implementation was particularly successful in practices where the needs of people with intellectual disability was a specific practice focus. The authors conclude this helped to foster shared learning and a clear impetus for health check implementation.

Although the issues discussed here cause some problems with the implementation and sustainability of health checks to people with intellectual and learning disability, a major concern is attendance, when individuals are invited for the check. Case Study 8.3 describes a situation where attendance at a health check required staff to take the initiative and provide direct support. While this area is recognised as under-researched, Chapman and colleagues (2017), in their narrative review, found that although people with intellectual and developmental disability had begun to benefit from the health checks, attendance was low and provision inconsistent. They go on to note that this may be due to the experiences people have, but this has not been investigated with any commentary with regards to identifying the root of the problem or what solutions can be established. Without this it is difficult to conclusively establish the success or otherwise of these checks. However, it is clear that a whole system approach is required to continue to minimise health inequality for people with intellectual and developmental disability for the future.

The following are examples of health check assessments in current use in the UK and Australia:

- Cardiff Health Check – Available at: www.wales.nhs.uk/sites3/Documents/480/LD_DES-Health_Check_UP.doc
- The OK Health check (children) – Available at: www.st-annes.org.uk/wp-content/uploads/2015/04/Appendix%2021%20-%20OK%20health%20check.pdf
- Comprehensive Health Assessment Profile (CHAP) – Available at: www.communities.qld.gov.au/disability-connect-queensland/service-providers/comprehensive-health-assessment-program-chap

CASE STUDY 8.3

A CASE STUDY ABOUT HEALTH CHECKS

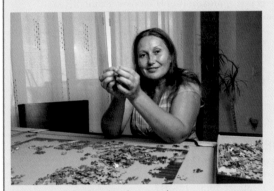

Shutterstock/andres barrionuevo lopez

Tracy is a 30-year-old woman with Autism Spectrum Disorder (ASD) who has her own tenancy and is supported by a small team of support staff. Tracy has good communication skills, but often has difficulty building relationships with people and can become worried about new situations. Support staff sometimes struggle to interpret Tracy's needs and are concerned that they are not always able to react quickly to changes in her health.

On a visit to Tracy's apartment, a support worker finds a letter from the local GP practice asking Tracy to attend for a health check with the practice nurse.

CASE STUDY QUESTIONS

1. How might the health check benefit Tracy?
2. What does the support worker need to know prior to Tracy's health check?
3. How might the support worker help to best prepare Tracy for the health check?

ROLE OF THE NURSE FOR PEOPLE WITH INTELLECTUAL AND DEVELOPMENTAL DISABILITY

As highlighted in the previous section, the UK and the Republic of Ireland are the only countries that continue to provide specialist practitioners for people with intellectual and developmental disability. Most relevant here is the training of specialist nurses at undergraduate level. In addition to basic nursing skills, the specialist nurse is often involved in a myriad of roles that cover the lifespan, for the person with intellectual disability and their family, and include many complex disabilities and co-morbidities (Northway et al 2017). Roles are often varied and are dependent on the group of people with intellectual

and developmental disability represented in services. In the study by Northway and colleagues (2017), functions of the specialist nurse that emerged were accessing healthcare; health promotion and education; development of roles across settings; awareness raising; rights and empowerment. Central to the implementation of these core skills is a relationship-centred model of nursing care that works collaboratively with the person, their family, caregivers and the myriad of health and social services needed to promote the best outcomes (Wilson, Wiese et al 2019). Most importantly, these nurses are an essential link between the health needs of the individual and mainstream health provision, as they are often required to ensure equal access to health services. In recent years, the specific roles in health liaison have been established to offer advice, work strategically across specialist and mainstream health services and raise awareness among medical and nursing staff in relation to the specific health needs of people with intellectual and developmental disability (Harris et al 2012). Despite their rarity across the developed world, these nurses play an essential part in the lives of this group and are often considered to be essential components in the holistic care of people with intellectual and developmental disability. Work to investigate the importance of this new role for the specialist nurse has provided positive accounts of their effectiveness in helping people with intellectual and developmental disability access and receive equitable healthcare (MacArthur et al 2015; Morton-Nance 2015).

Future Practice in Australia

Service delivery to people with more severe intellectual and developmental disability under the age of 65 in Australia is currently undergoing a major transformation. Previously, all funded services were provided on a block-funding basis (i.e. X number of beds or Y numbers at a day program), but are now transforming to an individualised model where each eligible person receives an individualised package to spend on the services and supports they want to prioritise. For the first time in Australia, this has opened the door to for-profit traders or businesses to tender and/or advertise to provide services. This means that nurses with skills in working with and supporting people with intellectual and developmental disability can advertise their expertise and provide practitioner-type services direct to individuals. Based on what has been covered so far in this chapter, the types of practitioner services could not only include health promotion and health screening activities, but also specific nursing care, such as training in gastrostomy and tracheostomy care, medication management, and diabetes and nutrition education. This critical juncture offers greater self-determination for people with intellectual and developmental disability and immense opportunities for skilled and innovative disability nurse practitioners.

CONCLUSION

People with intellectual and developmental disability have poorer health and need more support to attain better health than the general population. Emerson and Hatton (2014) argue there are two key challenges that lie ahead to improve the health and wellbeing of people with intellectual and developmental disability and reduce the health inequalities they face. These are to: 1) build a relevant knowledge base; and 2) change policy and practice. Although this chapter has cited some of the latest research in the field, including some innovative health promotion interventions, much more needs to be done and health professionals – particularly nurses – have a significant role to play to build the evidence base. For example, a recent audit of all disability research in Australia found that far too much research describes problems with far too little intervention or evaluation research that actually reports on what works, for whom and in what contexts (Centre for Disability Research and Policy 2014). It is incumbent upon all health professionals to embed evidence-based practice into their everyday work – now is the time for specialist disability nurses to heed the challenges outlined by Emerson and Hatton and start working with people with intellectual and developmental disability and their families to generate the evidence and drive the policy and practice changes that will lead to better health and wellbeing for people with intellectual and developmental disability.

Reflective Questions

1. How do you feel about the difference in life expectancy for people with intellectual and developmental disability?

2. If you could influence access to healthcare for people with intellectual and developmental disability, what key messages would you offer to healthcare practitioners?

3. After reading this chapter, what would you now do differently to facilitate better health for people with intellectual and developmental disability?

RECOMMENDED READING

Betz CL, Nehring WM (eds) 2010. Nursing care for individuals with intellectual and developmental disabilities: an integrated approach. Paul H Brookes, Baltimore, MA.

Emerson E, Hatton C 2014. Health inequalities and people with intellectual disabilities. Cambridge University Press, Cambridge, UK.

Taggart L, Cousins W (eds) 2014. Health promotion for people with intellectual and developmental disabilities. Open University Press, Maidenhead, UK.

REFERENCES

Anders PL, Davis EL 2010. Oral health of patients with intellectual disabilities: a systematic review. Special Care in Dentistry 30(3), 110–117.

Australian Institute of Health and Welfare (AIHW) 2008. Disability in Australia: intellectual disability. Cat. No. AUS 110. AIHW, Canberra.

Beange H, McElduff A, Baker W 1995. Medical disorders of adults with mental retardation: a population study. American Journal of Mental Retardation 99, 595–604.

Bhaumik S, Watson JM, Thorp CF et al 2008. Body mass index in adults with intellectual disability: distribution, associations and service implications: a population-based prevalence study. Journal of Intellectual Disability Research 52, 287–298.

Bigby C, Wilson NJ, Stancliffe RJ et al 2014. Transition to retirement: an effective program design to support older workers with intellectual disability participate individually in community groups. Journal of Policy and Practice in Intellectual Disabilities 11(2), 117–127.

Bosch J, Bass-Ringdahl SM 2010. Sensory impairment. In: CL Betz, WM Nehring (eds), Nursing care for individuals with intellectual and developmental disabilities: an integrated approach. Paul H Brookes, Baltimore, MA.

Boyle CA, Boulet S, Schieve LA et al 2011. Trends in the prevalence of developmental disabilities in US children, 1997–2008. Pediatrics 127(6), 1034–1042.

Bray GA 1987. Obesity: a disease of nutrient or energy balance? Nutrition Reviews 45, 129.

Brotherton M, Stancliffe RJ, Wilson, NJ et al 2020. Australians with intellectual disability share their experiences of retirement from mainstream employment. Journal of Applied Research in Intellectual Disabilities. Online. Available: https://doi.org/10.1111/jar.12712.

Bryant LD, Russell AM, Walwyn REA et al 2018 Characterizing adults with type 2 diabetes mellitus and intellectual disability: outcomes of a case-finding study. Diabetic Medicine 35, 352–359.

Centre for Disability Research and Policy 2014. Report of audit of disability research in Australia. The University of Sydney, Centre for Disability Research and Policy, Sydney.

Chapman J 2012. Annual health checks for people with learning disabilities. Learning Disability Practice 15(1), 22–24.

Chapman J, Iobell A, Bramwell R 2017. Do health consultations for people with learning disabilities meet expectations? A narrative literature review. British Journal of Learning Disabilities 46, 118–135.

Davis R, Proulx R, van Schrojenstein Lantman-de Valk H 2014. Health issues for people with intellectual disabilities: the evidence base. In: L Taggart, W Cousins (eds), Health promotion for people with intellectual and developmental disabilities. McGraw Hill Education, Maidenhead, Berkshire.

Denton M, Plenderleith J, Chowan J 2013. Health and disability as determinants for involuntary retirement of people with disabilities. Canadian Journal on Aging 32(2), 159–172.

Department of Agriculture 2016. Choose my plate. Online. Available: www.choosemyplate.gov/.

Department of Health 2001. Valuing people: a new strategy for learning disability for the 21st century. Author, London.

Dunkley AJ, Tyler F, Doherty Y et al 2017. Development of a multi-component lifestyle intervention for preventing type 2 diabetes and cardiovascular risk factors in adults with intellectual disabilities. Journal of Public Health 40(2), 141–150.

Durbin J, Selick A, Casson I et al 2016. Evaluating the implementation of health checks for adults with intellectual developmental disabilities in primary care: the importance of organizational context. Intellectual and Developmental Disabilities 54(2), 136–150.

Durvasula S, Beange H, Baker W 2002. Mortality in people with intellectual disability in northern Sydney. Journal of Intellectual and Developmental Disability 27, 255–264.

Eastgate G, Moyle J 2014. Sexual health. In: L Taggart, W Cousins (eds), Health promotion for people with intellectual and developmental disabilities. McGraw Hill Education, Maidenhead, Berkshire.

Emerson E, Hatton C 2014. Health inequalities and people with intellectual disabilities. Cambridge University Press, Cambridge, UK.

Emerson E, Honey A, Llewellyn G 2013. Left behind: monitoring the social inclusion of young Australians with self-reported long term health conditions, impairments or disabilities 2001–2009. Centre for Disability Research and Policy, University of Sydney.

Florio T, Trollor J 2015. Mortality among a cohort of persons with an intellectual disability in New South Wales, Australia. Journal of Applied Research in Intellectual Disabilities 28, 383–393.

Flygare Wallén E, Ljunggren G, Carlsson AC et al 2018. High prevalence of diabetes mellitus, hypertension and obesity among persons with a recorded diagnosis of intellectual disability or autism spectrum disorder. Journal of Intellectual Disabilities Research 62(4), 269–280.

Frawley P, Slattery J, Stokoe L et al 2011. Living safer sexual lives: respectful relationships. Peer educator and co-facilitator manual. Australian Research Centre in Sex, Health and Society, La Trobe University, Melbourne.

Frawley P, Wilson NJ 2016. Young people with intellectual disability talking about sexuality education and information. Sexuality and Disability 34(4), 469–484.

Fryers T 1993. Epidemiological thinking in mental retardation: issues in taxonomy and population frequency. International Review of Research in Mental Retardation 19, 97–133.

Glover G, Williams R, Heslop P et al 2016. Mortality in people with intellectual disabilities in England. Journal of Intellectual Disability Research 61(1), 62–74.

Hale LA, Trip H, Whitehead L et al 2011. Self-management abilities of diabetes in people with an intellectual disability living in New Zealand. Journal of Policy and Practice in Intellectual Disabilities 8(4), 223–230.

Hallawell B, Stephens J, Charnock D 2013. Physical activity and learning disability. The British Journal of Nursing 21 (10), 609–612.

Harris J, Abbott L, Jukes M 2012. Improving care for children with Down's syndrome. Learning Disability Practice 15 (6), 25–29.

Hellings JA, Butler MG, Grant JA 2010. Congenital causes. In: J O'Hara, J McCarthy, N Bouras (eds), Intellectual disability and ill health: a review of the evidence. Cambridge University Press, Cambridge.

Humphries K, Traci MA, Seekins T 2009. Nutrition and adults with intellectual or developmental disabilities: systematic literature review results. Intellectual and Developmental Disabilities 47(3), 163–185.

International Diabetes Federation 2020. About Diabetes. Online. Available: www.idf.org/aboutdiabetes/what-is-diabetes

Lante K, Stancliffe R, Bauman A et al 2014. Embedding sustainable physical activities into the everyday lives of adults with intellectual disabilities: a randomised controlled trial. BMC Public Health 14(1), 1–6.

Lennox N, Robertson J 2014. Health checks. In: L Taggart, W Cousins (eds), Health promotion for people with intellectual and developmental disabilities. McGraw Hill Education, Maidenhead, Berkshire.

MacArthur J, Brown M, McKechanie A et al 2015. Making reasonable and achievable adjustments: the contributions of learning disability liaison nurses in 'Getting it right' for people with learning disabilities receiving general hospital care. Journal of Advanced Nursing 71(7), 1552–1563.

Macdonald S, Morrison J, Melville CA et al 2018. Embedding routine health checks for adults with intellectual disabilities in primary health care: primary nurse perceptions. Journal of Intellectual Disability Research 62(4), 349–357.

Mac Giolla PC, Guerin S, Nunn J 2013. Train the trainer? A randomized controlled trial of a multi-tiered oral health education programme in community-based residential services for adults with intellectual disability. Community Dentist and Oral Epidemiology 41(2), 182–192.

Maine A, Brown MJ, Dickson A et al 2018. Pilot feasibility study of the Walking Away from Diabetes programme for adults with intellectual disabilities in two further education colleges: process evaluation findings. Journal of

Applied Research in intellectual Disabilities 32, 1034–1046.

Maine A, Brown MJ, Dickson A et al 2017. An evaluation of mainstream type 2 diabetes educational programmes in relation to the needs of people with intellectual disabilities: a systematic review of the literature. Journal of Applied Research in intellectual Disabilities 32, 256–279.

Maine A, Dickson A, Truesdale M et al 2017. An application of Bandura's 'Four Sources of Self Efficacy' to the self-management of type 2 diabetes in people with intellectual disability: an inductive and deductive thematic analysis. Research in Developmental Disabilities 70, 75–84.

Marks B, Sisirak J 2014. Health promotion and people with intellectual disabilities. In: L Taggart, W Cousins (eds), Health promotion for people with intellectual and developmental disabilities. McGraw Hill Education, Maidenhead, Berkshire.

Marks B, Sisirak J, Heller T 2010. Health matters for people with developmental disabilities: creating a sustainable health promotion program. Paul H Brookes, Baltimore, MA.

Martin D, Roy A, Wells M 1997. Health gain through healthchecks: improving access to primary health care for people with intellectual disability. Journal of Intellectual Disability Research 41, 401–408.

Maulik PK, Mascarenhas MN, Mathers CD et al 2011. Prevalence of intellectual disability: a meta-analysis of population-based studies. Research in Developmental Disabilities 32, 419–436.

McCarthy M, Hunt S, Milne-Skillman K 2016. 'I know it was every week, but I can't be sure if it was every day': domestic violence and women with learning disabilities. Journal of Applied Research in Intellectual Disabilities. Online. Available: https://doi:10.1111/jar.12237.

McVilly K, McGillivray J, Curtis A et al 2014. Systematic review of meta-analysis diabetes in people with an intellectual disability: a systematic review of prevalence, incidence and impact. Diabetic Medicine 31, 897–904.

MENCAP 2012. Death by indifference: 74 deaths and counting: a progress report 5 years on. MENCAP, London.

Merzel C, D'Afflitti J 2003. Reconsidering community-based health promotion: promise, performance and potential. American Journal of Public Health 93(4), 557–574.

Morton-Nance S 2015. Unique role of learning disability liaison nurses. Learning Disability Practice 18(7), 30–34.

National Center on Birth Defects and Developmental Disabilities 2016. Facts about developmental disabilities. Centers for Disease Control and Prevention. Online. Available: www.cdc.gov/ncbddd/developmentaldisabilities/facts.html.

Nehring WM 2010. Historical perspectives and emerging trends. In: CL Betz, WM Nehring (eds), Nursing care for individuals with intellectual and developmental disabilities: an integrated approach. Paul H Brookes, Baltimore, MA.

Northway R, Cushing K, Duffin S et al 2017. Supporting people across the lifespan: the role of learning disability nurses. Learning Disability Practice 20(3), 22–27.

Phillips A 2016. Vulnerable adults with diabetes: improving access to care. Practice Nursing 27(6), 287–290.

Radhakrishnan V 2010. Otorhinolaryngological disorders. In: J O'Hara, J McCarthy, N Bouras (eds), Intellectual disability and ill health: a review of the evidence. Cambridge University Press, Cambridge.

Robertson J, Hatton C, Emerson E et al 2014. The impact of health checks for people with intellectual disabilities: an updated systematic review of evidence. Research in Developmental Disabilities 35, 2450–2462.

Robertson J, Roberts H, Emerson E et al 2011. The impact of health checks for people with intellectual disabilities: a systematic review of evidence. Journal of Intellectual Disabilities Research 55(2), 1009–1019.

Rouse L, Finlay WML 2016. Repertoires of responsibility for diabetes management by adults with intellectual disabilities and those who support them. Sociology of Health and Illness 38(8), 1243–1257.

Schalock RL, Borthwick-Duffy SA, Bradley VJ et al 2010. Intellectual disability: definition, classification and systems of supports, 11th edn. American Association on Intellectual and Developmental Disabilities, Washington DC.

Schalock RL, Luckasson RA, Shogren KA 2007. The renaming of mental retardation: understanding the change to the term intellectual disability. Intellectual and Developmental Disabilities 45(2), 116–124.

SeeAbility 2016. SeeAbility facts. Online. Available: www.seeability.org/

Slevin E, Northway R 2014. Obesity. In: L Taggart, W Cousins (eds), Health promotion for people with intellectual and developmental disabilities. McGraw Hill Education, Maidenhead, Berkshire.

Slowie D, Martin G 2014. Narrowing the health inequality gap by annual health checks for patients with intellectual disability. The British Journal of General Practice 64, 101–102.

Stancliffe RJ, Bigby C, Balandin S et al 2015. Transition to retirement and participation in mainstream community groups using active mentoring: a feasibility and outcomes evaluation with a matched comparison group. Journal of Intellectual Disability Research 59(8), 703–718.

Stancliffe R, Lakin K, Larson S et al 2011. Overweight and obesity among adults with intellectual disabilities who use intellectual disability/developmental disability services in 20 US states. Intellectual and Developmental Disabilities 116(6), 401–418.

Stancliffe R, Lante K, Davis G et al 2014. Psychosocial outcomes following participation in a physical activity and exercise intervention. Journal of Applied Research in Intellectual Disabilities 27(4), 326.

Stancliffe RJ, Wilson NJ, Gambin N et al 2013. Transition to retirement: a guide to inclusive practice. Sydney University Press, Sydney.

Sullivan SG, Slack-Smith LM et al 2004. Understanding the use of breast cancer screening services by women with intellectual disabilities. Social and Preventative Medicine 49(6), 398–405.

Taggart L, Coates V, Truesdale-Kennedy M 2013. Management and quality indicators of diabetes mellitus in people with intellectual disabilities. Journal of Intellectual Disability Research 57(12), 1152–1163.

Trip H, Conder J, Hale L et al 2016. The role of key workers in supporting people with intellectual disability in the self-management of their diabetes: a qualitative New Zealand study. Health and Social Care in the Community 24(6), 789–798.

Trollor JN, Srasuebkul P, Xu H et al 2017. Cause of death and potentially avoidable deaths in Australian adults with intellectual disability using retrospective linked data. BMJ Open, 7, e013489.

Tyler F, Ling S, Bhaumik S et al 2020. Diabetes in adults with intellectual disability: prevalence and associated demographics, lifestyle, independence and health factors. Journal of Intellectual Disabilities Research 64(4), 287–295.

United Nations 2006. United Nations Convention on the Rights of Persons with Disabilities. Online. Available: www.un.org/development/desa/disabilities/convention-on-the-rights-of-persons-with-disabilities.html.

Walmsley J 2011. An investigation into the implementation of annual health checks for people with intellectual disabilities. Journal of Intellectual Disabilities 15(3), 157–166.

Ware RS, Lennox NG 2016. Characteristics influencing attendance at a primary care health check for people with intellectual disability: an individual participant data meta-analysis. Research in Development Disabilities 55, 235–241.

Whitehead LC, Trip HT, Hale LA et al 2016. Negotiating autonomy in diabetes self-management: the experiences of adults with intellectual disability and their support workers. Journal of intellectual Disability Research 60(4), 389–397.

Wilson NJ, Frawley P 2016. Transition staff discuss sex education and support for young men and women with intellectual and developmental disability. Journal of Intellectual and Developmental Disability 41(3) 209–221.

Wilson NJ, Lin Z, Villarosa A, George A 2019. Oral health status and reported oral health problems in people with intellectual disability: a literature review. Journal of Intellectual and Developmental Disability 44(3), 292–304.

Wilson NJ, Lin Z, Villarosa A, Lewis P et al 2019. Countering the poor oral health of people with intellectual and developmental disability: a scoping literature review. BMC: Public Health 19, 1530.

Wilson NJ, Parmenter TR, Stancliffe RJ et al 2010. A masculine perspective of gendered topics in the research literature on males and females with intellectual disability. Journal of Intellectual and Developmental Disability 35(1), 1–8.

Wilson NJ, Shuttleworth RP, Stancliffe RJ et al 2012. Masculinity theory in applied research with men and boys with intellectual disability. Intellectual and Developmental Disabilities 50(3), 261–272.

Wilson NJ, Wiese M, Lewis P et al 2019. Nurses working in intellectual disability-specific settings talk about the uniqueness of their role: a qualitative study. Journal of Advanced Nursing 75(4), 812–822.

Wilson-Jones M, Morgan E 2010. Cerebral palsy. In: CL Betz, WM Nehring (eds), Nursing care for individuals with intellectual and developmental disabilities: an integrated approach. Paul H Brookes, Baltimore, MA.

Woodhouse MJ 2010. Eye diseases and visual impairment. In: J O'Hara, J McCarthy, N Bouras (eds), Intellectual disability and ill health: a review of the evidence. Cambridge University Press, Cambridge.

World Health Organization (WHO) 2020. Diabetes fact sheet. Online. Available: www.who.int/news-room/fact-sheets/detail/diabetes/.

World Health Organization (WHO) 2002. Active ageing: a policy framework. WHO, Geneva.

Wullink M, Widdershoven G, van Schrojenstein Lantman-de Valk H et al 2009. Autonomy in relation to health among people with intellectual disability: a literature review. Journal of Intellectual Disability Research 53(9), 816–826.

Yang Q, Rasmussen SA, Friedman JM 2002. Mortality associated with Down's syndrome in the USA from 1983 to 1997: a population-based study. Lancet 359, 1019–1025.

CHAPTER 9

Management of Chronic Pain

CHRISTINE CHISENGANTAMBU • PAUL McDONALD

LEARNING OBJECTIVES

When you have completed this chapter you will be able to:

- identify the scope and impact of chronic pain in Australia
- discuss the relevance of a biopsychosocial model of chronic pain for persons with chronic illness and disability
- identify key components of pain assessment
- acknowledge the central role the person with chronic pain takes in the management of their health
- identify a range of therapies available for the management of chronic pain
- identify factors influencing managing pain in co-morbidity and substance abuse patients.

KEY WORDS

biopsychosocial model

chronic pain

disability-related pain

pain assessment

pain management

INTRODUCTION

Chronic pain is a global condition which is highly prevalent and is a major leading cause of physical and psychosocial disability. Chronic pain leads to loss of employment, interference with daily activities, emotional distress, depression and social isolation from family and friends (Backe et al 2018; World Health Organization [WHO] 2018). According to Pain Australia (2019a), in 2018 3.24 million Australians were living with chronic pain, of whom 1.50 million were male and 1.74 million were female. On the other hand, 2.21 million Australians of working age were living with chronic pain, accounting for more than 68% of the total figure. Furthermore, 1.03 million older Australians (65 years and over) were living with chronic pain, with rates almost twice as high as the working age population (Pain Australia 2019). The total financial cost associated with chronic pain was estimated to be $73.2 billion in 2018, which equates to $22,588 per person with chronic pain (Pain Australia 2019). The clinical significance of chronic pain in the context of a disabling disease is underscored by the negative impact of pain on a person's level of functioning. Chronic pain can cause severe physical, emotional, social and economic problems for affected individuals and their significant others.

The International Association of the Study of Pain (IASP) and WHO have included a classification of pain in the International Classification of Disease (ICD) – ICD-11, and recognise chronic pain as a cluster of chronic pain conditions (Sukel 2019; WHO 2018). Based on this classification, chronic pain is recognised as a health condition and a disorder in its own right, as well as a symptom that is secondary to an underlying disease, and has its own taxonomy and its own definition (Mills et al 2019; Sukel 2019).

This chapter is written for nurses and other health professionals to provide a broad overview of what is a complex topic. It briefly reviews the scope and nature of chronic pain with a particular focus on chronic pain secondary to chronic illness and disability. It argues the relevance of a biopsychosocial model of chronic disability-related pain and discusses the important role of some key psychosocial factors in shaping the pain experience. Key components of pain assessment and the array of therapies available are also briefly outlined.

CHRONIC PAIN DEFINED

Pain is a major symptom of many medical conditions and is one of the most cited reasons for seeking medical attention. However, chronic pain has been noted to be difficult to operationalise (Pitcher et al 2019). Nevertheless, chronic pain is characterised by pain that persists beyond the normal expected time of healing or injury and that lasts approximately beyond 3 months (The Australian Pain Society 2019). Commonly, pain has been defined to include unpleasant sensation. Although this definition has come under criticism, the most commonly used and the most oft-cited definition of pain and the one accepted by the International Association for the Study of Pain (IASP) (IASP 1979/2011) is:

Pain is an unpleasant sensory and emotional experience associated with actual or potential tissue damage or described in terms of such damage.

It is strongly postulated that the definition of pain should include a social view, which supports the most widely accepted and clinically useful definition of pain, 'Pain is whatever the experiencing person says it is, existing whenever the experiencing person say it does' (McCaffery 1968, p. 95). Supporting this definition is the understanding that pain is a subjective experience that exists in the person that feels it (Treede 2018).

Both of the above definitions highlight the fact that pain is what the person perceives pain to be. Secondly, both of the definitions underscore the inherent subjectivity of pain and acknowledge the importance of emotional as well as sensory factors in the pain experience. Arguably though, the McCaffery (1968) definition highlights the need to believe what the patient says about the pain and eliminates the personal biases of the nurse or practitioner in interpreting how pain is assessed and managed. It is important to note that although pain is usually considered to be a warning signal of actual or potential tissue damage, it can occur in the absence of tissue damage, even though the experience may be described as if the damage has occurred.

Before exploring chronic pain, it is important to understand acute pain. In evolutionary terms, *acute pain* can be understood as an important biological protective mechanism to warn the body of injury or disease. It directs immediate attention to the situation, promotes reflexive withdrawal and fosters other actions that prevent further damage and enhance healing.

Acute pain usually stops long before healing has occurred, which may take days or a few weeks. The mechanisms underlying the transition from acute to chronic pain include a complex interaction of physiological, emotional, cognitive, social and environmental factors. Thus, in contrast to acute pain, chronic pain persists constantly or intermittently past the normal time of healing and serves no biological purpose. It refers to pain that persists for extended periods of time (i.e. months or years), that accompanies a disease process, or that is associated with an injury that has not resolved within an expected time (IASP 2019; Salduker et al 2019). Chronic pain is simply defined as pain lasting longer than 3 months or past the standard time for tissue to heal (Salduker et al 2019).

The IASP (2019) argue that chronic pain should be recognised as a condition in its own right, underpinned by an agreed set of definitions and taxonomy (Treede et al 2019). In addition, pain is recognised as a form of disability for conditions such as back pain (Doody & Bailey 2017). It is therefore important to understand chronic pain and the need to take into account not only the intensity of pain but also pain-related disability and distress, along with psychosocial factors that contribute to the experience of pain (Mills et al 2019; Sukel 2019).

CAUSES OF CHRONIC PAIN

The causes of chronic pain are multifactorial and attributed to modifiable and non-modifiable factors; neuropathic and non-neuropathic and an interplay of biological, clinical, psychological, social, cultural, behavioural and lifestyles (Mills et al 2019). Arguably, the causes of chronic pain have taken a broader scope and contextual view of its complex pathophysiological aetiologies (Frenkel & Swartz 2017).

One of the most salient contributors to the pathophysiology of chronic pain is the neuroplasticity of the nervous system. This refers to the ability of neurons throughout the peripheral and central nervous systems to change their structure and function as a result of nociceptive input. In sum, chronic pain is perpetuated by a combination of multiple factors that are both pathogenetically and physically remote from the originating cause (Bruggink et al 2019; Doody & Bailey 2017; Linton et al 2018; Mill et al 2019).

Although pain problems are often classified by duration, another approach is to categorise pain problems based on underlying mechanisms. Nociceptive (physiological) pain is sustained by ongoing activation of the sensory system that subserves the perception of noxious stimuli. It implies the existence of damage to somatic or visceral tissues sufficient to activate the nociceptive system (Sneddon 2018). On the other hand, neuropathic (pathophysiological) pain is sustained by a set of mechanisms that are driven by damage to, or dysfunction of, the peripheral or central nervous systems (Treede et al 2019; Yam et al 2018). Neuropathic pain problems are common in diseases that affect the nervous system, such as multiple sclerosis, diabetes mellitus and herpes zoster. It may also result from surgery or trauma to nervous tissue. These divergent views reflect the theoretical perspectives of researchers based on the presumed aetiology of chronic pain. Consistent with this view, Woessner (2019) points to the fundamentally different assumptions relating to pain based on its pathology and that there are multitudes of pain-pathology referral patterns. Woessner (2019, p. 2) postulates that 'chronic pain most likely, involves all three types of pain — nociceptive, neuropathic, and central. Varying degrees and patterns of these dysfunctions occur to result in the different pain conditions'.

Pain in general is considered the fifth vital sign (Levy et al 2018; Tompkins et al 2017) and chronic pain on the other hand is considered a primary condition in its own right that needs specific tailored interventions. Woessner (2019, p. 3) asserts that:

> No matter how complex the pain problems of any individual patient, patterns of pathology do emerge and treatment options can be chosen.

THE ECONOMIC AND SOCIAL IMPACT OF CHRONIC PAIN

Much less is known about the specific impact of pain on physical and psychosocial functioning among people who already have a physical disability. Although there are significant gaps in the literature, the available evidence indicates that chronic disability-related pain is associated with poorer adjustment and reduced quality of life, independent of the effects of the disease itself. Overall, the literature demonstrates that chronic pain adversely affects the daily functioning and quality of life (Hadi et al 2019; Grabovac & Dorner 2019; Mills et al 2019; Stompór et al 2019). Notably, chronic pain is a prevalent major health problem which is often under-recognised in people with chronic conditions and disability, exacting a substantial social and economic burden on the affected individual (Mills et al 2019). A global epidemialogical study of chronic diseases found that 1.9 billion people were affected by common symptomatic chronic conditions, such as tension headaches, low back and neck pain (Mills et al

2019). According to AIHW (2019), back pain is the second leading cause of disease burden in Australia, with one in six Australians (16%) suffering from back problems. Further, additional studies indicate that pain is prevalent in conditions such as stroke (Churchill et al 2019), multiple sclerosis (Murphy et al 2017) and kidney failure (Davison 2019), to mention a few. A consistent observation to note in these studies is that individuals often report multiple types of pain and a significant subset experience moderate-to-severe pain intensity on a daily basis. What has also been noted in many conditions is that once pain develops in chronic conditions it often becomes a chronic problem across the illness trajectory. In making this observation, as the life expectancy of individuals with chronic illness increases, the prevalence of pain problems over the entire disease span worsens in the absence of reversible causes. When this happens, it is suggestive of disability-related pain, which is often best conceptualised as a chronic pain condition (van Hecke et al 2013).

Pain is a common and often under-recognised problem among people with chronic illness and disability. Literature on pain has documented the profound effects that chronic pain has on mood, personality and social relationships, as well as the concomitant experiences of depression, sleep disturbance and decrease in overall function. A study on lower back pain revealed overall limited functioning, poorer self-reported health, lower quality of life and depression, as well as more workplace absenteeism (Grabovac & Dorner 2019; Stompór et al 2019). Much less is known about the specific impact of pain on physical and psychosocial functioning among people who already have a physical disability.

For most of those affected, the presence of chronic pain compromises all aspects of their lives and the lives of their significant others. Enduring pain can create a sense of hopelessness and helplessness, also increasing feelings of depression (Sheng et al 2017). Wallis's (2005) words capture the pervasive impact of chronic pain (p. 46):

> Chronic pain is a thief. It breaks into your body and robs you blind. With lightning fingers, it can take away your livelihood, your marriage, your friends, your favourite pastimes and big chunks of your personality. Left unapprehended, it will steal your days and your nights until the world has collapsed into a cramped cell of suffering.

The increasing burden of pain, as well as the growing insight by clinicians that pain affects the person as a whole, has seen the rapid development of a large body of literature on pain and quality of life (QOL) in varying conditions (Adewusi et al 2019; Hadi et al 2018; Lemos et al 2019; Zis, Sarrigiannis et al 2019; Zis, Varrassi et al 2019). Observations from these studies denote pain as having a significant adverse effect on QOL. This effect exists despite the different types of pain, diseases, cultures and individuals. Secondly, the effect is pervasive and is manifested in many domains of life. The body domains most affected are the physical, followed by the emotional, social and cognitive functioning. Thirdly, the degree and kind of impact on QOL is often associated with features of pain such as its duration, intensity, present activation and salience of affective and evaluative components, as well as the disease that contributes to modulating the meaning of the pain and characteristics of the patients themselves – demographic and psychological issues.

When all facts are put together, it is clear that chronic pain is poorly understood by the general community, including many health professionals. The next section deals with these important conceptual issues.

UNDERSTANDING CHRONIC PAIN SECONDARY TO DISABILITY

The early theories of pain primarily focused on understanding the biological and pathophysiological components of pain, and there is an extensive literature examining the utility of these models (Gatchel & Howard 2019). Much of this work, however, focused on illness and biological processes and on individuals suffering from chronic non-malignant pain as a primary condition (e.g. chronic low back pain, headaches). In contrast, very little has been written about the experience of chronic pain secondary to a disabling disease, despite pain being a prominent characteristic of many chronic diseases and having the potential to compound distress and disability (Summers et al 2019). This is particularly the case for rehabilitation populations such as people with multiple sclerosis, spinal cord injury and cerebral palsy. Nevertheless, little is known, for example, about how pain contributes to disability, distress and QOL in these populations. Several studies point out the relationship between chronic pain and disability. There is also recognition of the impact of psychosocial and psychological aspects of chronic pain conditions linked to chronic diseases such as arthritis, cancer and sickle cell disease. It is recognised that this also impacts on a person's level of resilience when experiencing chronic pain (Ferrari et al 2019; Summers et al 2019).

A major contributor to the current situation is the failure of the prevailing biomedical model of pain to provide an adequate conceptualisation of chronic pain complicating disability. Although the dominant theoretical model in the chronic pain literature is a biopsychosocial model, most health professionals and laypersons continue to view disability-related pain from a traditional biomedical model (Gatchel & Howard 2019). According to this view, chronic pain is a symptom of underlying disease activity that can be treated only by identifying and correcting underlying tissue pathology. And as such, psychological and social factors are viewed as reactions to pain; once the underlying disease is successfully treated the associated psychosocial complications are also believed to supposedly disappear. While this model has proved useful in producing a number of important insights into pathophysiological mechanisms and the development of pharmacological treatments for clinical pain, it falls short when faced with the complexity of chronic pain (Hulla et al 2019).

Investigators' loyalty to the biomedical model can in part be attributed to the prevalent assumption that chronic pain secondary to chronic illness and disability is uniquely different to chronic pain as a primary condition. The putative distinction between these conditions implies that, since they are unique, the principles that are important to each differ and thus they should be viewed and treated differently. This distinction is based primarily on the belief that disability-related pain is closely tied to disease activity or tissue damage, whereas the association between reports of pain and tissue damage in people with chronic pain as a primary condition is of lower magnitude and, in some cases, largely non-existent. Thus, researchers concerned with disability-related pain have attempted to explain it in terms of disease activity and pathological pain mechanisms. Conversely, literature on chronic pain as a primary condition has paid greater attention to the role of psychosocial and environmental contributors to pain.

What has not been argued so cogently, however, is that even when a disease process is identifiable and treatable, psychosocial factors remain central to the development and perpetuation of chronic pain and may provide fruitful targets for intervention.

It could therefore be argued that although over the past few decades a major paradigm shift has occurred in the conceptualisation of chronic pain from a biopsychosocial perspective, pain experienced by individuals with a disability continues to be understood largely from a traditional biomedical model, despite its inherent limitations. Instead, an integrative model of chronic pain which attends to the multiple physical, psychosocial and behavioural factors involved is a more useful perspective to guide the study, assessment and treatment of disability-related pain.

TOWARDS A BIOPSYCHOSOCIAL MODEL OF CHRONIC DISABILITY-RELATED PAIN

Understanding chronic pain requires an understanding of psychological factors, including the emotional beliefs and mood factors related to the pain experience. This is because pain is regarded to be not only a sensation which is related to tissue damage but also an individualised perception that is strongly associated with and is perceived from a biopsychosocial model standpoint view and person's attitudes towards, as well as their pain-specific coping strategies (Tracy 2017; Vadivelu et al 2017).

Despite this association of a biomedical conceptualisation of disability-related pain, the assumption that there exists a simple one-to-one relationship between tissue pathology and pain has been convincingly refuted in the general pain literature. Over time, it is far more likely that psychosocial and behavioural factors interact with tissue damage to influence adjustment to pain (Woessner 2019). Thus, it is argued here that disability-related pain may best be viewed from a biopsychosocial perspective that seeks to incorporate the interrelationships among physical, psychological and social factors and the changes that occur among these relationships over time.

Biopsychosocial theorists draw attention to the distinction between disease and illness in understanding chronic pain (Gatchel & Howard 2019). Whereas the biomedical model has focused on disease, an objective, disruptive biological event caused by pathological, anatomic or physiological changes, the biopsychosocial model instead emphasises illness (Gatchel & Howard 2019; Woessner 2019). Illness is subjectively interpreted as an undesirable state of health based on the patient's concrete experiences. This, in turn, has a considerable influence on health-related behaviours, which include emotional, functional and psychosocial aspects of self (Seidlein & Salloch 2019).

The conceptual view of the biopsychosocial model is presented in Fig. 9.1. These nested circles within the model demonstrate the interdependent relationships among processes that culminate in the person's perception of pain and overt pain behaviours. For example, biological factors may initiate and maintain nociceptive input, psychological factors influence the interpretation and perception of pain, and social factors shape the person's behavioural responses.

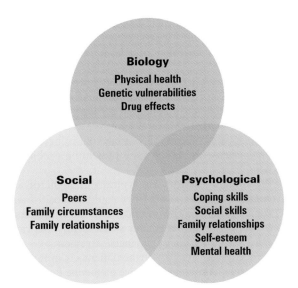

FIG. 9.1 **Biopsychosocial Model of Pain.**
Turk & Burwinkle 2006.

Several key assumptions characterise the biopsychosocial model of pain (Gatchel & Howard 2019). A central premise of the model is the multidimensional nature of chronic pain. From this perspective, pain is never solely somatically or psychologically based. Instead, the model posits that neurobiological, psychological and sociocultural factors interact to contribute to the development and perpetuation of pain. According to the model, it is this dynamic and reciprocal interplay among biomedical, psychosocial and behavioural factors that produces the individual's subjective experience of, and responses to, pain. Nociceptive stimulation, for example, can cause biological, psychological and social changes, which, in turn, affect future responses to pain. Moreover, psychological and social mechanisms can modulate nociceptive input and the response to treatment (Gatchel & Howard 2019; Walters & Williams 2019; Woessner 2019). The model also explicitly acknowledges that during the evolution of a pain problem, the relative level of impact of physical, psychological and social factors may shift. Thus, although biomedical factors may initiate the report of pain and predominate during the acute phase, over time they play an increasingly important role in the maintenance of and adjustment to pain (Hulla et al 2019).

The biopsychosocial model advocates a wider view that extends beyond treating disease to treating factors that contribute to illness (Gatchel & Howard 2019). By using the biopsychosocial model, different ways of understanding and managing chronic pain, which include, initiate, maintain and modulate physical, as well as individuals' perceptions about their pain, determine how they cope and manage the pain (Murphy et al n.d.).

In summary, the biopsychosocial conceptualisation of pain views a patient as being more than a diagnostic label and it takes into account the 4Ps (Bolton & Gillett 2019; PsycDB 2020).

1. **Predisposing factors** are areas of vulnerability that increase the risk for the presenting problem/pain.
2. **Precipitating factors** are typically thought of as stressors or other events (they could be positive or negative) that may be precipitants of the symptoms.
3. **Perpetuating factors** are any social factors that can exacerbate the pain, e.g. financial stress, etc.
4. **Protective factors** include the patient's own insight into their pain and supportive elements. Protective factors counteract the predisposing, precipitating and perpetuating factors.

In summary, the dominant biomedical model of disability-related pain, whose emphasis is on underlying disease activity and tissue damage alone, is too narrow in scope to accommodate the complexity of chronic pain.

Although there is a large body of evidence to support a biopsychosocial model in understanding and treating chronic pain as a primary condition, only recently have researchers begun to examine its utility among persons with disability-related pain (Martinez-Calderon et al 2018).

CULTURAL DETERMINANTS OF THE EXPERIENCE OF CHRONIC PAIN

Culture is a significant factor in shaping beliefs about pain and it affects how people interpret and respond to pain, determining acceptable pain behaviours and giving meaning to the pain experience (Givle & Maani-Fogelma 2020; Liao et al 2016). There is a lot of research examining the impact of racial, ethnic and cultural influence on understanding the meaning of how pain is perceived and managed (Orhan et al 2018). According to Mittinty and colleagues (2018), cultural and social environment, which is inclusive of beliefs, customs, languages, relationships with self, society and environment, significantly influences how an individual experiences and expresses pain and is central to interpretation of behaviour by healthcare providers. Thus, culture affects the individual's perception, report and expression of pain. Pain assessment and management strategies put in place can easily fail

if cultural considerations are not addressed between the individual and the healthcare provider.

A system review study looked at the understanding of pain among Australian Aboriginal and Torres Strait Islander peoples. They found that beliefs of both patients and practitioners are important in considering effective approaches for assessment and management of pain. This study insists that if pain is to be managed effectively, health professionals must appreciate their own, as well as their client's, beliefs, culture and influence on the patient's perceptions of pain (Arthur & Rolan 2019).

There is a paucity of research examining the pain experience of Australian Aboriginal and Torres Strait Islander peoples. Various studies have looked at cultural and communication misconceptions about interpretation of pain among Indigenous people. Research studies carried out by Fenwick (2006), and Fenwick and Stevens (2004) cited by Arthur and Rolan (2019), state that the misconception that Aboriginal people have a high pain tolerance requiring less pain relief is outdated and erroneous. On the other hand, the cultural misunderstanding and misinterpretation of Indigenous people being quiet and withdrawn requires healthcare professionals to understand sociocultural aspects and to respect and to have knowledge of cultural issues (Lin et al 2017). The key message is the importance of those involved in pain management being aware of the complexity of cultural social issues. Given that communication is the main component of culture, ineffective communication leads to ineffective care delivery and healthcare outcomes (LiLi 2017).

Givle and Maani-Fogelma (2020) and Arthur and Rolan (2019) state cultural factors which should be considered when caring for people in pain from diverse cultural backgrounds. They recommend several key strategies to assist in culturally appropriate assessment and management, namely: (1) utilising assessment tools to assist in measuring pain underlined by assessing beliefs and norms that influence the perception of pain; (2) appreciating variations in affective response to pain; (3) being sensitive to variations in communication styles; (4) recognising that communication of pain may not be acceptable within a culture; (5) appreciating that the meaning of pain varies between cultures; (6) utilising the knowledge of biological variations; (7) developing a personal awareness of values and beliefs that may affect responses to pain; (8) incorporating effective cultural practices into care; (9) using a family-centred approach, as family plays an important role in care; and (10) using interpreter services to ensure effective communication.

According to Laverty and colleagues (2017), and Bainbridge and colleagues (2015), in Australia, ensuring culturally safe care requires embedding Closing the Gap measures, which suggests that health practitioners need to provide culturally competent care if they are to be responsive to healthcare needs of diverse cultural groups. Undoubtedly, cultural competency is one of the key strategies for reducing inequalities for access to health-care services and contributes to improving the quality and effectiveness of care delivered. Cultural competency involves respect and ensures that 'the cultural diversity, rights, views, values and expectations of Aboriginal and Torres Strait Islander peoples are respected in the delivery of culturally appropriate health services' (Bainbridge et al 2015, p. 4). This means that mainstream nurses working within rich cultural environments need to listen to Indigenous people and respect the differences that exist. Furthermore, health professionals need to adopt culturally safe pain assessment and management strategies, and, wherever possible, defer to the person with chronic pain, as well as to their family and friends for cultural interpretations. Wherever possible, help should be sought from professionals with inside understanding of cultural norms; an obvious example is of Indigenous health workers in Australia.

Developing and using culturally appropriate management tools that build trust between health professionals and Aboriginal people is reported as one of the most important strategies for addressing such issues (Arthur & Rolan 2019).

PAIN BELIEFS AND COPING STRATEGIES

People with chronic pain develop underlying beliefs, attitudes and assumptions in an attempt to make sense of their pain condition. These include attributions about the cause, meaning and appropriate treatment of pain, as well as perceptions of the degree of control over pain and personal coping efficacy (Järemo et al 2017). Although certain beliefs may be adaptive and promote positive adjustment, others are likely to contribute to heightened pain, distress and disability. A large and growing body of research shows that pain-related beliefs are strongly associated with various measures of pain severity, physical and psychosocial functioning (Meints & Edwards 2018), as well as response and adherence to multidisciplinary pain treatments (Tompkins et al 2017). For example, beliefs that one does not have control over pain, that pain signifies harm and that one is disabled by pain are particularly problematic for people with chronic pain; however, increases in self-efficacy beliefs for managing pain appear to be beneficial

(Karasawa et al 2019). Observably, people who have high levels of self-efficacy, expectations of recovery, better control and management of their lives are able to confront situations that minimise the potential impact of the negative psychological factors, for example, pain catastrophising (Martinez-Calderon et al 2018). Evidently, high levels of self-efficacy predict greater physical functioning, physical activity participation, health status and seemingly, self-efficacy has a significant reverse association with disability, emotional distress and pain severity (Martinez-Calderon et al 2018). Undoubtedly, beliefs, appraisals and expectancies held by individuals regarding the possible consequences of pain and their abilities to deal with them, are hypothesised to affect functioning directly by influencing mood, as well as indirectly influencing coping efforts (Karasawa et al 2019).

Faced with ongoing pain, individuals also learn and utilise a variety of strategies to help cope or deal with their pain (Jones 2019). Pain-coping is defined as purposeful cognitive and behavioural efforts to manage or negate the negative impact of pain (Chen & Jackson 2019; Ho 2019). Gandhi and colleagues (2017) state that coping with chronic pain refers to accepting responsibility for dealing with one's pain and to be actively engaged in developing strategies for pain reduction and the pursuit of other life goals. Thus, the strategies utilised to cope with chronic pain require embracing lifestyle adaptations and self-management. Some of these adaptive functioning and passive coping strategies include lifestyle changes, such as exercising, resting or medication use and relaxation techniques (Murphy et al n.d., p. 23).

Pain Catastrophising

One specific maladaptive coping response that has consistently demonstrated robust associations with virtually all pain outcomes investigated, is termed catastrophising. Pain catastrophising is an exaggerated negative cascade of cognitive and emotional responses to actual or anticipated pain, which involves feelings of magnification, rumination and hopelessness (Gatchel & Neblett 2020). In confronting catastrophising, negative and non-constructive thinking can be transformed into more constructive, positive self-talk and thinking, which is considered to reduce negative emotional components.

Literature reveals pain catastrophising to be associated with higher levels of pain intensity, distress and disability and fear avoidance (Gatchel & Neblett 2020). Arguably, pain catastrophising involves distorted cognitions and misinterpretations of pain management information. It is therefore highly suggestive that adoptive coping strategies be used to change maladaptive beliefs about pain-inclusive cognitive behaviour therapy (CBT) and that interdisciplinary pain management approaches based upon the biopsychosoci model of pain be applied (Gatchel & Neblett 2020).

In summary, strong and consistent associations between psychosocial factors and adjustment to pain have been observed in disability groups, including catastrophising cognitions, task persistence, guarding and coping responses.

STIGMA AND CHRONIC PAIN

The broader social context of the individual also profoundly shapes chronic pain experience. One of the most important social aspects, from the perspective of people with chronic pain, is stigmatisation of chronic pain. Frequently, a person with chronic pain faces not only the negative personal impact of pain, but also the potent social dilemma of not being believed or having their experience delegitimised by others. Indeed, it is the very nature of chronic pain – its invisibility, its subjectivity and gender biases – which create such a challenge to both the healthcare provider and the sufferer (Samulowitz et al 2018). Pain simply cannot be proved or disproved. In contrast to the visible manifestations of disease, pain is privately experienced, demonstrable to others only through the individual's self-report or other non-verbal pain behaviours. Heshusius (2009, p. 14) states that:

> We appear normal. That is our liability. One can wince and moan only for so long. There comes a point where giving expression to one's pain takes energy one no longer has. One becomes quiet and pain becomes internalised ... Also, wincing and moaning when in acute pain are instinctive behaviours to which others respond with sympathy. When it becomes clear the pain will not go away, others may feel helpless. They may start to think you are exaggerating. They may be overwhelmed. They change the subject. The person in pain withdraws. You try to keep your composure, to stay coherent, not fall apart. Others will see exhaustion and depression in your face before they see pain.

The invisibility and often lack of known physical basis for chronic pain frequently invites speculation and judgement from others about its legitimacy. In the past, this has led to labelling individuals as fraudulent when they claim pain over time for which there is no medical explanation. This stigma, attached to those who report pain without an identifiable pathological basis, occurs in part because their illness falls outside of the socially sanctioned biomedical model of healthcare (Lies & Kenneth 2016). Literature reviews noted that there was a high prevalence of stigmatisation in people with pain, and there was a significant correlation between the type of stigma experienced, the level of pain intensity and other psychological factors, including self-esteem, anxiety and depression (Carr 2016). Given such a scenario, over time people with disabilities tend to keep pain hidden from others to avoid negative responses and the threat of stigma. Roman emperor and philosopher, Marcus Aurelius, wrote:

> When in pain, always be prompt to remind yourself that there is nothing shameful about it. Bear in mind also that, though we do not realize it, many other things which we find uncomfortable are, in fact, of the same nature as pain: feelings of lethargy, for example, or loss of appetite (quoted in Carr 2016).

In contrast to visible impairments, pain problems may be dismissed or discredited by friends, family, co-workers and others. People with physical disabilities are often particularly aware of the contested nature of their pain experience during encounters with healthcare providers (Craig et al 2020; Dubin et al 2017; Goldberg 2017, 2020). From their perspective, pain is often trivialised by healthcare providers as a natural or expected part of their disease, or dismissed altogether, and in some instances, pain is misunderstood. For example, a study examining the views of patients and health professionals on managing fibromyalgia revealed that the care provided by doctors and other healthcare professionals was perceived as deficient. Patients described being misunderstood by the professionals caring for them; consequently, there was a lack of understanding and support by healthcare providers (Dubin et al 2017; Scott et al 2019).

To address this issue, health professionals need to critically reflect on their own, often inadvertent, potential to contribute to the stigmatisation of people with chronic pain and to develop and adopt culturally sensitive stigma reduction measures (Rivera-Segarra et al 2019).

ASSESSMENT OF CHRONIC PAIN

Assessment of pain is an essential step to successful pain management. Nevertheless, many factors need to be considered when assessing pain as these factors have a bearing on how pain is managed. Pain assessment provides a baseline yardstick against which to measure a patient's progress during the course of treatment.

A biopsychosocial assessment of chronic pain is the key to developing an effective management plan.

Assessment begins with a comprehensive pain history (using the PQRST mnemonic), including provoking/palliative factors, quality, region (location) and radiation, severity and temporal pattern (onset, duration, pattern) for each individual pain problem. Evaluation of psychosocial factors, such as pain beliefs and coping strategies, mood and social interactions, should be undertaken. In addition, assessment of the impact of pain on functioning and QOL is also an essential component to direct treatment. Finally, a physical assessment should be completed that focuses on neurological and musculoskeletal body systems.

This section provides a brief introduction to some key pain assessment tools. For a comprehensive review of chronic pain assessment please refer to Fillingim and colleagues (2016) and McCormick and Law (2016).

Pain Rating Scales

Pain intensity is a quantitative estimate of the severity or magnitude of perceived pain. Pain intensity is without a doubt the most salient dimension of pain and a variety of pain-rating scales have been developed to measure it. Most of these tools are highly correlated with each other and therefore they can be used in most situations (McCormick & Law 2016; Pathak et al 2018). What is important is that the assessment tool is selected based on the individual's needs (e.g. developmental, cognitive, language and cultural factors) with consideration for the particular strengths and weaknesses of each tool.

The numerical rating scale (NRS) is the most established, reliable and widely used measure of pain intensity in clinical practice (McCormick & Law 2016; Pathak et al 2018). An NRS asks the client to rate their pain from 0 to 10 (an 11-point scale) or 0 to 100 (a 101-point scale), with the understanding that 0 represents one end of the pain intensity continuum ('no pain') and 10 or 100 represents extreme pain intensity ('pain as bad as it can be'). Clients simply state or circle the number on written versions of the scale that best represents their pain intensity, when asked: 'On a scale of 0 to 10, with 0 being no pain and 10 being the worst possible, where is your pain score?' Based on their study of pain, Pathak and colleagues (2018) and McCormick and Law (2016) recommend a combined NRS and FACES Scale as the preferred pain-rating scale in most clinical settings.

The FACES Pain Scale is a tool that was originally developed for children but has been found to be useful and popular among adults, especially those with cognitive or communication difficulties. Several variations of the FACES Scale concept include cartoon faces

(Wong-Baker FACES Pain Rating Scale; Wong & Baker 1988), hand-drawn realistic depictions (The FACES Pain Scale Revised; Hicks et al 2001) and photographs of actual children in distress (Oucher Scale; Beyer et al 1992). The Wong-Baker FACES Pain Rating Scale, for example, contains six cartoon faces (ranging from 'smiling' to 'crying') and is recommended for persons aged 3 years and older. An explanation is given to the client that each face is a person who feels happy because he has no pain (hurt) or sad because he has some or a lot of pain. Instructions are read to the client and they are asked to choose the face that best describes their pain intensity. There is also the FLACC behavioural pain scale used to assess pain in children: F – Face; L – Legs; A – Activity; C – Cry and C – Consolability (The Royal Children's Hospital Melbourne 2019; Beltramini et al 2017).

A verbal descriptor scale (VDS) simply consists of a list of adjectives describing different levels of pain intensity. Clients are asked to read over the list of descriptors and choose the word that best describes their pain intensity on the scale. A simple and clinically useful example is no pain, mild, moderate and severe pain (scored numerically from 0 to 3).

The visual analogue scale (VAS) consists of a 10 cm horizontal line, representing a continuum of pain intensity, with verbal descriptors at each end (e.g. 'no pain' to 'pain as bad as it can be' or 'worst possible pain'). The client is asked to indicate which point along the line best represents their pain intensity. The distance measured from the 'no pain' end to the mark made by the client is the pain intensity score. The VAS is commonly used in research as a measure of pain intensity.

Quality

Unidimensional measures of pain intensity alone do not capture the other qualitative aspects of pain. Asking the client to describe the quality of their pain using their own words is important. Providing a list of possible descriptors can sometimes be helpful if clients find it difficult to do this.

Although used more for research than clinical practice, the McGill Pain Questionnaire (MPQ), developed by Melzack in 1975, is used as a multidimensional measure of the sensory, affective and evaluative aspects of the pain experience, based on the gate-control theory (Boyle et al 2015).

The MPQ consists of 78 pain descriptors categorised into: (1) sensory-discriminative; (2) motivational-affective; (3) cognitive evaluative; and (4) the miscellaneous dimension (Boyle et al 2015). Twenty groups evaluating the major dimensions of pain quality are used to assess pain. Clients are read each list of descriptors or, using the Likert Scale, they can rate their pain frequency and select one word from each group if it is applicable to their pain. Each of the 78 words has been assigned a rank value within its group. From this data, it is possible to derive a Pain Rating Index (PRI) for the sensory, affective, evaluative and miscellaneous subscales, as well as a total PRI (Boyle et al 2015). The MPQ tool is supported by other pain questions embracing similar but varying sets of pain questions (Victoria Pain Specialists 2019). The psychometric properties of the MPQ have been well established and it is often utilised as the gold standard against which to validate pain measures (Edirisinghe et al 2019). Nevertheless, during assessment, the types of words chosen can also provide valuable information about the underlying pain mechanisms. For example, it has been demonstrated clinically that individuals with neuropathic pain are significantly more likely to use particular sensory adjectives (e.g. electric-shock, burning, tingling, cold, pricking and itching) to describe their pain. A Short-Form MPQ has been developed and recently expanded and revised as the Short-Form MPQ–2 (Dworkin et al 2016; Edirisinghe et al 2019; Jumbo 2019) capable of discriminating between neuropathic and non-neuropathic pain. Other specifically designed measures, such as the Neuropathic Pain Scale (Lape et al 2020), can be useful when a neuropathic component is suspected.

In addition to the tools used to assess chronic pain, three central questions need to be asked to determine how the pain is affecting the functionality of the person and how they are coping with the pain. Turk and colleagues (2016) cover a range of areas: psychosocial and behavioural factors (e.g. mood/affect, coping resources, expectations, sleep quality, physical function and pain-related interference with daily activities).

To answer these questions, the practitioner should use information gathered from the patient's history, physical examination and clinical interviews.

Onset and Duration

Information should be elicited about the onset, duration and pattern of pain. When did the pain begin? How long has it lasted? Does it occur at the same time each day? How often does it recur? Is it intermittent or constant?

Location

To assess pain location, the client is asked to describe or point to all areas of discomfort. Pain sites can be documented on a body diagram. A pain drawing consists of outline drawings of the human body, front and back, on which the participant indicates the location of pain by shading the painful area (see Fig. 9.2 and Case Study 9.1).

Exacerbating/Relieving Factors

The client is asked to describe provoking factors, such as physical movement or position, certain activities or environmental factors. For example, with a ruptured intervertebral disc, low back pain and radiating leg pain is usually aggravated by bending over or lifting objects. When exacerbating factors are identified, it is easier to plan interventions to prevent pain from occurring or worsening. People with chronic pain have usually tried a number of pain management techniques, so it is informative to know whether the client has found effective ways of relieving pain. These can include medication and non-medication pain management techniques. These strategies can then be incorporated into the management plan if appropriate.

Impact of Pain

An assessment of the impact of pain on QOL domains is particularly useful to determine treatment priorities. Several pain assessment instruments incorporate most of the relevant questions and can help standardise pain assessment. Developed in 1989, the Brief Pain Inventory (BPI) was developed initially to assess cancer pain (Cleeland 1989). The BPI has become a measurement tool for assessing clinical pain (Stanhope 2016) and is, for example, widely used to measure pain severity, and for clinical and research purposes (see Fig. 9.2). It is relatively short, easy for patients to complete and is sensitive to changes in pain over time or in response to treatment. The BPI scale assesses the extent to which pain interferes with mood, walking, general activity, work, relations with other people, sleep and enjoyment of life. Using validated, brief screening tools such as the BPI is useful for identifying problems, which can then be more comprehensively assessed by the nurse and/or referred for specialist assessment and management.

Pain Diaries

Pain diaries are effective tools to assess the peaks and troughs of pain, identify triggers and help to determine the effectiveness of treatments (see Fig. 9.3). A common problem is that people fail to fill them out progressively or complete them just before an appointment 'for the nurse'. The client and family should receive explanations of the purpose of using the pain

Brief Pain Inventory

Date ____ / ____ / ____   Time: _____

Name: _____ _____ _____
            Last   First   Middle Initial

1) Throughout our lives, most of us have had pain from time to time (such as minor headaches, sprains and toothaches). Have you had pain other than these everyday kinds of pain today?
   1. Yes   2. No

2) On the diagram, shade in the areas where you feel pain. Put an X on the area that hurts the most.

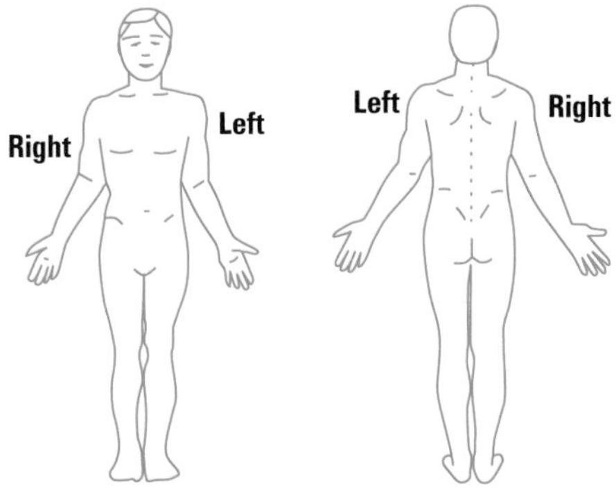

3) Please rate your pain by circling the one number that best describes your pain at its **worst** in the past 24 hours.
   0   1   2   3   4   5   6   7   8   9   10
   No   Pain as bad as
   pain   you can imagine

4) Please rate your pain by circling the one number that best describes your pain at its **least** in the past 24 hours.
   0   1   2   3   4   5   6   7   8   9   10
   No   Pain as bad as
   pain   you can imagine

5) Please rate your pain by circling the one number that best describes your pain on the **average**.
   0   1   2   3   4   5   6   7   8   9   10
   No   Pain as bad as
   pain   you can imagine

6) Please rate your pain by circling the one number that tells how much pain you have **right now**.
   0   1   2   3   4   5   6   7   8   9   10
   No   Pain as bad as
   pain   you can imagine

7) What treatments or medications are you receiving for your pain?
   _____
   _____

8) In the past 24 hours, how much **relief** have pain treatments or medications provided? Please circle the one percentage that most shows how much relief you have received.
   0% 10 20 30 40 50 60 70 80 90 100%
   No   Complete
   relief   relief

9) Circle the one number that describes how, during the past 24 hours, pain has **interfered** with your:

   A. General activity
   0   1   2   3   4   5   6   7   8   9   10
   Does not   Completely
   interfere   interferes

   B. Mood
   0   1   2   3   4   5   6   7   8   9   10
   Does not   Completely
   interfere   interferes

   C. Walking ability
   0   1   2   3   4   5   6   7   8   9   10
   Does not   Completely
   interfere   interferes

   D. Normal work (includes both work outside the home and housework)
   0   1   2   3   4   5   6   7   8   9   10
   Does not   Completely
   interfere   interferes

   E. Relations with other people
   0   1   2   3   4   5   6   7   8   9   10
   Does not   Completely
   interfere   interferes

   F. Sleep
   0   1   2   3   4   5   6   7   8   9   10
   Does not   Completely
   interfere   interferes

   G. Enjoyment of life
   0   1   2   3   4   5   6   7   8   9   10
   Does not   Completely
   interfere   interferes

FIG. 9.2 **Brief Pain Inventory.** Pasero & McCaffery 2011.

CASE STUDY 9.1

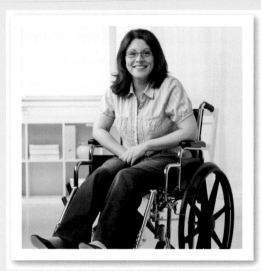

iStockphoto/AVAVA.

The following case study is an example of a nursing assessment of an individual with chronic disability-related pain drawn from research on the impact of pain on the quality of life of people with multiple sclerosis (Harrison et al 2015).

HISTORY

Mrs L is a 41-year-old married woman living in south-east Queensland, who presents with worsening pain in her hands. She has secondary progressive multiple sclerosis, diagnosed 2 years ago. Mrs L was employed as an office worker, but has been unable to continue working because of increasing pain and fatigue.

Mrs L reports pain and fatigue as her worst MS-related problems. She has minor difficulties with memory and speech. There is some upper extremity involvement with difficult clothing with zips, handling small coins and washing her hair. She also reports bladder incontinence and sexual dysfunction.

Current medications for pain include Avonex, sertraline and gabapentin.

PAIN CHARACTERISTICS

- Using a 0–10 numerical rating scale, Mrs L reported her pain was 2/10 on assessment. Over the past 2 weeks Mrs L rates her pain as 10/10 at its worst, 2/10 at its least and 8/10 on average.
- Mrs L indicated she experiences pain in both hands and right leg, shown on the pain drawings below.
- She completed the McGill Pain Questionnaire and endorsed the following: sensory descriptors were flickering, shooting, lancinating, cramping, searing, hurting and taut; affective descriptors were exhausting, terrifying, punishing and wretched; evaluative descriptor chosen was unbearable; miscellaneous descriptors chosen were radiating, numb, freezing and torturing.
- She describes the pain as constant over the past year and a half.
- Provoking factors identified were heat, stress and friction. She manages her pain best by controlling the temperature (keeping cool) and avoiding stress.

PSYCHOSOCIAL RESPONSES TO PAIN

- On the Pain Beliefs and Perceptions Inventory, Mrs L endorses beliefs about pain constancy and pain permanence, but scores low on beliefs about self-blame or that pain is a mystery.
- The Coping Strategies Questionnaire was administered and scores demonstrate frequent use of catastrophising, praying/hoping and ignoring pain, low scores for coping self-statements or increasing behavioural activities and no use of reinterpreting pain or diverting attention.
- Her perceived self-efficacy was low with perceived control over pain scored as 1/6 and ability to decrease pain 2/6 on the CSQ.

IMPACT OF PAIN

- Mrs L completed the Brief Pain Inventory pain interference scales (0 = does not interfere, 10 = completely interferes) indicating: mood 5/10, walking 0/10, general activity 8/10, work 10/10, relations with other people 3/10, sleep 3/10 and enjoyment of life 5/10.

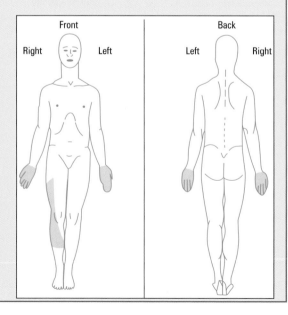

CASE STUDY QUESTIONS

1. What factors should be considered when assessing Mrs L?

2. What type of assessment tool can be used in this situation?

3. Why is it important to consider impact of pain on QOL?

Developed by Christine Chisengantambu.

Pain Control Diary: Patient Example

This is a record of how your pain medicines are working. Please keep this record until you and your nurse/ doctor find the dose and frequency of medicine that provides satisfactory pain relief for you most of the time. After that, you only need to keep this record when you have problems related to your pain medicines.

Name: _____Martin_____   Date: __Friday__

GOALS Satisfactory pain rating: ___3___   **Activities:** _sleep through the night; walk around the house_

Analgesics: _ibuprofen 400 mg 8 am, 2 pm, 8 pm; dulonetine 30 mg 8 am,_

8 pm; MS Contin 100 mg 8 am, 8 pm; MSIR 30 mg every 2 hours if needed

My pain rating scale:

```
  |----|----|----|----|----|----|----|----|----|----|
  0    1    2    3    4    5    6    7    8    9    10
 No                        Moderate               Worst
pain                         pain                possible
                                                  pain
```

Directions: Rate your pain before you take pain medicine and 1 to 2 hours later.

Time	Pain Rating	Pain Medicine I Took	Side Effects (drowsy? upset stomach?)	Other
12:15 am	6	30 MSIR	No	
3	6	30 MSIR		can't sleep
5:15	6	30 MSIR		
8	6	30 MSIR + ibuprofen + MS Contin 100 mg + dulonetine		staying in bed
10	5			talk with nurse
10:30	6	MSIR 45 mg MS Contin 30 mg		
12:30 pm	3			planning to nap

If pain is greater than ___5___ , or if you have other problems with your pain medicine, call:

Nurse: Name/phone   _C. Adams   555-1234_

Doctor: Name/phone   _Jancs   555-4321_

FIG. 9.3 **Pain Diary.** (Yang J, Bauer BA, et al. The Modified WHO Analgesic Ladder: is it appropriate for chronic non-cancer pain?, Journal of Pain Research 2020:13, 411–417. Reprinted with permission from Dove Medical Press Ltd.)

diary, along with information about how and when to complete the diary. The discussion also helps the nurse to establish the degree to which the person is committed to collecting the information.

There is increasing clinical and research interest in the use of electronic pain diaries (e.g. digital pens, palmtop computers, mobile phones) to improve compliance and satisfaction. Research thus far suggests electronic pain assessment tools are preferable as they are easily implemented. They also have been shown to have a high reliability, validity and utility, as their use allows patients to monitor fluctuation of their daily pain levels as well as the effect of therapeutic interventions. Ultimately, the use of pain diaries can enhance in patients the sense of self-control and facilitate communication with caregivers (Charoenpol et al 2019).

CHRONIC PAIN AND CO-MORBIDITIES

Pain is a multidimensional, complex, subjective, perceptual phenomenon, a cardinal sign of many conditions (Lapkin et al 2019). Pain can be brought on by many other conditions and, equally, too many other conditions can bring on pain, affecting its aetiologies and manifestations (Crofford 2015).

Co-morbidity occurs when a person has two or more health conditions at the same time (AIHW 2016). Sufferers of chronic pain can also share co-morbidities and underlying mechanisms for chronic conditions; it can exist in an existing medical condition or because of some direct or indirect causal relationships between existing conditions. Co-morbidities may have profound implications on the degree of physical and social disability which arise with the co-existing condition. Co-morbidities are known to be associated with higher mortality and reduced quality of life and health providers need to take co-morbid diseases into account when treating patients with chronic pain (Ramanathan et al 2018). Chronic conditions compound on pain and play a significant role in the persistence of chronic pain. Equally too, pain appears to be a co-morbid factor of a number of disorders and pain is likely to make these disorders more serious and lead to their chronicity (Brennstuhl et al 2015; Dahan et al 2014; Ramanathan et al 2018). For example, there is a strong association between the presence of chronic pain and mental health conditions, such as depression and anxiety (Brennstuhl et al 2015; Dahan et al 2014; Gatchel et al 2015; Sheng et al 2017). A systematic literature review by IsHak and colleagues (2018) indicates that pain and depression are highly intertwined and may co-exacerbate physical and psychological symptoms. These

symptoms could lead to poor physical functional outcomes and longer duration of symptoms.

Pain also slows recovery from depression, and depression makes pain more difficult to treat. Other chronic conditions in which chronic pain has a significant role and is a common feature include: mental health disorders, diabetes mellitus (DM) with its various pain syndromes, such as peripheral neuropathic, rheumatic diseases and end-stage renal disease (ESRD), to mention a few (Gatchel et al 2015; Hsu et al 2014; Liberman et al 2014; Schreiber et al 2015; Simoes et al 2017).

Chronic pain in co-morbidity contributes to its morbidity, and its effects can be both severe and persistent, contributing significantly to levels of ill-health, loss of QOL, and limiting the general level of functioning and social activities.

The management of chronic pain in people with co-morbidities can be complex and time-consuming, more so than for those with single conditions. The existence of co-morbidity often complicates treatment and management of the existing medical condition, which may need to be understood in view of the physical changes and its associated impact on the co-morbidity conditions and of the management of chronic pain. All co-existing medical conditions need to be understood and managed effectively.

Individuals with multiple chronic conditions have been found to utilise healthcare resources more and to have higher healthcare expenditures and medical care costs (Griffith et al 2019; Hopman et al 2016; Hamar et al 2015). Given the fact that chronic pain is multifactorial in nature, a multimodal and interdisciplinary approach that includes physical and psychological treatment and patient support, together with the use of pharmacological and non-pharmacological therapies based on underlying condition, is vital to managing chronic pain. See Case Study 9.2 for an example of this.

Treatment Options

Treatment options for chronic pain broadly include pharmacological approaches; interventional techniques, including nerve blocks, surgery, implantable drug-delivery systems and spinal-cord stimulators; exercise and physical rehabilitation; psychological treatments; interdisciplinary treatment; and complementary and alternative treatments (American Society of Regional Anaesthesia Pain Medicine 2020). It is beyond the scope of this chapter to provide a detailed discussion of the various treatment options. Nevertheless, various approaches are used for the management of chronic non-cancer pain. These approaches for pain management start with those with lowest risk and least

CASE STUDY 9.2

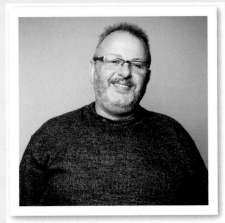

iStockphoto/SilviaJansen.

CHRONIC PAIN AND CO-MORBIDITY

This case study shows a typical professional approach to management of a patient with co-morbidities and chronic pain. It illustrates the challenges and at the same time the importance of using a multimodal, multidisciplinary and holistic approach. Many factors need to be considered in order not only to manage the chronic pain but the increase in pain. These factors include: a) the new medical diagnosis impacting on chronic pain; b) the pharmaceutical therapy that needs to be considered in light of his medical diagnosis; and c) physiological changes (e.g. de-rearranged liver function tests). All these factors need to be considered in light of the demands being made by the patient to increase her/his pain relief medications. Therefore, the nursing role is not only challenged, but is expanded and versatile to ensure coordination of care activities that takes on a broad view in consideration of the patient's medical conditions and social issues.

Social History

Mr W is a 52-year-old Caucasian male, unemployed and separated from his wife. He has two children who live interstate. He currently lives in a two-bedroom housing commission flat on the second floor. He has been trying to lose weight and increase his exercise for the past 6 months without success. He drinks two bottles of beer every night and a glass of red wine with dinner. He also smokes 8 cigarettes a day.

Relevant Medical History

- Diabetes mellitus type 1, end-stage renal disease (ESRD) on haemodialysis × 3 times a week
- Chronic back pain which he sustained 10 years ago on a building site
- Depression

- Substance dependence
- Coronary artery disease (CAD), diagnosed 3 months ago
- Obesity

Presenting Problem

Mr W has been referred by his GP for uncontrolled pain, de-rearranged liver function tests and a gangrenous toe on the right leg. He also complained of having severe pain in his feet and legs, with burning, sharp stabbing, and numbness. He reports his pain as 7–8/10 decreasing to 5 with opioid medication. The pain has worsened in the past 2 weeks and is exacerbated by almost everything and ameliorated by medications. The GP increased his oxycontin and prescribed a fentanyl patch a week ago.

Prior to presenting to his GP, Mr W noticed a black discolouration on his right big toe, which his doctor has put down as gangrenous. His medications at this stage include:

Oxycontin SR 10 mg BD

Gabapentin 50 mg BD

Aspirin 300 mg daily

Fentanyl path 25 mg changed every 3/7

Metformin 1000 mg BD

Isosorbide dinitrate 40 mg daily

Metoprolol 50 mg OD

Warfarin 3 mg daily

Lisinopril 5 mg daily

Atorvastatin 20 mg nocte

Prozac 20 mg daily

Docusate 2 tablets BD

The overall goal is to control the pain and reach a therapeutic level of drug administration where pain is kept at an acceptable level, manage the gangrenous toe and normalise liver function. Pain management strategies are developed in conjunction with the pharmacist, pain team and the treating doctor. As part of the team approach, Mr W is referred to a clinical psychiatrist. During consultation it is revealed that Mr W has given up hope and he has stopped taking his antidepressant medications. Mr W has indicated that he is not in a good relationship with his two sons and that he has not seen either of them for the past 3 years. Mr W has also indicated that he is lonely since he does not go out due to mobility issues. Mr W has been referred to the vascular team for the gangrenous toe and he has also been referred to the physiotherapist, occupational therapist, social worker and discharge planner.

CASE STUDY QUESTIONS

1. How do co-morbidities impact on Mr W?
2. What role will the multidisciplinary/multimodal team play in managing Mr W?
3. What strategies can be used to manage co-morbidities?

Developed by Christine Chisengantambu.

invasiveness to those that are opioid laden and invasive procedures (Duarte et al 2016; Thong 2018).

Analgesics

Analgesia is the first line of management for effective use of pain in either acute or chronic medical conditions, even though the success rate accounts for only 30% (Borsook et al 2011).

There are three classes of analgesics: non-opioids (paracetamol, non-steroidal anti-inflammatory drugs (NSAIDs)), opioids and adjuvant drugs. Developed in 1986, the WHO analgesic pain ladder (Fig. 9.4), which consists of a stepwise approach to administering analgesics depending on pain severity, is a well-known treatment model developed to manage pain in patients with cancer pain, but broadly relevant to either acute and chronic pain problems (Vergne-Salle 2016). The three steps of the analgesic ladder address different pain intensities, beginning with a non-opioid analgesic such as paracetamol or an NSAID and possibly an adjuvant, then adding so-called 'mild' opioids such as codeine and eventually 'strong' opioids such as morphine. A fourth step has been added to the WHO ladder of chronic pain which involves the use of strong opioid analgesic administered in various routes such as nerve block, epidurals, patient-controlled analgesia (PCA) pump, neurolytic block therapy and spinal stimulators (Vargas-Schaffer 2010). Nevertheless, administration of analgesics should be undertaken whenever possible and around the clock, rather than as needed. Adjuvant analgesics are drugs that have a primary indication other than pain, but are analgesic for some painful conditions. They include anticonvulsants, antidepressants, sodium channel blockers or muscle relaxants. Pharmacological management of chronic pain is a complex area and beyond the remit of this chapter.

Impact of Chronic Pain on Sleep

Various studies indicate a strong association between chronic pain and sleep disorders. Chronic pain increases sleep disturbance and insomnia and equally too, lack of sleep increases pain and worsens existing pain in conditions such as headaches, migraine and musculoskeletal pain, and contributes to irritability and mood changes (Dueñas et al 2016; Hadi et al 2019; Jank et al 2017; Finan et al 2013). It is therefore important that management of pain should be directed towards addressing the impact of pain on QOL, particularly mood and sleep (Dueñas et al 2016; Hadi et al 2019).

Sleep promotion interventions, such as teaching the individual and partner about the need for stimulus control, progressive muscle relaxation and sleep practice measures, are the first-line management strategies. Sleep practice measures include establishing a sleep routine, environmental control, limiting caffeine and alcohol (and for some, fluids) during the evening. Other routines may include establishing the bedroom as a sleep room (not for reading, working or hobbies), physical comfort (temperature, perhaps a warm bath

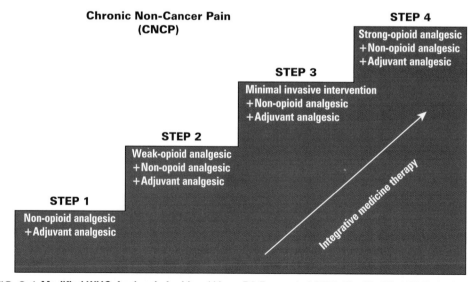

FIG. 9.4 Modified WHO Analgesic Ladder. J Yang, BA Bauer et al 2020. The Modified WHO Analgesic Ladder: is it appropriate for chronic non-cancer pain? Journal of Pain Research 13, 411–417.

just prior to bedtime, planning analgesia so the effects are peaking at the time of falling asleep) and promoting relaxation. If these are ineffective, the assistance of the multidisciplinary team must be sought for additional measures such as hypnotic medication, biofeedback and cognitive behavioural therapy; in summary a multimodal approach is essential (Borys et al 2015).

MANAGEMENT OF CHRONIC PAIN – MULTIMODAL AND MULTIDISCIPLINARY APPROACHES

Recognising that chronic pain and disability are not only influenced by tissue pathology, but also by psychological and social factors, mandates the use of multidisciplinary teams.

Clinical approaches to the treatment of disability-related pain therefore reflect the dominance of a biomedical paradigm and a multimodal approach (Alles & Smith 2018; Tompkins et al 2017; Woessner 2019). Notably though, there is an absence of research examining the effectiveness of multidisciplinary pain programs for chronic disability-related pain. Nevertheless, multimodal and multidisciplinary teams emphasise a range of strategies aimed at maximising pain reduction, improving health-related quality of life, independence and mobility, enhancing psychological wellbeing and preventing secondary dysfunction. Furthermore, the use of a multimodal and multidisciplinary approach supports a biopsychosocial approach and views the client from all angles of their social, emotional and physical wellbeing (Fancourt & Steptoe 2018; Gauntlett-Gilbert & Brook 2018).

It is therefore no wonder that multidisciplinary interventions for chronic pain have become more accepted with various comprehensive approaches and have rapidly increased in number over the last few decades. This is coupled with strong evidence supporting the fact that multidisciplinary pain programs that address both the physical and psychosocial components of pain seem to be a promising approach to reducing pain and disability and are considered to be the most effective means of treating chronic pain (Gauntlett-Gilbert & Brook 2018; Nees et al 2020).

A multimodal approach is an individualised, dynamic and multicomponent approach to managing chronic pain. This approach involves choosing among a wide range of options included in several categories: pharmacologic, physical medicine, education and behavioural approaches, interventional and surgical modalities. Thus, management of chronic pain requires involvement of a multimodal and multidisciplinary team which combines resources based on the patient's needs, while at the same time this enables the use of pharmacological and nonpharmacological modalities of pain management (Cascella 2019). In addition, the use of multimodal and multidisciplinary approaches has been seen to combine a variety of therapeutic modalities and utilise a team approach consisting of but not limited to physicians, behavioural specialists, nurse case managers and physical therapists to help patients develop skills to actively cope with and self-manage their pain (DeBar et al 2018; Fancourt & Steptoe 2018).

The use of multidisciplinary and multimodal approaches is not without its challenges. Patient–provider interactions in the management of chronic pain in primary care have been identified, including insufficient knowledge of pain management, time constraints, differing goals, attitudes and misconceptions concerning treatment, and debate surrounding the use of opioids for chronic pain (Cheatle 2016).

To effect a multimodal and multidisciplinary approach of clinical management should include dialogue with the client about realistic expectations of pain relief and the need to focus on improving the client's functionality. Effective management often necessitates the use of a blend of different approaches based on the individual's response to treatment.

IMPACT OF RELATIONSHIPS ON CHRONIC PAIN

Doctor–patient relationships play a vital role in how pain is assessed and managed. In a study carried out by Sherman and colleagues (2018), it was found that 82% of the patients with chronic pain trusted their doctor's judgement in managing their opiate pain medicine. NSW Health (2018) postulates that patients who have good relationships with their doctors tend to be more satisfied with their care. Furthermore, in other studies, good doctor–patient relationships revealed patients gain control over their decisions and were enabled to voice their views. This in turn enables doctors to review the efficacy of the pain management (Canovas et al 2018; Pavlin et al 2019; Strauss 2020). That said, new trends on the management of pain focus on promoting doctor–patient relationships.

People with chronic pain and their families are the primary managers of chronic pain. With this view, the family, as part of the multidisciplinary team, has a central role of support if effective management outcomes are to be realised (Akbari et al 2016; Cosio 2020). This support is encouraged when the partners and family are included in the pain management education and are supported to learn the principles of self-management.

Two studies carried out by Campbell and colleagues (2018) and Derbyshire and colleagues (2013) on the impact of family on pain found that family members had a significant level of effect on how pain was managed and vice versa. For example, when the client indicates pain, there was a 30% increase in family-level effect, of shared pain between the client and family.

Negative impacts of chronic pain on relationships include friction between partners, resentment related to the impact of the pain, decrease in intimacy and, ultimately, erosion of the relationship, which can end in separation and divorce (Fu et al 2016; Golics et al 2013). Golics and colleagues (2013) also found that personal friendships were strained as pain or a chronic condition interfered with visiting, social outings and movement. Holidays become a pleasure of the past, and planned activities are frequently cancelled due to pain. In addition, family members described their own existing medical conditions as worsening at the expense of looking after their partners. Other elements include having perceptions of sadness in the family, mood swings, and the deterioration in leisure activities, along with sleep disturbances (Dueñas et al 2016). The families studied also indicated experiencing financial burden, often compounded by the patient giving up work, and many also indicated that looking after a patient with a chronic condition is expensive in many ways. Consequently, because of these impacting factors over time, many partners developed depression and anxiety in the long run (Dueñas et al 2016). However, not all family relationships are 'doom and gloom'; some family members felt closer to the patient with pain through supporting each other in difficult times, and others described making more effort to spend time as a family. This in turn has enhanced cohesion and resilience as everyone works together to adapt to the demands of chronic pain (Cosio 2020). Family relationships are not only supportive but improve engagement in care and promote effective management of chronic pain (Paterick et al 2017).

COMMUNICATION AND PATIENT EDUCATION

Effective communication and a trusting relationship are fundamental to helping the person in pain to achieve their goals. It is vital for nurses to give the person in pain the opportunity to talk about their pain and pain-related concerns, validate their experiences and provide interventions that enable self-management. Good communication with the multidisciplinary team

and mutual respect for their specialist contributions are also essential. Developing a trusting, therapeutic relationship with the person involves accepting the person's report of pain, actively listening, displaying empathy and using effective verbal and non-verbal communication skills. Good communication also entails close communication about the pain experience between partners, and is also vitally important, not only for supportive measures but is also seen to improve family engagement in care (Paterick et al 2017). Furthermore, close communication about the pain experiences improves knowledge and exploration of strategies that enhance self-management. Overall, communication among clinicians, patients and their families is essential and plays an important role towards improving patient quality healthcare and attaining positive outcomes.

Patient education on the other hand has been defined as 'any set of planned activities designed to improve a patient's health behaviours, health status, or both' (Lorig 2001, p. xiii cited by Masters 2017). Thus, patient education aims to facilitate patient knowledge and understanding in order to help the client make sense of their pain and guide them towards effective ongoing self-management. Education about the illness, its manifestations, diagnostic studies and the treatment regimen can help to diminish anxiety, reduce stress and assist the person to cope with ongoing pain, self-manage pain, enhance feelings of control and adhere to the treatment plan (Rod 2016).

While many of the specific treatment options for chronic pain are outlined below, there are some important generic principles of practice that are relevant to all health professionals working with people with chronic pain. Unruh and Harman (2002) provide an excellent discussion of these guiding principles, which are summarised in Box 9.1.

To promote accessibility and utilisation of pain services and trust in the services offered, health professionals need to be seen to be exploring all options to find a diagnosis and treatment. Furthermore, the utilisation model notes that enabling factors that predict healthcare use by chronic pain sufferers should include consultation with pain specialists in which interprofessional relationships play a huge part (Mann et al 2017).

The reader is encouraged to reflect on their past experience of working with clients with chronic pain as a health professional or student, or perhaps personal experience of pain and interaction with health professionals and consider how these principles might facilitate therapeutic intervention.

BOX 9.1
Generic Principles of Practice

- Believe the client's description of her or his pain and suffering.
- Treat acute pain aggressively.
- Always assess the client's pain and its impact on daily life before planning intervention.
- Avoid 'leaps to the head' to explain the client's pain.
- Determine whether the primary goal of intervention is pain reduction or improvement in function.
- Incorporate evidence-based decision-making into practice.
- Combine medical, pharmacological, cognitive behavioural, occupational and physical strategies.

- Understand and correct misconceptions about the use of pain medication and addiction risks.
- Recognise that a positive response to a cognitive behavioural intervention does not mean that the client's pain has a psychological cause.
- Help the client to make long-term lifestyle changes.
- Involve the client's family whenever possible.
- Recognise dual responsibilities and obligations.
- Create a positive therapeutic milieu.
- Conduct an ethical practice.
- Participate in research, education and professional pain associations.

Paradigm Shift in Pain Treatment

Despite the scope and impact of chronic pain, management of pain is yet to be achieved. A study carried out in 10 countries showed that chronic pain is inadequately treated around the world (Cheung et al 2019). In addition, other studies have shown poor pain management practices among different ethnographic backgrounds (Webster et al 2019). Imminent in literature also are the complexities of understanding and managing chronic pain in elderly patients (Holloway et al 2018). Given this background, the use of opioids has been observed to be on the increase for cancer, non-cancer indications and for social use. Literature reveals that the global trends for opioid use such as heroin is on the increase, with the United States showing a double rise in numbers since 2015 (Phillips et al 2017; Ritchie & Roser 2020; Strang et al 2015). For Australia, 11% of Australians aged 14 used drugs for either illicit or non-medical purposes. An AIHW (2018) report indicates that opioid deaths rose by 62% between 2007 and 2016.

According to the United Nations Office on Drugs and Crime (2015), globally 35 million people suffer from drug-use disorders and require treatment services. The trends for substance abuse, either due to recreational or therapeutic use, are on the rise and are attributed to many factors, which include the evolution of the opiate epidemic, social elements such as music festivals, drug trafficking and the growth in illegal use of drugs such as heroin and amphetamines for social use. This has consequently led to an increase in the number of patients with drug dependence problems. And equally too many public health strategies and clinical management approaches have contributed to

multifaceted control and deterrence measures; for example, the harm minimisation program, such as the needle and syringe program and the methadone program and drug testing have given some understanding of how to manage substance abuse.

Consequently, because of the increase in demand for opioid use, there is improved knowledge in the context of pain management such as being aware of the pseudo addiction, a syndrome associated with the undertreatment of pain, characterised by problem behaviours around seeking more opioid analgesia (Quinlan & Cox 2017).

Understanding the concepts of pain intolerance, opioid dependence and withdrawal prevention are essential to deliver effective pain management in patients with substance abuse disorders. Opioid-dependent patients have a measurable degree of pain intolerance and increased sensitivity. These changes may lead to increased opioid requirements for effective pain relief in such patients, and because of this, they are at increased risk of receiving inadequate pain management. Nevertheless, according to Quinlan and Cox (2017), the goals of treating acute pain in patients using opioids are to provide adequate analgesia, prevent withdrawal, and avoid triggering a relapse or worsening of the addiction disorder. Overall, literature reveals a lack of understanding and research-supported guidance on how to manage these patients.

According to Quinlan and Cox (2017), the principle of treating pain in opioid dependence in a patient should include:
- creating a supportive, non-judgemental environment
- establishing whether other drugs are misused

- an analgesic plan:
  - optimise non-opioid analgesia
  - use increased doses of opioids compared with opioid-naive patients but with careful monitoring for side effects
  - change from parenteral to oral formulations of opioids as soon as possible
- a withdrawal management plan
  - continue opioid substitution therapy or replace with an appropriate opioid
  - consider withdrawal syndromes of other drugs taken
- minimise stress
  - allow for multidisciplinary discharge planning.

Managing clients who have chronic pain and are also substance abusers has its own challenges, as illustrated in Case Study 9.3.

It is not possible within this overview to provide the details of management of acute and chronic pain in substance-dependent patients. However, the skills

---

CASE STUDY 9.3

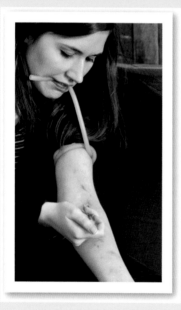

iStockphoto/MikeCherim.

SUBSTANCE ABUSE

The following scenario occurs at the emergency department (ED) at 2300 hours on a Saturday night. This case study demonstrates the challenges of managing a patient with aggressive behaviour, who has a history of substance abuse and chronic pain. The aggressive behaviour makes it hard to determine if the patient is in pain or is demonstrating signs and symptoms of withdrawal.

Social History

Ms Sue is a 22-year-old single woman who has been living with her boyfriend James in the inner suburbs of a major city for the past 3 years. Sue has an 18-month-old child.

When Sue was 11 years old, her father, whom she says was a very heavy drinker, abused her mother constantly and domestic violence was part of the household. Sue's father left her mother and the kids, and she has never seen her father since then. At 14 she started drinking and smoking marijuana. At 16 she had dropped out of high school and at 18 she ran away from home and moved from one state to another with different boyfriends. At 20 she returned home, but did not stay for long; then she moved in with James who is a drug dealer. At 21 she had her child with James. James introduced her to heroin. She reports using about a 1/2 gram of heroin per day just to be able to function and feel comfortable. Sue wants to stop using heroin for the sake of her child.

MEDICAL HISTORY

- Sue claims to suffer from migraine headaches for which she takes Endone 5 mg prn.
- She also states that she suffers from dysmenorrhoea.
- At 21 years she had a laparoscopic appendectomy for which she claims she still has severe abdominal pains periodically.

Medications

Endone 5 mg BD

Multivitamins 1 tablet daily

Smokes 10–15 cigarettes day

Heroine and marijuana user

For the sake of her child, Sue wants to stop using heroin. Sue was BIB (brought in by ambulance) after she was found on the floor sweaty and disoriented by James. While in ED Sue suddenly becomes violent and aggressive; she takes her clothes off and shouts and kicks the nurses. In order to manage Sue, a psychologist is sent to review her and a referral is made to the drug and alcohol nurse. Sue is completely disoriented; however, she claims to have a severe headache and she states her pain score is 10/10. The doctors have withheld further administration of pain relief until they can perform a head CT. Sue is also demanding to see her child. A urine test and blood sample have been taken and the patient is awaiting psychiatric review. Pain score chart and withdrawal scales should be used to monitor the patient. Her withdrawal score is 5 and valium 5 mg has been given, but the patient is demanding something stronger.

Lately she has noticed that her breasts have become swollen and more tender. She also hasn't had her period in the last 12 weeks. She is pretty sure she is pregnant. However, she is not sure she can stop using drugs to have a second child, even though James wants her to keep the pregnancy. All these factors may be compounding her pain and behaviour.

CASE STUDY QUESTIONS

1. How would you determine drug/alcohol withdrawal from chronic pain?
2. What management strategies can be used?
3. What pain management regime can be developed for this client?

Developed by Christine Chisengantambu.

needed when managing and prescribing opioids in substance abuse patients, as stated by the skills and principles needed to treat opioid drug addiction, are (Leach 2018; NPS 2016):

- an understanding of the pharmacology of opioids
- a knowledge of the underlying conditions and their effect on health
- an understanding of dependence
- knowledge of alternative ways of relieving pain and distress
- the ability to help patients change their attitudes and behaviour
- taking a thorough drug history and making a comprehensive assessment of pain and risk
- implementing multimodal treatment therapies that maximise non-opioid analgesics, adjuvant medicines and non-drug therapies and avoid sole reliance on opioids
- never continuing claimed previous treatment without independently verifying the claims directly with the previous prescriber, and making your own thorough assessment of the patient
- using risk management strategies that monitor compliance, aberrant behaviour and supply and diversion, and include specialist support
- providing patient communication and information that is non-judgemental and empathic, framed as your concern for the patient's safety.

It is important to be aware that in patients with addiction and dependence the occurrence of psychological distress and physical discomfort in the form of opioid withdrawal symptoms is a common feature if opioid use is not adequately managed. Clinical settings have withdrawal charts/tools that can assist clinicians to identify and manage substance withdrawal manifestations. It is the clinician's responsibility to be familiar with the tool used in their clinical setting.

Nurses are required to understand the actions and side effects of analgesic medications. Such knowledge can assist both clients and carers to better use and understand their medications. In addition, it is important that those who prescribe and administer medications consider the following CDC opioid prescribing guidelines (CDC 2016):

- Use non-opioid therapies for the most extended time possible.
- Use first-line medication options by preference.
- Implement multimodal treatment therapies that maximise non-opioid analgesics and use interdisciplinary rehabilitation for patients who have failed standard treatments, have severe functional deficits, or psychosocial risk factors.
- Identify and address co-existing mental health conditions (e.g. depression, anxiety, post-traumatic stress disorder [PTSD]).
- Focus on functional goals and improvements, engaging patients actively in their pain management.
- Use risk management strategies that monitor compliance, aberrant behaviour, provide diversion, and include specialist support.
- Provide patient communication and information that is non-judgemental and empathic, framed as your concern about the patient's safety.
- Use disease-specific treatments when available (e.g. triptans for migraines, gabapentin/pregabalin/duloxetine for neuropathic pain).
- Consider interventional therapies (e.g. corticosteroid injections) in patients who fail standard non-invasive therapies.

The greatest barriers to adequate and timely pain management for people with chronic pain remain those fears and misconceptions that have been reported for decades, such as the side effects of opioids, fear of addiction and the belief that pain indicates disease progression.

Non-Drug Interventions

Non-pharmaceutical interventions can bring relief from chronic pain and give people a sense of control. Relaxation therapy, cutaneous stimulation, such as heat and cold, massage, guided imagery, music therapy, self-hypnosis and biofeedback are some examples.

A critical review of the domain of psychological interventions for chronic pain includes: self-regulatory, behavioural, CBT and acceptance and commitment therapy (Cano-García et al 2017).

Several studies have found that CBT, whether administered alone or in combination with medical treatment, improves pain. The primary aims of CBT are to help patients alter beliefs that are detrimental to their self-management of the pain; monitor their thoughts, emotions and behaviours, and link these to environmental events, pain, emotional distress and psychosocial difficulties. This supports the person to develop and maintain effective and adaptive ways of thinking, feeling and responding; and perform behaviours that assist them to cope with pain, emotional distress and psychosocial difficulties (Cano-García et al 2017; Black 2016). Interventions that influence the person's cognition, such as education, reassurance, coping strategy training, stress management, cognitive restructuring, distraction, problem-solving, changing pain behaviours, increasing physical activity, goal setting and pacing, are all part of CBT (Cianfrini & Doleys 2017).

People living with chronic pain often fear that they will increase the pain and cause further damage by movement and exercise; or that there is an underlying pathology that has not yet been discovered. Reassurance and education can assist the person to understand the fallacy of these beliefs and develop more realistic strategies, such as exercise and pacing to prevent further deterioration in their physical capabilities. Acceptance that chronic pain is not curable nor able to be explained is difficult and the individual with chronic pain needs professional as well as personal support to come to this acceptance.

Complementary Therapies

The use of complementary therapies plays an important role in both acute and chronic pain, and as a result people who suffer from chronic pain are increasingly turning to complementary and alternative therapies. The philosophical orientation of these therapists is opposite to the reductive stance taken by conventional Western medicine. They take a holistic perspective and, according to their particular tradition, treat the person rather than the causative pathology.

The emphasis is on total wellbeing rather than the control or, some would say, masking of symptoms; in this particular case, pain. Of course, as the sciences of complementary therapy and Western medicine advance, their boundaries overlap. Indeed, in many general practices medical practitioners and complementary therapists work from the same centre. Some registered nurses also bring their expertise in complementary therapies to the management of chronic pain and have led research in developing an evidence base for these approaches.

Given the increasing use of complementary therapies for chronic pain, health professionals require knowledge about the use and effectiveness of these specific practices so that they can assist clients to make informed, evidence-based decisions about their use. The reader is referred to the systematic reviews by Kong and colleagues (2016) of the effectiveness of commonly used complementary therapies for chronic pain. Palliation and pain are discussed in Chapter 12.

CONCLUSION

Chronic pain is a common problem experienced among people with chronic illness and disability. Despite significant gaps in the literature, the available evidence demonstrates the negative impact of pain on QOL, over and above the effects of the disease itself. It is argued here that the biopsychosocial model offers the most heuristic approach to chronic disability-related pain. From this perspective it is the person in pain, rather than the underlying disease process, that is the focus of assessment and management.

Chronic pain is also invisible to others. Health professionals are encouraged to routinely screen for pain problems during each interaction with people with physical disabilities. Elicitation of a pain problem should prompt a comprehensive pain assessment, as well as the need to assess its potential impact on the person's QOL. Many of the strategies for adequately managing and adapting to chronic pain are educational – self-management, coping skills, knowledge of the condition and effective use of analgesia – and registered nurses have a significant role in this education (Howarth & Poole 2019; Morales-Fernandez et al 2016).

Timely referral to and collaboration with specialist pain management services will also enhance the care of people with chronic pain and ensure they receive the best available therapies.

Reflective Questions

1. Pain is an under-recognised and under-treated problem among people with disabilities. Why do you think this is so? What are the potential barriers?

2. Revisit Case Study 9.2 and determine the clinical priorities in this case. What strategies could you utilise to promote the client's self-management of pain in this situation?

3. What are your experiences of working with people with chronic pain as a student or health professional? Did you feel adequately prepared? What knowledge gaps have you identified that would have assisted you in working with these people which require your further study?

Acknowledgement

This chapter was adapted from the previous edition based on the work of Clint Douglas. Any errors or omissions are the author's own.

RECOMMENDED READING

Austin P 2017. Chronic pain: a resource for effective manual therapy. Handspring Publishing, East Lothian, Scotland.

Raffaeli W, Arnaudo E 2017. Pain as a disease: an overview. Journal of Pain Research 10, 1–6.

Stannard C, Kalso E et al 2016. Evidenced-based chronic pain management. Wiley-Blackwell. BMJ, Oxford.

REFERENCES

Adewusi JK, Hadjivassiliou M, Vinagre-Aragon A et al 2018. Peripheral neuropathic pain in idiopathic Parkinson's disease: prevalence and impact on quality of life; a case controlled study. Journal of the Neurological Sciences, 392, 3–7.

Akbari F, Dehghani M, Khatibi A et al 2016. Incorporating family function into chronic pain disability: the role of catastrophizing. Pain Research Management. ID 6838596.

Alles SRA, Smith PA 2018. Etiology and pharmacology of neuropathic pain. Pharmacological Reviews, 70(2), 315–347.

American Society of Regional Anesthesia Pain Medicine 2020. Treatment options for chronic pain. Online. Available: www.asra.com/page/46/treatment-options-for-chronic-pain.

Arthur L, Rolan P 2019. A systematic review of western medicine's understanding of pain experience, expression, assessment, and management for Australian Aboriginal and Torres Strait Islander Peoples. Pain Reports 4(6), e764.

Australian Institute of Health and Welfare (AIHW) (2018–April 2020). Opioid harm in Australia: and comparisons between Australia and Canada. Cat. no. HSE 210. AIHW, Canberra. Online. Available: www.aihw.gov.au/getmedia/605a6cf8-6e53-488e-ac6e-925e9086df33/aihw-hse-210.pdf.aspx?inline=true.

Australian Institute of Health and Welfare (AIHW) 2019. Back problems. Online. Available: www.aihw.gov.au/reports/chronic-musculoskeletal-conditions/back-problems/contents/what-are-back-problems.

Australian Pain Society 2019. New sensation: chronic pain as a new concept for the international classification of diseases. Australian Pain Society Newsletter 39(5), 9–11.

Backe IF, Patila GG, Nes RB et al 2018. The relationship between physical functional limitations, and psychological distress: considering a possible mediating role of pain, social support and sense of mastery. SSM Population Health 4, 153–163.

Bainbridge R, McCalman J, Clifford A et al 2015. Closing the Gap. Cultural competency in the delivery of health services for Indigenous people. Issues paper no.13. Closing the Gap Clearinghouse, Australian Government. Online. Available: www.aihw.gov.au/uploadedFiles/ClosingTheGap/Content/Our_publications/2015/ctgc-ip13.pdf.

Beltramini A, Milojevic K, Pateron D 2017. Pain assessment in newborns, infants, and children. Pediatric Annals 46(10), e387–e395.

Beyer JE, Denyes MJ, Villarruel AM 1992. The creation, validation, and continuing development of the Oucher: a measure of pain intensity in children. Journal of Pediatric Nursing 7(5), 335–346.

Black R, Clark MR, Dinoff B 2016. CBT and ACT therapy for chronic pain: how does psychotherapy help? Practical Pain Management (PPM). Online. Available: www.practicalpainmanagement.com/patient/treatments/mental-and-emotional-therapy/cbt-act-therapy-chronic-pain-how-does-psychotherapy.

Bolton DG, Gillett G 2019. Biopsychosocial conditions of health and disease. In: The biopsychosocial model of health and disease. Palgrave Pivot, Cham. https://doi.org/10.1007/978-3-030-11899-0_4.

Borsook D, Becerra L, Hargreaves R 2011. Biomarkers for chronic pain and analgesia. Part 1: the need, reality, challenges, and solutions. Discovery Medicine 11(58) 197–207.

Borys C, Lutz J, Strauss B et al 2015. Effectiveness of a multimodal therapy for patients with chronic low back pain regarding pre-admission healthcare utilization. PLoS ONE 10(11), e0143139.

Boyle GJ, Boerresen BH, Jang DM 2015. Patients' factor analyses of the McGill Pain Questionnaire (MPQ) in acute and chronic pain. Psychological Reports: Measures and Statistics 116(3), 797–820.

Brennstuhl MJ, Tarquinio C, Montel S 2015. Chronic pain and PTSD: evolving views on their comorbidity. Perspective in Psychiatric Care 51(4), 295–304. Online. Available: http://onlinelibrary.wiley.com/doi/10.1111/ppc.12093/pdf.

Bruggink L, Hayes C, Lawrence G et al 2019. Chronic pain: overlap and specificity in multimorbidity management. Australian Journal of General Practice (AJGP) 48(10), 689–669.

Campbell P, Jordan KP, Smith BH et al 2018. Chronic pain in families: a cross-sectional study of shared social, behavioural, and environmental influences. Pain 159(1), 41–47.

Cano-García FJ, González-Ortega MC, Sanduvete-Chaves S et al 2017. Evaluation of a psychological intervention for patients with chronic pain in primary care. Frontier in Psychology 8, 435.

Canovas L, Carrascosa AJ, García M et al 2018. Impact of empathy in the patient-doctor relationship on chronic pain relief and quality of life: a prospective study in Spanish pain clinics. Pain Medicine 19, 1304–1314.

Carr DB 2016. Patients with pain need less stigma, not more. Pain Medicine 17(8), 1391–1393.

Cascella M 2019. The rationale for a multimodal approach to pain treatment. In: M Cascella (ed.) From conventional to innovative approaches for pain treatment. Online. Available: www.intechopen.com/books/from-conventional-to-innovative-approaches-for-pain-treatment/introductory-chapter-the-rationale-for-a-multimodal-approach-to-pain-treatment.

Centers for Disease Control and Prevention (CDC) 2016. CDC Guideline for prescribing opioids for chronic pain – United States, 2016. Online. Available: www.cdc.gov/mmwr/volumes/65/rr/rr6501e1.htm.

Charoenpol FN, Tontisirin N, Leerapan B et al 2019. Pain experiences and intrapersonal change among patients with chronic non-cancer pain after using a pain diary: a mixed-methods study. The Journal of Research Pain 12, 477–487.

Cheatle MD 2016. Facing the challenge of pain management and opioid misuse, abuse and opioid-related fatalities. Expert Review of Clinical Pharmacology 9(6), 751–754.

Chen S, Jackson T 2019. Causal effects of challenge and threat appraisals on pain self-efficacy, pain coping, and tolerance for laboratory pain: an experimental path analysis study. PLoS ONE 14(4): e0215087.

Cheung CW, Choo CY, Kim YC et al 2019. Inadequate management of chronic non-cancer pain and treatment-related adverse events in Asia: perspectives from patients from 10 countries/regions. SN Comprehensive Clinical Medicine (2019), 442–450.

Churchill G, Madddy E, Ray Z et al 2019. Effective interventions for post-stroke shoulder subluxation and pain. Practical Pain Management (PPM) 19(7), 40–42.

Cianfrini LR, Doleys DM 2017. The role of psychology in pain management. Practical Pain Management (PPM) 6(1). Online. Available: www.practicalpainmanagement.com/treatments/psychological/role-psychology-pain-management.

Cleeland CS 1989. Measurement of pain by subjective report. In: CR Chapman, JD Loeser (eds), Issues in pain measurement. Raven Press, New York.

Cosio D 2020. Family: their role and impact on pain management. Practical Pain Management (PPM) 19(7), 18–22.

Craig KD, Holmes C, Hudspith M et al 2020. Pain in persons who are marginalized by social conditions. Pain 161(2), 261–265.

Crofford LJ 2015. Chronic pain: where the body meets the brain. Transactions of the American Clinical and Climatological Association 126, 167–183.

Dahan A, van Velzen M, Niesters M 2014. Comorbidities and the complexities of chronic pain. Anesthesiology 121, 675–677.

Davison SN 2019. Clinical pharmacology considerations in pain management in patients with advanced kidney failure. Nephropharmacology for the Clinician CJASN 14, 917–931.

DeBar L, Benes L, Bonifay A et al 2018. Patients with chronic pain on long-term opioid treatment in primary care (PPACT) – protocol for a pragmatic cluster randomized trial. Contemporary Clinical Trials 67, 91–99.

Derbyshire SWG, Osborn J, Brown S 2013. Feeling the pain of others is associated with self-other confusion and prior pain experience. Frontiers in Human Neurosciences. Online. Available: https://doi.org/10.3389/fnhum.2013.00470.

Doody O, Bailey ME 2017. Interventions in pain management for persons with an intellectual disability. Journal of Intellectual Disabilities 3(1). Online. Available: https://doi.org/10.1177/1744629517708679.

Duarte RV, Lambe T, Raphael JH et al 2016. Intrathecal drug delivery systems for the management of chronic non-cancer pain: protocol for a systematic review of economic evaluations. British Medical Journal. 6:e012285.

Dubin RE, Kaplan A, Graves L et al 2017. Acknowledging stigma: its presence in patient care and medical education. Canadian Family Physician 63(12), 906–908.

Dueñas M, Ojeda B, Salzar A et al 2016. A review of chronic pain impact on patients, their social environment and the health care system. Journal of Pain Research 9, 456–467.

Dworkin RH, Bruehl S, Fillingim RB et al 2016. Multidimensional diagnostic criteria for chronic pain: introduction to the ACTTION–American Pain Society Pain Taxonomy (AAPT). The Journal of Pain 17(9), Supplement T1–T9.

Edirisinghe NP, Makuloluwa TR, Amarasekara TD et al 2019. Psychometric properties of Sinhala Version of Short-Form McGill Pain Questionnaire-2 (SF MPQ-2-Sin) among patients with cancer pain in Sri Lanka. Pain Research and Management. Online. Available: http://downloads.hindawi.com/journals/prm/2019/5050979.pdf.

Fancourt D, Steptoe A 2018. Physical and psychosocial factors in the prevention of chronic pain in older age. The Journal of Pain 19(12), 1385–1391.

Fenwick C 2006. Assessing pain across the cultural gap: central Australian indigenous peoples pain assessment. Contemporary Nurse 2, 218–227.

Fenwick C, Stevens J 2004. Postoperative pain experiences of Central Australian Aboriginal women. What do we understand? Australian Journal of Rural Health 12, 22–27.

Ferrari S, Vanit C, Pellizer M et al 2019. Is there a relationship between self-efficacy, disability, pain and sociodemographic characteristics in chronic low back pain? A multicenter retrospective analysis. Archives of Physiotherapy 9(9), 1–9.

Fillingim RB, Loeser JD, Baron R et al 2016. Assessment of chronic pain: domains, methods, and mechanisms. The Journal of Pain 17(9 Suppl), T10–T20.

Finan PH, Godin BR, Michael T et al 2013. The association of sleep and pain: an update and a path forward. Journal of Pain 14(12), 1539–1552.

Frenkel L, Swartz L 2017. Chronic pain as a human rights issue: setting an agenda for preventative action. Global Health Action 10(1), 1348691.

Fu Y, McNichol E, Marczewski K et al 2016. Patient–professional partnerships and chronic back pain self-management: a qualitative systematic review and synthesis. Health and Social Care in the Community 24(3), 247–259.

Gandhi W, Morrison I, Schweinhardt P 2017. How accurate appraisal of behavioral costs and benefits guides adaptive pain coping. Frontiers in Psychiatry. Online. Available: https://doi.org/10.3389/fpsyt.2017.00103.

Gatchel R, Neblett R 2020. Pain catastrophizing: what clinicians need to know. Practical Pain Management (PPM) 20(2). Online. Available: www.practicalpainmanagement.com/pain/other/co-morbidities/pain-catastrophizing-what-clinicians-need-know.

Gatchel RJ, Howard KJ 2019. The biopsychosocial approach. Practical Pain Management (PPM) 8(4). Online. Available: www.practicalpainmanagement.com/treatments/psychological/biopsychosocial-approach.

Gatchel RJ, Worzer W, Brede E et al 2015. Etiology of chronic pain and mental illness: how to assess both. Practical Pain Management (PPM) 11(9). Online. Available: www.practicalpainmanagement.com/pain/other/co-morbidities/etiology-chronic-pain-mental-illness-how-assess-both.

Gauntlett-Gilbert JP, Brook P 2018. Living well with chronic pain: the role of pain-management programmes. BJA Education 18(1), 3–7.

Givle A, Maani-Fogelma P 2020. The importance of cultural competence in pain and palliative care. Online. Available: www.statpearls.com/kb/viewarticle/41271.

Goldberg DS 2020. Pain doesn't stigmatize people. We do that to each other. STAT Reports. Online. Available: www.statnews.com/2020/01/23/pain-doesnt-cause-stigma-we-do-that-to-each-other/.

Goldberg DS 2017. Introduction on stigma and health. Journal of Law, Medicine & Ethics 45, 475–483.

Golics CJ, Khurshid M, Basra A et al 2013. The impact of patients' chronic disease on family quality of life: an experience from 26 specialties. International Journal of General Medicine 2013 (6), 787–798.

Grabovac I, Dorner ET 2019. Association between low back pain and various everyday performances: activities of daily living, ability to work and sexual function. Wien Klin Wochenschr 13, 541–549.

Griffith LE, Gruneir A, Fisher K et al 2019. Insights on multimorbidity and associated health service use and costs from three population-based studies of older adults in Ontario with diabetes, dementia and stroke. BMC Health Services Research 19(313), 1–11.

Hadi MA, McHugh GA, Closs SJ 2019. Impact of chronic pain on patients' quality of life: a comparative mixed-methods study. Journal of Patient Experience 6(2), 133–141.

Hamar GB, Rula ER, Coberley G et al 2015. Long-term impact of a chronic disease management program on hospital utilization and cost in an Australian population with heart disease or diabetes. BMC Health Services Research 15(174), 1–9.

Heshusius L 2009. Inside chronic pain: an intimate and critical account. Cornell University Press, New York.

Hicks CL, von Baeyer CL, Spafford PA et al 2001. The Faces Pain Scale – revised: toward a common metric in pediatric pain measurement. Pain 93(2), 173–183.

Ho LYW 2019. A concept analysis of coping with chronic pain in older adults. Pain Management Nursing 20, 563–571.

Holloway H, Parker D, McCutcheon H 2018. The complexity of pain in aged care. Contemporary Nurse 54(2), 121–125.

Hopman P, Heins MJ, Korevaar JC et al 2016. Health care utilization of patients with multiple chronic diseases in the Netherlands: differences and underlying factors. European Federation of Internal Medicine 26(3), 190–196.

Howarth A, Poole D 2019. Assessment and management of chronic pain. Nursing Standard. doi:10.7748/ns.2019.e11395. Online. Available: https://journals.rcni.com/nursing-standard/cpd/assessment-and-management-of-chronic-pain-ns.2019.e11395/full.

Hsu HJ, Yen CH, Hsu KH et al 2014. Factors associated with chronic musculoskeletal pain in patients with chronic kidney disease. British Medical Nephrology 5(6), 1–9.

Hulla R, Brecht D, Stephens J et al 2019. The biopsychosocial approach and considerations involved in chronic pain. Healthy Aging Research 8(6), 1–4.

International Association for the Study of Pain (IASP) 2019. Chronic pain has arrived in the ICD-11. Online. Available: www.iasp-pain.org/PublicationsNews/NewsDetail.aspx?ItemNumber=8340.

IsHak WW, Wen RY, Naghdechi L et al 2018. Pain and depression: a systematic review. Harvard Review of Psychiatry 26(6), 352–363.

Jank R, Gallee A, Boeckle M et al 2017. Chronic pain and sleep disorders in primary care. Pain Research and Treatment 1–9. Online. Available: www.hindawi.com/journals/prt/2017/9081802/.

Järemo P, Arman M, Gerdle B et al 2017. Illness beliefs among patients with chronic widespread pain–associations with self-reported health status, anxiety and depressive symptoms and impact of pain. BMC Psychology 5(24), 1–10.

Jones T 2019. The 5 coping skills every chronic pain patient needs. Practical Pain Management (PPM) 19(17). Online. Available: www.practicalpainmanagement.com/treatments/complementary/biobehavioral/5-coping-skills-every-chronic-pain-patient-needs.

Jumbo SO 2019. Psychometric properties of the Brief Pain Inventory-Short Form and Revised Short McGill Pain Questionnaire Version-2 in Musculoskeletal Conditions. Western Libraries. Western Graduate and Postdoctoral Studies Electronic Thesis and Dissertation Repository. 6490. Online. Available: https://ir.lib.uwo.ca/etd/6490.

Karasawa Y, Yamada K, Iseki M et al 2019. Association between change in self-efficacy and reduction in disability among patients with chronic pain. PLoS ONE 14(4), e0215404.

Kong LJ, Lauche R, Klose P et al 2016. Tai Chi for chronic pain conditions: a systematic review and meta analysis of randomized controlled trials. Scientific Report 6(25325), 1–9.

Lape EC, Selzer F, Davi AM et al 2020. Psychometric properties of the Neuropathic Pain Scale (NPS) in a knee osteoarthritis population. Osteoarthritis and Cartilage Open 2(1), 1–10.

Lapkin S, Fernandez R, Ellwood L et al 2019. Reliability, validity and generalizability of multidimensional pain assessment tools used in postoperative adult patients: a systematic review protocol. The JBI Database of Systematic Reviews and Implementation Reports 17(7), 1334–1340.

Laverty M, McDermot DR, Calm T 2017. Embedding cultural safety in Australia's main health care standards (editorial). Perspective. Online. Available: www.mja.com.au/system/files/2017-06/10.5694mja17.00328.pdf.

Leach JM 2018. Managing addiction to prescribed opioids: the job of general practice. British Journal of General Practice 68(674), 426–427.

Lemos OB, da Cunha AMR, Cesarino CB et al 2019. The impact of chronic pain on functionality and quality of life of the elderly. Brazilian Journal of Pain (BrJP) São Paulo 2(3), 237–241.

Levy N, Sturgess J, Mills P 2018. Pain as the fifth vital sign and dependence on the 'numerical pain scale' is being abandoned in the US: Why? British Journal of Anaesthesia 120(3), 435–438.

Liao KYH, Henceroth M, Lu Q et al 2016. Cultural differences in pain experience among four ethnic groups: a qualitative pilot study. Journal of Behavioral Health 5(2), 55–81.

Liberman O, Roni Peleg R, Shvartzman R 2014. Chronic pain in type 2 diabetic patients: a cross-sectional study in primary care setting. European Journal of General Practice 20, 260–267.

Lies DR, Kenneth C 2016. Understanding stigma and chronic pain: a state-of-the-art review. International Association for the Study of Pain 157(8), 1607–1610.

LiLi J 2017. Cultural barriers lead to inequitable healthcare access for Aboriginal Australians and Torres Strait Islanders. Chinese Nursing Research 4(4), 207–210.

Lin IB, Ryder K, Coffin J et al 2017. Addressing disparities in low back pain care by developing culturally appropriate information for Aboriginal Australians: 'My back on track, my future'. Pain Medicine 18(11), 2070–2080.

Linton SJ, Flink IK, Vlaeyen JWS 2018. Understanding the etiology of chronic pain from a psychological perspective. Physical Therapy 98(5), 315–324.

Mann EG, Johnson A, Gilro A et al 2017. Pain management strategies and health care use in community-dwelling individuals living with chronic pain. Pain Medicine 18, 2267–2279.

Martinez-Calderon J, Meeus M, Struyf F et al 2018. The role of psychological factors in the perpetuation of pain intensity and disability in people with chronic shoulder pain: a systematic review. British Medical Journal (BMJ) 8, e020703.

Masters K 2017. Role development in professional nursing practice, 4th edn. Jones & Bartlett Learning, USA.

McCaffery M 1968. Nursing practice theories related to cognition, bodily pain, and man-environment interactions. University of California Students' Store, Los Angeles.

McCormick T, Law S 2016. Assessment of acute and chronic pain. Anaesthesia & Intensive Care Medicine 17(9), 421–424.

McGrath P 2006. 'The biggest worry' research findings on pain management for Aboriginal peoples in Northern Territory, Australia. Rural and Remote Health 6, 549.

Meints SM, Edwards RR 2018. Evaluating psychosocial contributions to chronic pain outcomes. Progress in Neuropsychopharmacology and Biological Psychiatry 87(Pt B), 168–182.

Melzack R 1987. The short-form McGill Pain questionnaire. Pain 30, 191–197.

Mills SEE, Nicolson KP, Smith BH 2019. Chronic pain: a review of its epidemiology and associated factors in population-based studies. British Journal of Anaesthesia 123(2), e273–e283.

Mittinty MM, McNeil DW, Jamieson LM 2018. Limited evidence to measure the impact of chronic pain on health outcomes of Indigenous people. Journal of Psychosomatic Research 107, 53–54.

Morales-Fernandez A, Morales-Asencio JM, Canca-Sanchez JC et al 2016. Impact on quality of life of a nursing intervention programme for patients with chronic non-cancer pain: an open, randomized controlled parallel study protocol. Journal of Advanced Nursing 72(5), 965–1216.

Murphy JL, McKellar JD, Raffa SD et al (n.d.). Cognitive behavioral therapy for chronic pain among veterans: therapist manual. Washington, DC: U.S. Department of Veterans Affairs. Online. Available: https://www.va.gov/PAINMANAGEMENT/docs/CBT-CP_Therapist_Manual.pdf.

Murphy KL, Bethea JR, Fischer R 2017. Neuropathic pain in multiple sclerosis–current therapeutic intervention and future treatment perspectives. In: IS Zagon, PJ McLaughlin (eds), Multiple sclerosis perspectives in treatment and pathogenesis. Codon Publishers, Brisbane.

National Prescribing Service (NPS) MedicineWise 2016. Pain management in patients with a history of opioid dependence. Information for health professionals. Online. Available: www2.health.vic.gov.au/-/media/health/files/collections/policies-and-guidelines/safe-opiod-use/pain-management-in-patients-with-a-history-of-opioid-dependence---for-health-professionals.pdf.

Nees TA, Riewe E, Waschke D et al 2020. Multidisciplinary pain management of chronic back pain: helpful treatments from the patients' perspective. Journal of Clinical Medicine 99(145), 1–18.

New South Wales (NSW) Health 2018. Chronic pain management. Online. Available: www.health.nsw.gov.au/pharmaceutical/doctors/Pages/chronic-pain-medical-practitioners.aspx#bookmark3.

Orhan C, Van Looveren E, Cagnie B et al 2018. Are pain beliefs, cognitions, and behaviors influenced by race, ethnicity, and culture in patients with chronic musculoskeletal pain: a systematic review. Pain Physician 21, 541–558.

Pain Australia 2019. The cost of pain in Australia. Deloitte Access Economics. Online. Available: www.painaustralia.org.au/static/uploads/files/the-cost-of-pain-in-australia-final-report-12mar-wfxbrfyboams.pdf.

Paterick TE, Patel N, Tajik J et al 2017. Improving health outcomes through patient education and partnerships with patient. Proceedings Baylor University Medical Centre 30(1), 112–113.

Pathak A, Sharma S, Mark P et al 2018. The utility and validity of pain intensity rating scales for use in developing countries. PAIN Reports 3(5), e672.

Pavlin K, Lazar MB, Bolle N 2019. Automatic thoughts of chronic pain patients regarding their medical doctor–patient relationship. The EFIC – 2019, Pain in Europe XI Conference. 11th Congress Of The European Pain Federation EFIC 4–7 September 2019.

Phillips JK, Ford MA, Bonnie RJ 2017. Pain management and the opioid epidemic: balancing societal and individual benefits and risks of prescription opioid use. National Academies of Sciences, Engineering, and Medicine; Health and Medicine Division; Board on Health Sciences Policy; Committee on Pain Management and Regulatory Strategies to Address Prescription Opioid Abuse; National Academies Press (US); Washington DC. Online. Available: www.ncbi.nlm.nih.gov/books/NBK458661/.

Pitcher MH, Von Korff M, Bushnell CM et al 2019. Prevalence and profile of high-impact chronic pain in the United States. Journal of Pain 20(2), 146–160.

Psychiatry DataBase (PsycDB) 2020 Biopsychosocial Model and case formulation. Online. Available: www.psychdb.com/teaching/intermediate/biopsychosocial-formulation.

Quinlan J, Cox F 2017. Acute pain management in patients with drug dependence syndrome. PAIN Reports 2(4), e611.

Ramanathan S, Hibbert P, Wiles L et al 2018. What is the association between the presence of comorbidities and the appropriateness of care for low back pain? A population-based medical record review study. BMC Musculoskeletal Disorders, 19, Art no. 391, https://doi.org/10.1186/s12891-018-2316-z.

Ritchie H, Roser M 2020. Drug use. OurWorldInData.org. Online. Available: https://ourworldindata.org/drug-use

Rivera-Segarra E, Varas-Díaz N, Santos-Figueroa A 2019. 'That's all fake': health professionals stigma and physical healthcare of people living with serious mental illness. PLoS ONE 14(12), e0226401.

Rod K 2016. Finding ways to lift barriers to care for chronic pain patients: outcomes of using internet-based self-management activities to reduce pain and improve quality of life. Pain Research and Management Article ID 8714785.

Salduker S, Allers E, Bechan S et al 2019. Practical approach to a patient with chronic pain of uncertain etiology in primary care. Journal of Pain Research 12, 2651–2662.

Samulowitz A, Gremyr I, Eriksson E et al 2018. 'Brave men' and 'emotional women': a theory-guided literature review on gender bias in health care and gendered norms towards patients with chronic pain. Hindawi Pain Research and Management. Online. Available: www.ncbi.nlm.nih.gov/pmc/articles/PMC5845507/pdf/PRM2018-6358624.pdf.

Schreiber AK, Nones, CF, Reis RC et al 2015. Diabetic neuropathic pain: physiopathology and treatment. World Journal of Diabetes 6(3), 432–444.

Scott W, Yu L, Patel S et al 2019. Measuring stigma in chronic pain: preliminary investigation of instrument psychometrics, correlates, and magnitude of change in a prospective cohort attending interdisciplinary treatment. The Journal of Pain. Online. Available: https://doi.org/10.1016/j.jpain.2019.03.011.

Seidlein AH, Salloch S 2019. Illness and disease: an empirical–ethical viewpoint. BMC Medical Ethics 20(5), 1–10, Online.

Sheng J, Liu S, Wang Y et al 2017. The link between depression and chronic pain: neural mechanisms in the brain. Neural Plasticity. Online. doi: 10.1155/2017/9724371. PMCID: PMC5494581.

Sherman KJ, Walker RL, Saunder SM et al 2018. Doctor–patient trust among chronic pain patients on chronic opioid therapy after opioid risk reduction initiatives: a survey. The Journal of the American Board of Family Medicine (JABFM) 31(4), 578–587.

Simoes D, Araujo F, Severo M et al 2017. Patterns and consequences of multimorbidity in the general population: there is no chronic disease management without rheumatic disease management. Arthritis Care & Research 69(1), 12–20.

Sneddon LU 2018. Comparative physiology of nociception and pain. American Physiology Society 33(1), 63–73. Online. Available: https://journals.physiology.org/doi/full/10.1152/physiol.00022.2017.

Stanhope J 2016. Brief pain inventory review. Occupational Medicine 1–2.

Stompór M, Grodzicki T, Stompór T et al 2019. Prevalence of chronic pain, particularly with neuropathic component, and its effect on overall functioning of elderly patients. Medical Science Monitor, 25, 2695–2701.

Strang J, Groshkova T, Uchtenhagen A et al 2015. Heroin on trial: systematic review and meta-analysis of randomised trials of diamorphine-prescribing as treatment for refractory heroin addiction. British Journal of Psychiatry 207(1), 5–14.

Strauss A 2020. The psychiatric model of treating chronic pain. Practical Pain Management (PPM) 20(1). Online. Available: www.practicalpainmanagement.com/treatments/psychological/psychiatric-model-treating-chronic-pain

Sukel K 2019. A new classification of chronic pain for better patient care and research. IASP: Pain Research forum. Online. Available: www.painresearchforum.org/news/109900-new-classification-chronic-pain-better-patient-care-and-research.

Summers SJ, Higgins NC, Te M et al 2019. The effect of implicit theories of pain on pain and disability in people with chronic low back pain. Musculoskeletal Science and Practice 40, 65–71.

The Royal Children's Hospital Melbourne 2019. Pain assessment and measurement. Online. Available: https://www.rch.org.au/rchcpg/hospital_clinical_guideline_index/Pain_assessment_and_measurement/.

Thong I 2018. Safely managing chronic noncancer pain in general practice. Medicine Today 19(2), 55–60.

Tompkins DA, Hobelmanna JG, Compton P 2017. Providing chronic pain management in the 'fifth vital sign' era: historical and treatment perspectives on a modern-day medical dilemma. Drug Alcohol Dependency 173(Suppl 1), S11–S21.

Toye F, Seers K, Allcock A et al 2013. A meta-ethnography of patients' experience of chronic non-malignant musculoskeletal pain. Health Services and Delivery Research 1(12). Online. Available: www.ncbi.nlm.nih.gov/books/NBK262987/pdf/Bookshelf_NBK262987.pdf.

Tracy LM 2017. Psychosocial factors and their influence on the experience of pain. Pain Reports 2(4): e60.

Treede RD 2018. The International Association for the Study of Pain definition of pain: as valid in 2018 as in 1979, but in need of regularly updated footnotes. Pain Report 3(2), e643.

Treede RD, Rief W, Barke A et al 2019. Chronic pain as a symptom or a disease: the IASP Classification Chronic Pain for the International Classification of Diseases (ICD-11). Nature Review 160, 19–27.

Turk DC, Burwinkle TM 2006. Coping with chronic pain. In: A Carr, M McNulty (eds), The handbook of adult clinical psychology: an evidence-based practice approach. Routledge, London.

Turk DC, Fillingim RB, Ohrbach R et al 2016. Assessment of psychosocial and functional impact of chronic pain. The Journal of Pain 17(9), Suppl. 2, T21–T49.

United Nations Office on Drugs and Crime 2015. World Drug Report. Online. Available: www.unodc.org/documents/wdr2015/World_Drug_Report_2015.pdf.

Unruh AM, Harman K 2002. Generic principles of practice. In: J Strong, AM Unruh, A Wright et al (eds), Pain: a textbook for therapists. Churchill Livingstone, Edinburgh.

Vadivelu N, Kai AM, Kodumudi G et al 2017. Pain and psychology – a reciprocal relationship. Ochsner Journal 17, 173–180.

van Hecke O, Torrance N, Smith BH 2013. Chronic pain epidemiology and its clinical relevance. British Journal of Anaesthesia 111(1), 13–18.

Vargas-Schaffer G 2010. Commentary is the WHO analgesic ladder still valid? Twenty-four years of experience. Canadian Family Physician 56 (June), 514–517.

Vergne-Salle P 2016. WHO analgesic ladder: is it appropriate for joint pain? From NSAIDS to Opioids Fact Sheet No. 18. International Association for the Study of Pain. Online. Available: www.apsoc.org.au/PDF/GYAP/2016_GYAP/Fact_Sheet_18_WHO_Analgesic_Ladder.pdf.

Wallis C 2005. The right (and wrong) way to treat chronic pain. Time, February 20. Online. Available: http://med.stanford.edu/content/dam/sm/pain/documents/press/TIME_reduced.pdf.

Walters ET, Williams A C de C 2019. Evolution of mechanisms and behaviour important for pain. Philosophical Transactions Royal Society B 374, 1–8.

Webster F, Rice K, Katz J et al 2019. An ethnography of chronic pain management in primary care: the social organization of physicians' work in the midst of the opioid crisis. PLoS ONE 14(5), e0215148.

Woessner J 2019. A conceptual model of pain: treatment modalities. Practical Pain Management (PPM) 3(1) Online. Available: www.practicalpainmanagement.com/treatments/conceptual-model-pain-treatment-modalities?page=0,1.

Wong DL, Baker CM 1988. Pain in children: comparison of assessment scales. Pediatric Nursing 14(1), 9–17.

World Health Organization 2018. ICD-11 international classification of diseases for mortality and morbidity statistics. Online. Available: https://icd.who.int/browse11/l-m/en.

Yam MF, Loh YC, Tan CS et al 2018. General pathways of pain sensation and the major neurotransmitters involved in pain regulation. International Journal of Molecular Sciences 19(2164), 1–23.

Zis P, Sarrigiannis PG, Rao DG et al 2019. Chronic idiopathic axonal polyneuropathy: prevalence of pain and impact on quality of life. Brain Behaviour 9(1), article e01171.

Zis P, Varrassi G, Vadalouka A et al 2019. Psychological aspects and quality of life in chronic pain. Hindawi Pain Research and Management ID 8346161.

CHAPTER 10

Rehabilitation for the Individual and Family

JULIE PRYOR • KATE O'REILLY • MELISSA BONSER • GILLIAN
GARRETT • DUNCAN McKECHNIE

LEARNING OBJECTIVES

When you have completed this chapter you will be able to:

- conceptualise rehabilitation as a personal journey undertaken by the person experiencing disability, their family and friends
- understand the importance of rehabilitation interventions across the continuum of care
- understand rehabilitation as a co-production that requires synergistic teamwork
- design, deliver and evaluate person-centred nursing care in line with the International Classification of Functioning Disability and Health
- discuss the nurse's role in the rehabilitation journey of the person experiencing disability, their family and friends.

KEY WORDS

brain injury	rehabilitation
disability	spinal cord injury
goal setting	

INTRODUCTION

As a result of disability associated with injury or illness, many persons embark on a rehabilitation journey, an 'individual, active and dynamic process' (Barnes & Ward 2000, p. 6), aimed at regaining control over their bodies and their lives (Ozer 1999). For some people, especially many of whom have lifelong chronic conditions, this necessitates biographical adjustment (Bourke et al 2015; Sveen et al 2016) and 'the holistic reconstruction of the "self"' (Siegert et al 2007, p. 1609). This process is driven by self-reflective meaning-making (Thomas et al 2014).

Rehabilitation is a personal journey that can differ significantly from one person to another (Legg et al 2019). Due to the complex nature of illness, injury and impairment, a person's awareness of their rehabilitation needs can evolve over time. Furthermore, each person's journey is unique in that the experience of injury or illness is assigned personal significance in accordance with the individual's context (Scheel-Sailer et al 2017). Family members, friends and colleagues also embark on a journey of their own as they seek to make sense of what has happened and integrate this into their lives.

Nursing's role in rehabilitation begins at the person's first point of contact with health services, and rehabilitation informs nursing decision-making thereafter. Rehabilitation requires all healthcare professionals to possess, and act upon, an awareness of how what does and does not happen today affects the person's desired tomorrow (Plaisted 1978). As such, rehabilitation is more than a series of intermittent interventions done to patients by health professionals (Pryor 2005). It is a continuous and complex process of co-production (Pryor 2014), which:

- is underpinned by patient enablement (Baker et al 2019b)
- requires clinical staff to work actively to enhance therapeutic connection and engagement (Kayes et al 2015; Tyrrel & Pryor 2016)
- requires active patient participation (NSW Agency for Clinical Innovation 2019)

- is enhanced by a self-management approach (Scheel-Sailer et al 2017) that fosters a can-do attitude and the preservation of a positive sense of self.

Rehabilitation is about adaptation, reconstruction of self-identity and developing a sense of a new normal (Bourke et al 2015; Ellis-Hill 2011; Levack et al 2010; Sveen et al 2016). Both the person who is the patient and their family members are affected in this way. See Table 10.1 for examples of studies that give us some insights into this experience for individuals and their families.

TABLE 10.1
Examples of Studies Illustrating Biographical Adjustment Following Disability

Study Details	Summary of Findings
Amsters et al (2018), an Australian qualitative study of shared narratives following spinal cord injury (SCI)	Sharing stories of life after SCI led to the development of a framework for the promotion of participation to be used by the health professional. The three central aspects were: help me, encourage me and accept me as I am on this journey.
Bourke Hay-Smith et al (2015), a phenomenological study about the experience of rehabilitation following tetraplegia involving four people (3 males, 1 female) in New Zealand	SCI disrupts a person's life biography. Study participants worked 'to gain some form of mastery and control over their new set of circumstances. The dynamics of relationships with staff, being involved in decisions, having strong sources of support, interacting with peers, and learning through doing, were all influences on participants' sense of self-agency' (p. 299). 'To move forward with life, there was a need to "re" store, or "re" establish a sense of balance where the participants' changed physical self was integrated into their personal life and a coherent future visualized' (p. 300).
Levack Boland et al (2014), a grounded theory study of the impact of traumatic brain injury (TBI) on self-identity involving 49 people (34 males, 15 females) in New Zealand	The study findings suggest that 'in order to recover a robust, coherent and satisfying sense of self-identity after TBI, one needs to: (1) regain a strong internal sense of who one is, and to feel like a complete person, (2) be treated like a person of worth by other members of one's community and by society at large, and (3) feel like one has a place in the world where one "fits" and that one values' (p. 4).
Sveen et al (2016), a focus group study about returning to work following mild TBI involving 20 people (8 males, 12 females) in Norway	Life after brain injury 'manifests as a dynamic, unfolding and continuous temporal process of reconstructing daily life routines and occupations' (p. 5). Fatigue was 'the most pervasive impairment affecting occupational capacity and balance' (p. 4). Study participants felt 'estranged from their pre-injury selves and not comfortable with how they experienced themselves after the injury' (p. 4).
Conti Garrino et al (2016), a phenomenological study involving 11 (3 males, 8 females) family caregivers (including 8 spouses) of people with SCIs in Italy	Caregivers experienced 'absolute loneliness characterized by increased insecurity and feelings relating to the lack of support'. Because of their caregiving role, they experienced 'a sense of total cancellation of their own time and their personal self' (p. 162). Immediately before discharge was described as a 'delicate phase' (p. 164) and a strong link with the rehabilitation facility was important to caregivers as they navigated discharge and beyond and the associated mix of emotions. Some felt their 'lack of freedom as imprisonment' (p. 165).
Young, Lutz Creasy et al (2014), a grounded theory study involving 14 spousal carers (3 males, 11 females) in interviews, pre- and post-discharge from inpatient rehabilitation in Florida	Carers reported transition from hospital to home as very difficult or traumatic. They felt unprepared, 'totally overwhelmed, isolated, alone and abandoned', and didn't know what was expected of them (p. 1895).

Amsters et al 2018; Bourke Hay-Smith et al 2016; Conti Garrino et al 2016; Levack Boland et al 2014; Sveen et al 2016; Young et al 2014.

REHABILITATION AS A TYPE OF HEALTHCARE

Rehabilitation is a health strategy aimed at enabling human functioning, the importance of which is underlined by the World Health Organization (WHO), which has positioned functioning as the third health indicator following mortality and morbidity (WHO 2019). This positioning is underpinned by the estimated 66.2% global growth in Years Lived with Disability (YLD) between 1990 and 2017 (Jesus et al 2019). As an 'educational, problem-solving process' (Wade 2005, p. 814), rehabilitation is most effective when it starts as part of acute care.

Within the context of health, the terms functioning and disability are defined in the WHO International Classification of Functioning Disability and Health (ICF) (2001). *Functioning* is 'an umbrella term for body functions, body structures, activities and participation' (pp. 212–13). *Disability* is 'an umbrella term for impairments, activity limitations and participation restrictions' (p. 213). Of most importance in rehabilitation is *functional performance*, which is what an individual can do in their 'societal context', and includes 'all aspects of their physical, social and attitudinal world' (p. 15). The components of ICF are defined in Box 10.1.

The ICF is a biopsychosocial model of disability (WHO 2001). It highlights how functioning and disability at the personal level are created through dynamic interaction between a person's health conditions and contextual factors (see Fig. 10.1). This framework 'is about *all people*' (WHO 2001, p. 7, italics original).

The ICF facilitates selection of rehabilitation interventions that address the full impact of a health condition on a person's life (Kearney & Pryor 2004). That is, rehabilitation interventions target:

- impairments of body structures and functions
- activity limitations
- participation restrictions
- environmental factors
- personal factors.

While rehabilitation is commonly understood to be about the return of physical function, the *re* in rehabilitation can also mean *to do again*; this creates opportunities for doing things in different ways (Pryor & Dean 2012); for example, washing one's body using different techniques and equipment. This is particularly important when return to a previous level of function is not likely, either in the short term or at all. The central process of change in rehabilitation is 'learning by the patient and also often by family members and significant others of how to achieve wanted activities in

> **BOX 10.1**
> **Components of ICF**
>
> **DEFINITIONS**
> In the context of health (p. 10):
> **Body functions** are the physiological functions of body systems (including psychological functions).
> **Body structures** are anatomical parts of the body such as organs, limbs and their components.
> **Impairments** are problems in body function or structure such as a significant deviation or loss.
> **Activity** is the execution of a task or action by an individual.
> **Participation** is involvement in a life situation.
> **Activity limitations** are difficulties an individual may have in executing activities.
> **Participation restrictions** are problems an individual may experience in involvement in life situations.
> **Environmental factors** make up the physical, social and attitudinal environment in which people live and conduct their lives.
> **Personal factors** are the particular background of an individual's life and living, and comprise features of the individual that are not part of a health condition or health states (p. 17).

WHO 2001. International Classification of Functioning Disability and Health (ICF).

the presence of altered or limited skills and abilities' (Wade 2015, p. 1151).

In rehabilitation there is a strong emphasis on the restoration of individual functioning and independence, as evidenced in the following WHO (2016a) definition:

> *Rehabilitation of people with disabilities is a process aimed at enabling them to reach and maintain their optimal physical, sensory, intellectual, psychological and social functional levels. Rehabilitation provides disabled people with the tools they need to attain independence and self-determination.*

While initially thought of as the third phase of medicine (Rusk 1960), rehabilitation is now understood as an important component of healthcare across the continuum of care (Wade 2016). This has come about as awareness of the benefits of rehabilitation as an intervention and service type has grown. Therefore, rehabilitation is provided to persons experiencing functional performance limitations associated with a wide range of illnesses and injuries, as well as limitations associated with the ageing process.

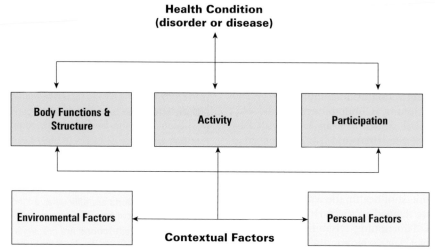

FIG. 10.1 **Interactions Between the Components of ICF.** WHO 2001. International Classification of Functioning Disability and Health (ICF).

There is a stereotype that often depicts a person with a disability as being in a wheelchair or requiring a walking aid. This misconception within our community is far from the reality of many people who have impairments from injury or illness. Prince (2017) highlights that it is estimated 40% of people who live with disability have invisible impairments. People who survive catastrophic spinal cord injury (SCI) and traumatic brain injury (TBI) often have several hidden impairments, such as living with debilitating fatigue, headaches, limb spasticity, anxiety, neurogenic bladder and bowel, depression and impaired memory (Curvis et al 2018; Piatt et al 2016). Unfortunately, the significant impact of hidden disabilities is often not well understood (Kattari et al 2018).

The hidden impairments previously highlighted are far reaching and may impact on a person's employment, their ability to maintain social relationships and their self-identity (Carr et al 2017; O'Reilly et al 2018; Olkin et al 2019). This chapter encourages you in your nursing role to consider the far-reaching impact of hidden impairments for those with whom you work. Getting to know a person and their individual context is essential for fostering individualised rehabilitation that strives for meaningful participation.

Rehabilitation is a complex intervention (Cameron 2010), using four different, but equally important types of rehabilitation interventions: recovery, adaptation, compensation and prevention (NSW Agency for Clinical Innovation 2019). Recovery relates to regaining function to as close to premorbid level as possible,

adaptation is about changing what or how tasks are completed to achieve an intended outcome, compensation involves implementing assistive strategies to complete tasks, and prevention, which includes health promotion, focuses on reducing the risks of poor outcomes.

Integral to the success of these treatment approaches is a deep appreciation that rehabilitation goals cannot be achieved without active patient participation and that a person's physical, cognitive, emotional, psychosocial, cultural and spiritual needs impinge on each other (Ellis-Hill et al 2008) and relate to all aspects of the person's rehabilitation. It is important to remember that a person experiencing disability also retains many abilities (Pryor & Lingane 2017); nurses play a key role in preserving these abilities.

ICF supports the move away from an impairment-oriented approach in rehabilitation to a functional or task-oriented approach. It also facilitates teamwork by providing a common language for all disciplines (WHO 2001). This is important because rehabilitation is about more than healthcare.

REHABILITATION IS EVERYONE'S BUSINESS

While there has been a growing body of scholarship about rehabilitation as a health strategy, including the benefits of early rehabilitation, our understanding of rehabilitation should not be limited to that. Rehabilitation is everyone's business because many different people, services and organisations can help a person regain control over their body and their life. This has long been recognised by the WHO in their work on community-based rehabilitation (CBR) (WHO 2010). CBR is:

> a multisectoral approach working to improve the equalization of opportunities and social inclusion of people with disabilities while combating the perpetual cycle of poverty and disability. CBR is implemented through the combined efforts of people with disabilities, their families and communities, and relevant government and non-government health, education, vocational, social and other services (WHO 2016b).

Appreciation of the relevance of this approach for the developed world has been slow to develop, but that is set to change with national positioning at policy level of rehabilitation as everyone's business (National Health Service England 2016). Like several early nursing commentators (e.g. Dittmar 1989; Pryor 2001), the National Health Service England (2016, p. 5) reinforces that rehabilitation is 'a philosophy of care that helps to ensure people are included in their communities, employment and education'.

They rightly situate the person as playing a key role in their rehabilitation and position community assets, such as 'parks, cycle paths, outdoor gyms, swimming pools, leisure facilities, scouts/guides, play areas, smart phone apps etc.', and 'structured peer support' (p. 13) as major contributors to rehabilitation. Harnessing such disparate sources of support can be challenging; therefore, goals can be an effective tool for focusing and coordinating effort.

THE USE OF GOALS

Most human behaviour is goal-directed, regardless of how 'nebulous or unconsidered the behaviour may be' (Wade 2009, p. 291). The use of goals has become a hallmark of rehabilitation, and is recommended within clinical guidelines (e.g. Stroke Foundation 2019) and models of care (e.g. Central Adelaide Local Health Network 2016). Current literature certainly discusses the challenges in regard to the robustness of evidence about the relationship between goals and health outcomes (Levack et al 2015); nevertheless there is consensus that goal setting is a core component of rehabilitation.

The setting of goals is said to facilitate self-determination and engagement in the activities of rehabilitation. As described by Playford and colleagues (2009), goals may not necessarily have to be achievable, but may reflect a person's ambitions; this is integral to person-centredness. Goals represent why the patient is engaging in rehabilitation and why clinicians are providing interventions.

Wade's (2009) caution that goals should not be used to predict outcomes of rehabilitation, but rather that goals should be identified to guide rehabilitation interventions, is worth remembering.

In the rehabilitation context, goals can be set by any member of the rehabilitation team: the patient, significant others, treatment team members or relevant external stakeholders (such as funding agencies). Case and family conferencing and individual patient goal-setting meetings are mechanisms used by many rehabilitation teams to set goals. It is helpful to think of goals in two ways: long-term personal goals and short-term clinical goals.

Long-Term Personal Goals

The long-term goal of most patients is to return to their pre-injury or pre-illness life (Hafsteinsdottir & Grypdonck 1997). Regardless of whether or not this is possible, this goal identifies what is important to a person and provides the rationale for the interventions of healthcare professionals. In relation to ICF (WHO 2001), pre-injury or pre-illness life is often understood in terms of a person's participation in meaningful life situations (Thomas et al 2015), for example, recreational athlete, book lover, parent, teacher, gardener or builder.

Following biographical disruption (Bourke Hay-Smith et al 2015), re-establishment of a 'person's sense of control over his or her body and life' (Ozer 1999, p. 43) is an essential first step in rehabilitation. 'Restoring a sense of personal narrative' (Bourke et al 2015, p. 300) and 'the development of a resilient, intrinsic, spiritually based self' (Faull & Hills 2006, p. 729) are central to rehabilitation effectiveness. This can be particularly challenging following brain injury due to impaired cognition (Levack et al 2014), SCI and stroke. The person needing to use a wheelchair following SCI needs to come to see the chair as an extension of self (Papadimitriou 2008). Ellis-Hill (2011) explains that this re-establishment is a process and recognises the role of nurses in the journey, as the often-protracted transition to a new normal begins in hospital. Effective goal setting can assist in this process. Firstly, goals can help patients to move from pre-contemplation to action (van den Broek 2005). Secondly, goals can be a powerful mechanism for enhancing patient ownership of, and engagement in, their rehabilitation (Levack et al 2006). Thirdly, goal achievement can be a reference point for evaluating rehabilitation outcomes (NSW ACI 2019).

Short-Term Clinical Goals

The conversion of a person's long-term personal goals into short-term clinical goals that healthcare professionals can contribute to directly requires negotiation;

many short-term goals may underpin one long-term goal. We are reminded by Levack Kayes and Fadyl (2010) that depending on whose perspective is being considered (be it the person who is the patient, their family or clinicians), what are identified as problems in need of rehabilitation can differ. Discussion with and education of patients and families about the use of goals in rehabilitation is an essential first step towards developing a shared understanding (Bowen et al 2010). Demystifying the goal-setting process enables patients to re-establish decisional autonomy over their situation (Cardol DeJong & Ward 2002). Mutual goal setting should also ensure that the needs of both service users and service providers are best served, rather than rehabilitation being viewed as 'a product to be dispensed' (Stewart & Bhagwanjee 1999, p. 339) 'by one party to another' (Clapton & Kendall 2002, p. 990). Clinicians need to consider the values and preferences of patients and families and significant others, their own clinical judgement, the time and resources required to work towards stated goals and the consequences of pursuing that goal (Levack 2009). The consequences of not pursuing a particular goal may also need to be considered.

Short-term clinical goals can be most useful when articulated as S(specific) M(measurable) A(agreed) R(relevant) T(time-limited) goals. The relevance of SMART clinical goals is highlighted by Hill (1999), who herself has experienced traumatic brain injury; she notes that rehabilitation needs to assist injured persons to 're-orient or rebuild their life using a new set of "maps" with which to navigate life' (p. 839). SMART goals can contribute to the creation of these new maps.

In the short term, rehabilitation outcomes are evaluated by way of achievement of SMART goals. Healthcare professionals, however, need to be mindful that patients often evaluate their progress in relation to their pre-injury or pre-illness lifestyle and satisfaction with their reconstructed personal identity, not the small steps along the way (Ellis-Hill 2011). As a discipline, nursing is ideally situated to ensure that the benefits of rehabilitation are available to all consumers of healthcare.

NURSING AND REHABILITATION

Rehabilitation is central to nursing practice across the continuum of care, regardless of a person's age, diagnosis or setting (Pryor 2002). The overarching goal of rehabilitation, namely maximising human potential, is synonymous with the goal of nursing. Dittmar (1989, p. 2) describes rehabilitation as 'an approach, a philosophy, an attitude and a process', which can be woven into nursing practice, regardless of the clinical setting. Hickey and Thomas (2020) reinforce this point in noting the principles of rehabilitation are an integral component of independent nursing practice.

Kirkevold's (1997) description of four nursing functions is one way to understand nursing's rehabilitation role. These functions, while derived from a Norwegian study of stroke nursing, are relevant to rehabilitative nursing practice, regardless of diagnosis or setting (see Table 10.2). Several aspects of other rehabilitation studies complement Kirkevold's (1997) work, with four particular aspects relevant to the practice of all nurses. Firstly, adopting a rehabilitative approach requires nurses to 'focus on a person's ability in order to see possibilities rather than focusing on disabilities' and to adopt 'a wellness model of care' (Pryor & Smith 2002, p. 253). These are essential components for the person with an impairment in the reconstruction of their identity (Levack et al 2010) and could also be described as a humanised approach to care that encourages active participation in rehabilitation and healthcare (St-Germain et al 2011; Todres et al 2009).

Secondly, viewing 'every nurse–patient interaction as a teaching/learning opportunity' (Pryor & Smith 2002, p. 253) ensures that nurses assess patient readiness, ability and potential to be coached to self-care. This often starts with teaching patients about rehabilitation and how the rehabilitation roles of patients and nurses differ from their acute care roles (Pryor 2005).

Thirdly, like Kirkevold (1997) who reports that nurses create an atmosphere of positivity and optimism for each client, Pryor (2000) refers to a *rehabilitative*

TABLE 10.2 Four Rehabilitative Nursing Functions	
Interpretive function	Nurses help patients and families make sense of what has happened to them, what is happening to them and what may happen in the future
Consoling function	Nurses develop trusting relationships with patients and family members and provide emotional support
Conserving function	Nurses are involved in maintaining normal bodily functions with a heavy emphasis on prevention and physical protection
Integrative function	Nurses help patients integrate new learning, in relation to their activities of daily living, into their daily lives

Kirkevold 1997.

milieu that is contributed to by all people and activities on the unit. Tyrrell and colleagues (2012) found that partnerships are formed between nurses, patients and families, and in so doing, nurses facilitate self-determination and motivation, the ultimate aim being for patients to regain control over their own lives. Most importantly, nurses need to accept responsibility for creating therapeutic relationships (Tyrrell & Pryor 2016) to enable patients to engage 'with' as well as engage 'in' rehabilitation (Bright et al 2015).

Three knowledge types, identified by Liaschenko and Fisher (1999), are central to the effectiveness of nursing in supporting patients on their rehabilitation journey:

1. Case knowledge (generalised and objective knowledge, such as anatomy and physiology, disease processes and pharmacology)
2. Patient knowledge (knowledge of how a person is responding to their clinical situation)
3. Person knowledge (understanding each person as unique, knowing their personal and private biography and understanding how actions make sense for that person).

While all three types of knowledge are essential, person knowledge is of particular importance for rehabilitation. It is through knowing a person that relevant, person-specific goals and motivators can be identified (Levack et al 2010). Getting to know the patient, as a person, also communicates to their family and friends that they are valued by healthcare workers as a person, not just a patient (Youngson 2012).

In the remainder of this chapter, rehabilitation as a personal journey following injury or illness and as an intervention is illuminated through discussion of Karen's story (see Case Study 10.1, part 1). This case study illustrates how trauma can result in lifelong disability that is a chronic condition.

SPINAL CORD INJURY – WHAT IS IT?

The spinal cord is 'an elongated mass of nerve tissue that occupies the upper two-thirds of the vertebral canal and usually measures 42 to 45 cm long and about 1 cm in diameter at its widest point in the adult' (Hickey 2020b, p. 74). It 'extends from the upper borders of the atlas (first cervical vertebra) to the lower border of the first lumbar vertebra' (Hickey 2020b, p. 74). The spinal cord communicates messages and is the main pathway for transmitting information between the brain and the nerves that lead to muscles, skin, internal organs and glands (Raymond 2017a). The spinal cord is surrounded by the spinal column. This flexible bony

CASE STUDY

PART 1

Karen is a 45-year-old registered nurse; she is married and has 2 children. Both Karen and her husband work full-time as they are paying off their mortgage in Sydney. Outside of work Karen enjoys spending time with her family, which includes her parents and her in-laws. She enjoys watching her daughters participate in a variety of sports and is the fitness trainer for both of her daughters' netball teams. Karen likes cycling and running and trains with a small but close group of friends throughout the week and on weekends. Karen and her husband both have hectic schedules; they equally share their parenting roles and the home tasks such as washing, cooking and cleaning, and the children have designated chores they are responsible for.

While Karen was out riding her bicycle with a friend, it is thought that she may have hit a pothole as she was descending a hill causing her to fall from her bike. She had a loss of consciousness of less than 30 minutes and was responsive when an ambulance arrived at the scene; her Glasgow Coma Score was recorded as 14/15 as she showed some disorientation. Karen was taken by road ambulance directly to a tertiary hospital for specialist care, where she spent 35 days in acute care.

A CT brain showed a small frontal subdural hematoma that was managed conservatively. A CT spine revealed fracture dislocation at C5/6. An AIS exam diagnosed T6 AIS D SCI. As a result, she has a neurogenic bladder and bowel.

structure is made up of 33 vertebral bodies (7 cervical, 12 thoracic, 5 lumbar, 5 sacral and 4 coccygeal), separated by discs but held together by ligaments and supported by muscles (Raymond 2017a). There are 31 pairs of spinal nerves (8 cervical, 12 thoracic, 5 lumbar, 5 sacral and 1 coccygeal) that exit the spinal cord through openings in the vertebral column (Hickey 2020b).

Any external force to the spinal column, such as from a motor vehicle accident, fall or violent attack, can result in damage to the spinal cord (Australian Institute of Health and Welfare [AIHW]: Tovell 2019; Merritt et al 2019). The forces can displace bone fragments or exert pressure resulting in bruises or tears of the spinal cord tissue (Raymond 2017a). Transport-related injuries and falls accounted for more than three-quarters of traumatic spinal cord injuries (TSCIs) in Australia in 2015–2016 (AIHW: Tovell 2019). Non-traumatic causes of spinal cord injury are increasing as our population ages; these include infections, tumours, degenerative changes and embolic events (Davis et al 2019; Sauri et al 2017).

An injury to the spinal cord can disrupt movement, sensation and function below the level of injury (Vernese et al 2019). The extent of disability is dependent upon the level and completeness of injury to the spinal cord. The higher and more complete the level of injury, the greater the deficit will be in terms of impairments of bodily functions. An impairment scale developed by the American Spinal Injury Association (ASIA) (2019) is widely used to classify spinal cord injury by level and type (see Table 10.3). Using this scale, the patient with a spinal cord injury receives a diagnosis inclusive of the level of injury and ASIA Impairment Scale (AIS) (ASIA 2019), for example, in Karen's case T6 AIS D.

The range of impairments experienced by a person with SCI may present as numerous activity limitations and participation restrictions. In addition to the loss of movement and sensation, physical functional deficits often include bladder, bowel and sexual dysfunction. SCI requires ongoing management of these impairments to prevent or manage related problems, such as skin breakdown, pain and spasticity. SCI can impact on many aspects of a person's life; hence, the ability to work, study, socialise and participate in leisure activities may be altered. The psychological impact of SCI can also be great, with many people experiencing biographical disruption (Hickey 2020a; Raymond 2017b) and adverse social consequences, including high risk of divorce, social discrimination and unemployment (WHO 2013).

In the following sections of the chapter, rehabilitation in acute care, inpatient rehabilitation and the community will be discussed. Karen's story will be used to illuminate rehabilitation as an intervention in each of these settings, but more importantly as an ongoing personal journey.

ACUTE CARE – WHERE REHABILITATION BEGINS

In an instant, life as Karen knew it changed as a consequence of trauma to her body. Participation in valued life roles, such as working as a nurse, being a wife and mother, as well as playing sport, were interrupted. The complexity of physical impairments and psychological adjustment to disability challenged Karen and those around her (Bibi et al 2018), as they embarked on a journey of biographical reconstruction (Bourke et al 2015). For participants in the study by Bourke and colleagues (2015), this entailed acquiring information, regaining control and restoring a sense of personal narrative. Central for supporting this process is connecting a past that lacks experience of being disabled with a future that lacks access to tangible future possibilities (Papadimitriou & Stone 2011). Morse's (1997) five-stage model provides further insight into this process (Table 10.4).

In all acute care settings (emergency, high dependency and the ward), nurses actively facilitate Karen's rehabilitation, with the preservation of her integrity and dignity as a person being central to this. In ICF (WHO 2001) terms, Karen has significant impairments of body structures and functions, activity limitations and participation restrictions.

Throughout her post-injury journey Karen's goal is to return to her pre-injury life. This goal guides the co-production of her rehabilitation through synergistic

---

TABLE 10.3
ASIA Impairment Scale (AIS)

A = complete	No sensory or motor function is preserved in the sacral segments S4–S5
B = sensory incomplete	Sensory but not motor function is preserved below the neurological level and includes the sacral segments S4–S5 (light touch, pinprick at S4–S5: or deep anal pressure (DAP)) AND no motor function is preserved more than three levels below the motor level on either side of the body
C = motor incomplete	Motor function is preserved at the most caudal sacral segments for voluntary anal contraction (VAC) OR the patient meets the criteria for sensory incomplete status (sensory function preserved at the most caudal sacral segments (S4–S5) by light touch, pinprick or DAP), and has some sparing of motor function more than three levels below the ipsilateral motor level on either side of the body
D = motor incomplete	Motor incomplete status as defined above, with at least half (half or more) of key muscle functions below the single neurological level of injury having a muscle grade ≥ 3
E = normal	If sensation and motor function as tested with the ISNCSCI are graded as normal in all segments, and the patient had prior deficits, then the AIS grade is E. Someone without an initial SCI does not receive an AIS grade

American Spinal Injury Association 2019. International standards for neurological classification of spinal cord injury. Retrieved from:https://asia-spinalinjury.org/wp-content/uploads/2019/10/ASIA-ISCOS-Worksheet_10.2019_PRINT-Page-1-2.pdf © 2019 American Spinal Injury Association. Reprinted with permission.

TABLE 10.4
Five Stages of Responding to Threats to Integrity

1. Vigilance	'The first changes in the onset of acute or chronic illness bring about a dis-ease, with the individuals suspecting that something is wrong' (p. 28).
2. Disruption: Enduring to Survive	'The major task of the critically ill is to hold on to life' (p. 31).
3. Enduring to Live: Striving to Regain Self	'Once the acute crisis has been resolved, the real work derived from illness or the injury must begin' (p. 31).
4. Suffering: Striving to Restore Self	The person 'begins to struggle with grief, mourning what has been lost and the altered future' (p. 32).
5. Learning to Live With the Altered Self	'The person must get to know and to trust the altered body' (p. 33).

Morse 1997.

teamwork (Pryor 2014). As nurses spend the most time with patients, they have a unique opportunity to ensure that the relationship between each healthcare intervention and Karen's long-term goal are clearly understood by Karen and her family. This is an essential aspect of nursing's interpretive function, as is explaining to Karen and her family the nature of Karen's injuries and the processes and rationale for the various treatments. Understanding how the interventions of health workers relate to a person's everyday life assists people to integrate what is happening into their lives.

The consequences of injuries like Karen's on family and friends are significant, with several authors describing how these reverberate throughout the entire family and social network (Dickson et al 2012; Flemming et al 2012). Pratt and Baldry (2002, p. 291) describe this reverberation as follows:

It is during this journey from intensive care to a rehabilitation unit or ward that a metamorphosis occurs – relatives become 'carers'. As such, certain expectations are made and roles placed upon them by professional staff and by others in their environment. Carers, meanwhile, will have little time to adjust to this new role and will perceive themselves in their pre-injury condition.

As healthcare workers we often focus on the transfer of care to family and our role in the development of the skills required to provide that care. As illustrated in

two studies included in Table 10.1 (Conti et al 2016; Young et al 2014), families need much more from us. Family members need support as many experience biographical disruption and a rollercoaster of emotions associated with their experiences.

Karen and her family members will probably be emotionally and physically compromised learners. They are unlikely to be self-directed learners, because at this time it is common to experience difficulty in knowing what needs to be learned (Pryor & Jannings 2004). While education helps people to cope, we need to appreciate that not all learning takes place within an inpatient setting (Olinzock 2004). Much of a person's learning will be about how imparted information is integrated in line with their own values, physical environments and personal contexts (Schipper et al 2011). Therefore, many patients and their family members benefit from written as well as verbal information (Mateer et al 2005).

While nurses address all the components of ICF in acute care settings, a major aspect of acute care is maintaining normal bodily functions. With a heavy emphasis on prevention and physical protection (the conserving function), nurses make a significant contribution to patient rehabilitation through 'the management and promotion of homeostasis' (McPherson 2006, p. 788). Unfortunately, overlooking the maintenance of existing function, a central aspect of rehabilitation (Pryor 1999), can result in iatrogenic complications, such as joint contractures and imposed dependence (Gignac & Cott 1998).

In the early acute stage Karen cannot actively contribute to maintaining homeostasis. Therefore, nurses provide wholly compensatory care, shifting to partially compensatory care, then educative–supportive care (Orem 1995) as Karen's condition allows. Knowing when to adopt a hands-on (wholly or partially compensatory) or hands-off (educative–supportive) approach is a hallmark of rehabilitation nursing expertise (Pryor & Smith 2002). Table 10.5 provides examples of how nurses conserve Karen's function.

PRE-TRANSFER EDUCATION

Pre-transfer education about what rehabilitation is and how it differs from acute care is vital for patients and their families (Pryor & O'Connell 2008). Unless previously exposed to rehabilitation, most people do not understand it (Miller 2003); nurses who have not worked in rehabilitation services commonly possess little rehabilitation knowledge. Therefore, staff from the rehabilitation unit should deliver this education to

TABLE 10.5
Example Goals and How Nurses Conserve Karen's Function in Acute Care

Short-Term Goals	Nursing Interventions
Conserve function and prevent complications of immobility, such as deep vein thrombosis, pressure injury, joint contractures, pneumonia, constipation	• Regular range of motion exercises for all joints • Regular inspection of pressure points • Use of pressure-relieving mattresses • Airway management • Ensure adequate nutritional and fluid intake • Management of bowel and bladder elimination • Early identification of potential complications • Timely reporting of unexpected changes
Conserve function and prevent secondary spinal injury due to unstable fracture site that may cause further cord damage	• Immobilising the spine when moving and handling Karen
Conserve function and prevent secondary injury due to spinal shock, such as paralytic ileus and neurogenic bladder	• Management of intravenous line and fluids • Insertion and management of nasogastric tube • Monitoring for vomiting and abdominal distension • Monitoring oral intake, bowel sounds and flatus • Insertion and management of indwelling urinary catheter • Prevention and management of urinary tract infection • Accurate observation and recording of fluid intake and output
Conserve function and prevent secondary injury due to autonomic dysreflexia (AD)	• Monitoring for signs of AD (pounding headache, flushing above the level of injury, profuse sweating) • Managing any episodes of AD (determine cause, measure BP, administer medication as required)

allow for the provision of accurate information and to answer questions. Whenever possible, pre-transfer education should include written information and a visit to the rehabilitation unit by patient and family and significant others. These measures enhance the likelihood of informed decision-making.

The importance of pre-transfer education is highlighted in studies that found pre-transfer preparation of patients for rehabilitation to be inadequate (Gibbon 2004; Pryor & O'Connell 2008). Inadequate preparation can be detrimental to patient progress, because patients need time to adjust their expectations of hospitalisation to enable them to fully access the benefits of rehabilitation. Nurses are ideally situated to ensure that patients, their family and friends have timely access to accurate information.

INPATIENT REHABILITATION

Inpatient rehabilitation differs significantly from acute care. In the rehabilitation unit, patients are encouraged to work hard, be as independent as possible and interact with other patients as the momentum of rehabilitation increases. Each patient has an individualised

rehabilitation plan consisting of short-term clinical goals that are linked to the patient's longer-term personal goals. All goals are reviewed regularly.

Patients do the work of rehabilitation, with members of the clinical team guiding and supporting the process. The patient and family are central team members; other members include specialist rehabilitation nurses, specialist rehabilitation doctors, recreation therapists, physiotherapists, case managers, occupational therapists, speech pathologists, psychologists, social workers, dietitians, pharmacists and rehabilitation assistants, as well as cleaning, administration and catering staff.

All family, friends and staff have the potential to make a valuable contribution to patient rehabilitation, but optimal teamwork can be a major challenge. The role of nursing overlaps with the roles of all the other disciplines, and 'integrated action is a pre-requisite for successful rehabilitation' (Gutenbrunner et al 2011, p. 760). This means nurses, medical and allied health staff need to work synergistically to assess, plan, intervene and evaluate together, dialoguing, valuing and respecting each other's contribution. The coordination of patient, family and staff effort is a primary nursing responsibility (Pryor & Smith 2002). Furthermore, as Low (2003) explains, nurses are well positioned to ascertain a person's suitability for working with allied health staff and whether such participation will be of benefit in light of the person's other medical and nursing needs at a given time. This is central to ensuring a patient's health and functional goals are addressed (Pryor 2005).

Transfer to an inpatient rehabilitation unit does not guarantee patient readiness for active participation in rehabilitation. Despite the best efforts of clinicians to ease patients into rehabilitation, patients are not always ready for the demands of an inpatient rehabilitation program. On the other hand, failure by the clinical team to understand the patient and family perspective following trauma may inhibit rehabilitation that is truly person-centred (Ellis-Hill et al 2008; Youngson 2012). Anxiety, grief, loneliness, boredom and restricted visitors can lead to a lack of patient motivation (Flemming et al 2012). Frustration (Hafsteinsdottir & Grypdonck 1997) and lack of confidence (Pryor 2005) have also been recognised as factors that impact on patient engagement with rehabilitation activities, although rehabilitation nurses who understand their vital role have been found to enhance patient engagement (Pryor & Buzio 2010).

One group that has particular needs is patients with cognitive impairments. Neurorehabilitation is often difficult when patients lack insight that they have an impairment that would benefit from rehabilitation (van den Broek 2005). In this pre-contemplation stage of the transtheoretical model of change (Prochaska et al 1992), problem identification by the patient is a primary goal of rehabilitation (see Case Study 10.1, part 2).

BRAIN INJURY – WHAT IS IT?

The human brain is a complex organ made up of approximately 100 billion cells (Hickey 2020b), the functioning of which can be impacted by traumatic and non-traumatic injuries. Traumatic brain injury (TBI) is the result of an external force to the brain from a penetrating projectile, a blast force or from acceleration–deceleration forces (Kreutzer et al 2016; O'Phelan 2016). Examples of these forces which result in trauma to the brain are a gunshot, falls, a sporting accident, assault, or injury from a motor vehicle accident (O'Reilly et al 2018). Non-traumatic aetiologies may include hypoxia, vascular complications, a disease or degeneration process, infection, cancer or drug abuse.

Worldwide, TBI is a significant healthcare problem and is often referred to as the silent epidemic (Faul et al 2010). The heterogeneous nature of TBI neurotrauma

---

CASE STUDY

PART 2

During Karen's rehabilitation, admission nursing staff identified Karen's significant fatigue. This was initially identified after her morning showering routine and was confirmed with allied health staff. Staff were noticing that Karen did not always reliably recall information from previous information sessions, such as education regarding self-administration of medication, intermittent self-catheterising (ISC) and bowel routines. This impacted on her ability to complete these tasks independently. Nursing staff also identified that Karen was having difficulty in initiating what she needed to complete her morning routine, such as preparing her clothing and toiletries. The nursing and allied health staff recognised that Karen was not following her timetable and required prompting to attend appointments.

Nursing staff identified the need for a neuropsychological assessment as they suspected that Karen's presentation suggested a mild TBI sustained in the bicycle accident. This assessment confirmed that Karen had slowed information processing and her ability to retain new information was reduced. Having this information was a way to enable staff to develop cueing systems which Karen could implement to improve her independence. Adjusting Karen's timetable to allow for rest periods dispersed throughout her day was an important strategy to ensure she had the ability to be an active participant in her rehabilitation.

---

can result in a diverse and complex array of sequalae ranging from subtle, to debilitating and enduring, including cognitive, physical, neurobehavioural, neuropsychological and executive functions. Personality, communication, language, sensory and emotional disorders are also commonly associated with TBI' (McKechnie et al 2014, p. 16).

Severity of injury is classified using various assessment tools with the Glasgow Coma Scale (GCS) the most commonly used in the acute phase (O'Phelan 2016). As Karen had a very brief loss of consciousness of unknown duration (although less than 30 minutes) and her GCS was assessed as 14/15 at the scene, her injury is classified as a mild TBI (Kreutzer et al 2016; Silverberg, Lange & Iverson 2016). Post Traumatic Amnesia (PTA) testing is also another severity of injury tool commonly used; however, as Karen was oriented to time, person and place within 24 hours of her injury this also classifies her injury as a mild TBI (Silverberg et al 2016) and PTA testing was not commenced.

Establishing Routines

Structure and routine are important aspects of rehabilitation. Patients with memory impairment, fatigue, neurobehavioural concerns (such as adynamia) and depression or anxiety as a result of brain or spinal cord injury, benefit greatly from sequencing tasks. The family and significant others also benefit as it provides a general guide of a patient's rehabilitation program facilitating visiting, as well as leisure and community activities. Nurses work with patients to establish routines for personal activities of daily living (ADLs). Of particular importance is the establishment of routines for urinary and faecal elimination as this will support patients to gain the most benefit from rehabilitation programs and function more independently in the community (Carr et al 2017; Piatt et al 2016). In Karen's case, timetabling is an effective tool for establishing routines for intermittent self-catheterisation that can help to prevent urinary leakage, highlighted as particularly anxiety-provoking for people following SCI (Carr et al 2017; Piatt et al 2016).

The goals for Karen's ongoing bladder management are to:
- prevent overstretching of the bladder
- prevent or minimise UTIs
- control bladder spasm
- minimise risk of vesicoureteric reflux, and
- minimise volume of residual urine in bladder.

To achieve these goals and maintain renal health Karen needs to follow the following steps:
- Clean hands using handwash
- Clean genital areas
- Remove catheter from packaging without touching the catheter
- Spread labia apart gently with thumb and index finger
- With the other hand, gently insert the catheter into the urethra; urine will flow once the catheter reaches the bladder
- When the urine stops flowing slowly remove catheter
- Discard catheter into bin
- Clean hands

The goals of Karen's bowel routine are to:
- Have a reliable and predictable bowel routine
- Avoid bowel accidents, and
- Avoid complications, such as constipation and diarrhea.

To achieve these goals and maintain a healthy bowel Karen needs to complete the following tasks daily:
- Have breakfast or a hot drink to initiate the gastrocolic reflex

- Wait 15–30 minutes
- Check for faeces in rectum – if some present remove a small amount
- Insert a Microlax enema
- Wait 10 minutes
- Check rectum, if faeces still present carry out digital stimulation
- Wait 10 minutes – if no result repeat step above
- Repeat a maximum of 3 times
- If no faeces present after any of the checks, clean up
- Make a note of amount and type of stool passed or if no stool passed.

See Box 10.2 for examples of Karen's long-term rehabilitation goals.

Timetabling

In inpatient rehabilitation, the flow of a patient's day should resemble, as far as possible, that of their usual lifestyle. Patients actively participate in all aspects of their personal care, dress in day clothes and commonly eat meals in a dining room. A combination of individual and group sessions with various disciplines is common. Karen's mutually agreed timetable for week 4 of her inpatient rehabilitation program is presented in Table 10.6. Note the progression from less to more independence in some self-care activities, for example, self-administration of medications.

As each rehabilitation journey is unique, we must remember that although some patients appear to transition through these stages seamlessly, others may falter or vacillate. It may take some patients more time to regain self-efficacy to direct their life given the catastrophic event and challenging process of integrating this into a new way of living (Craig et al 2019). Therefore, timetabling can also be used as a cueing system, a method for behaviour support and, if patients are to independently attend to their own therapy appointments, a mechanism for cognitive assessment.

Box 10.2
Examples of Karen's Long-Term Rehabilitation Goals

Karen wants to:
- return to part-time employment
- resume her fitness trainer role for her children's sports
- resume cycling with her friends
- independently cook two family meals each week.

TABLE 10.6
Karen's Timetable for Week 4

Time	Monday	Tuesday	Wednesday	Thursday	Friday	Saturday	Sunday
06.00	CISC with nurse supervising	CISC with nurse supervising	CISC with nurse supervising	CISC with nurse supervising	Independent CISC	Independent CISC	Independent CISC
06.30	Sleep	Sleep	Sleep	Sleep	Sleep	Sleep	Sleep
07.30	Breakfast	Breakfast	Breakfast	Breakfast	Breakfast	Breakfast	Breakfast
08.00	Medication education	Medication education	SAM using Webster pack with nurse supervising	SAM using Webster pack with nurse supervising	Independent SAM using a Webster pack	Independent SAM using a Webster pack	Independent SAM using a Webster pack
	Bowel care supervised by nurse	Bowel care supervised by nurse	Bowel care supervised by nurse	Bowel care supervised by nurse	Independent bowel care using flowchart	Independent bowel care using flowchart	Independent bowel care using flowchart
08.30	Shower independently	Shower independently	Shower independently	Shower independently	Shower independently	Shower independently	Shower independently
09.00	Free time or rest	Free time or rest	Free time or rest	Free time or rest	Free time or rest	Free time or rest	Free time or rest
10.00	CISC with nurse supervising	CISC with nurse supervising	CISC with nurse supervising	CISC with nurse supervising	Independent CISC	Independent CISC	Independent CISC
10.30	WC skills outside with RT	Session in the gym with physio	Communication group with SP	Group community access trip on buses & ferry with RT	Coffee group supported by nurses	Independent exercises in gym	Independent exercises in gym
11.00	Car transfer practice with OT	Counselling session with clin psych	Free time or rest	Group community access trip on buses & ferry with RT	Session in the gym with physio	Independent exercises in gym	Free time or rest
12.00	Free time or rest	Free time or rest	Free time or rest	Group community access trip on buses & ferry with RT	Free time or rest	Free time or rest	Free time or rest
12.30	Lunch	Lunch	Lunch	Lunch in the community	Cook hot meal for lunch with supervision from OT	Lunch	Cook lunch for wife with support as required
13.00	Meeting with keyworker to discuss progress and new goals	Peer support with local spinal injuries support group	Goal planning meeting with whole team to confirm next set of goals and actions	Group community access trip on buses & ferry with RT	Cardio group with physiotherapy assistant	Trip out with husband and children mobilising independently	Cook lunch with family with support as required

Continued

TABLE 10.6
Karen's Timetable for Week 4 – cont'd

Time	Monday	Tuesday	Wednesday	Thursday	Friday	Saturday	Sunday
14.00	CISC with nurse supervising	CISC with nurse supervising	CISC with nurse supervising	Independent CISC	Independent CISC in community	Independent CISC	Independent CISC
14.30	Medication education	Medication education	SAM using Webster pack with nurse supervising	SAM using Webster pack with nurse supervising	SAM using Webster pack with nurse supervising	Independent SAM using Webster pack	Independent SAM using Webster pack
15.00	Hydrotherapy with physio	Return to work discussion with VT	WC skills outside with RT	Free time or rest	Physiotherapy session in the gym	Out with family	Sunday afternoon film club supported by nurses
16.00	Hydrotherapy with physio	Free time or rest	Free time or rest	Free time or rest	Free time or rest	Out with family	Sunday afternoon film club supported by nurses
17.00	Free time or rest	Physiotherapy session in the gym	Free time or rest	Free time or rest	WC skills outside with RT	Out with family	Free time or rest
18.00	CISC with nurse supervising	CISC with nurse supervising	CISC with nurse supervising	Independent CISC	Independent CISC in community	Independent CISC	Independent CISC
18.30	Dinner	Dinner	Dinner	Dinner	Dinner	Dinner	Dinner
19.30	Phone children	Phone friend	Skype sister and nephews	Phone mum and dad	Phone husband	Phone children	Skype brother and nieces
20.00	Medication education	Medication education	SAM using Webster pack with nurse supervising	SAM using Webster pack with nurse supervising	Independent SAM using Webster pack	Independent SAM using Webster pack	Independent SAM using Webster pack
21.00	Free time or bed	Free time or bed	Free time or bed	Free time or bed	Free time or bed	Free time or bed	Free time or bed
22.00	CISC with nurse supervising	CISC with nurse supervising	CISC with nurse supervising	Independent CISC	Independent CISC in community	Independent CISC	Independent CISC
22.30	Sleep	Sleep	Sleep	Sleep	Sleep	Sleep	Sleep
02.00	CISC with nurse supervising	CISC with nurse supervising	CISC with nurse supervising	Independent CISC	Independent CISC in community	Independent CISC	Independent CISC
02.30	Sleep	Sleep	Sleep	Sleep	Sleep	Sleep	Sleep

Abbreviations: CISC = clean intermittent self-catheterisation; SAM = self-administration of medications; physio = physiotherapist; RT = recreation therapist; OT = occupational therapist; clin psych = clinical psychologist; WC = wheelchair skills; SP = speech pathologist; VT = vocational therapist.

By the end of week 4 rehabilitation, Karen was able to:

- independently mobilise short distances indoors with Canadian crutches
- independently mobilise outdoors in a manual wheelchair
- independently perform ISC with cueing from a memory aid
- independently perform bowel care with cueing from a memory aid
- with supervision, use a hand cycle
- with prompting, recognise and manage signs of cognitive fatigue
- cook two different family meals (tacos and spaghetti bolognaise).

While Karen is independent with self-catheterisation, bowel care and preparing some simple meals, transferring these skills to her home environment may take some time. This transition will benefit from consultation with a community rehabilitation service.

Cueing systems

For persons who are cognitively impaired, routine is supported by the use of cueing systems. Cueing systems involve the use of an external stimulus (alarms, signage or timetable) to notify someone that something needs to be done. Assistive technologies within smart phones are increasingly being used as cueing systems. When effective training is provided, these technologies can help patients with poor initiation and memory problems (Wong et al 2017). Cueing systems allow the patient to work collaboratively with others to decide what actions are to be prompted. Cueing systems also provide some structure and assistance for family members in encouraging safe participation in rehabilitation (such as always using a frame to mobilise or self-catheterisation).

Nursing's Contribution to Karen's Rehabilitation

Nursing interventions, like other rehabilitation interventions, need to focus on maintaining and restoring function, promoting health and preventing and minimising disability. As with all interventions, nurses assess, plan, implement and evaluate their intervention.

Two recent articles reporting on a review of literature provide frameworks for understanding the nature (Baker et al 2019a) and mechanisms (Baker et al 2019b) of nursing's contribution to Karen's rehabilitation. Nurses provided nurse-initiated care, such as managing patients' health conditions and providing technical care to maintain patient safety and nursing care to support patients' goals, which includes assisting with personal ADLs and providing carry-on therapy (Baker et al 2019a). Nurses also provided emotional care to support biographical adjustment (Baker et al 2019a), which for Karen was a major undertaking. The mechanisms nurses used were building therapeutic nurse–patient relationships, coaching patients to self-care, creating a rehabilitative milieu and coordinating patient care (Baker et al 2019b). These nursing roles fit well with the core influencing activities in the NSW program logic for rehabilitation, in particular enabling self-management, providing a facilitatory environment and person-centred assessment, treatment, education and care (NSW ACI 2019). Table 10.7 lists examples of interventions that nurses could use to support Karen to achieve her rehabilitation goals.

LIFE AFTER INPATIENT REHABILITATION

A seamless transition from the inpatient rehabilitation setting to the community is ideal for maintaining the momentum of rehabilitation for the person and their family. To facilitate this transition, rehabilitation inpatients commonly access the local community and their home with an inpatient treatment team member in preparation for overnight leave and eventual discharge. However, the environment in which this occurs is usually well structured, contained and controlled.

Transition from an inpatient to community setting can involve new challenges for the patient, their family and friends, as well as those working with them. Commonly, a person leaving inpatient rehabilitation believes they can get on with their life and things will return to normal quite quickly after discharge. The impact of an injury is often felt most when the person returns home. Here the reality of the altered body and altered life is most apparent (O'Brien et al 2002).

While in the inpatient rehabilitation setting, engagement of a community case manager and a community rehabilitation service can be key for community reintegration and a seamless rehabilitation program. Case management is a 'collaborative process that assesses, plans, implements, coordinates, monitors and evaluates the options and services required to meet an individual's health needs using communication and available resources to promote quality, cost effective outcomes' (Snowden 2001, p. 3). Case management has an element of advocacy as a case manager assists the person, their family and friends to identify solutions to activity limitations and participation restrictions (Snowden 2001). As such, the case manager helps individuals structure their rehabilitation in ways that are meaningful to them.

TABLE 10.7
Example Nursing Interventions

Goal	Example Interventions
Patient self-management of urinary elimination	• Education of patient regarding bladder function pre- and post-SCI (including bladder management methods) • Prepare and educate patient about bladder investigations • Support patient through trial of void, including maintaining record of input and output • Education regarding CISC • Practise CISC under supervision • Gauge readiness for independence in CISC • Educate and encourage patient to set alarms on memory aid for CISC timing • Coordinate and document team evaluation of urinary elimination • Modify bladder management program as required • Education of family as/if required
Patient self-management of faecal elimination	• Obtain a pre-injury history regarding faecal elimination • Education regarding bowel management before and after SCI (including nutrition and medication) • Education regarding bowel movement classification (Bristol Stool Chart) • Education regarding assisted bowel evacuation – PR check, enema administration, abdominal massage and digital stimulation • Attend to bowel care under supervision, prompts and support • Support to problem-solve around bowel problems using flowchart • Gauge readiness for independent bowel care • Document and coordinate team evaluation of bowel management • Education of family as/if required
Patient self-management of skin	• Education regarding SCI and how this affects skin and pressure area management • Education regarding skin checks, what to look for and actions to take • Education regarding techniques for pressure relief (devices, chair positions, frequency) • Support patient to problem-solve around potential or real problems using flowchart • Support in decision-making around pressure-relieving devices – cushions, mattresses • Advice regarding appropriate clothing • Education of family as/if required

In the community, the nature of rehabilitation changes. The intensity of clinical sessions with health professionals is reduced or ceased as rehabilitation is integrated more into daily life. Increased self-reliance and the support of family and friends are crucial to goal achievement at this stage (Ylvisaker et al 2003). Here the multi-agency and multi-sectorial nature of rehabilitation is more evident, illuminating how rehabilitation is everyone's business. Every person, agency and service that Karen interacts with has the potential to enable her rehabilitation. Unfortunately, it is also true that these same interactions can become barriers. This means that each of us has a responsibility to ensure that in our personal as well as our professional lives we are socially inclusive and enable human functioning and participation.

Part 3 of Case Study 10.1 presents an overview of Karen's progress after her return home.

CONCLUSION

Understanding rehabilitation as a co-production that is everyone's business positions nurses to optimise their contribution to patient rehabilitation. This understanding tells nurses that they are key influencers of the process and outcomes of patient rehabilitation. Being person-centred means that over time we hand over responsibility to the person who is the patient and their family. Preparing patients, families and significant others for this is a key nursing responsibility. Values-based goal setting is a useful skill that nurses need to use to facilitate this process.

CASE STUDY

PART 3

As a registered nurse, Karen is registered with the Australian Health Practitioners Registration Agency (AHPRA). On return home Karen remained unable to return to work due to both her physical and cognitive impairments, which were reportable to AHPRA due to the mandatory reporting requirements. Being unable to work, drive or participate in sport in the way she had before her injury impacted significantly on Karen's self-esteem and she felt she was becoming socially isolated. Karen worked hard on her physical recovery, attending three weekly gym sessions and one hydrotherapy session. Karen sustained her injuries on a road in NSW and was therefore on the icare scheme, which provides lifelong funding for equipment, home modifications and care, including ongoing therapy as long as these are demonstrated to be reasonable and necessary. Examples of items that are funded are Karen's mobility aids, such as a wheelchair she uses when needing to mobilise over longer distances or in crowded spaces such as at school pick-up, and continence equipment such as catheters.

Both Karen and her husband were anxious about their financial future as they had been reliant on both incomes to meet their mortgage payments and family living expenses. Karen had started seeing a vocational rehabilitation provider to consider what her future employment options could be.

For Karen, many of the impairments she lives with, such as debilitating fatigue, headaches, limb spasticity, spasm, anxiety, neurogenic bladder and bowel, depression and impaired memory, are not visible. The hidden impairments that Karen lives with are likely to impact on her ability to earn an income, participate in her sports, her sexual relationship and self-identity, her parenting role and her ability to support her aging parents.

Reflective Questions

1. Select one of the short outcomes in the Principles to Support Rehabilitation Care document (NSW Agency for Clinical Innovation 2019) and identify what nursing interventions you could use to achieve this outcome.
2. Describe nursing interventions that could be used to support biographical adjustment and explain how each is expected to work.
3. Identify 10 ways in which nurses can create a rehabilitative milieu.

RECOMMENDED READING

Baker MJ, Pryor J, Fisher MJ 2019a. Nursing practice in inpatient rehabilitation: a narrative review – part 1. JARNA (Journal of the Australasian Rehabilitation Nurses' Association) 22(2), 7–21.

Baker MJ, Pryor J, Fisher MJ 2019b. Nursing practice in inpatient rehabilitation: a narrative review – part 2. JARNA (Journal of the Australasian Rehabilitation Nurses' Association) 22(3), 7–15.

NSW Agency for Clinical Innovation 2019. Principles to support rehabilitation care. Rehabilitation Network ACI_0241 [07/19]. Online. Available: www.aci.health.nsw.gov.au/__data/assets/pdf_file/0014/500900/rehabilitation-principles.pdf.

REFERENCES

American Spinal Injury Association (ASIA) 2019. International Standards for neurological classification of spinal cord injury. Online. Available: https://asia-spinalinjury.org/wp-content/uploads/2019/10/ASIA-ISCOS-Worksheet_10.2019_PRINT-Page-1-2.pdf.

Amsters D et al 2018. Determinants of participating in life after spinal cord injury – advice for health professionals arising from an examination of shared narratives. Disability and Rehabilitation 40(25), 3030–3040.

Australian Institute of Health and Welfare (AIHW): Tovell A 2019. Spinal cord injury Australia 2015–16. Injury research and statistics series no.122. Cat. No. INJCAT 202. AIHW, Canberra.

Baker MJ, Pryor J, Fisher MJ 2019a. Nursing practice in inpatient rehabilitation: a narrative review – part 1. JARNA (Journal of the Australasian Rehabilitation Nurses' Association) 22(2), 7–21.

Baker MJ, Pryor J, Fisher MJ 2019b. Nursing practice in inpatient rehabilitation: a narrative review – part 2. JARNA (Journal of the Australasian Rehabilitation Nurses' Association) 22(3), 7–15.

Barnes MP, Ward AB 2000. Textbook of rehabilitation medicine. Oxford University Press, Oxford.

Bibi S, Rasmussen P, McLiesh P 2018. The lived experience: nurses' experience of caring for patients with a traumatic spinal cord injury. International Journal of Orthopaedic and Trauma Nursing 30, 31–38.

Bourke JA, Hay-Smith EJC, Snell DL et al 2015. Attending to biographical disruption: the experience of rehabilitation following tetraplegia due to spinal cord injury. Disability and Rehabilitation 37(4), 296–303.

Bowen C, Yeates G, Palmer S 2010. Brain injuries series. A relational approach to rehabilitation: thinking about relationships after brain injury. Karnac Books.

Bright FAS, Kayes NM, Worrell L et al 2015. A conceptual review of engagement in healthcare and rehabilitation. Disability and Rehabilitation 37(8), 643–654.

Cameron ID 2010. Models of rehabilitation – commonalities of interventions that work and of those that do not. Disability and Rehabilitation 32(12), 1051–1058.

Cardol M, DeJong B, Ward D 2002. On autonomy and participation rehabilitation. Disability & Rehabilitation 24(18), 970–974.

Carr J, Kendall M, Amsters D et al 2017. Community participation for individuals with spinal cord injury living in Queensland Australia. Spinal Cord 55, 192–197.

Central Adelaide Local Health Network 2016. General rehabilitation sub-acute model of care. Online. Available: www.cpsu.asn.au/upload/2016-Info-Updates/UPDATED-General-Rehabilitation-SubAcute-Model-of-Care-30-Nov-2016.pdf.

Clapton J, Kendall E 2002. Autonomy and participation in rehabilitation: time for a new paradigm? Disability and Rehabilitation 24(18), 987–991.

Conti A, Garrino L, Montanari P et al 2016. Informal caregivers' needs on discharge from the spinal cord unit: analysis of perceptions and lived experiences. Disability and Rehabilitation 38(2), 159–167.

Craig A, Tran Y, Guest R et al 2019. Trajectories of self-efficacy and depressed mood and their relationship in the first 12 months following spinal cord injury. Archives of Physical Medicine and Rehabilitation 100, 441–447.

Curvis W, Simpson J, Hampson N 2018. Social anxiety following traumatic brain injury: an exploration of associated factors. Neuropsychological Rehabilitation 28(4), 527–547.

Davis M, Allam A, Korupolu R 2019. An overview of nontraumatic spinal cord injury and dysfunction. In: R Mitra (ed.), Principles of rehabilitation medicine. McGraw Hill Education, New York.

Dickson A, O'Brien G, Ward R et al 2012. Adjustment and coping in spousal caregivers following a traumatic spinal cord injury: an interpretive phenomenological analysis. Journal of Health Psychology 17(2), 247–257.

Dittmar S 1989. Scope of rehabilitation. In: S Dittmar (ed.), Rehabilitation nursing: process and application. CV Mosby, St Louis.

Ellis-Hill C 2011. Identity and sense of self: the significance of personhood in rehabilitation. Journal of the Australasian Rehabilitation Nurses' Association 14(1), 6–13.

Ellis-Hill C, Payne S, Ward C 2008. Using stroke to explore the life thread model: an alternative approach to understanding rehabilitation following acquired disability. Disability and Rehabilitation 30(2), 150–159.

Faul M, Xu L, Wald M et al 2010. Traumatic brain injury in the United States: emergency department visits hospitalizations and deaths 2002–2006. Center for Disease Control and Prevention, National Center for Injury Prevention and Control Atlanta (GA). Online. Available: www.cdc.gov/traumaticbraininjury/pdf/blue_book.pdf.

Faull K, Hills MD 2006. The role of the spiritual dimension of the self as the prime determinant of health. Disability and Rehabilitation 28(11), 729–740.

Flemming J, Sampson J, Cornwell P et al 2012. Brain injury rehabilitation: the lived experience of inpatients and their family caregivers. Scandinavian Journal of Occupational Therapy 19, 184–193.

Gibbon B 2004. Service user involvement: the impact of stroke and the meaning of rehabilitation. Journal of the Australasian Rehabilitation Nurses' Association 7(2), 8–12.

Gignac MA, Cott C 1998. A conceptual model of independence and dependence for adults with chronic physical illness and disability. Social Science Medicine 47(6), 739–753.

Gutenbrunner C, Meyer T, Melvin J et al 2011. Towards a conceptual description of physical and rehabilitation medicine. Journal of Rehabilitation Medicine 43, 760–764.

Hafsteinsdottir TB, Grypdonck M 1997. Being a stroke patient. A review of the literature. Journal of Advanced Nursing 26, 580–588.

Hickey JV 2020a. Assessment and evaluation of neuroscience patients. In: J Hickey, AL Stayer (eds), The clinical practice of neurological and neurosurgical nursing. Wolters Kluwer, Philadelphia.

Hickey JV 2020b. Overview of neuroanatomy and neurophysiology. In: J Hickey, AL Stayer (eds), The clinical practice of neurological and neurosurgical nursing, 9th edn. Lippincott, Williams and Wilkins, Philadelphia.

Hickey JV, Thomas LW 2020. Rehabilitation of patients with neurological disorders. In: J Hickey, A Stayer (eds), The clinical practice of neurological and neurosurgical nursing, 8th edn. Wolters Kluwer, Philadelphia.

Hill H 1999. Traumatic brain injury: a view from the inside. Brain Injury 13(11), 839–844.

Jesus T, Landry MD, Hoenig H 2019. Global need for physical rehabilitation: systemic analysis from the Global Burden of Disease Study 2017. International Journal of Environmental Research and Public Health 16, 980–998.

Kattari S, Olzman M, Hanna M 2018. 'You look fine!': ableist experiences by people with invisible disabilities. Journal of Women and Social Work 33(4), 477–492.

Kayes NM, Mudge S, Bright FAS et al 2015. Whose behavior matters? Rethinking practitioner behavior and its influence on rehabilitation outcomes. In: K McPherson, BE Gibson, A Leplege (eds), Rethinking rehabilitation: theory and practice. CRC Press, Boca Raton.

Kearney P, Pryor J 2004. The international classification of functioning, disability and health (ICF) and nursing. Journal of Advanced Nursing 46(2), 162–170.

Kirkevold M 1997. The role of nursing in the rehabilitation of acute stroke patients: toward a unified theoretical perspective. Advances in Nursing Science 19(4), 55–64. © Wolters Kluwer Health.

Kreutzer J, Mills A, Marwitz J 2016. Ambiguous loss and emotional recovery after traumatic brain injury. Journal of Family Theory & Review 8, 386–397.

Legg M, Foster M, Parakh S et al 2019. Trajectories of rehabilitation across complex environments (TRaCE): design and baseline characteristics for a prospective cohort study on spinal cord injury and acquired brain injury. BMC Health Services Research 19. Art no. 700 (2019).

Levack WMM 2009. Ethics in goal planning for rehabilitation: a utilitarian perspective. Clinical Rehabilitation 23, 345–351.

Levack WMM, Boland P, Taylor WJ et al 2014. Establishing a person-centred framework of self-identity after traumatic brain injury: a grounded theory study to inform measure development. BMJ Open 4, e004630.

Levack WMM, Kayes NM et al 2010. Experience of recovery and outcome following traumatic brain injury: a metasynthesis of qualitative research. Disability and Rehabilitation 32 (12), 986–999.

Levack WMM, Taylor K, Siegert R et al 2006. Is goal planning in rehabilitation effective? A systematic review. Clinical Rehabilitation 20, 739–755.

Levack WMM, Weatherall M, Hay-Smith EJC et al 2015. Goal setting and strategies to enhance goal pursuit for adults with acquired disability participating in rehabilitation. Cochrane Database of Systematic Reviews 20(7), CD009727.

Liaschenko J, Fisher A 1999. Theorising the knowledge that nurses use in the conduct of their work. Scholarly Inquiry for Nursing Practice. An International Journal 13(1), 29–41.

Low G 2003. Developing the nurse's role in rehabilitation. Nursing Standard 17(45), 33–38.

Mateer C, Sira CS, O'Connell ME 2005. Putting humpty dumpty together again. The importance of integrating cognitive and emotional interventions. Journal of Head Trauma Rehabilitation 20(1), 62–75.

McKechnie D, Pryor J, Fisher MJ 2014. Falls in inpatient TBI rehabilitation. Journal of Australasian Rehabilitation Nurses' Association 17, 14–18.

McPherson K 2006. Rehabilitation nursing – a final frontier? International Journal of Nursing Studies 43, 787–789.

Merritt C, Taylor M, Yelton C et al 2019. Economic impact of traumatic spinal cord injuries in the United States. Neuroimmunology and Neuroinflammation, 6, 9 DOI: 10.20517/2347-8659.2019.15.

Miller E 2003. Rehabilitation nursing in a consumer-driven world. Rehabilitation Nursing 28(5), 139–163.

Morse J 1997. Responding to threats to integrity of self. Advances in Nursing Science 19(4), 21–36. © Wolters Kluwer Health.

National Health Service England 2016. Commissioning guidance for rehabilitation. Online. Available: www.england.nhs.uk/wp-content/uploads/2016/04/rehabilitation-comms-guid-16-17.pdf.

NSW Agency for Clinical Innovation 2019. Principles to support rehabilitation care. Rehabilitation Network ACI_0241 [07/19]. Online. Available: www.aci.health.nsw.gov.au/__data/assets/pdf_file/0014/500900/rehabilitation-principles.pdf.

O'Brien J, Nicholson P, Johnson R et al 2002. Introduction. In: R Gravell, R Johnson (eds), Head injury rehabilitation: a community team perspective. Whurr Publishers, London.

O'Phelan K 2016. Traumatic brain injury: definitions and nomenclature. In: F Zollman (ed.), Manual of traumatic brain injury: assessment and management, 2nd edn. Springer, New York.

O'Reilly K, Wilson NJ, Peters K 2018. Narrative literature review: health, activity and participation issues for women following traumatic brain injury. Disability and Rehabilitation 40(19), 2331–2342.

Olinzock B 2004. A model for assessing learning readiness for self direction of care in individuals with spinal cord injuries: a qualitative study. SCI Nursing 21(2), 69–74.

Olkin R, Hayward H, Abbene M et al 2019. The experience of microaggressions against women with visible and invisible disabilities. Journal of Social Issues 75(3), 757–785.

Orem DE 1995. Nursing: concepts of practice, 5th edn. Elsevier, Philadelphia.

Ozer MN 1999. Patient participation in the management of stroke rehabilitation. Topics in Stroke Rehabilitation 6(1), 43–59.

Papadimitriou C 2008. Becoming en-wheeled: the situated accomplishment of re-embodiment as a wheelchair user after spinal cord injury. Disability & Society 23(7), 691–704.

Papadimitriou C, Stone DA 2011. Addressing existential disruption in traumatic spinal cord injury: a new approach to human temporality in inpatient rehabilitation. Disability and Rehabilitation 33(21–22), 2121–2133.

Piatt J, Nagata S, Zahl M et al 2016. Problematic secondary health conditions among people with spinal cord injury and its impact on social participation and daily life. The Journal of Spinal Cord Medicine 39(6), 693–698.

Plaisted LM 1978. Rehabilitation nurse. In: RM Goldenson (ed.), Disability and rehabilitation handbook. McGraw-Hill, New York.

Playford ED, Siegert R, Levack W et al 2009. Areas of consensus and controversy about goal setting in rehabilitation: a conference report. Clinical Rehabilitation 23, 334–344.

Pratt C, Baldry K 2002. Families and carers. In: R Gravell, R Johnson (eds), Head injury rehabilitation: a community team perspective. Whurr Publishers, London.

Prince M 2017. Persons with invisible disabilities and workplace accommodation: findings from a scoping literature review. Journal of Vocational Rehabilitation 24, 75–86.

Prochaska JO, DiClemente CC, Norcross J 1992. In search of how people change. American Psychologist 47(9), 1102–1114.

Pryor J 2014. Editorial. JARNA (Official Journal of the Australasian Rehabilitation Nurses' Association) 17(1), 2–3.

Pryor J 2005. A grounded theory of nursing's contribution to inpatient rehabilitation. PhD thesis. Deakin University, Melbourne.

Pryor J 2002. Rehabilitative nursing: a core nursing function across all settings. Collegian (Royal College of Nursing Australia) 9(2), 11–15.

Pryor J 2001. Rehabilitation nursing in Australia: a valid and valued specialty. Contemporary Nurse 11(2–3), 125–132.

Pryor J 2000. Creating a rehabilitative milieu. Rehabilitation Nursing 25(4), 141–144.

Pryor J 1999. Goals and focus. In: J Pryor (ed.), Rehabilitation – a vital nursing function. Royal College of Nursing, Canberra.

Pryor J, Buzio A 2010. Enhancing inpatient rehabilitation through the engagement of patients and nurses. Journal of Advanced Nursing 66(5), 978–987.

Pryor J, Dean S 2012. The person in context. In: S Dean, R Seigert, W Taylor (eds), Interprofessional rehabilitation: a person centred approach. Wiley-Blackwell, Oxford.

Pryor J, Jannings W 2004. Preparing patients to self manage faecal continence following spinal cord injury. International Journal of Therapy and Rehabilitation 11(2), 79–82.

Pryor J, Lingane B 2017. Rehabilitation, co-morbidity and complex care. In: A Johnson, E Chang (eds), Caring for older people in Australia: principles for nursing practice, 2nd edn. Wiley, Sydney.

Pryor J, O'Connell B 2008. Incongruence between nurses' and patients' understandings and expectations of rehabilitation. Journal of Clinical Nursing 18, 1766–1774.

Pryor J, Smith C 2002. A framework for the role of registered nurses in the specialty practice of rehabilitation nursing in Australia. Journal of Advanced Nursing 39(2), 249–257.

Raymond D 2017a. A person centred approach to assessing the nervous system. In: P LeMone et al. Medical–surgical nursing: critical thinking for person-centred care. Pearson Australia, Melbourne.

Raymond D 2017b. Nursing care of people with intracranial disorders. In: P LeMone et al. Medical–surgical nursing: critical thinking for person-centred care. Pearson Australia, Melbourne.

Rusk HA 1960. Rehabilitation: the third phase of medicine. Rhode Island Medical Journal 43, 385–387.

Sauri J, Chamarro A, Gilabery et al 2017. Depression in individuals with traumatic and nontraumatic spinal cord injury living in the community. Archives of Physical Medicine and Rehabilitation 98, 1165–1173.

Scheel-Sailer A, Post M, Michel F et al 2017. Patients' views on their decision making during inpatient rehabilitation after newly acquired spinal cord injury – a qualitative interview-based study. Health Expectations 20, 113–1142.

Schipper K, Widdrshoven G, Abma T 2011. Citizenship and autonomy in acquired brain injury. Nursing Ethics 18(4), 526–536.

Siegert RL, Ward T, Levack WM et al 2007. A Good Lives Model of clinical and community rehabilitation. Disability and Rehabilitation 29(20–21), 1604–1615.

Silverberg N, Lange R, Iverson G 2016. Concussion and mild traumatic brain injury: definitions, distinctions and diagnostic criteria. In: F Zollman, Manual of traumatic brain injury: assessment and management, 2nd edn. Springer Publishing Company, New York.

Snowden F 2001. Case manager's desk reference, 2nd edn. Aspen Publishers, Gaithersburg.

St-Germain D, Boivin B, Fougeyrollas P 2011. The caring-disability creation process model: a new way of combining 'care' in nursing and 'rehabilitation' for better quality of services and patient safety. Disability and Rehabilitation 33(21–22), 2105–2113.

Stewart R, Bhagwanjee A 1999. Promoting group empowerment and self reliance through participatory research: a case study of people with physical disability. Disability and Rehabilitation 21(7), 338–345.

Stroke Foundation 2019. Clinical Guidelines for Stroke Management. Online. Available: https://informme.org.au/en/Guidelines/Clinical-Guidelines-for-Stroke-Management.

Sveen U, Soberg HL, Ostensjo S 2016. Biographical disruption, adjustment and reconstruction of everyday occupations and work participation after mild traumatic brain injury. A focus group study. Disability and Rehabilitation 38(23), 2296–2304.

Thomas EJ, Levack WMM, Taylor WJ 2015. Rehabilitation and recovery of self-identity. In: K McPherson, BE Gibson, A Leplege (eds), Rethinking rehabilitation: theory and practice. CRC Press, Boca Raton.

Thomas EJ, Levack WMM, Taylor WJ 2014. Self-reflective meaning making in troubled times: changes in self-identity after traumatic brain injury. Qualitative Health Research 24(8), 1033–1047.

Todres L, Galvin K, Holloway I 2009. The humanization of healthcare: a value framework for qualitative research. International Journal of Qualitative Studies on Health and Well-being 4, 68–77.

Tyrrell E, Levack W, Ritchie L et al 2012. Nursing contribution to the rehabilitation of older patients: patient and family perspectives. Journal of Advanced Nursing 68(11), 2466–2476.

Tyrrell EF, Pryor J 2016. Nurses as agent of change in the rehabilitation process. JARNA (Official Journal of the Australasian Rehabilitation Nurses' Association) 19(1), 13–20.

van den Broek MD 2005. Why does neurorehabilitation fail? Journal of Head Trauma Rehabilitation 20(5), 464–473.

Vernese L, Kessler A, McCormick K et al 2019. Traumatic myelopathy. In: R Mitra. Principles of rehabilitation medicine. McGraw Hill Education, New York.

Wade D 2016. Rehabilitation – a new approach. Part four: a new paradigm, and its implications. Clinical Rehabilitation 30(2), 109–118.

Wade D 2015. Rehabilitation – a new approach. Part two: the underlying theories. Clinical Rehabilitation 29(12), 1045–1054.

Wade D 2009. Goal setting in rehabilitation: an overview of what, why and how. Clinical Rehabilitation 23, 291–295.

Wade D 2005. Describing rehabilitation interventions. Clinical Rehabilitation 19, 811–818.

Wong D, Sinclair K, Seabrook E et al 2017. Smartphones as assistive technology following traumatic brain injury: a preliminary study of what helps and what hinders. Disability & Rehabilitation 39(23), 2387–2394.

World Health Organization (WHO) 2019. Rehabilitation 2030. Health policy and systems research agenda for rehabilitation 10 and 11 July 2019. Online. Available: www.who.int/rehabilitation/Global-HSPR-Rehabilitation-Concept-Note.pdf.

World Health Organization (WHO) 2016a. Rehabilitation. Online. Available: www.who.int/topics/rehabilitation/en/.

World Health Organization (WHO) 2016b. Community based rehabilitation. Online. Available: www.who.int/disabilities/cbr/en/.

World Health Organization (WHO) 2013. International perspectives on spinal cord injury. Online. Available: http://apps.who.int/iris/bitstream/10665/94190/1/9789241564663_eng.pdf.

World Health Organization (WHO) 2010. Community based rehabilitation. Online. Available: http://apps.who.int/iris/bitstream/10665/44405/7/9789241548052_health_eng.pdf.

World Health Organization (WHO) 2001. International Classification of Functioning Disability and Health. WHO, Geneva.

Ylvisaker M, Jacobs H, Feeney T 2003. Positive supports for people who experience behavioural and cognitive disability after brain injury: a review. Journal of Head Trauma Rehabilitation 8(1), 7–32.

Young ME, Lutz BJ, Creasy KR et al 2014. a comprehensive assessment of family caregivers of stroke survivors during inpatient rehabilitation. Disability and Rehabilitation 36(22), 1892–1902.

Youngson R 2012. Time to care: how to love your patients and your job. Rebelheart Publishers, New Zealand.

CHAPTER 11

Impact of Obesity

SHARON CROXFORD • DIANNE REIDLINGER

LEARNING OBJECTIVES

When you have completed this chapter you will be able to:

- understand the relationship between obesity and chronic disease and disability
- define healthy weight, overweight and obesity in adults and children
- identify individuals at risk and discuss the role of lifestyle modification for reducing the impact of obesity
- be aware of evidence-based guidelines for obesity in Australia and New Zealand
- understand the nurse's role in managing obesity as part of a multidisciplinary/interdisciplinary team.

KEY WORDS

body mass index	obesity
diet	overweight
lifestyle change	physical activity

INTRODUCTION

This chapter describes the impact of overweight and obesity on chronic disease and disability. The definitions of overweight and obesity and prevalence are described, as well as how these are measured and assessed in research compared with practice. This chapter begins with prevalence and the determinants of obesity, followed by complications and associated chronic conditions, and finally describes weight-management approaches and strategies.

WHY IS OBESITY A CONCERN?

Obesity is a serious public health issue in Australia, New Zealand and worldwide, contributing greatly to the risk and complications of chronic disease and disability. Obesity is associated with serious health issues including hypertension, type 2 diabetes mellitus, hyperlipidaemia and cardiovascular disease (CVD), infertility and cancer (Jiang et al 2016). Further, it directly and indirectly affects health related to the renal and musculoskeletal systems, and is associated with poorer

mental health and quality of life (Poirier et al 2006). Obesity, particularly central obesity, is a defining feature of metabolic syndrome which involves a cluster of conditions involving dyslipidaemia, hypertension, insulin resistance and elevated blood glucose, and a pro-thrombotic and pro-inflammatory state, which are all modifiable risk factors for heart disease (Grundy 2016). Central obesity is responsible for 65–75% of risk of essential hypertension (Hall et al 2015) and dyslipidaemia, characterised by increased plasma triglycerides and free fatty acids, decreased high-density lipoprotein cholesterol and altered low-density lipoprotein cholesterol (Klop et al 2013). In addition to the direct impact on disease in Australia and New Zealand, obese individuals often have low physical activity, high alcohol use, and a diet that is low in fruit and vegetables – further increasing risks to their health.

In 2017–18, 31.3% of Australian adults were obese and an additional 35.6% were overweight (ABS 2019). More than 1 in 10 (11.0%) had a BMI > 35.0 kg/m^2 (AIHW 2017). More men (42.0%) were overweight than women (29.6%), with the prevalence of obesity similar (32.5% men, 30.2% women) (ABS 2019). Sixty per cent of men and 66.0% of women had a waist circumference associated with the greatest risk of health complications (AIHW 2017). One-quarter (24.9%) of Australian children aged 2–17 years were overweight or obese in 2017–18, with 17.0% categorised as overweight and 8.2% obese. Rates were similar between girls and boys and have remained stable over the past 10 years (ABS 2019).

Obesity prevalence is similar in New Zealand, with 31% of adults classified as obese in 2018–19 (Ministry of Health NZ 2019a). The 2018–19 New Zealand Health Survey results showed the proportion of children aged 2–14 years that were overweight or obese was 31.1%, with 19.8% overweight and 11.3% obese, with rates fairly static over the past 10 years.

While total prevalence appears to be increasing only slightly, the proportion of people with a BMI of 40.0 kg/m^2 or more is expected to rise (PwC Australia 2015). The current prevalence and predicted shift towards more people being more obese will have a significant impact on healthcare costs. The direct cost of obesity to the Australian health system in 2011–12 was AU$3.8 billion, with indirect costs totalling over AU$4.8 billion a year, discounting costs related to diminished wellbeing and lost income (PwC Australia 2015). In New Zealand

in 2012 it was estimated that obesity cost between NZ$722 million and NZ$849 million in healthcare costs and lost productivity (Lal et al 2012).

WHAT IS OBESITY?

Obesity is a condition of excess body fat. The location and amount of body fat a person stores will depend on their ethnicity, gender, life-stage and lifestyle, and these all need to be considered when assessing weight status. Central obesity, also referred to as visceral obesity, is an accumulation of intraperitoneal fat around the abdomen, the upper body, and carries the greatest health risk, although excess subcutaneous fat also increases risk (Grundy 2016). The most frequently used anthropometric measure of fat mass is BMI. Body mass index is defined as weight divided by height^2 (with weight in kilograms and height in metres). Adults with a BMI between 25.0 and 29.9 kg/m^2 are defined as overweight and those with a BMI over 30.0 kg/m^2 as obese (WHO Regional Office for Europe 2020) (see Table 11.1). This classification is not appropriate for all ethnic groups and adult thresholds are not suitable for children. Modified BMI classifications are used for Asia-Pacific peoples where these groups typically have a distribution of body fat that results in central obesity (see Table 11.1). A more useful

TABLE 11.1
Body Mass Index and Waist Circumference Classifications for Adults

| | BMI PRINCIPAL CUT-OFF POINTS (kg/m²) | |
	General Population	Asia-Pacific Peoples
Underweight	<18.5	<18.5
Normal range	18.5–24.9	18.5–22.9
Overweight	≥25.0	23.0–24.9
Pre-obese	25.0–29.9	
Obese	≥ 30.0	≥25.0
Obese class I	30.0–34.9	
Obese class II	35.0–39.9	
Obese class III	≥40.0	

| | WAIST CIRCUMFERENCE PRINCIPAL CUT-OFF POINTS (cm) | | | |
| | General Population | | Asian Peoples | |
	Males	Females	Males	Females
Low risk	<94 cm	<80 cm		
Increased risk	94– <102	80– <88		
Greatly increased risk	≥ 102	≥ 88	≥ 90	≥ 80

Harris 2013; Lim, Lee et al 2017; WHO Europe 2020.

anthropometric measure is waist circumference (cm), a surrogate of visceral fat stores and indicative of chronic disease risk. A waist circumference of < 94 cm in men and < 80 cm in women is associated with lowest risk, where a measurement ≥ 102 cm in men and 88 cm in women is linked with greatly increased risk. Again, cut-offs for ethnic groups differ with measurements ≥ 90 cm in men and ≥ 80 cm in women associated with the greatest risk in Asian populations (see Table 11.1) (Harris 2013). BMI does not accurately represent healthy weights of people with a high proportion of lean muscle mass with low body fat, for example, elite athletes, or people with decreased muscle mass, for example, severely undernourished, or people who are dehydrated or over-hydrated. Other anthropometric measures are used to assess weights status in these groups.

In children, overweight and obesity are defined by different BMI cut-offs. Information gathered using the percentile ranking takes into consideration the child's age and gender, recognising that the amount of body fat regularly changes with gender and age. There are a number of cut-offs in use internationally, and there is ongoing debate about appropriate use of BMI in childhood to define overweight and obesity. In New Zealand growth charts are recommended based on the WHO age- and sex-specific charts; overweight is classified as above the 91st centile and obesity as above the 98th centile for all children (Ministry of Health NZ 2016). In Australia there are no nationally developed charts for children up to the age of 18 years. For children 0–2 years the WHO growth charts are recommended and the US Centers for Disease Control (CDC) charts are recommended for children over 2 years. A BMI above the 85th centile is considered overweight and above the 95th centile is obese on the CDC charts (Figs 11.1 a and b). Somewhat confusingly, the WHO growth charts use different cut-off points compared to the CDC charts with obesity indicated above the 97th percentile. The important practice point is that children are consistently monitored using the same chart over time (The Royal Children's Hospital 2020).

WHO ARE THE HIGH-RISK GROUPS FOR OBESITY?

There are a range of influences on health and obesity, including gender, culture, genetics and social determinants. Culture has both a direct and indirect health impact, affecting belief systems directly while also resulting in the marginalisation of some groups and stigmatisation, which in turn is exacerbated by culturally unsafe health services. Social determinants encompass income, education level, level of social support, occupation, societal values and the environment where we live and work (Smith 2016). These factors are largely outside of an individual's control, but impact on beliefs and attitudes to, and control over, health and health-promoting behaviours.

Although obesity prevalence is of concern across the Australian and New Zealand populations, the rates of obesity differ according to geographical location and socioeconomic status. Generally, those who are living with greater disadvantage also have higher levels of obesity. While these indicators alone do not determine an individual's risk of developing obesity, they are often associated with a greater number of barriers to individuals pursuing healthy eating and activity. The burden of chronic illnesses, including CVD, is known to disproportionately affect populations from lower incomes (Bambra et al 2010). It is estimated that around half of the variation in CVD morbidity and mortality between the least and most deprived populations is explained by modifiable risk factors such as smoking, high alcohol consumption, obesity, physical inactivity and poor diet (Scarborough et al 2011).

Australians and New Zealanders who are living with a disability, and those from specific culturally and linguistically diverse (CALD) groups, are known to be at a high risk of obesity (AIHW 2018a). Also at great risk are Aboriginal and/or Torres Strait Islander peoples, Māori and Pacific Islanders, along with those from lower socioeconomic backgrounds. Additional specific strategies are needed for obesity prevention and management in these groups.

Aboriginal and/or Torres Strait Islander peoples have higher rates of obesity than non-Indigenous people across almost every age group, with 69.0% classified as either overweight or obese in those aged 18 years and over (AIHW 2019). The prevalence of obesity for Aboriginal and/or Torres Strait Islander adults was 40.0% in 2012–13 (ABS 2019) compared with 31.3% in the general Australian population in 2017–18 (AIHW 2019). Prevalence rates in Aboriginal and Torres Strait Islander children aged 2–14 years are higher than that of the non-Indigenous Australian child population. In 2012–13, 19.6% of Aboriginal and Torres Strait Islander children were overweight and 10.2% obese and, alarmingly, 35% aged 15–17 years were overweight or obese (ABS 2014). Obesity is estimated to contribute to 14.1% of the health gap between Aboriginal and/or Torres Strait Islander peoples and the total Australian population, with high body mass contributing to the burden of endocrine disorders (62%), kidney and urinary diseases (37%), CVD (34%)

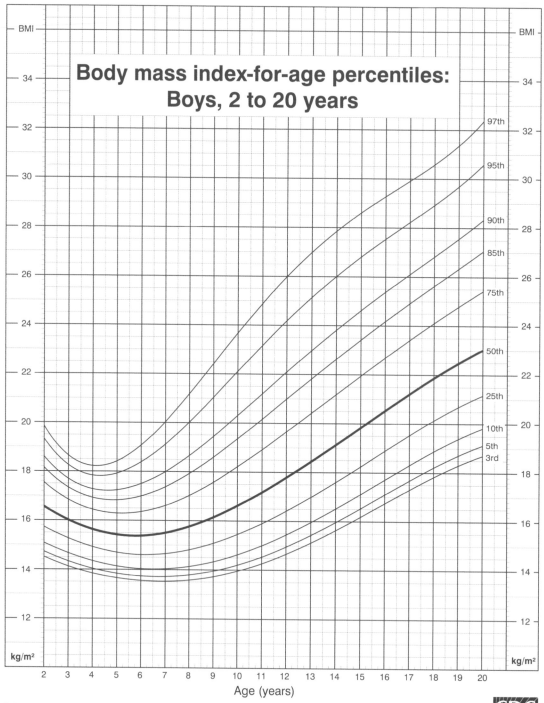

Body mass index-for-age percentiles: Boys, 2 to 20 years

Age (years)

Published May 30, 2000.
SOURCE: Developed by the National Center for Health Statistics in collaboration with
the National Center for Chronic Disease Prevention and Health Promotion

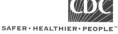

SAFER · HEALTHIER · PEOPLE™

FIG. 11.1a **Body mass index-for-age percentiles, boys 2–20 years.** Kuczmarski et al 2000.

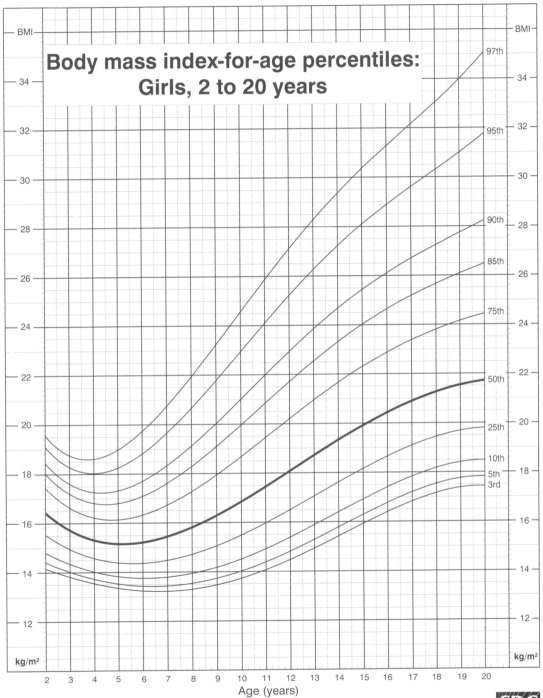

Body mass index-for-age percentiles:
Girls, 2 to 20 years

Published May 30, 2000.
SOURCE: Developed by the National Center for Health Statistics in collaboration with
the National Center for Chronic Disease Prevention and Health Promotion (2000).

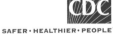

SAFER · HEALTHIER · PEOPLE™

FIG. 11.1b **Body Mass index-for-age percentiles, girls 2–20 years.**

and cancer (5%) (AIHW 2016). Obesity rates for Aboriginal and/or Torres Strait Islander peoples vary geographically, with the highest rates found in inner regional areas (40%) compared with the lowest rates in very remote areas (32%) (Australian Health Ministers Advisory Council 2015). In all geographical locations across Australia, Aboriginal and/or Torres Strait Islander peoples were more overweight and obese than non-Indigenous Australians (AIHW 2018b). Socioeconomic disadvantage is responsible for 42–54% of the gap in life expectancy between Aboriginal and/or Torres Strait Islander peoples and non-Indigenous Australians, with obesity responsible for an additional 9–17%, or 1–3 years (Zhao et al 2013). The continued disparities in obesity-related health of Aboriginal and/or Torres Strait Islander peoples compared with non-Indigenous Australia warrants urgent and persistent attention. 'Closing the Gap' is an Australian government strategy, conceived in 2007, to address the inequities and inequality in health and life expectancy. In 2018, with life expectancy around 8–9 years less for Indigenous Australians compared to non-Indigenous Australians and in light of only two of the seven targets being on track, the government re-committed to the next phase (COAG 2018). Tackling obesity will be critical to increasing life expectancy.

In New Zealand, there is evidence of significant health inequalities for Māori who die 6 to 7 years earlier, on average, than the non-Māori New Zealand population (Ministry of Health NZ 2018). In New Zealand in 2018–19, 48.2% of Māori and 66.5% of Pacific Islander adults 15 years and over, were classified as obese (Ministry of Health NZ 2019a), with Māori people 1.8 times more likely to be obese than non-Māori people, and Pacific Islanders 2.5 times more likely than non-Pacific Islanders (Ministry of Health NZ 2019b). These prevalence rates are among the highest in the world. The higher obesity rates contribute to the higher incidence of diabetes in Māori and Pacific Islanders compared with the non-Māori/Pacific Islander populations (7.1%, 11.2%, 4.6% respectively) (Ministry of Health NZ 2019c) and the younger age at diagnosis for diabetes (43 years vs 55 years). The higher prevalence of diabetes and the younger age at diagnosis contributes significantly to the concomitantly higher rates of chronic kidney disease and greater need for dialysis in these groups (St George 2013). There was a marked difference in obesity prevalence rates between ethnicities in both adults and children. Almost one-third (28.4%) of Pacific children, 15.5% of Māori children, and 9.9% of Asian children are obese, compared to 8.2% of European/other children (Ministry of Health NZ 2019d).

Socioeconomic disadvantage is also associated with higher rates of obesity in both adults and children (Backholer et al 2012; O'Dea & Dibley 2014). Socioeconomic disadvantage is measured by a number of characteristics, including language spoken, family unit, educational attainment, employment, housing, car ownership and income (ABS 2013). The inverse relationship between income, education and obesity has long been recognised (Pavela et al 2016), and both the lack of, and expense of, healthy foods in lower income areas is negatively associated with diet quality (AIHW 2017). Disadvantage is associated with poverty and food insecurity, with food insecurity linked to obesity. Buying cheaper foods, by necessity, often results in poor diet quality. Highly refined foods with added fats and sugars are often inexpensive and/or easy to access in areas of socioeconomic disadvantage (Croxford 2015).

In New Zealand in 2015 adults living in deprived areas were 1.6 times more likely to be obese, with the difference for women greater than men (1.8 and 1.4 respectively) (Ministry of Health NZ 2019e). Data from Australian adults in 2014–15 also showed a disparity, with 61% of women in the lowest socioeconomic group obese compared to 48% women in the highest socioeconomic group, with little difference for men (AIHW 2017). Interestingly, research in Brisbane proposed that BMI in disadvantaged neighbourhoods did not change with individual socioeconomic status, suggesting that environmental factors were important (Rachele et al 2019). In tackling obesity, community-based strategies aimed at changing the environment may be more successful than targeting individuals for behaviour change in more disadvantaged groups (Beauchamp et al 2014).

Despite the overwhelming need for action on obesity in these population groups, the evidence base for interventions for addressing obesity in Aboriginal and/or Torres Strait Islander peoples, as well as people from socioeconomically disadvantaged backgrounds, is disappointing (Laws et al 2014). Some evidence is available that demonstrates the effectiveness for primary care-delivered, tailored weight-loss and community-based weight-loss interventions in socioeconomically disadvantaged populations, particularly for low-income women (Bambra et al 2015).

In addition to the Aboriginal and Torres Strait Islander populations, a significant proportion of the Australian community come from other CALD backgrounds. Approximately 29% of the Australian population are born overseas, and 27.3% speak a language other than English at home (ABS 2017). Similarly, in New Zealand, around a quarter of the population are born overseas. Migration from China, India, South Africa, Fiji, Samoa, the Philippines, the Republic of Korea and Australia has resulted in increasing ethnic diversity, with India, China and the Philippines recently overtaking the UK and Ireland as the most common birthplace for those born outside of New Zealand (Ministry of Business, Innovation & Employment 2019). Although grouped together due to diversity, the reality is that these groups are by their nature quite diverse – including age, socioeconomic status, cultural norms, dietary patterns and physical activity preferences. Due to the different 'waves' of immigration throughout the history of Australia and New Zealand, the age structure of different cultural groups is not uniform. Older people from CALD backgrounds may experience greater socioeconomic disadvantage (although this varies across groups). Language, cultural translation, lack of familiarity with healthcare services and systems and a preference for family to provide care may impact on the effectiveness of interventions to prevent obesity (FECCA 2015). Change in weight status following migration will differ across migrant groups. Research in Australia has indicated that male migrants from North Africa, the Middle East and Oceania are at greatest risk, irrespective of their socioeconomic status (Menigoz et al 2016). Ensuring culturally competent, gender and age-specific healthcare and weight management advice to meet the needs of these groups is important.

Children and adults with limited mobility and intellectual or learning disabilities are at high risk of developing obesity (CDC 2019). Approximately 18% of the Australian population have a disability, with 72% of people over 2 years of age with a disability overweight or obese, compared to 52% of the Australian population without a disability (AIHW 2019). The proportion of Aboriginal and/or Torres Strait Islander peoples who report living with a disability was 24% in 2015, compared to 18% of non-Indigenous Australians. Disabilities reported were physical disability (29%), vision, hearing or speech impairment (21%), psychological (9%) and intellectual (8%) impairment (Australian Indigenous HealthInfoNet 2019). In New Zealand, 24% of the population identified as living with a disability, with higher than average prevalence for Māori and Pacific Islanders (Statistics NZ 2014). Increased weight in people with disabilities can be more problematic than for people living without disability, creating an additional health burden. Low physical activity and fewer opportunities to engage in programs that promote physical activity can exacerbate

the problem (Froehlich-Grobe & Lollar 2011). While people with disabilities are at high risk of becoming obese, obesity increases the risk of disability. Predictions of the impact of obesity and diabetes on the prevalence of disability in older Australians suggests that as the obesity trend continues its trajectory of 1980–2000, by 2025 an additional 13% of the population will be living with avoidable disability (Wong et al 2016).

There is increasing recognition of the role of nurses in the provision of preventative health advice for the management of chronic disease risk factors such as weight, blood pressure, cholesterol, and behaviour change, including diet and physical activity (Sargent et al 2012). Nurses themselves have identified lifestyle advice as an important topic in their interactions with patients in the primary care setting (Martin et al 2013). A survey of Australian nurses across hospital, community and other facilities demonstrated that most of their patients would benefit from such support (Kable et al 2015). This highlights the opportunity for nurses to deliver healthy lifestyle advice to support weight management. Likewise, opportunities exist for obesity prevention in young children through practice nurse brief interventions (Denney-Wilson et al 2014).

Case Study 11.1 illustrates the interactions between a nurse in general practice and a young adult living with disability with recent weight gain. The case study identifies the multiple factors that contribute to overweight and obesity, and potential strategies available to support sustained improvement in physical and mental health.

HOW IS WEIGHT STATUS MEASURED?

Measurement of weight and height to calculate BMI and waist circumference are often key components in monitoring weight status. Accurate measurement requires a standard approach to collecting the data. Table 11.2 summarises the important steps in measuring height, weight and waist circumference in children and adults who are able to stand. Recumbent length and weight are measured in infants. For people with disabilities who cannot stand, alternative methods are used to take anthropometric measures; for example, for people in wheelchairs, the person and wheelchair are weighed on an accessible scale, the person is moved from the wheelchair to a safe place and the wheelchair weighed on its own. The person's weight is the difference between the two. Height can be calculated from predictive equations that use knee-height in adults. For those over 65 years

CASE STUDY 11.1

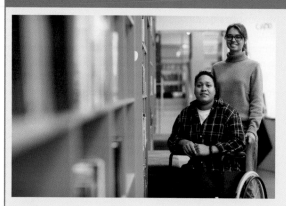

Shutterstock/SeventyFour.

Mr Liam O'Reilly is a 22-year-old who was born with my-elomeningocele spina bifida present in the lumbar-sacral region of his spinal cord. He has altered bowel and bladder function, and difficulty walking due to poor innervation and muscle weakness in his legs. As an adolescent, he wore knee-ankle orthoses to stabilise his gait while walking, but now relies only on heel insert orthotics.

Two years ago, Liam had surgery on his left foot due to severe infection as a result of a pressure injury. Following the surgery, his mobility was severely reduced and he gained a significant amount of weight. At a recent appointment with his doctor, he raised the ongoing pain and frequent ulceration in his feet that occur when he walks further than the distance of a few houses from his home. The doctor noted that he was overweight, with high blood cholesterol and triglycerides, so he requested the practice nurse to see him to provide some lifestyle advice.

Michelle, the nurse, measured his height at 165 cm and weight at 85 kg, and calculated his body mass index to be 30.6 kg/m^2 (see Table 11.1, p. 184). During the consultation, she noticed that Liam appeared unhappy with having these measurements taken. Michelle discussed with him the many benefits of even a small amount of weight loss, which would help his mobility and take some of the strain off his feet. Liam opened up to Michelle that he did not believe he could ever lose weight, and that he had 'lost faith' in even trying. He told her that he is frequently preoccupied with the pain in his legs and feet, his difference to other people of his age, and that food and alcohol was a source of comfort to him when he felt 'down' about his situation.

Michelle decided to talk further with Liam to find out more about his lifestyle and experiences. She found out that Liam receives disability income support and is unemployed. He lives independently but relies on his father to help him financially. His father visits him daily to help with household chores, including cooking and cleaning. He has previously tried to get work in a local café but was unsuccessful. He described that social situations often make him anxious, as he feels judged because of his differences, including his disability and larger body. Other than when his father visits each afternoon, he spends his days watching television or playing video games, and has few friends.

Liam identified that he was interested in food and preparing tasty meals, but confided that he did not have the skills to cook complicated recipes. His eating patterns were irregular, he often skipped breakfast and lunch, snacking for most of the afternoon before eating a large evening meal, often from the local fast food outlet. He stated his preference to eat bread, chips, eggs and meat and that he has little patience with vegetables and fruit. He was frustrated with his inability to increase his physical activity, but his previous efforts had caused him pain and embarrassment. As a young person, he expressed that he would dearly like more social interactions but he did not feel safe meeting new people.

Michelle focused on the issues that Liam had raised, as she had identified his behaviours did not support good mental or physical health, including his weight. She requested a referral from the doctor for a podiatrist to review his feet. She discussed some ideas to encourage him to include physical activity in his daily routine, including engaging a personal trainer for strength training and hydrotherapy classes at the local council pool.

He agreed to try three changes to his food intake, which were to:

- eat a breakfast of cereal with banana and milk each morning
- include one or two spoons of cooked frozen vegetables with his evening meal, slowly increasing his vegetable intake as his confidence with cooking improved
- plan to have a healthy lunch meal every day of a sandwich and fruit, using an educational handout from the Queensland Health website which Michelle gave to him: www.health.qld.gov.au/__data/assets/pdf_file/0015/150063/wtmgt_mealplan.pdf

Liam came in every 2 weeks to see Michelle, and they decided not to keep track of his weight, but rather to monitor the agreed changes to his food intake and attempts at physical activity. At each visit, Michelle checked with Liam on his strength training sessions with his personal trainer, and whether he had been able to make the dietary changes they had discussed. As Liam often talked about watching cookery programs on television, she suggested that he enrol in a local community cooking class run by 'Jamie's Ministry of Food'. Liam did so, and developed basic cooking skills that allowed him to prepare

CASE STUDY 11.1 – cont'd

better home cooked foods. He also met some other young people at the class, which gave him a little more confidence in his social skills. The regular check-ins with Michelle were a helpful way to keep on track, and Liam appreciated the interest that Michelle showed, as well as having someone to 'bounce ideas off' when he struggled to make some of the changes.

After 4 months, Liam had made some good progress and wanted to weigh himself on the practice scales. He now weighed 80 kg, which represented a small weight loss. He had new orthotics with less pain in his feet, and was now able to do some walking each day in addition to the hydrotherapy classes which he had managed to keep

up. He felt more optimistic about his life and had made a friend whom he now saw regularly. The GP was very happy with the changes to Liam's blood lipids, noting improvements to his blood cholesterol and fasting blood triglyceride levels.

CASE STUDY QUESTIONS

1. What are the potential risk factors associated with Liam's high BMI?
2. What lifestyle modification recommendations would you continue to encourage?
3. What outcomes would you continue to monitor and how would you encourage Liam to remain motivated?

TABLE 11.2
Tips for Anthropometric Measures

Weight (kg)	Using calibrated, zeroed scales on a firm surface (not carpet), measure the client in light clothing without shoes, jackets, heavy clothing or jewellery, and with empty pockets standing with their hands at sides looking straight ahead.
Height (m)	Using a stadiometer, measure the client standing straight with arms by sides, and ankles, buttocks, shoulder blades and head touching the backboard. Eyes should look straight ahead, feet flat and pointed out at 60° angle, heels together, legs straight and knees together. The client should take a deep breath and the measuring device brought down to rest on the top of the head.
Waist circumference (cm)	Using a tape measure, take a measurement at the midpoint between the lower rib and iliac crest using a tape measure. The client should fold their arms as if giving themselves a light hug, or have their hands loosely at their sides and breathe normally.

CDC 2019.

the most commonly used proxy is ulna length, the length between the point of the elbow (olecranon process) to the midpoint of the bony point of the wrist (styloid process). Conversion tables are used to estimate height. Nurses, in particular primary healthcare nurses, play an essential role in helping to measure, monitor and support treatment of the obesity crisis in Australia and New Zealand.

WHAT ARE THE STRATEGIES FOR ACHIEVING HEALTHY WEIGHT?

Given its links with socioeconomic and cultural disadvantage, effective prevention and management of obesity requires interventions that consider a range of sociocultural factors. While many effective strategies to address these rely on policy level actions across health and non-health sectors to address structural contributors, nurses

and other health professionals are well placed to assist individuals with obesity to make positive changes to improve their health.

Body weight stigma is increasingly recognised as a consequence and potential determinant of obesity in our society (Tomiyama et al 2018). Weight stigma refers to the social devaluation of people who do not conform to prevailing social expectations of body weight and shape (Tomiyama et al 2018; Phelan et al 2015). Research over many years has demonstrated stigmatised reactions to people with obesity, such as disgust and blame (Vartanian 2010), with stigmatisation occurring in the community as well as by health professionals during patient care (Phelan et al 2015; Puhl & Heuer 2009). Such stigma is stressful and leads to physiological stress responses, further resulting in many of the emotional, cognitive and behavioural changes associated with weight gain. These responses in turn may cause poorer health and greater weight gain (Tomiyama et al 2018). Health professionals, including nurses, should be mindful of patient preferences and avoid stigmatising language when suggesting weight-related interventions to improve health.

Lifestyle Modifications

The most recent government-endorsed guidance for weight management in both Australia (NHMRC 2013a) and New Zealand (Ministry of Health NZ 2017) highlights the importance of lifestyle modification to achieve and maintain healthy weight. Modifiable factors for obesity include improved dietary choices, increased physical activity (according to an individual's ability and control), and reduction of psychological stressors (see Case Study 11.1, p. 190, for examples of strategies). In an individual already carrying excess weight, the health benefits associated with lifestyle interventions include both mental and physical health improvements. The intentional weight loss resulting from such interventions confers some of these benefits, although the lifestyle changes themselves have also been independently associated with greater wellbeing.

A range of chronic disease risk factors have shown improvement with weight loss in people with a higher BMI, positively impacting cardiovascular disease and diabetes risk. Randomised controlled trials have demonstrated that weight loss results in a long-term decrease in serum total cholesterol, low-density lipoprotein (LDL) cholesterol and triglycerides (TGs), and smaller reductions in high-density lipoprotein (HDL) cholesterol in the obese population (Poobalan et al 2004). The evidence supports a greater improvement in blood lipids with a larger weight loss, with individuals who lose around 10% of initial body weight showing more improvement across more lipid outcomes than those who lose around 5% of body weight (Brown et al 2016). Intervention studies have also demonstrated a reduction in blood pressure (BP) with weight loss, irrespective of whether a BMI in the 'healthy range' (18.5–25 kg/m^2) is achieved. Based on a meta-analysis of 17 trials, it has been estimated that a weight loss of 5.1 kg can reduce systolic and diastolic BP by 4.4 and 3.6 mmHg, respectively (Neter et al 2003), and further benefits are experienced with greater weight loss (Appel et al 2006).

Improvements in blood glycaemia with weight loss is well established in individuals with 'pre-diabetes' (impaired fasting glucose and impaired glucose tolerance), with a meta-analysis of randomised controlled trials demonstrating a reduction in progression to type

2 diabetes of 30% seven years after the intervention (Haw et al 2017). More recent research has demonstrated weight loss in early diagnosed type 2 diabetes to induce remission of the disease (Lim et al 2011). The impact appears to be sustained 2 years following weight loss, with remission rates of around 60% for individuals who maintained at least 10 kg of their weight loss after the intervention (Lean et al 2019). Importantly, diabetes reversal was recently identified as the top research priority by people with type 2 diabetes in the United Kingdom (Taylor & Barnes 2018), highlighting the importance of discussing with patients the potential impact of successful weight loss, particularly for those patients who are newly or recently diagnosed with type 2 diabetes.

Despite these positive impacts on chronic disease risk, and the prevailing view that weight loss is a positive outcome for many overweight individuals, the limited control that people actually have over their weight, and the potential for negative health consequences should not be overlooked. In particular, many individuals with larger bodies may have a range of external social and environmental factors that are not within their control. Additionally, the human body's weight homeostasis mechanisms are complex and generally lead to weight maintenance in the longer term (Muller et al 2018). In many cases, an emphasis on weight reduction for a person who has been exposed to weight stigma over the years may lead to reduced motivation and disillusionment. Ensuring that individuals have access to non-weight focused interventions with an emphasis on lifestyle changes that are genuinely modifiable, is important for adopting a person-centred approach.

Dietary Modifications

There are many variations of healthy eating patterns that promote health and wellbeing. The best dietary pattern for an individual is one that fits their lifestyle and goals, and can be sustained. Most of the diet-related conditions in Australia are associated with excessive intake of energy-dense and nutrient-poor foods and fluids, alcohol, added sugars and salt, and inadequate intake of fruits, vegetables and whole grain cereals (NHMRC 2013a). The Australian Eat for Health Program uses the latest scientific evidence to develop public health, educator and consumer resources to promote health and wellbeing (NHMRC 2013a). These dietary recommendations can be effective in guiding food consumption; however, it is important to be aware that overconsumption of even healthy food can lead to excessive energy intake compared with requirements and hence a gain in body weight (NHMRC 2013a).

The Australian Dietary Guidelines (Table 11.3) and the New Zealand Eating and Activity Guidelines have been developed to guide selection on the type and amounts of foods from the core food groups and to encourage dietary patterns that reduce the risk of chronic conditions (Ministry of Health NZ 2015; NHMRC 2013b). The New Zealand guidelines also incorporate physical activity guidelines; however, in Australia there is separate activity guidance outlined in Australia's Physical Activity and Sedentary Behaviour Guidelines (Department of Health 2014) These are useful resources for health professionals, including nurses; however, they do not apply to those who require specialised advice in relation to a medical condition or to the frail elderly; these patients should be referred for medical review and consultation with an Accredited Practising Dietitian (APD) in Australia, or a Registered Dietitian (RD) in New Zealand.

For a useful food selection guide based on these dietary guidelines, the Australian Guide to Healthy Eating can be downloaded from www.eatforhealth.gov.au. Australia's Physical Activity and Sedentary Behaviour Guidelines (specifically for children, adults and older adults), with supporting resources, can be downloaded from www1.health.gov.au.

Healthy Eating and Activity Guidelines for New Zealand Adults (Ministry of Health NZ 2015) include statements on healthy eating, physical activity and body weight (Figure 11.2). A series of resources are available, which are suitable for the general public and health professionals, including the rationale and scientific evidence underpinning the recommendations. These are available on www.health.govt.nz.

Evidence Surrounding Other Dietary Patterns

There are many different dietary patterns associated with good health. Common characteristics of healthier dietary patterns include consuming plenty of vegetables, legumes and fruits and limiting processed foods and items with low nutritional benefit. In the development of national dietary guidelines, the Australian and New Zealand governments have reviewed available scientific evidence to support their guidance for limiting overweight and obesity and diet-related chronic disease (NHMRC 2011). However, other dietary patterns with some evidence to support their use include moderate fat diets such as the Mediterranean diet. The Mediterranean diet includes a large proportion of vegetables, legumes and whole grains. It is not a low fat diet as typically 30–40% of energy comes from fat; however, the fat is predominantly monounsaturated fatty acids in the form of olive oil. Replacing butter with healthy fats such as olive oil and canola oil and including nuts and seeds are strategies to achieve a dietary fat profile similar to the Mediterranean diet. Herbs and spices are used instead of salt to add flavour. Several randomised controlled trials have demonstrated that the Mediterranean diet is an alternative to

---

TABLE 11.3
Australian Dietary Guidelines

Guideline 1	To achieve and maintain a healthy body weight, be physically active and choose the quantity of nutritious food and fluids to meet your energy needs.
Guideline 2	Enjoy a wide variety of nutritious foods from the five food groups every day: • plenty of different types and colours of vegetables and legumes/beans • fruits • whole grains and high fibre cereals, e.g. oats, rice, couscous • lean meats, poultry, seafood, eggs and meat alternatives such as soy products, tofu • milk, yoghurt, cheese and their dairy-free alternatives, mostly reduced fat (reduced fat milks are not suitable for children < 2 years). And drink plenty of water.
Guideline 3	Limit high-energy, low nutrition foods and fluids, such as those containing saturated fat, added salt, sugar and alcohol
Guideline 4	Encourage and support breastfeeding
Guideline 5	Prepare and store food safely

NHMRC 2013.

Eating and Activity Guidelines Statements for New Zealand Adults

Making good choices about what and how much you eat and drink and being physically active are important for good health.

Eating Statements

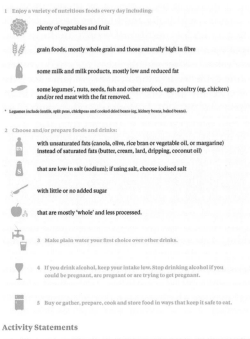

1 Enjoy a variety of nutritious foods every day including:

plenty of vegetables and fruit

grain foods, mostly whole grain and those naturally high in fibre

some milk and milk products, mostly low and reduced fat

some legumes*, nuts, seeds, fish and other seafood, eggs, poultry (eg, chicken) and/or red meat with the fat removed.

* Legumes include lentils, split peas, chickpeas and cooked dried beans (eg, kidney beans, baked beans).

2 Choose and/or prepare foods and drinks:

with unsaturated fats (canola, olive, rice bran or vegetable oil, or margarine) instead of saturated fats (butter, cream, lard, dripping, coconut oil)

that are low in salt (sodium); if using salt, choose iodised salt

with little or no added sugar

that are mostly 'whole' and less processed.

3 Make plain water your first choice over other drinks.

4 If you drink alcohol, keep your intake low. Stop drinking alcohol if you could be pregnant, are pregnant or are trying to get pregnant.

5 Buy or gather, prepare, cook and store food in ways that keep it safe to eat.

Activity Statements

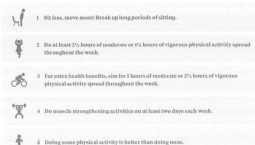

1 Sit less, move more! Break up long periods of sitting.

2 Do at least 2½ hours of moderate or 1¼ hours of vigorous physical activity spread throughout the week.

3 For extra health benefits, aim for 5 hours of moderate or 2½ hours of vigorous physical activity spread throughout the week.

4 Do muscle strengthening activities on at least two days each week.

5 Doing some physical activity is better than doing none.

Body Weight Statement

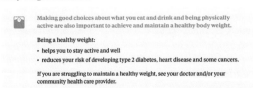

Making good choices about what you eat and drink and being physically active are also important to achieve and maintain a healthy body weight.

Being a healthy weight:
• helps you to stay active and well
• reduces your risk of developing type 2 diabetes, heart disease and some cancers.

If you are struggling to maintain a healthy weight, see your doctor and/or your community health care provider.

FIG. 11.2 **Eating statements** Ministry of Health NZ 2020.

low fat diets in helping to reduce overweight and obesity as well as improve metabolic markers (DAA 2012; Garaulet 2015).

A plant-based dietary pattern does not eliminate animal foods, but may include smaller amounts of dairy, fish and meat in addition to a predominance of plant-based foods. The Mediterranean diet fits within an overarching 'plant-based dietary pattern'. The term reflects a more flexible dietary approach than vegetarianism and veganism, and confers similar health benefits. Plant-based diets are characterised by a lower intake of animal products and higher intake of plant-based foods, including vegetables, legumes, fruits, whole grains, nuts and seeds (Hemler & Hu 2019). Adopting such a dietary approach, while also limiting sweetened beverages and juices, refined grains, fried potatoes and sweets, has been linked to a reduced risk of obesity, coronary heart disease, type 2 diabetes and cancer (Hemler & Hu 2019).

SCREENING FOR OBESITY

Given the extent of the obesity problem, and associated co-morbidities, it is important that all health practitioners are involved in the prevention and management of overweight and obesity across the spectrum of health service provision. Nurses, in particular primary healthcare nurses, play an essential role in helping to address the obesity crisis in Australia and New Zealand. This role includes the identification and diagnosis of overweight and obesity; development of a respectful therapeutic relationship that enables effective communication about the problem, and its wider risks for the individual; assistance in setting achievable activity- and food-related goals that focus on long-term behavioural change and health improvement; provision of support and regular monitoring of the individual's progress towards behavioural goals and weight targets; acting as a resource to correct misinformation and dietary fads; giving basic evidence-based advice to support health for individuals who are overweight or obese; and facilitating referrals to dietitians and other health professionals to address weight loss in the context of other co-morbidities.

KEY POINTS FOR NURSES IN MANAGING OBESITY

• Screen and assess for overweight and obesity.
• Assist in achieving appropriate health-related goals.
• Provide support and motivation regarding beneficial behaviour change.

- Give basic evidence-based nutrition advice.
- Facilitate referrals to Accredited Practising Dietitians (in Australia), Registered Dietitians (in New Zealand) and other health professionals when there are multi-morbidities.

Nurses are in an ideal position to facilitate the early identification and management of weight problems (Phillips et al 2014). Most nurses understand the importance of healthy weight; however, they may feel underconfident or not adequately trained to address the issue with their patients. They have a key role in identifying and managing overweight and obese patients, beginning with the measurement of weight, height and waist circumference. For effective weight management, consideration should be given to the wider sociocultural and psychological determinants of lifestyle and health (Lazarou & Couter 2010). Health-promoting advice from nurses can assist individuals in the obese category, as well as those in the overweight category, as there is a greater risk of obesity for individuals who are already overweight.

There is evidence that obesity is underdiagnosed in primary healthcare for men more than women (Walsh & Fahy 2012). If not identified in the first instance, it is not surprising that patients then do not get the counselling they need to assist them to reduce their weight, prevent further deterioration in their health and improve the management of their chronic disease/s. With training in the accurate measurement of weight, height and waist circumference, nurses who are in regular contact with patients for their chronic disease management and care are ideally placed to ensure the early identification of overweight and obesity, and can provide opportunistic advice and ongoing support in the context of an existing therapeutic relationship.

For successful weight loss, nurses can provide assistance and motivation to patients to eat a bit less and be more active. They should be encouraged to adopt realistic goals, as very few obese individuals will be able to lose enough weight to achieve a BMI less than 25 kg/m^2 (i.e. in the healthy weight range). Instead, a goal of around 5% weight loss in 3 months and 10% in 6 months is much more achievable and is associated with clinically significant health outcomes, particularly if the weight loss is maintained (Aucott et al 2005). Nurses can help patients to identify ways to achieve greater physical activity in their day-to-day lives, and to understand their own dietary habits so they can substitute lower energy, higher quality foods for more discretionary food choices. In particular, water can be substituted for alcohol, sugar-sweetened beverages and juices to encourage a lower energy (calorie or kilojoule) intake. Other discretionary foods consumed (such as biscuits, cakes, chips and lollies) should be identified using the Australian Guide to Healthy Eating as a resource and the individual encouraged to replace these with fresh fruit and vegetables, whole grain cereals, milk, yoghurt, fish and small amounts of lean meats.

VERY LOW CALORIE DIETS

A Very Low Calorie Diet (VLCD) is defined as a medically supervised weight-loss plan that uses commercially prepared formulas (usually shakes and/or bars) to achieve significant short-term weight loss. The shakes or bars typically replace all food consumption for a period of weeks to months and the plan requires regular medical sessions with a medical team and dietitian. There is strong evidence (NHMRC level A) that meal replacements monitored by health professionals provide greater weight loss in obese adults than general dietary advice for a period of 1 to 12 months (DAA 2012). There is some evidence (NHMRC level C) that VLCD (< 4.2 MJ/d) incorporating meal replacements that are monitored by health professionals is as effective in achieving weight loss in overweight and obese adults as a low energy diet without meal replacements for periods of time varying from 3 months to 5 years (DAA 2012).

ALTERNATIVES TO WEIGHT LOSS

Weight-normative (also known as weight-centric) interventions focus on weight loss to achieve health and wellbeing. By contrast, weight-inclusive approaches aim to reduce weight stigma and improve health access (Tylka et al 2014). The cycle of weight loss followed by regain is a well-known phenomenon associated with weight-normative practice and one that imbues a sense of failure on the recipient with the potential to do further health harm. Poor body image is a widespread issue, and associated with serious health concerns including disordered eating, harmful dieting practices and other negative health behaviours (de Freitas 2018). The World Health Organization (WHO) has recognised the potential harm from weight bias, including consequences for individuals, such as body dissatisfaction, low self-esteem, suicidal thoughts and acts, depression and other psychological disorders (WHO Regional Office for Europe 2017). Consequently, there has been a shift from weight-normative to weight-inclusive interventions, greater acceptance of body diversity and specific programs targeting behaviour changes to improve health rather than alter body weight (Bombak 2014).

Weight-loss interventions have relatively limited evidence of long-term success (Fildes et al 2015) and there is the potential for harm from dieting practices that result in weight cycling (Montani et al 2015). Along with alternative non-diet approaches, the evidence for a more weight-inclusive approach to improve health has grown in recent years. In an investigation into mortality and lifestyle behaviours in a cohort of around 40,000 individuals in the United States, higher intakes of fruit and vegetables, reduced alcohol intake, increased physical activity and reduced smoking were associated with a significantly lower mortality regardless of body mass index (Matheson et al 2012). Intervention trials suggest that shifting the focus away from weight does not result in poorer health outcomes than weight-loss interventions, with some reporting improved outcomes for weight-inclusive practice. In particular, psychological outcomes (disordered eating, self-esteem and depression) are often improved in non-diet interventions compared to weight-focused interventions (Clifford et al 2015).

It is very likely that dietary modification and physical activity exert independent health effects conferring additional benefits to individuals using these strategies for weight loss. Individuals may prefer to focus on improving their dietary behaviours and physical activity as elements within their control, rather than their weight and their preference for non-weight-focused goals should be respected given the evidence supporting behaviourally based interventions.

CONCLUSION

Obesity is a major public health issue for both adults and children across Australia, New Zealand and worldwide, contributing greatly to the risk and complications of chronic disease. Prevalence rates are high in the general population, but are even higher for people with a disability, Aboriginal and Torres Strait Islander people, Māori, and other CALD backgrounds, as well as those from socioeconomically disadvantaged backgrounds. There is an increasing recognition of the role of nurses in the provision of preventative health advice for the management of chronic disease risk, including diet and physical activity for weight management and obesity prevention. There is good evidence that weight loss in people who are overweight to reduce the risk factors for chronic disease, and lifestyle modification (improving dietary intake and increasing physical activity), is more effective if it is supported by all healthcare practitioners.

In particular, nurses are in an ideal position to facilitate the early identification and management of weight problems, and to adopt an accepting, person-centred approach when setting health goals. This includes screening individuals for overweight and obesity, assisting them to achieve appropriate weight goals, support and motivation to promote beneficial lifestyle changes, regardless of the impact on body weight, providing basic evidence-based advice, and facilitating referrals to Accredited Practising Dietitians (in Australia), Registered Dietitians (in New Zealand) and other specialist health professionals when there are multiple co-morbidities.

REFERENCES

Appel LJ, Brands MW, Daniels SR et al 2006. Dietary approaches to prevent and treat hypertension. A scientific statement from the American Heart Association. Hypertension 47, 296–308.

Aucott L, Poobalan A, Cairns W et al 2005. Effects of weight loss in overweight/obese individuals and long-term hypertension outcomes. Hypertension 45, 1035–1041.

Australian Bureau of Statistics (ABS) 2019. National Health Survey: first results 2017–18. ABS cat. no. 4364.0.55.001. ABS, Canberra.

Australian Bureau of Statistics (ABS) 2016. Cultural diversity in Australia 2016. 2017.0 Census of Population and Housing: Reflecting Australia – Stories from the Census 2016. Online. Available: www.abs.gov.au/ausstats/abs@.nsf/Lookup/by%20Subject/2071.0~2016~Main%20Features~Cultural%20Diversity%20Article~60.

Australian Bureau of Statistics (ABS) 2014. Australian Aboriginal and Torres Strait Islander Health Survey: updated results 2012–13. ABS cat. no. 4727.0.55.006. ABS, Canberra.

Australian Bureau of Statistics (ABS) 2013. Census of Population and Housing: Socio-Economic Indexes for Areas (SEIFA), Australia 2011. Online. Available: www.abs.gov.au/ausstats/abs@.nsf/Lookup/2033.0.55.001main+features100052011.

Australian Health Ministers' Advisory Council 2015. Aboriginal and Torres Strait Islander Health Performance Framework 2014 Report. AHMAC, Canberra.

Australian Indigenous HealthInfoNet 2019. Overview of Aboriginal and Torres Strait Islander health status 2018. Online. Available: https://healthinfonet.ecu.edu.au/healthinfonet/getContent.php?linkid=617557&title=Overview+of+Aboriginal+and+Torres+Strait+Islander+health+status+2018&contentid=36501_1.

Australian Institute of Health and Welfare (AIHW) 2019. People with disability in Australia 2019: in brief. Cat. no. DIS 74. AIHW, Canberra.

Australian Institute of Health and Welfare (AIHW) 2018a. Australia's health 2018. Australia's health series no. 16. AUS 221. AIHW, Canberra.

Australian Institute of Health and Welfare (AIHW) 2018b. Aboriginal and Torres Strait Islander Health Performance

Framework (HPF) report 2017. Online. Available: www.aihw.gov.au/reports/indigenous-australians/health-performance-framework/contents/tier-2-determinants-of-health/2-22-overweight-and-obesity.

Australian Institute of Health and Welfare (AIHW) 2017. A picture of overweight and obesity in Australia 2017. Cat. no. PHE 216. AIHW, Canberra.

Australian Institute of Health and Welfare (AIHW) 2016. Australian Burden of Disease Study: impact and causes of illness and death in Aboriginal and Torres Strait Islander people 2011. Australian Burden of Disease Study series no. 6. Cat. no. BOD 7. AIHW, Canberra.

Backholer K, Mannan HR, Magliano DJ et al 2012. Projected socioeconomic disparities in the prevalence of obesity among Australian adults. Australian and New Zealand Journal of Public Health 36, 557–563.

Bambra C, Gibson M, Sowden A et al 2010. Tackling the wider social determinants of health and health inequalities: evidence from systematic reviews. Journal of Epidemiology and Community Health 64(4), 284–291.

Bambra CL, Hillier FC, Cairns JM et al 2015. How effective are interventions at reducing socioeconomic inequalities in obesity among children and adults? Two systematic reviews. Public Health Research 3(1).

Beauchamp AJ, Backholer K, Magliano DJ et al 2014. The effect of obesity prevention interventions according to socioeconomic position: a systematic review. Obesity Reviews 15(7), 65–66.

Bombak A 2014. Obesity, health at every size and public health policy. American Journal of Public Health 104(2), e60–e67.

Brown JD, Busemi J, Milson V et al 2016. Effects on cardiovascular risk factors of weight losses limited to 5–10%. Translational Behavioral Medicine 6(3), 339–346.

Centers for Disease Control (CDC) 2019. Disability and obesity. Online. Available: www.cdc.gov/ncbddd/disabilityandhealth/obesity.html.

Clifford D, Ozier A, Bundros J et al 2015. Impact of non-diet approaches on attitudes, behaviors, and health outcomes: a systematic review. Journal of Nutrition Education and Behavior 47(2), 143–155.

Council of Australian Governments 2018. COAG statement on the Closing the Gap Refresh. Council of Australian Governments, Canberra. Online. Available: www.coag.gov.au/sites/default/files/communique/coag-statement-closing-the-gap-refresh.pdf.

Croxford S 2015. Poverty, disadvantage and food insecurity. In: S Croxford, C Itsiopoulos, AA Forsyth et al (eds), Food and nutrition throughout life. Allen & Unwin, Crow's Nest.

de Freitas C, Jordan H, Hughes EK 2018. Body image diversity in the media: a content analysis of women's fashion magazines. Health Promotion Journal of Australia 29, 251–256.

Denney-Wilson E, Robinson A, Laws R et al 2014. Development and feasibility of a child obesity prevention intervention in general practice: the Healthy 4 Life pilot study. Journal of Paediatrics and Child Health 50(11), 890–894.

Department of Health 2014. Australia's Physical Activity and Sedentary Behaviour Guidelines. Commonwealth Department of Health, Canberra.

Dietitians Association of Australia (DAA) 2012. Best Practice Guidelines for the Treatment of Overweight and Obesity in Adults. DAA, Canberra.

Federation of Ethnic Communities Councils of Australia (FECCA) 2015. Review of Australian Research on Older People from Culturally and Linguistically Diverse Backgrounds. FECCA, Canberra.

Fildes A, Charlton J, Rudisill C 2015. Probability of an obese person attaining normal body weight: cohort study using electronic health records. American Journal of Public Health 105, e54–e59.

Froehlich-Grobe K, Lollar D 2011. Obesity and disability. American Journal of Preventive Medicine 41(5), 541–545.

Garaulet M 2015. The Mediterranean diet and obesity from a nutrigenetic and epigenetics perspective. In: VR Preedy, RR Watson (eds), The Mediterranean diet: an evidence-based approach. Elsevier, London.

Grundy SM 2016. Metabolic syndrome update. Trends in Cardiovascular Medicine 26, 364–373.

Hall JE, do Carmo JM, da Silva AA et al 2015. Obesity-induced hypertension. Interaction of neurohumoral and renal mechanisms. Circulation Research 116(6), 991–1006.

Harris MF 2013. The metabolic syndrome. Australian Family Physician. Online. Available: www.racgp.org.au/afp/2013/august/the-metabolic-syndrome/.

Haw JS, Galaviz KI, Straus AN et al 2017. Long-term sustainability of diabetes prevention approaches: a systematic review and meta-analysis of randomized clinical trials. JAMA Internal Medicine 177(12), 1808–1817.

Hemler EC, Hu FB 2019. Plant-based diets for personal, population, and planetary health. Advances in Nutrition 10(Suppl 4), S275–S283.

Jiang S-Z, Lu W, Zong X-F et al 2016. Obesity and hypertension. Experimental and Therapeutic Medicine 12(4), 2395–2399.

Kable A, James C, Snodgrass S et al 2015. Nurse provision of healthy lifestyle advice to people who are overweight or obese. Nursing and Health Sciences 17(4), 451–459.

Klop B, Elte JMF, Cabezas MC 2013. Dyslipidemia in obesity: mechanisms and potential targets. Nutrients 5(4), 1218–1240.

Kuczmarski RJ, Ogden CL, Guo SS et al 2000. CDC growth charts for the United States: methods and development. Department of Health and Human Services. Vital Health Stat 11(246). 2002. Figures 13, 14. Online. Available: www.cdc.gov/nchs/data/series/sr_11/sr11_246.pdf.

Lal A, Moodie M, Ashton T et al 2012. Health care and lost productivity costs of overweight and obesity in New Zealand. Australia and New Zealand Journal of Public Health 36, 550–556.

Laws R, Campbell KJ, van der Pligt P et al 2014. The impact of interventions to prevent obesity or improve obesity related behaviours in children (0–5 years) from socioeconomically disadvantaged and/or indigenous families: a systematic review. BMC Public Health 14, 779.

Lazarou C, Couter C 2010. The role of nurses in the prevention and management of obesity. British Journal of Nursing 19(10), 641–647.

Lean MEJ, Leslie WS, Barnes AC et al 2019. Durability of a primary care-led weight management intervention for remission of type 2 diabetes: 2-year results of the DiRECT open-label, cluster-randomised trial. Lancet Diabetes and Endocrinology 7(5), 344–355.

Lim EL, Hollingsworth KG, Aribisala BS et al 2011. Reversal of type 2 diabetes: normalization of beta cell function in association with decreased pancreas and liver triacylglycerol. Diabetologia 54(10), 2506–2514.

Lim SU, Lee JH, Kim JS et al 2017. Comparison of World Health Organization and Asia-Pacific body mass index classifications in COPD patients. International Journal of Chronic Obstructive Pulmonary Disease 12, 2465–2475.

Martin L, Leveritt MD, Desbrow B et al 2013. The self-perceived knowledge, skills and attitudes of Australian practice nurses in providing nutrition care to patients with chronic disease. Family Practice 31, 201–208.

Matheson EM, King DE, Everett CJ 2012. Healthy lifestyle habits and mortality in overweight and obese individuals. Journal of the American Board of Family Medicine 25(1), 9–15.

Menigoz K, Nathan A, Turrell G 2016. Ethnic differences in overweight and obesity and the influence of acculturation on immigrant bodyweight: evidence from a national sample of Australian adults. BMC Public Health 16, 932.

Ministry of Business, Innovation & Employment 2019. Migration data explorer. Online. Available: https://mbienz.shinyapps.io/migration_data_explorer/#.

Ministry of Health NZ 2019a. Obesity statistics. Online. Available: https://www.health.govt.nz/nz-health-statistics/health-statistics-and-data-sets/obesity-statistics.

Ministry of Health NZ 2019b. Data Explorer Indicator: Obese: BMI of 30.0 or greater (or IOTF equivalent for 15-17 years). Online. Available: https://minhealthnz.shinyapps.io/nz-health-survey-2018-19-annual-data-explorer/_w_6e82b379/#!/explore-indicators.

Ministry of Health NZ 2019c. Data Explorer Adults Topic: Other health conditions. Online. Available: https://minhealthnz.shinyapps.io/nz-health-survey-2018-19-annual-data-explorer/_w_67d1131b/#!/explore-topics.

Ministry of Health NZ 2019d. New Zealand Health Survey Annual Data Explorer. Online. Available: https://minhealthnz.shinyapps.io/nz-health-survey-2019-20-annual-data-explorer/_w_4614b1fd/#!/.

Ministry of Health NZ 2019e. Data Explorer Indicator: Obese: BMI of 30.0 or greater (or IOTF equivalent for 15–17 years). Online. Available: https://minhealthnz.shinyapps.io/nz-health-survey-2018-19-annual-data-explorer/_w_6e82b379/#!/explore-indicators.

Ministry of Health NZ 2018. Life expectancy. Online. Available: www.health.govt.nz/our-work/populations/maori-health/tatau-kahukura-maori-health-statistics/nga-mana-hauora-tutohu-health-status-indicators/life-expectancy.

Ministry of Health NZ 2017. Clinical guidelines for weight management in New Zealand. Ministry of Health, Wellington.

Ministry of Health NZ 2016. Clinical guidelines for weight management in New Zealand children and young people. Ministry of Health, Wellington. Online. Available: www.health.govt.nz/publication/clinical-guidelines-weight-management-new-zealand-children-and-young-people.

Ministry of Health NZ 2015. Eating and activity guidelines for New Zealand adults. Ministry of Health, Wellington. CC BY 4.0.

Montani JP, Schutz Y, Dulloo AG 2015. Dieting and weight cycling as risk factors for cardiometabolic diseases: who is really at risk? Obesity Reviews 16(Suppl 1), S7–S18.

Muller MJ, Geisler C, Heymsfield SB et al 2018. Recent advances in understanding body weight homeostasis in humans. F1000Research 7, 1025.

National Health and Medical Research Council (NHMRC) 2013a. Clinical Practice Guidelines for the Management of Overweight and Obesity in adults, adolescents and children. NHMRC, Melbourne.

National Health and Medical Research Council (NHMRC) 2013b. Australian Dietary Guidelines. NHMRC, Canberra.

National Health and Medical Research Council (NHMRC) 2011. A review of the evidence to address targeted questions to inform the revision of the Australian Dietary Guidelines. Commonwealth of Australia, Canberra.

Neter JE, Stam BE, Kok FJ et al 2003. Influence of weight reduction on blood pressure: a meta-analysis of randomized controlled trials. Hypertension 42, 878–884.

O'Dea JA, Dibley MJ 2014. Prevalence of obesity, overweight and thinness in Australian children and adolescents by socioeconomic status and ethnic/cultural group in 2006 and 2012. International Journal of Public Health 59(5), 819–828.

Pavela G, Lewis DW, Locher J et al 2016. Socioeconomic status, risk of obesity, and the importance of Albert J. Stunkard. Current Obesity Reports 5(1), 132–139.

Phelan SM, Burgess DJ, Yeazel MW et al 2015. Impact of weight bias and stigma on quality of care and outcomes for patients with obesity. Obesity Reviews 16(4), 319–326.

Phillips K, Wood F, Kinnersley P 2014. Tackling obesity: the challenge of obesity management for practice nurses in primary care. Family Practice 31(1), 51–59.

Poirier P, Giles TD, Bray GA et al 2006. Obesity and cardiovascular disease: pathophysiology, evaluation, and effect of weight loss: an update of the 1997 American Heart Association Scientific Statement on Obesity and Heart Disease from the Obesity Committee of the Council on Nutrition, Physical Activity, and Metabolism. Circulation 113, 898–918.

Poobalan A, Aucott L, Smith WCS et al 2004. Effects of weight loss in overweight/obese individuals and long-term lipid outcomes – a systematic review. Obesity Reviews 5, 43–50.

Puhl RM, Heuer CA 2009. The stigma of obesity: a review and update. Obesity 17(5): 941–964.

PwC Australia 2015. Weighing the cost of obesity: a case for action. PwC Australia, Australia. Online. Available: www.pwc.com.au/pdf/weighing-the-cost-of-obesity-final.pdf.

Rachele JN, Schmid CJ, Brown WJ et al 2019. A multilevel study of neighborhood disadvantage, individual socioeconomic position, and body mass index: exploring cross-level interaction effects. Preventative Medicine Reports 14 (100844).

Sargent GM, Forrest LM, Parker RM 2012. Nurse delivered lifestyle interventions in primary health care to treat chronic disease risk factors associated with obesity: a systematic review. Obesity Reviews: An Official Journal of the International Association for the Study of Obesity 13, 1148–1171.

Scarborough P, Bhatnagar P, Wickramasinghe KK et al 2011. The economic burden of ill health due to diet, physical inactivity, smoking, alcohol and obesity in the UK: an update to 2006–07 NHS costs. Journal of Public Health (Oxford) 33(4), 527–535.

Smith JD 2016. Australia's rural, remote and Indigenous health. Elsevier Australia, Chatswood.

St George I (ed.) 2013. Coles' medical practice in New Zealand. Medical Council of New Zealand, Wellington.

Statistics NZ 2014. Disability Survey: 2013 key facts. Online. Available: http://archive.stats.govt.nz/browse_for_stats/health/disabilities/DisabilitySurvey_HOTP2013.aspx.

Taylor R, Barnes AC 2019. Can type 2 diabetes be reversed and how can this best be achieved? James Lind Alliance research priority number one. Diabetic Medicine 36, 308–315.

The Royal Children's Hospital 2020. Growth charts. Online. Available: https://www.rch.org.au/childgrowth/Growth_Charts/.

Tomiyama AJ, Carr D, Granberg EM et al 2018. How and why weight stigma drives the obesity 'epidemic' and harms health. BMC Medicine 16, 123.

Tylka TL, Annunziato RA, Burgard D et al 2014. The weight-inclusive versus weight-normative approach to health: evaluating the evidence for prioritizing well-being over weight loss. Journal of Obesity 2014, ID: 983495.

Vartanian LR 2010. Disgust and perceived control in attitudes toward obese people. International Journal of Obesity 34, 1302–1307.

Walsh MAF, Fahy KM 2012. Interaction between primary health care professionals and people who are overweight or obese: a critical review. Australian Journal of Advanced Nursing 29(2), 23–29.

Wong E, Woodward M, Stevenson C et al 2016. Prevalence of disability in Australian elderly: impact of trends in obesity and diabetes. Preventive Medicine 82, 105–110.

World Health Organization (WHO) Regional Office for Europe 2020. Body mass index – BMI. Online. Available: www.euro.who.int/en/health-topics/disease-prevention/nutrition/a-healthy-lifestyle/body-mass-index-bmi.

World Health Organization (WHO) Regional Office for Europe 2017. Weight bias and obesity stigma: considerations for the WHO European Region. Online. Available: www.euro.who.int/__data/assets/pdf_file/0017/351026/WeightBias.pdf?ua=1

Zhao Y, Wright J, Begg S et al 2013. Decomposing Indigenous life expectancy gap by risk factors: a life table analysis. Population Health Metrics, 11:1. Online. Available: https://pophealthmetrics.biomedcentral.com/track/pdf/10.1186/1478-7954-11-1.

CHAPTER 12

Palliation in Chronic Illness

JANE L. PHILLIPS • CLAIRE FRASER • CLAUDIA VIRDUN

LEARNING OBJECTIVES

When you have completed this chapter you will be able to:

- understand the historical factors that have shaped the development of current palliative care services and practices
- describe the philosophy and identify principles that inform the provision of palliative care to people living with a life-limiting illness
- identify the challenges and opportunities to integrate palliative care principles into nursing practice
- identify the nurse's role within the interdisciplinary palliative care team
- describe the core nursing capabilities required to provide best evidence-based palliative care to people living with a life-limiting illness.

KEY WORDS

carers	palliative care
end of life	quality of life
interdisciplinary team	

INTRODUCTION

Nursing is integral to the provision of high-quality evidence-based palliative care for people living with an advanced, progressive life-limiting illness, as well as for their family and carers. It is now widely acknowledged that palliative care is indicated for people living with a range of progressive life-limiting illnesses, including but not limited to: cancer, chronic obstructive pulmonary disease (COPD), advanced dementia, Parkinson's disease, multiple sclerosis, end-stage kidney disease and heart disease. As a life-limiting illness can occur at any age, palliative care is relevant across the lifespan, including: neonates, children, adolescents and young people, working age people and older people.

Optimal palliative care occurs when an individualised interdisciplinary team is created for each person with palliative care needs. This interdisciplinary team ought to include all relevant health and social support personnel with the expertise to meet the needs of the person and their carers. Nurses play a key role within the interdisciplinary team, with the intensity of nursing care often increasing as the person approaches the last days of their life. Palliative care nursing shares many of the same principles and practices of nursing more broadly, namely a commitment to addressing the physical, psychological, emotional, cultural, social, practical, spiritual and informational aspects of a person's health and wellbeing (Phillips et al 2018). It is nursing care that is focused on optimising quality of life by maintaining the person's function, minimising their suffering, and attending to their needs in a compassionate and appropriate way during their last year of life (Palliative Care Australia 2016; Phillips et al 2018).

This chapter commences with a brief overview of the historical development of palliative care before focusing on the contemporary issues and challenges of providing care to people living with a progressive life-limiting illness who have unmet palliative care needs. The management of any progressive life-limiting illness is often complex, as many people have other co-morbidities and can present with a range of symptoms. This complexity requires an individualised approach to planning and delivering palliative nursing care, which is demonstrated in the case studies included in this chapter. These case studies illustrate how the philosophy and principles of palliative care can be readily individualised for people with different life-limiting illnesses, care settings and palliative care needs. Applying these principles ensures that individualised patient-centred palliative care is available for all, regardless of their underlying disease, their age or place of care. These case studies also highlight the core palliative care capabilities required by *'all nurses'* caring for people with a life-limiting illness as part of the multi-professional, interdisciplinary team.

THE DEVELOPMENT OF PALLIATIVE CARE

Palliative care has existed in many different forms for well over 200 years. During this time there have been three major phases of development, as summarised below:

- **Religious care of the dying:** Up until the twentieth century, palliative care was largely limited to care provided by religious organisations in hospices for the destitute and dying (Phillips et al 2015). This contributed to palliative care being viewed as 'terminal care', or care provided to a person in the last days to weeks of their life. As death occurred within the confines of the hospice, it contributed to death and dying being 'hidden' from wider society, so that death was no longer seen as a normal part of life.
- **The modern palliative care phase:** The next phase of development occurred largely as a social movement that emerged in the 1970s. This social movement emerged in response to growing concerns about the focus on aggressive and often medically futile cancer treatments for people with advanced cancer and the lack of symptom management provided to people with cancer who were imminently dying (Phillips et al 2015). Dame Cicely Saunders (1918–2005), a nurse, social worker and doctor, was one of the key champions of improving care for the dying and led the establishment of St Christopher's Hospice in North London. Within this hospice, the focus of care was on the physical, psychological and spiritual needs of dying patients (Pace & Lunsford 2011). This interdisciplinary model of palliative care was subsequently adopted by other Commonwealth countries, such as Canada and Australia. The impetus to establish palliative care services in the United States occurred much later and was largely in response to the landmark 'SUPPORT study' (Connors et al 1995), which identified that people dying in acute care had significant unmet needs. Shortly after these results were reported, the 'Approaching death:

improving care at the end-of-life' guidance document statement was published (Institute of Medicine 1997). Since the development of modern palliative care, the specialty has continued to evolve rapidly (Phillips et al 2015).
- **A population-based model of care:** The current phase of development is focused on implementing a population-based model of palliative care to ensure that everyone with unmet palliative care needs has access to the level and intensity of care they require, regardless of their diagnosis, age, geographical location, care setting or age (Palliative Care Australia 2018b).

DEFINING PALLIATIVE CARE

The importance of a population-based approach is reflected in the current World Health Organization (WHO) (2016) definition of palliative care (see Box 12.1). This contemporary definition ensures that palliative care principles remain at the core of treatment and that patients' individualised needs are central to the outcomes. It also highlights the importance of robust assessment and proactive planning to prevent distress and unnecessary suffering. The underpinning principles inform and guide palliative care nursing practice.

Changing Epidemiology Profile of People with Palliative Care Needs

While the modern palliative care movement may have had its genesis in cancer, a number of epidemiological changes are reshaping the delivery of palliative care services in Australia and New Zealand, as detailed below.

Children with life-limiting conditions

Fortunately, in high-income countries like Australia and New Zealand only a very small number of children will have a life-limiting illness spanning a wide range of different illnesses, and only a few will die from their disease. For example, in a population of 250,000 people where 50,000 are children, in a one-year period, approximately eight children will die from a life-limiting illness (three from cancer, five from non-malignant disease); 70 children will have a life-limiting condition; and 35 children will require specialist palliative care (EAPC Taskforce for Palliative Care in Children 2009).

Paediatric palliative care is derived from adult palliative care, and is the active total care of the child's body, mind and spirit, and supports their family (see Box 12.1). Palliative care ought to begin when the child's life-limiting illness is diagnosed and continues

BOX 12.1
WHO's Definition of Palliative Care

ADULTS

Palliative care is an approach that improves quality of life of patients and their family facing the problems associated with life-threatening illness, through the prevention and relief of suffering by means of early identification and impeccable assessment and treatment of pain and other problems, physical, psychological and spiritual. Palliative care:

- provides relief from pain and other distressing symptoms
- affirms life and regards dying as a normal process
- intends neither to hasten nor postpone death
- integrates the psychology and spiritual aspects of patient care
- offers a support system to help patients live as actively as possible until death
- offers a support system to help the family cope during the patient's illness and in their own bereavement
- uses a team approach to address the needs of patients and their families, including bereavement counselling if indicated
- will enhance quality of life, and may also positively influence the course of illness; and
- is applicable early in the course of the illness, in conjunction with other therapies that are intended to prolong life, such as chemotherapy or radiation therapy, and includes those investigations needed to better understand and manage distressing clinical complications.

CHILDREN

Palliative care for children represents a special, albeit closely related field to adult palliative care. WHO's definition of palliative care appropriate for children and their families is as follows: The principles apply to other paediatric chronic disorders:

- Palliative care for children is the active total care of the child's body, mind and spirit, and also involves giving support to the family
- It begins when illness is diagnosed, and continues regardless of whether or not a child receives treatment directed at the disease
- Health providers must evaluate and alleviate a child's physical, psychological and social distress
- Effective palliative care requires a broad multidisciplinary approach that includes the family and makes use of available community resources; it can be successfully implemented even if resources are limited; and
- It can be provided in tertiary care facilities, in community health centres and even in children's homes.

WHO 2018a, 2018b.

regardless of whether or not a child receives active treatment or not (WHO 2018b). Timely introduction of palliative care requires health professionals to evaluate and alleviate the child's physical, psychological, and social distress, and requires an interdisciplinary approach that includes the family. Palliative care for children also needs to make use of all relevant and available community resources. Adopting this approach ensures that palliative care is successfully implemented even if resources are limited.

It also focuses on the child's physical and cognitive development, including their language, and endeavours to optimise their ability to understand and be involved in decision-making. Paediatric palliative care also focuses on the needs of the parents, carers and siblings, and the implications of the child's condition on family-functioning and decision-making (Battista & LaRagione 2019). In an Australian and New Zealand context, palliative care for a progressive life-limiting illness in children mainly takes place in the home,

hospital or in specialist hospices. Children with non-malignant progressive life-limiting illnesses often have complex needs and experience various illness trajectories complicated by prognostic uncertainty (Virdun, Brown et al 2015). Many have progressively deteriorating diseases requiring longer term palliative care (Battista & LaRagione 2019).

Importantly, palliative care can be provided alongside life-prolonging treatments or it can focus purely on symptom relief and quality of life (Virdun, Brown et al 2015). The stigma attached to the phrase 'palliative care', which is associated with death and giving up, can often be a barrier to parents accepting early referral to the specialist palliative care team (Battista & LaRagione 2019). In addition to dispelling this myth, there are a number of other actions nurses need to consider when working with children with palliative care needs and their families, including:

- assisting parents, who are often struggling to cope with the diagnosis, to learn the necessary skills to provide technical care and navigate the health and social care systems for relevant services and information

- understanding the family dynamics and the impact these dynamics have on their willingness to accept palliative care and engage with the team
- appraising the child's developmental age, their level of understanding, along with the family's acceptance, which assists the team to determine the degree to which the child can participate in decision-making related to treatment options and death and dying discussions
- determining the degree to which the siblings and the family are keen to be involved in the child's care and then tailoring individualised support and education to equip them for this role
- understanding that education support may be required so that a child's teachers are able to adequately support the child, their peers and sensitively answer any questions they may have; and
- appreciating that family members/friends are at risk of experiencing a complicated bereavement and will therefore need close follow-up after the death of the child (Battista & LaRagione 2019).

Similar to adults, children often experience sub-optimal symptom control due to a lack of assessment; misconceptions by the child, their families or health professionals about pain and its management; and various healthcare system-related issues (Battista & LaRagione 2019). Low incidence coupled with rarity of disease and prognostic uncertainty makes paediatric palliative care challenging, especially when most healthcare professionals, outside of specialist paediatric palliative care services, have limited exposure to caring for these children and their parents. As a result, this population is often underserved (Virdun, Brown et al 2015a).

Increasing burden of non-communicable diseases

Although the philosophy of palliative care and its associated practices may have its genesis in cancer care, palliative care is now a component in the management of all progressive life-limiting illnesses, such as end-stage cardiac or pulmonary disease, advanced dementia, renal and liver failure, and other neurological conditions (Palliative Care Australia 2018b). Similar to other high-income countries, non-communicable diseases in Australia and New Zealand continue to exact a high toll on the health of individuals. People are now living longer with increasing levels of morbidity associated with one or more chronic illnesses (World Health Organization [WHO] 2018). In 2016, non-communicable diseases caused 71% of deaths globally, and accounted for 88% of the deaths in high-income countries (WHO 2018). Similarly, cardiovascular disease, dementia, cerebrovascular disease, including stroke, lung cancer and COPD were the top five leading underlying causes of death for Australian males and females of all ages combined in 2017 (Australian Institute of Health and Welfare [AIHW] 2019).

Population ageing

As the result of a number of significant medical and technological advances, much of the world's population is now ageing and living with one or more non-communicable diseases (WHO 2018). This longevity means that dementia is now the leading cause of death for women, and the second leading overall cause of death in Australia (Australian Bureau of Statistics [ABS] 2018a; AIHW 2019). Three in 10 people aged over 85 years, and one in 10 people aged over 65 years have dementia (The National Centre for Social and Economic Modelling 2017).

Dementia is a collection of symptoms caused by a range of neurocognitive disorders, leading to cognitive decline. Symptoms can include memory impairment and a decline in executive function, motor function, language ability and/or visuospatial cognitive function (Smits et al 2015). These diseases are complicated by a long, unpredictable course affecting decision-making capacity, communication and understanding (Palliative Care Australia 2018a, 2018b), requiring surrogate decision-makers to make decisions on the patient's behalf. An inability to advocate for oneself increases the vulnerability of older people, most of whom will spend their last year of life in a residential aged care facility. From a human rights perspective, older people living in aged care are entitled to the same liberties as those residing in their own homes and need to be provided with similar opportunities to receive high-quality palliative care. Such care requires access to assessment by general practitioners, advocacy and interdisciplinary collaboration tailored to meet the individual needs of each older person (Palliative Care Australia 2018a, 2018b).

The intercepting vulnerabilities of dementia, living in residential aged care, and the high percentage of multi-morbidity makes this population at risk of sub-optimal palliative care, which is often amplified if English is not the person's first language.

Indigenous populations

The Indigenous peoples of Australia and New Zealand are not a homogenous population but rather are comprised of a diverse group of people living in many different communities sharing different values.

The life expectancy of Aboriginal and Torres Strait Islander people is approximately 8.6 years lower than other Australians (AIHW 2019). An analysis of life expectancy and contributing factors to mortality reveal that chronic diseases, such as cardiovascular diseases and cancer, occurring in the 35–74-year age group, are responsible for the majority of the life expectancy gap (AIHW 2020). In 2017, cancer overtook circulatory disease as the leading cause of death in this population (AIHW 2020). Aboriginal and Torres Strait Islander people affected by cancer have a reduced 5-year survival rate (40%) compared to other Australians (52%) (AIHW 2020). When gender, age and geographical isolation are considered, this population has a 97% higher risk of death than other Australians (AIHW 2020).

It is currently estimated that an Aboriginal and Torres Strait Islander male born in 2005–07 is likely to live to 67.2 years, about 11.5 years less than other Australian males (who could expect to live to 78.7 years) (AIHW 2019). An Aboriginal and Torres Strait Islander female born in 2005–07 is likely to live to 72.9 years, which is almost 10 years less than other Australian females (82.6 years) (AIHW 2019).

The Māori experience is somewhat better, although still reflective of the Australian experience. Life expectancy from birth for non-Māori exceeded that of Māori by 8.6 years for males and by 7.9 years for females in 2005–07. For males, three-quarters of this difference was due to higher Māori death rates at ages 40–79 years; and for females, three-quarters of this difference was due to higher Māori death rates at ages 50–84 years (Stats NZ: Tatauranga Aotearoa 2020).

An important principle that underlies the delivery of all care provided to Indigenous peoples is 'cultural safety', a practice which respects, supports and empowers the cultural identity and wellbeing of an individual (Laverty et al 2017). While it is not expected that all nurses will fully understand Indigenous beliefs, there is an expectation that they will demonstrate respect and a commitment to providing culturally safe, individualised person-centred care (Taylor & Guerin Thompson 2019). Despite the diversity within Indigenous cultures, there are some common themes that need to be acknowledged and respected, including the isolation of some communities from major treatment centres; the belief of many in the importance of Country, along with an unwillingness to travel outside of Country for treatment; and the need for communication that is clear and easily understood. Also, Indigenous people have the same desire to die at home as other cultures, but enabling this to happen may be challenging in some circumstances or place an added burden on already stretched family networks, given their historical treatment. Aboriginal and Torres Strait Islander people often, and understandably, have a distrust of government agencies. The intergenerational trauma and decreased education and employment opportunities over past decades has led to a significant number of Aboriginal and Torres Strait Islander people having lower socio-economic status. While many Aboriginal and Torres Strait Islander people have a broader concept of family, which makes the input of significant others important, their lower socioeconomic status often impacts on their ability to call upon family and friends to assist with care at home (Shahid et al 2018). Aboriginal and Torres Strait Islander people health workers are often vital links between non-Indigenous healthcare providers and Indigenous communities, and can assist the palliative care team to more effectively and respectfully meet the patient and carer(s) needs.

Culturally and linguistically diverse (CALD) communities

Australia is a multicultural society, comprised of people belonging to 270 ancestries (Australian Human Rights Commission 2015). In Australia, the culturally and linguistically diverse (CALD) population is defined by country of birth, English proficiency, and main language other than English spoken at home (Department of Immigration and Multicultural Affairs 2001). Within Australia one in three people is born overseas; one in 10 children have one parent born overseas; one in three children have both parents born overseas; one in four people speak a language other than English at home; and one in three people aged over 65 years were born overseas (ABS 2016).

Culture influences how one views death and dying, choices at end of life and how people are cared for immediately following death (Givler & Maani-Fogelman 2020). Upholding these values at end of life is central to patient-centred care, family-centred care, autonomy and respect, and reflected in global palliative care policy. Person-centred palliative care is always responsive to the needs, preferences and values of the patient living with a life-limiting illness, their carers and families (Palliative Care Australia 2018a). Culture, education and language differences can alter the process and interpretation of communication (Rosas-Blum et al 2007). These differences can adversely affect medical care and decision-making and lead to suboptimal care and unnecessary patient and family suffering (Levetown 2008).

Impact of these epidemiological changes

These significant epidemiological changes illustrate the burden and impact that population ageing and non-communicable diseases are having on contemporary society and the changing patterns of death. Whereas once people died at a younger age of an unexpected death, increasingly people living in high-income countries, such as Australia and New Zealand, will have an expected death at an older age, as a result of one or more non-communicable diseases. Additionally, epidemiological change, the needs of younger people, Indigenous peoples and people from CALD communities all require special consideration to ensure that their palliative care, in addition to being timely and responsive, is person-centred and culturally and age appropriate.

PERSON-CENTRED CARE

Person-centred care is a key component of effective care for people living with and dying from progressive illness, in any clinical setting. Put simply, person-centred care occurs when the person with palliative care needs is at the centre of assessment, care planning and provision, as well as their family and carer(s).

The Picker Institute Europe (2017) identified eight essential characteristics of person-centred care relevant to palliative care. This population needs: 1) fast access to reliable healthcare advice; 2) effective treatment delivered by trusted professionals; 3) continuity of care and smooth transitions; 4) involvement of and support for family and carers; 5) clear, comprehensible information and support for self-care; 6) involvement in decisions and respect for patient preferences; 7) emotional support, empathy and respect; and 8) attention to physical and environmental needs.

The way nurses operationalise person-centred care for people with palliative care needs is best described by McCormack and McCance (2017) in the person-centred practice framework. This framework is composed of four constructs considered essential for person-centred nursing care, namely: 1) prerequisites and/or nursing attributes; 2) care environment and/or context of care; 3) person-centred processes of care; and 4) person-centred outcomes (Fig. 12.1).

Given nurses are the only healthcare professionals available 24 hours a day in most care settings, they are in a central position to lead and enable person-centred care for their patients. Developing a therapeutic relationship, listening carefully to the person's needs and working innovatively to enable this to occur within the context of advanced progressive illness, is important. A synthesis of research conducted over the past 30 years outlines key areas of importance which enable optimal care from the perspectives of patients with palliative care needs and their families (Virdun, Luckett et al 2015; Virdun et al 2017). These areas of importance include effective communication and shared decision-making; expert care; an adequate environment for care; family involvement in care provision; financial affairs; maintenance of sense of self and identity; minimising burden; respectful and compassionate care; trust and confidence in clinicians; and maintenance of patient safety and prevention of harm (Virdun, Luckett et al 2015; Virdun et al 2017). Building upon this work, a recent Australian study involving palliative care patients and their carers confirmed the importance of these domains and provided additional depth of understanding about how to enable this in practice (Virdun et al 2020). Person-centred care is the foundation for enabling optimal care by facilitating respectful and compassionate care; effective communication and shared decision-making; effective teamwork; enabling family involvement and maintaining role, meaning and identity for patients.

ADOPTING A PUBLIC HEALTH APPROACH TO PALLIATIVE CARE

Managing death and dying is not just a responsibility of the healthcare system but of the community at large because most people will live out their lives in their respective communities, and not within the healthcare environment. This realisation has led to the development of health-promoting palliative care, which is a population-based approach with direct links to the World Health Promotion guidelines, the Ottawa Charter (CareSearch 2012). These health and social care principles when applied to palliative care enhance the individual's quality of life by strengthening the community's inherent capacity to better support their needs (Kellehear & O'Connor 2008). A health-promoting model of palliative care focuses on building public policies that support dying, death, loss and grief; creating supportive environments (in particular, social supports); strengthening community action; developing personal skills in these areas; and re-orienting the health system (Kellehear 1999).

The promotion of quality of life in the face of a progressive life-limiting illness is firmly based on a person-centred approach that takes into account the physical, psychological, emotional and spiritual dimensions of the person (McCormack & McCance 2017; Picker Institute Europe 2017). This holistic model of care acknowledges the fact that people living with a progressive life-limiting illness live within a community and the

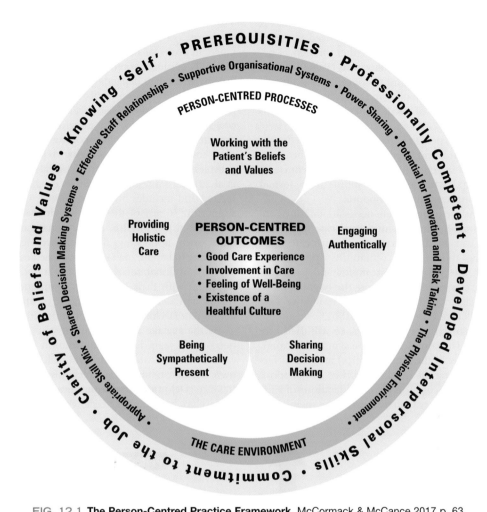

FIG. 12.1 **The Person-Centred Practice Framework.** McCormack & McCance 2017 p. 63.

presence or absence of community support greatly impacts on the quality of care that can be provided by informal and formal healthcare providers.

OPERATIONALISING A POPULATION-BASED MODEL OF PALLIATIVE CARE

Adopting a health-promoting model of palliative care provides the foundation for the delivery of a population-based model of palliative care which demands that palliative care becomes 'everybody's business'. Achieving this requires healthcare professionals from a wide range of disciplines, including medicine, nursing and allied health, to function as an interdisciplinary team and to work collaboratively with the patient and their carer(s) to address their unmet palliative care

needs. It also acknowledges that not everyone with palliative care needs will require the same level and intensity of palliative care. As diagnosis and prognosis are poor indicators of needs, health professionals are encouraged to formally assess their patient's needs using validated tools such as the 'Palliative Care Needs Assessment Tool' (PC-NAT) (Waller et al 2008). The PC–NAT not only helps to identify patients' and caregivers' specific palliative care needs, it also helps to facilitate early intervention and assists with prioritising the use of scarce resources and identifying the level and intensity of palliative care that people need at different times throughout their illness trajectory (Waller et al 2008). People with relatively straightforward palliative care needs can often be effectively managed by their usual team (sometimes referred to as the 'generalist palliative care team') (Palliative Care Australia 2018b). Whereas people with more complex needs will need to access the specialist palliative care team, either through a one-off consultation or on an ongoing basis (Palliative Care Australia 2018b). It is helpful to conceptualise a population-based model of palliative care as a triangle with three different levels of need, as described below and illustrated in Fig. 12.2.

- Level I: The person's palliative care needs are straightforward and predictable and can be managed by their generalist palliative care team and their carer(s) with additional inputs from formal and informal community supports.
- Level II: As the patient's care needs are intermediate and fluctuating, the patient's usual care team may need to consult the specialist palliative care team and engage more formal community supports.
- Level III: The patient has complex and persistent palliative care needs that require the ongoing input and management by the specialist palliative care team (Palliative Care Australia 2018b).

As the person's illness progresses, so will their care needs change. The complexity of the symptoms experienced and needs of the family/carer(s) are critical factors in determining the need for services and support. The next section focuses on the considerations of each of the interdisciplinary palliative care team members.

The Carer

A carer is '... a person who provides any informal assistance, in terms of help or supervision, to people with disability or older people (aged 65 years and over)' (ABS 2018b). Australia's dependency on the input of carers is increasing, with one in eight Australians (2.86 million people) in 2015 providing informal care (Deloitte Access Economics 2015). The caregiver role has changed dramatically from one of supporting the person during their convalescence to now being required to provide complex physical care and psychological support (Nuzzo et al 2015). As a result, the primary carer's role is multi-faceted and includes but is not limited to helping and supporting in any of the daily activities of the person being cared for; physical and personal care and assistance, such as dressing, lifting, showering, feeding or providing transport; management of medications; provision of emotional, social or financial support; and helping them with their day-to-day organisation, appointments and dealing with emergencies and managing equipment (Deloitte Access Economics 2015).

As the average age of a patient with palliative care needs is 75 years, it is not uncommon for the primary carer to also be older and have health issues of their own, which can impact on their ability to provide ongoing care (Deloitte Access Economics 2015). Many carers themselves have unmet needs which can be amplified

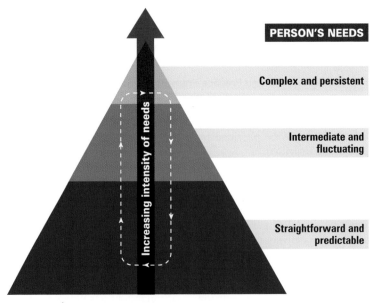

Person's movement between levels

FIG. 12.2 **Conceptual Model of Level of Palliative Care Needs.** Palliative Care Australia: Palliative Care Service Development Guidelines, Canberra 2018b. PCA. p.11.

by the caregiving role. While their caregiving experience may have both positive and negative elements, it places enormous physical, emotional and financial demands on the person assuming the carer role (Luckett et al 2019). Carers frequently experience depression and anxiety, and sleep deprivation, which adds to carer burden (Trevino et al 2018).

The Generalist Palliative Care Team

For those people with a palliative diagnosis and a relatively uncomplicated illness trajectory, care is most appropriately delivered by the generalist palliative care team. If a person is being cared for at home, this generalist palliative care team is likely to include the person's general practitioner (GP), other medical specialists, community nurses and allied health professionals. If the person is living within a residential aged care facility, the nurses and care assistants working within the facility and the GP will form the basis of the generalist palliative care team. Regardless of the care setting, the generalist palliative care team play a pivotal role in the management and coordination of services to support the person with the progressive life-limiting illness and their carer(s). To be effective, this team needs to have an open, honest, supportive relationship with the patient and their carer(s) and other team members; the ability to determine in partnership with the patient and carers the goals of care; the capabilities to assess and manage the symptoms commonly experienced by people with a palliative illness; and to identify when referral on to other specialist providers and/or services is indicated. It is important that the generalist palliative care team is aware of and utilises relevant informal and formal support networks available within the person's local community.

The Specialist Palliative Care Team

The specialist palliative care team provides care to those patients whose needs exceed the capacity and resources of the primary care provider(s) (Level II and III, see Fig. 12.2). Referral to a specialist palliative care service will in most cases be made through the patient's GP or other medical specialist, but can also be initiated by nurses in many care settings. Many specialist palliative care teams in Australia and New Zealand work within a consultative model of care and in close collaboration with the generalist palliative care team and the carer(s) (Luckett et al 2012). Specialist palliative care services have achieved much in raising the profile of the need for expert communication, exemplary pain and symptom management, psychosocial support and spiritual counselling for people faced with the prospect of dying (Ernecoff et al 2020).

The specialist palliative care team provides specialist palliative care for patients and their families where assessed needs exceed the resources and/or capability of the generalist palliative care team; assessment and care consistent with the needs of the patient, caregiver and family and, within available services, capability and resources; consultation and support to the primary care service managing the care of people with life-limiting illness in community, acute care hospitals and residential aged care facilities; ongoing care to patients with complex, unstable conditions not restricted to physical symptoms but including psycho-emotional, social and spiritual problems; and education to primary care providers and other professionals providing generalist palliative care (Palliative Care Australia 2018b).

Optimal Symptom Management

The relief and management of symptoms associated with a progressive life-limiting illness is one of the primary aims of palliative care. If symptoms are not well controlled the person's quality of life can quickly deteriorate and adversely impact on carer stress and wellbeing (Kavalieratos et al 2016). In the home setting, suboptimal symptom management can quickly escalate to a crisis, culminating in the person being transferred to hospital for assessment and management. Good symptom control is dependent upon a holistic, patient-centred approach. The WHY Framework is a very useful and practical model that supports clinical decision-making in regards to palliative care symptoms (Currow & Clark 2010). The essential elements and considerations of this approach to assessment are reproduced in Box 12.2.

BOX 12.2
Does This Person Have a Life-Limiting Illness?

An understanding of the natural course of the illness can help to make clearer the following questions.

Is today's new symptom:

- an expected manifestation of the illness?
- an unexpected manifestation of the illness?
- an exacerbation of a coexisting problem?
- a totally new problem?

Is this person unwell today because of overall progression in a (maximally) treated disease?
OR
Is this person unwell today because of the effects of an acute problem with an easily reversible cause?

Currow & Clark 2010.

Optimal symptom control is the responsibility of the interdisciplinary team working with the person. If symptoms become difficult to manage, the generalist palliative care providers need to alert the case manager (usually the GP) and a referral to the specialist palliative care team may be needed. Where there is any change made to the plan of care, particularly if there is any change made to medications, it is important that the person with palliative care needs and their carer are fully educated as to the reasons behind the change and the intended outcomes.

PREFERRED PLACE OF CARE VS PREFERRED PLACE OF DEATH

Most people with a progressive life-limiting illness who have palliative care needs will want to spend as many days as possible in their preferred place of care, supported by their carer(s) and the generalist palliative care team. It is important not to assume that their 'preferred place of care' will be the same as their 'preferred place of death', as these are two very different questions and need to be framed as such (Agar et al 2008). As care needs increase, the likelihood that the person will require hospitalisation becomes higher, especially if their symptoms and/or physical care needs exceed available community supports and the family's physical, emotional or financial capacity to care. The most common reasons for hospitalisation at the end of life are because the person requires acute medical or surgical care; better symptom control; does not wish to die at home; and/or their carer requires respite or is not comfortable managing a home death.

END-OF-LIFE CARE

Although not always easy to predict, recognising when the person with a progressive life-limiting illness has transitioned into the terminal phase of care is critical to confirming the agreed goals of care and ensuring that the patient and family are adequately prepared. The terminal phase of life is often unpredictable and can last days to sometimes weeks (although uncommon). As people approach death, they generally become increasingly weak, sleep for longer periods, have a reduced appetite and are less active. They often lose interest in visitors and may experience periods of restlessness or agitation. Screening and assessing for these needs is an important nursing activity that ought to be undertaken at the commencement of each eight-hour shift and on an ongoing basis. It is important that healthcare professionals sensitively communicate their observations that the person's status has changed, and that their deterioration is suggestive of actively dying, and to confirm the agreed goals of care. The carer(s) must be allowed time and space to be able to express any concerns they might have with this agreed plan of care and to spend time with the person. An important component of the nursing role at this time, in addition to patient care, is to check in with carers, show kindness, support and care, and understand if they have any outstanding concerns at this time. If they do have concerns, ensure these are addressed and that, if required, referrals are made to the other relevant team members, such as social work or psychology services. Carers appreciate nurses who demonstrate respect and compassion towards the person dying, both before and after death in relation to the care being provided.

As the person enters the terminal phase of their illness and swallowing ceases or becomes difficult, the prescribed medications need to be reassessed and ceased if they are not contributing to the person's comfort. Converting the essential medications (i.e. opioids for pain, anti-emetics for nausea and/or vomiting) from oral administration to subcutaneous delivery via the subcutaneous route, or via a subcutaneous syringe driver, helps to ensure that the person's comfort is maintained.

BEREAVEMENT AND GRIEF

Most people who experience the death of someone close to them will not need specialist counselling, but rather will benefit from the support of others who can acknowledge their loss, listen to their experience and provide or direct them to relevant information (Remedios et al 2011). Bereavement refers to death of a person with whom there has been an enduring relationship, while grief is how bereavement affects us at an emotional, cognitive, social, physical, financial and spiritual level (Remedios et al 2011). The way in which people will make the necessary psychological and emotional adaptations after the death of a significant other is often informed by past experiences, including the decedent's (person who has died) last weeks and days of life (Corless & Meisenhelder 2019). How well the transition to palliative care and the dying process is managed has a significant bearing on the quality of the bereavement of family and friends. For nurses supporting a grieving person or family, listening compassionately and responding in a genuine manner is a powerful therapeutic intervention, particularly if the nurse was involved in their care (Corless & Meisenhelder 2019).

A small proportion of people can experience an intense, long-lasting form of grief which can take over their lives and significantly impair their ability to cope (Neimeyer et al 2011). People in this group need to be referred to bereavement counsellors or other psychological/psychiatric services. Many palliative care teams have bereavement counsellors or social workers with experience in working with grief. Bereavement groups are very useful for those who do not have adequate social support or who prefer talking about their sadness with those who have experienced a similar loss.

The following two case studies portray the delivery of palliative care from a nursing perspective. The first case study involves a young mother in declining health with advanced metastatic breast cancer, receiving care in the community. The second case study refers to a patient with a life-limiting heart condition in a residential care facility. After each case study, a nursing response is provided based on the principles and practices of holistic person-centred palliative care.

CASE STUDY 12.1

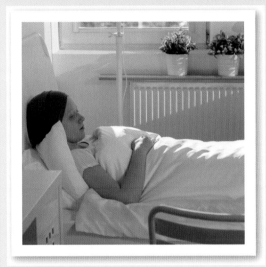

iStockphoto/KatarzynaBialasiewicz.

Laura is a 36-year-old mother of two children who was employed as a part-time medical receptionist in a busy rural practice. Laura's husband Tom owns his own business. Laura was diagnosed with an inflammatory breast cancer and after extensive surgical intervention, radiotherapy and chemotherapy, was progressing well. However, 9 months after completing her treatment, Laura developed pain in her hip, which on investigation was found to be due to bone metastases in her femur.

Laura was immediately referred to her radiation oncologist and subsequently received radiotherapy and commenced second-line chemotherapy. As a result of the chemotherapy, Laura experienced a number of distressing side-effects including nausea, vomiting, fatigue, hair loss, as well as significant anxiety, resulting in numerous hospital admissions. During these admissions Laura declined the medical team's suggestion of involving the palliative care team.

CASE STUDY QUESTIONS

1. As Laura does not want to be referred to the specialist palliative care team at this time, who else within the interdisciplinary team could assist her right now?

2. What is the hospital nurse's role in supporting Laura's family at this time?

3. Laura is anxious about her illness and what her future holds. How would you respond to her concerns?

Several weeks into her treatment, Laura developed a persistent headache and unsteady gait. A CT scan identified that she had brain and liver metastases. She was again reviewed by the radiation oncologist and received whole-brain irradiation. This initially provided some relief for her headaches and gait, but after some months her symptoms recurred. Laura was now spending most of her day in bed, and was experiencing a number of symptoms, including extreme fatigue, weakness, pain, poor appetite and feeling generally overwhelmed. It was evident Laura's disease was progressing despite treatment and after a consultation with her medical oncologist, Laura decided she would stop her chemotherapy and devote what time she had left to spend time with her husband, children, extended family and friends, and try to maintain some of her role as a mother and wife.

CASE STUDY QUESTION

4. As you start to plan Laura's discharge home, list what needs to be considered to enable Laura to achieve her goals and identify who else needs to be involved to support her at home.

During her second-line chemotherapy, Laura experienced overwhelming nausea and vomiting, fatigue and weakness, as well as bone and abdomen pain, related to her bone and liver metastasis. At this time, Laura had multiple conversations with her oncology team and her husband to agree on a plan of care. During these conversation, Laura decided to cease the chemotherapy as it was no longer controlling her cancer and was making her weak; focus on feeling stronger; and manage her anxiety. At the end of the meeting Laura was referred to the psychologist to assist with managing her anxiety. Laura knew she has advanced incurable cancer, but she wanted to focus on life and was not ready to talk about her future and death or dying.

CASE STUDY QUESTIONS

5. Do you think it is appropriate for Laura to focus on her quality of life at this time?

6. She has been referred to the psychologist working with the cancer care team. Who else could assist Laura and her family at this time?

7. Earlier in Laura's illness, she declined a referral to the specialist palliative care team. Do you think revisiting this conversation is appropriate? If so, how would you progress this?

On discharge home, her medical oncologist provided a comprehensive discharge summary to her GP. Laura visited her GP the day after she was discharged and together they discussed her goals and how they could work together to try and achieve these. The practice nurse also participated in this consultation with Laura's permission and the GP assessed Laura's symptoms, including her headaches, unsteady gait, back, shoulder and abdomen pain, and her profound weakness. Laura felt her anxiety was well supported at this time with ongoing input from the psychologist and with her transition home. However, Laura and her husband were very worried about how to talk with their children about Laura's illness.

CASE STUDY QUESTION

8. What can the practice nurse do to support Laura and her family at this time?

In an effort to palliate Laura's headache and unsteady gait, it was suggested that she be commenced on steroids to help reduce the intra-cranial pressure causing these symptoms. One of the roles of the nurse in this situation would be to reiterate possible side effects associated with the steroid use and to ensure that Laura understands how this medication works, the rationale for its use and how to minimise its many side effects (i.e. insomnia, increased appetite and muscle weakness). As a result of the spread of the cancer to her bones, Laura began to experience moderate to severe aching pains. During the assessment process a pain management plan was discussed and it was recommended by the specialist palliative care nurse that Laura be commenced on a combination of paracetamol, a non-steroidal anti-inflammatory (NSAID); and oral liquid morphine, for break-through pain. In case Laura experienced nausea with these medications it was also recommended that she be ordered prophylactic anti-nausea medications. At this stage a bowel management plan would be necessary to avoid constipation if regular use of opioids analgesia is used.

It must be stressed that at all levels of this debilitating disease, Laura will have sexual, physical and emotional needs. Laura is still relatively young and is in a long-term relationship with her husband. Both Laura and her husband may require counselling to assist them to maintain some level of intimacy. Sexuality is an important component of an individual's quality of life and palliative care staff struggle with limited use of assessment tools which would enhance ease of communication (Hjalmarsson & Lindroth 2020). The nurse will need to assess the importance Laura places on her own personal body image and sexuality, and be open to the appropriate communication skills required to allow Laura to voice her feelings.

Following a conversation with her GP, Laura accepted a referral to the specialist palliative care team and understood how they would work with her GP to manage her symptoms. The specialist palliative care team visited Laura and initially established a therapeutic relationship, reassuring her they would work with her to achieve her goals, as much as is possible. She was relieved to hear they would help her focus on living as well as she could.

Firstly, it is important to clarify patient goals and assess symptom and supportive needs. By utilising therapeutic communication skills, the patient and family and caregiver in consultation with the palliative team can reach a decision regarding their future care. Laura's desire to remain as independent as possible could be facilitated by referral to the other members of the interdisciplinary team such as physiotherapists and occupational therapists.

The following individuals may be identified as being helpful in supporting Laura to achieve her goals and meet these needs as they become evident during the palliative journey.

- *District and community nursing services:* Early referral to these services is vital to enable Laura to realise her goal to remain at home with family. Home nurses are in a unique position to provide long-term care and a holistic approach. Nursing services provide essential nursing support that may include:
  - personal care
  - ongoing assessment of symptoms and recommendation for changes to the management plan
  - monitoring medication requirements
  - liaising with other team members.
- *Medical practitioners:* The GP's role in this community-based scenario would be to support Laura's decision to remain at home by ensuring that she received the appropriate medical assessment for medication and community support. The knowledge that the GP may have regarding Laura's medical and social history will be invaluable for her future management.

- *Social worker:* Laura's situation can create significant emotional and financial distress. Social workers can play an invaluable role in mobilising financial assistance (i.e. sickness benefits, carers' allowances and liaising with previous employers). At some point, Laura's illness will most probably require some form of domiciliary support. They can also offer additional emotional support and counselling for her husband and children. Often where there are advanced cancers in younger people, it must be acknowledged that it creates increased stress for family, carers and the healthcare team.

- *School counsellor:* In this situation they would be an essential member of the team and provide essential support for Laura's children. This support may include the provision of academic assistance and specific counselling services for Laura's children and their friends.

- *Cancer support services:* Generic cancer support services offer a wide range of voluntary services and supportive networks. For example, body image workshops, Canteen, education pamphlets/DVDs and telephone counselling.

- *Mental health liaison team:* If depression and anxiety become a concern, then referral to the mental health team and/or a community-based psychologist would be appropriate. Medication and specific cognitive and behavioural therapies can promote wellness and improve quality of life in this situation.

- *Bereavement counsellor:* This form of counselling is focused on anticipatory grief and offers bereavement support to surviving family, friends and carers.

- *Pastoral care:* The spiritual dimension of Laura's life may require support and guidance. People facing death will often express a desire to explore the spiritual aspect of their beliefs or reconnect with a religious group.

- *Dietitian:* The dietitian assesses nutritional needs and develops a plan for maximising nutritional intake, but for this to be effective Laura ought to have been referred to the dietitian as soon as she started to lose weight.

- *Occupational therapist:* As Laura decided to be cared for at home for as long as possible, she would require specialised equipment and home medications as her illness progressed.

- *Physiotherapist:* Laura may also benefit from a physiotherapy review to help her manage her secondary bone pain and a gentle exercise program to help her maintain her strength.

As a result of the support provided by the extended palliative care team and the mobilisation of community support networks, Laura was able to maintain relative independence and autonomy at home. Laura's husband and children received both formal and informal support throughout this difficult time. Over the period leading up to her death, Laura was able to successfully adapt to her circumstances and participate in preparing family and friends. As Laura became progressively unwell, she decided she did not want to die in her home as she was worried about the effect this may have on her children. Her rural town did not have an inpatient specialist palliative care unit, but her local hospital had two private rooms that were set up to support dying patients if required. She discussed this with her specialist palliative care nurse and stated she would like to be transferred to this setting for her final days of life, if possible. She was hopeful her husband could stay with her and her children be cared for by her parents at this time. She wanted them to be able to visit, but also have time away from her illness and dying as needed. Laura was transferred to her local hospital three days before she died.

CASE STUDY QUESTIONS

9. What is your role as the nurse caring for Laura when she comes in for care on this last admission?

10. She is now struggling to swallow some of her medications. What can you do to help with this?

11. How can you help Laura's husband at this time?

12. Laura's husband asks what might happen over the next few hours/days. What do you say? (If you are not sure, you will find some useful tips here: https://palliativecare.org.au/resources/the-dying-process)

CASE STUDY 12.2

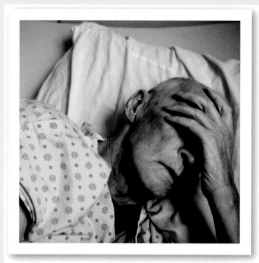

iStockphoto/Aguru.

John is a 74-year-old retired factory worker who is estranged from his immediate family. Fifteen years ago John's wife died suddenly and tragically. As a result, John became depressed and his consumption of alcohol increased considerably. In conjunction with his drinking, he smoked heavily and his nutritional intake became inadequate. John's health deteriorated and 13 years ago he was diagnosed with chronic dilated cardiomyopathy.

He was commenced on a combination of Angiotensin converting enzyme (ACE) inhibitors, diuretics, beta blockers and cardiac glycosides (i.e. digoxin). His underlying depression was treated with medications and counselling, and as a result he was able to make positive lifestyle changes. His condition stabilised and for some time he maintained his health with the help of nursing and allied health support and medical supervision, which necessitated a number of medication adjustments. However, the medications became less effective and his shortness of breath, oedema and fatigue increased, and he experienced more frequent chest pain.

John's health deteriorated significantly and he required an admission to hospital for acute shortness of breath. Once stabilised, John was transferred to a local residential aged care facility due to his care needs. However, John's cardiac condition continued to deteriorate and he developed irreversible left-sided heart failure, causing overwhelming pulmonary oedema. John entered the terminal phase of his illness and consented for the aged care nursing team to contact family members.

PALLIATIVE CARE NURSING RESPONSE

The importance of palliative nursing care as a core generic skill in nursing practice for patients with life-limiting illnesses has been highlighted earlier in this chapter. There is often a reluctance by some healthcare professionals to regard Stage IV heart failure as being palliative, which results in many older people with this condition not receiving a palliative approach to care or being referred to specialist palliative care services if they have complex care needs (Ezekowitz et al 2017). Prognostic uncertainty and the difficulty of explaining the mortality risk has led to recommendations that initiating a palliative approach ought to be needs based (Denvir et al 2015). Integrating the results of the PC-NAT (Waller et al 2008) and a comprehensive person-centred nursing assessment will ensure that the person living with a progressive life-limiting illness has access to the best palliative and end-of-life care, according to their needs.

Appropriate and sensitive communication is central to all palliative care nursing practices. Although many nurses find it challenging to discuss death in the initial assessment, this is exactly where discussion on the outcome of John's treatment should be addressed. People in John's condition require the opportunity to discuss their feelings and emotions in preparation for death. This is part of the groundwork when one is working towards 'a good death' and is guided by the WHO (2016) principle of affirming life and regarding dying as a normal process. In attempting to discuss death with John, the nurse must be aware of the impact of increasing hypoxia causing breathlessness and confusion, which may contribute to communication difficulties, as well as John's ability to understand what is being said.

The generalist nurse can play a significant role in John's care. Physical symptoms associated with heart failure, such as pain, breathlessness, weight loss (cardiac cachexia), nausea and vomiting, weakness and incontinence are common, and comparable with the symptoms of end-stage cancer. Although patients with heart failure and those with cancer exhibit similar disease-related burdens, patients with heart failure with worse health status experience greater physical and psychological symptom burdens (Kavalieratos et al 2016). Nurses are quite aware of the important role they play in the basic physical need requirements and can provide skilled care in assisting John to maintain some functionality and ability to self-care. Oxygen, opioids and diuretic drug therapy all remain essential medical elements of John's care and therefore require vigilant monitoring for effectiveness with the aim of maintaining comfort.

John's condition has clearly deteriorated to the point where medical treatment with a curative intent is not possible. Palliative care in this case study provides the necessary treatment to promote comfort levels and minimise suffering associated with his worsening chronic condition by:

- relieving distressing symptoms
- assisting John to come to terms with end-of-life issues
- maintaining a level of quality of life that is compliant with John's personal wishes.

Often, heart failure, like cancer, has a high level of unpredictability, where patients often experience sporadic improvements of health, but heart failure is more likely than cancer to end in sudden death due to arrhythmias. The nurse must be aware of the anxiety as a result of the uncertainty of the situation and particularly the breathlessness. In this situation a long-acting benzodiazepine in moderate doses can be helpful in ameliorating anxiety and helping to maximise respiratory function.

The instability of the situation can be addressed once the breathlessness has been stabilised and, when appropriate, the nurse can initiate dialogue, making inquiries regarding his future care. It is timely then to consider, in consultation with his GP, medical specialists and the specialist palliative care nurses:

- agreeing and documenting John's goals of care, and updating his care plan accordingly
- optimising John's symptom management
- contacting his family and friends
- adhering to his advance care plan
- considering and addressing his spiritual needs
- identifying what might assist John's comfort within his new aged care environment (e.g. his food preferences, window access, ability to get outside, music or other)
- revisiting his funeral arrangements.

Nurses can play a pivotal role in the coordination of each person's individualised interdisciplinary team. As a result of the information gathered through ongoing assessment and monitoring, nurses may find themselves providing leadership and direction to other members of the team. This could also require nurses playing an advocacy role in assisting John to meet his end-of-life goals. The following individuals may be identified as being helpful in supporting John to achieve his goals and meet his needs as they become evident.

- *Palliative care nurse specialist:* Provides expert advice on symptom management, education to the patient and staff, and liaises with generalist nursing and medical practitioners. If symptoms become very difficult to manage, the palliative care nurse specialist will usually have access to a palliative medicine specialist. The palliative care nurse specialist provides advice on the dying process and helps to ensure that appropriate assessments and medications are in place in case the situation deteriorates rapidly. They may also provide advice on other nursing interventions; opioid management and titration, if indicated; the prevention and management of delirium; appropriate bowel management; and strategies for ensuring that prn medications are available.
- *Medical practitioner:* GPs work as members of the interdisciplinary team helping to provide the necessary medical reviews, prescribing and intervention.
- *Social worker:* To help John with his financial and social needs. Liaises with social services and establishes contact with solicitors and funeral directors. Helps to liaise with family members and offers counselling and support for problematic or difficult family situations.
- *Mental health liaison team:* This community-based team is available for people experiencing emotional and psychological distress as a result of their condition. This may include the addition of antidepressant/anxiolytic medications and specific therapeutic interventions.
- *Bereavement counsellor:* Offers bereavement support for the grieving process to surviving family, friends and carers.
- *Pastoral care:* Spiritual leaders provide counselling for patients requiring spiritual guidance. Patients at this time are often re-evaluating the meaning and direction of their life.
- *Dietitian:* Can provide patient consultation: assess nutritional needs with the patient and develop a plan for maximising nutritional intake.
- *Physiotherapist:* Can be helpful in providing additional support in teaching patient and nursing staff in assisting John to maximise his cardio-pulmonary function.
- *Occupational therapist:* Can provide advice on minimising John's energy requirements by assessing his physical capabilities and providing appropriate equipment.

With thorough assessment and goal setting, John was able to remain in control with the assistance of interventions that enhanced the quality of his life. Six weeks following his transiting to the residential facility, John died peacefully.

CONCLUSION

Nurses are pivotal to ensuring that people with palliative care needs and their families have access to best-evidence-based palliative care. Every nurse, regardless of the care setting, will be called upon to provide palliative care. This reality makes palliative care a core nursing capability and demands that every nurse has the ability to identify the person's physical, psychological and spiritual needs through impeccable assessment(s) and to tailor their care accordingly, including time appropriate referrals to palliative care. Nurses also need to be able to communicate effectively with the person with palliative care needs and their families, and identify when to be their advocate. Having the knowledge and skills to act as a high functioning member of each interdisciplinary team configured for the person with palliative care needs is an important nursing attribute.

Reflective Questions

1. Using Palliative Care Australia's three levels of palliative care needs (Fig. 12.1), describe the type of palliative care a person with end-stage kidney disease would receive at each level and who is likely to be providing this care?

2. If you were the primary nurse caring for a patient with end-stage kidney disease, what would be the important considerations of care required to ensure their comfort?

3. Identify the role of the generalist nurse as a member of the interdisciplinary team supporting a patient with palliative care needs in the community, in an aged care setting, and in a hospital.

RECOMMENDED READING

Ernecoff NC, Check D, Bannon M et al 2020. Comparing specialty and primary palliative care interventions: analysis of a systematic review. Journal of Palliative Medicine 23(3), 389–396.

Health Quality and Safety Commission New Zealand 2020. Kia kōrero | Let's talk advance care planning campaign. Online. Available: www.hqsc.govt.nz/our-programmes/advance-care-planning/kia-korero-lets-talk-advance-care-planning/.

Palliative Care Australia 2018. Palliative care service development guidelines. PCA, Canberra.

REFERENCES

Agar M, Currow DC, Shelby-James TM et al 2008. Preference for place of care and place of death in palliative care: are these different questions? Palliative Medicine 22(7), 787–795.

Australian Bureau of Statistics (ABS) 2018a. Causes of death, Australia 2017. ABS, Canberra.

Australian Bureau of Statistics (ABS) 2018b. Disability, ageing and carers, Australia: summary of findings. Online. Available: www.abs.gov.au/statistics/health/disability/disability-ageing-and-carers-australia-summary-findings/latest-release.

Australian Bureau of Statistics (ABS) 2016. 2016 Census QuickStats. Online. Available: https://quickstats.censusdata.abs.gov.au/census_services/getproduct/census/2016/quickstat/036.

Australian Human Rights Commission 2015. Face the facts: cultural diversity. Online. Available: www.humanrights.gov.au/our-work/education/face-facts-cultural-diversity.

Australian Institute of Health and Welfare (AIHW) 2020. Indigenous life expectancy and deaths. AIHW, Canberra.

Australian Institute of Health and Welfare (AIHW) 2019. Deaths in Australia. Online. Available: www.aihw.gov.au/reports/life-expectancy-death/deaths-in-australia/contents/leading-causes-of-death.

Battista V, LaRagione G 2019. Paediatric hospice and palliative care. In: B Ferrell, J Paice (eds), Oxford textbook of palliative nursing. Oxford University Press, New York.

CareSearch 2012. Public health palliative care (health promoting palliative care). Online. Available: www.caresearch.com.au/caresearch/tabid/1477/Default.aspx.

Connors AF, Dawson NV, Desbiens NA et al 1995. A controlled trial to improve care for seriously ill hospitalized patients: The Study to Understand Prognoses and Preferences for Outcomes and Risks of Treatments (SUPPORT). Journal of American Medical Association 274(20), 1591–1598.

Corless IB, Meisenhelder JB 2019. Bereavement. In: B Ferrell, J Paice (eds), Oxford textbook of palliative nursing. Oxford University Press, New York.

Currow D, Clark K 2010. Emergencies in palliative and supportive care. Oxford University Press, Oxford.

Deloitte Access Economics 2015. The economic value of informal care in Australia in 2015. Carers Australia.

Denvir MA, Murray SA, Boyd KJ 2015. Future care planning: a first step to palliative care for all patients with advanced heart disease. Heart 101(13), 1002–1007.

Commonwealth Interdepartmental Committee on Multicultural Affairs 2001. The guide: implementing the standards for statistics on cultural and language diversity. Department of Immigration and Multicultural Affairs, Canberra.

EAPC Taskforce for Palliative Care in Children 2009. Palliative care for infants, children and young people: the facts. Online. Available: www.palliative.lv/wp-content/uploads/2013/01/The_Fact.pdf.

Ernecoff NC, Check D, Bannon M et al 2020. Comparing specialty and primary palliative care interventions: analysis of a systematic review. Journal of Palliative Medicine 23(3), 389–396.

Ezekowitz JA, O'Meara E, McDonald MA et al 2017. 2017 Comprehensive update of the Canadian Cardiovascular Society guidelines for the management of heart failure. Canadian Journal of Cardiology 33(11), 1342–1433.

Givler A, Maani-Fogelman PA 2020. The importance of cultural competence in pain and palliative care. StatPearls Publishing, Treasure Island, Florida.

Hjalmarsson E, Lindroth M 2020. 'To live until you die could actually include being intimate and having sex': a focus group study on nurses' experiences of their work with sexuality in palliative care. Journal of Clinical Nursing 29(15–16), 2979–2990.

Institute of Medicine (US) Committee on Care at the End of Life 1997. Review: approaching death: improving care at the end of life. MJ Field, CK Cassel (eds). National Academies Press, Washington, DC. PMID: 25121204.

Kavalieratos D, Corbelli J, Zhang D et al 2016. Association between palliative care and patient and caregiver outcomes: a systematic review and meta-analysis. Journal of American Medical Association 316(20), 2104–2114.

Kellehear A 1999. Health promoting palliative care. Oxford University Press, Melbourne.

Kellehear A, O'Connor D 2008. Health-promoting palliative care: a practice example. Critical Public Health 18(1), 111–115.

Laverty M, McDermott DR, Calma T 2017. Embedding cultural safety in Australia's main healthcare standards. Medical Journal of Australia 207(1),15–16.

Levetown M 2008. Communicating with children and families: from everyday interactions to skill in conveying distressing information. Pediatrics 121, e1441.

Luckett T, Phillips M, Agar M et al 2019. Elements of effective palliative care models: a rapid review. BMC Health Services Research 14(1), 1–22.

McCormack B, McCance T 2017. Person-centred practice in nursing and health care – theory and practice. Wiley Publishing, Oxford.

Neimeyer RA, Harris DL, Winokuer HR et al 2011. Grief and bereavement in contemporary society: bridging research and practice. Routledge/Taylor & Francis, New York, NY.

Nuzzo P, McCorkle R, Ercolano E 2015. Home care. In: B Ferrell, J Paice (eds), Oxford textbook of palliative nursing. Oxford University Press, New York.

Pace JC, Lunsford B 2011. The evolution of palliative care nursing education. Journal of Hospice & Palliative Nursing 13(6), S8–S19.

Palliative Care Australia 2018a. National Palliative Care Standards. PCA, Canberra.

Palliative Care Australia 2018b. Palliative Care Service Development Guidelines. PCA, Canberra.

Palliative Care Australia 2016. National standards assessment program quality report 2010–2015 Online. Available: http://palliativecare.org.au/wp-content/uploads/dlm_uploads/2016/03/2015-National-Report.pdf.

Phillips JL, Ingham J, McLeod R 2015. The development of palliative medicine in Australia and New Zealand, 2nd edn. Hodder Arnold, Sydney.

Phillips JL, Virdun C, Bhattarai P et al 2018. Nursing and palliative care. In: RD MacLeod, L van den Block (eds), Textbook of palliative care. Springer International Publishing, Cham.

Picker Institute Europe 2017. Principles of patient centred care. Online. Available: www.picker.org/about-us/principles-of-patient-centred-care/.

Remedios C, Thomas K, Hudson P 2011. Psychosocial and bereavement support for family caregivers of palliative care patients: a review of the empirical literature. Centre for Palliative Care, St Vincent's Hospital & Collaborative Centre of The University of Melbourne, Melbourne.

Rosas-Blum E, Shirsat P, Leiner M 2007. Communicating genetic information: a difficult challenge for future pediatricians. BMC Medical Education 7, 17–17.

Shahid S, Taylor EV, Cheetham S et al 2018. Key features of palliative care service delivery to Indigenous peoples in Australia, New Zealand, Canada and the United States: a comprehensive review. BMC Palliative Care 17(1), 72.

Smits LL, van Harten AC, Pijnenburg YAL et al 2015. Trajectories of cognitive decline in different types of dementia. Psychological Medicine 45(5), 1051–1059.

Stats NZ: Tatauranga Aotearoa 2020. Ethnic group summaries reveal New Zealand's multicultural make-up. Online. Available: www.stats.govt.nz/news/ethnic-group-summaries-reveal-new-zealands-multicultural-make-up.

Taylor K, Guerin Thompson P 2019. Healthcare and Indigenous Australians: cultural safety in practice, 3rd edn. MacMillan International Higher Education and Red Global Press, London, UK.

The National Centre for Social and Economic Modelling 2017. Economic cost of dementia in Australia 2016–2056. Institute for Governance and Policy Analysis (IGPA), University of Canberra, Canberra.

Trevino KM, Prigerson HG, Maciejewski PK 2018. Advanced cancer caregiving as a risk for major depressive episodes and generalized anxiety disorder. Psycho-Oncology 27(1), 243–249.

Virdun C, Brown N, Phillips J et al 2015. Elements of optimal paediatric palliative care for children and young people: an integrative review using a systematic approach. Collegian 22(4), 421–431.

Virdun C, Luckett T, Lorenz K et al 2020. Hospital patients' perspectives on what is essential to enable optimal palliative care: a qualitative study. Palliative Medicine 34(10), 1402–1415.

Virdun C, Luckett T, Lorenz K et al 2017. Dying in the hospital setting: a metasynthesis identifying the elements of end-of-life care that patients and their families describe as being important. Palliative Medicine 31(7), 587–601.

Virdun C, Luckett T, Davidson PM et al 2015. Dying in the hospital setting: a systematic review of quantitative studies identifying the elements of end-of-life care that patients and their families rank as being most important. Palliative Medicine 29(9), 774–796.

Waller A, Girgis A, Currow D et al 2008. Development of the Palliative Care Needs Assessment Tool (PC-NAT) for use by multi-disciplinary health professionals. Palliative Medicine 22(8), 956–964.

World Health Organization (WHO) 2018a. Integrating palliative care and symptom relief into primary health care: a

WHO guide for planners, implementers and managers. World Health Organization, Geneva. Licence: CC BY-NC-SA 3.0 IGO.

World Health Organization (WHO) 2018b. Integrating palliative care and symptom relief into paediatrics: a WHO guide for health care planners, implementers and managers. World Health Organization, Geneva. Licence: CC BY-NC-SA 3.0 IGO.

World Health Organization (WHO) 2018c. The top 10 causes of death. Online. Available: www.who.int/news-room/fact-sheets/detail/the-top-10-causes-of-death.

World Health Organization (WHO) 2016. Palliative care. Online. Available: www.who.int/ncds/management/palliative-care/introduction/en.

World Health Organization (WHO) 1998. Symptom relief in terminal illness. WHO, Geneva.

CHAPTER 13

Principles for Nursing Practice: Schizophrenia

ANDREA MCCLOUGHEN • NIELS BUUS

LEARNING OBJECTIVES

When you have completed this chapter you will be able to:

- describe the onset and course of schizophrenia
- identify the community beliefs about schizophrenia that lead to stigmatisation and self-stigmatisation
- discuss the concept of recovery in relation to schizophrenia
- identify the essential components of recovery-focused services for people with schizophrenia
- consider the role of the nurse in the recovery process for a person with schizophrenia.

KEY WORDS

psychosocial education	stigmatisation
recovery	therapeutic alliance
schizophrenia	

INTRODUCTION

Schizophrenia is a severe mental illness that can affect every facet of a person's life. In the past, schizophrenia was viewed as an inevitably deteriorating disorder marked by a declining ability to live and participate in the community. However, people who have had an acute episode of schizophrenia often recover from that episode, and for people who do not fully recover, or go on to have further episodes, their life is not necessarily marked by deterioration. This chapter will discuss the causes and course of schizophrenia, and its impact on quality of life. A focus of this chapter is the effect of stigmatisation and self-stigmatisation, as well as a focus on the recovery process and what this means for the delivery of mental health services and the role of the nurse.

DESCRIPTION OF THE DISORDER

Schizophrenia is often referred to as a severe or serious mental illness, which indicates a mental, behavioural

or emotional condition characterised by a severe intensity and duration of symptoms and disablement that can seriously impair social, personal, family and occupational functioning (Department of Health and Ageing 2013). Severe mental illness is associated with conditions like schizophrenia where pronounced psychotic phenomena such as hallucinations and delusions are experienced. The person has difficulty identifying reality, thinking, communicating, managing emotional responses and making judgements to the extent that their social functioning is impaired. Schizophrenia is identified as a leading cause of disability worldwide despite a low lifetime prevalence range of 0.26% to 0.67% of the population (Chong et al 2016). The onset of the illness is usually between 15 and 25 years of age.

Symptoms of Schizophrenia

The symptoms of schizophrenia are referred to as 'positive' or 'negative' symptoms. Positive symptoms are overt and observable experiences, which occur as excesses or distortions in thinking, emotions and behaviour, not typically experienced by people without schizophrenia. Positive symptoms occur at the onset and during the experience of schizophrenia and include symptoms associated with psychosis – hallucinations, delusions, thought disorder and disorganised behaviour. Positive symptoms tend to relapse and remit, although some people experience residual psychotic symptoms over the long term (Owen et al 2016):

- *Hallucinations*: hallucinations are a disturbance in sensory perception experienced when hearing, seeing, smelling, feeling or tasting things in the absence of external stimuli. Auditory hallucinations are the most common form of perceptual disturbance and may include hearing voices commenting on the person's behaviour, or hearing voices telling the person to act in particular ways.
- *Delusions*: delusions are a type of thought disturbance where people hold beliefs that are not in keeping with objective evidence, with strong conviction. The beliefs are not shared by other members of the same culture and are not based in the person's spiritual, educational or social experiences. The person may believe that there is a conspiracy to harm them, with a lack of evidence that this is so, and when other members of the same community do not see such a threat. Delusions are unable to be shifted by reasoning or presenting evidence to the contrary.
- *Thought disorder*: Thought disorder occurs when a person's thinking becomes disorganised and continuity of thoughts and information processing are disrupted. Thought disorder can significantly impair communication and is evident when a person's verbal expression is illogical and confused. The person's speech may not be understandable or speech patterns may seem disconnected to what is happening or being discussed. A person with thought disorder may also experience disruption to thoughts, such that they may feel that thoughts are being removed from their mind; that thoughts are being inserted into their mind; or that their thoughts are being broadcast aloud when they have not been spoken.
- *Disorganised behaviour*: disorganised behaviour can appear to be bizarre and unusual. A person may experience impaired motor behaviour, which can lead to difficulty executing activities of daily living (ADLs), or they may display repetitive behaviours that appear as movements which lack purpose and are repeatedly performed in the same way. Disorganised behaviour can reflect a chaotic mental state

and be illustrated in the form of dishevelled or inappropriate clothing and poor personal grooming.

Negative symptoms may be less obvious than positive symptoms and reflect a deficit or diminution in thinking, emotions and behaviour indicative of an absence or loss in feeling and ability that is typically present in most people. Negative symptoms are marked by lack of energy and motivation (avolition), social withdrawal, failure to initiate and maintain speech (alogia), lack of pleasure (anhedonia), decreased emotions and emotional expression (blunted/flat affect), and responses to the environment that are inappropriate (Barabassy et al 2018). Negative symptoms tend to be more chronic than positive symptoms and are associated with long-term impact on social function (Owen et al 2016).

THE DIAGNOSIS OF SCHIZOPHRENIA

According to the Diagnostic and Statistical Manual of Mental Disorders, Fifth Edition (DSM-V) (American Psychiatric Association 2013) schizophrenia is diagnosed in the presence of at least two of the following symptoms: hallucinations, delusions, disorganised speech, disorganised behaviour, negative symptoms. In addition, the presence of these symptoms is accompanied by disruption to social and occupational functioning and the duration of the symptoms and dysfunction is at least 6 months, although if treated this may be shorter. Other disorders, such as mood disorders, substance abuse and physical illness, need to have been ruled out (American Psychiatric Association 2013; Galletly et al 2016).

WHAT CAUSES SCHIZOPHRENIA?

A specific cause of schizophrenia has not yet been determined. However, the risk of developing schizophrenia is likely to be influenced by a complex interaction of a number of factors (Cunningham & Peters 2014). Factors that have been implicated in individual vulnerability to develop schizophrenia include genetic predisposition, whereby a person inherits risk for psychosis or schizophrenia rather than inheriting the condition. While twin studies have demonstrated high genetic risk for schizophrenia, they also show that illness vulnerability is not solely indicated by genetic factors (Hilker et al 2018). The heritable characteristics may increase the likelihood to experience schizophrenia if the person is exposed to particular stressful life events (Cooke 2014). Neuroanatomical abnormalities are also associated with schizophrenia. It is thought that prenatal exposure to maternal stress and medical illness, intrauterine infections, birth trauma and head injury in childhood may impact on brain development and function, increasing the risk of schizophrenia in later life (Pugliese et al 2019). In addition, social factors and environmental stress, such as change in role or relationships, drug use, abuse and trauma, particularly occurring at times of neurodevelopmental vulnerability, income inequality and urbanicity, are all believed to interact with vulnerability to precipitate a psychotic episode (Davis et al 2016; Fusar-Poli et al 2017; van Nierop et al 2015). A number of protective factors may mitigate the impact of the vulnerability and environmental stress. People who report psychotic experiences but have low levels of social and environmental adversity, and protective factors of intact IQ, spirituality and psychological and emotional wellbeing, have a reduced likelihood of pathological outcomes (Peters et al 2016), and people with good pre-morbid functioning in a number of areas, such as peer and family relationships and employment, social support and effective coping strategies, tend to have better outcomes (Cheng et al 2016).

THE COURSE OF SCHIZOPHRENIA
The Prodromal Phase
Before the onset of acute psychotic symptoms (delusions and hallucinations, disordered speech and thoughts), the person may experience a number of poorly defined signs indicating subtle changes in volition, thinking and perception, which may be evident to the person, but not others (Madaan et al 2014). Subsequently, the person may experience further changes from previous functioning that occur as a decline in school or occupational performance and withdrawal from social relationships. However, these signs may be attributed by others to developmental issues (e.g. adolescent behaviours) or to changes in the environment (stress related to family, social relationships, school or work). In addition to these negative symptoms, the person may also develop transient, sub-threshold forms of psychotic symptoms characterised by beliefs and interests that are seen as strange or out of character, odd ritualistic behaviours or they may begin talking to themselves.

The Active Phase
The active phase describes the onset of psychotic features of hallucinations and delusions, accompanied by disturbances in thinking and behaving. Mood symptoms are regularly experienced and may be evident in a dysphoric mood where the person feels highly anxious, frightened, angry or depressed. Psychosis can involve intense emotional distress and has been described as a shattering experience where trust in the world is lost (Bögle & Boden 2019). Cognitive deficits are also common, and may include diminished memory, reduced attention and slowed processing (APA 2013). They may have difficulty thinking through the most mundane of tasks, but because this experience is so frightening, they may have difficulty admitting that there is a problem. Delusions can be undermining of trust in others, even the closest of family and friends (Cavelti et al 2016).

The Residual Phase
This phase is marked by a diminution of active symptoms. However, the extent to which active psychotic symptoms resolve is variable. The onset of the active psychotic phase may take considerable time to resolve. The person may be left with a number of symptoms that do not seem to be responsive to medication. Similar to the prodromal phase, these residual symptoms commonly comprise of negative symptoms, marked by a lack of energy, failure to be able to initiate interest and engagement with others, and lack of motivation. It may be difficult to differentiate between the residual symptoms of the illness, the effects of medication and the effect of the trauma of the acute psychotic illness. People who have experienced an acute psychotic episode may see their future as unpredictable, have little confidence in the reliability of their own mind and continue to fear that the illness will return.

The recovery style of people who have experienced a psychotic illness varies and several models have been put forward to explain the process. Based on the early work of Thomas McGlashan, it has been argued that people recovering from psychosis will use one of two contrasting styles: an 'integrative' style or a 'sealing-over' style, or a mixture of both (Espinosa et al 2016). The integrative style is characterised by awareness of self before, during and after the psychotic experience, because the person has the ability to accept the psychotic illness as part of their life experience and incorporate it into their identity. Through the psychotic experience, the person becomes aware of the continuity between their thoughts and feelings (Zizolfi et al 2019). This style requires a level of flexibility in thinking, accepting the psychosis as a life experience that need not be viewed negatively. The sealing-over style utilises encapsulation of the psychotic experience, viewing it as a negative intrusion and avoiding thinking about the experience. Detachment and removal are used to exclude and separate psychotic mental events from awareness (Zizolfi et al 2019). Some people use a mix of the two styles and for some people their recovery styles may change over time, moving from sealing-over to integration and vice versa. It is noted that people with a sealing-over style of recovery have a significantly more debilitating psychotic illness, which tends to be associated with poorer social functioning and quality of life and higher levels of depression (Espinosa et al 2016). In addition, the style of recovery appears to be related to insight and understanding of the illness. A study of the relationship between a personal sense of recovery and cognitive insight indicated that low levels of cognitive insight were related to a higher personal sense of recovery and this may reflect the value of the 'sealing-over' of the psychotic experience. More strongly related to a sense of personal recovery was the presence of hope (Giusti et al 2015). Jose and colleagues (2015) systematically reviewed both qualitative and quantitative literature on consumer perspectives of recovery in schizophrenia. This review indicated that consumers considered recovery to be a 'long-term process' with a variable pathway. In addition, recovery was seen as an outcome where the person felt 'better about self, family and social functioning and … able to live with the disability or overcome the effects of symptoms'. These issues have implications for education about illness and sensitivity about the timing and style of education. Sealing-over style of recovery may be self-protective against being overwhelmed by the psychotic experience and by stigmatisation, which is discussed later in this chapter.

The length and severity of each phase of the illness is highly variable, as is the outcome. It has been proposed that for about 75% of people with schizophrenia the course is characterised by remissions alternating with relapses, and less than one in seven people meet the criteria for recovery (Vita & Barlati 2018). However, numerous studies have identified that schizophrenia has heterogeneous outcomes, comprising of severe cases requiring multiple hospital admissions, to those cases where a single episode is followed by complete remission. It should also be noted that people with persistent symptoms can recover in later phases of the illness (Galletti et al 2016). A number of studies have reported around 50% of participants experiencing recovery or long-term significant improvement, suggesting that stable remission may be more achievable than previously considered (Vita & Barlati 2018; Zipursky & Agid 2015).

SCHIZOPHRENIA AND CHRONICITY

Chronicity has been associated with schizophrenia since Kraepelin, in 1896, classified a group of mental disorders as dementia praecox and predicted that the recovery rate for this disorder was between 2.6% and 4.1%. Bleuler, in the early 1900s, further developed the definition of the illnesses, labelled them 'the schizophrenias', identified primary and secondary symptoms and also suggested that people never fully recovered (Glynn 2014). The idea that schizophrenia is a progressive deteriorating illness has pervaded medical and research literature since the time of Kraepelin (Zipursky & Agid 2015).

This view of schizophrenia, as an inevitably chronic illness, has since been questioned in long-term follow-up studies (Davidson 2020), and it has been suggested that the course of the illness is sensitive not only to biological vulnerability but also to social development, culture, social networks and stress and coping (Cavelti et al 2016). Coping with the effects of the illness is compounded by the fact that people with long-term mental health problems face additional difficulties in coping with social systems. People with chronic schizophrenia have lives that are often marked by stress and impoverishment. Problems relate to role transition, living arrangements and financial concerns, as well as loneliness and difficulty in negotiating satisfactory relationships. Even in the face of an unhelpful social context, people with long-term mental illness have been shown not to inevitably decline into a deteriorating condition.

EFFECT OF SCHIZOPHRENIA ON THE ACTIVITIES OF DAILY LIVING

Schizophrenia can have a huge impact on the ADLs and all parts of the person's life are likely to be affected by the experience of having a psychotic illness. The difficulty of living with a mental illness such as schizophrenia is one of dealing with ongoing symptoms, managing the problems of taking medication and receiving other treatments and suffering alienation, isolation and loneliness. Relating to others is difficult, in that although there may be a need for contact with people, there may also be a fear of closeness and the problem of managing the stress that closeness might create.

The extent of difficulties related to ADLs depends not solely on the severity of the illness, nor on the residual symptoms, but also on the extent of developmental delay caused by the onset of the illness. Young people who develop psychotic illness may not have well-developed social and practical skills for daily living prior to the onset of the illness. Poor judgement and disordered thinking patterns make daily decision-making difficult.

Thus, the person with schizophrenia may need support for, and education about, organising hygiene, clothing, shopping, cooking and house-cleaning, managing finances, developing social relationships and managing time. Employment may present a significant challenge for people with severe mental illness and many people with schizophrenia are unemployed, even when they wish to work (Gammelgaard et al 2017). When they do have employment, they may need support related to the management of medication and work, and disclosure of their health status (Bennett et al 2012). Studies of the impact of supported employment programs for people with schizophrenia indicate that participants experience improved quality of life and wellbeing, and a reduction in symptoms, particularly negative ones, and those in long-term employment may experience clinical benefits in terms of protection against relapse and rehospitalisation (Charzyńska et al 2015; Mueser et al 2016). In Gammelgaard and colleagues' (2017) qualitative study of a supported employment intervention, participants experienced increased self-esteem, confidence and hope, life skills, stability and normality in everyday life, and expanded networks.

STIGMA AND SCHIZOPHRENIA

Stereotyping is a way of organising information about groups of people. Stereotypes typically involve negative beliefs about a group and are associated with prejudice (agreement with stereotypical beliefs) and discrimination (behavioural consequences of prejudice) (Thornicroft et al 2016). Stigma refers to negative and stereotypical attitudes and beliefs about people and is present when stereotyping, labelling, separation, loss of status and discrimination co-occur (SANE 2019; Thornicroft 2016). There are a number of negative stereotypes associated with mental illness and particularly with schizophrenia. Beliefs that mental illness is a lifelong, deteriorating disease, that people with mental illness are violent and that people with mental illness cannot live on their own, or hold a job, or be in a relationship, pervade societal thinking. These stereotypes are perpetuated by inaccurate and offensive media reports that link mental illness with violence and crime, fear and the need for exclusion or patronising care (Oliveira et al 2015; SANE 2019). Mental health stigma influences self-perception and interpersonal relationships and leads to discrimination in relation to basic needs associated with housing, employment and health services (Sickel et al 2014). The social messages inherent in the stigma are powerful and strongly linked with poor self-image, a lack of self-esteem and self-stigmatisation.

IMAGE OF SELF

The effect on the sense of self of a person who develops schizophrenia may be one of the most profound aspects of the illness (Davidson 2020; Parnas & Henriksen 2014). The onset of the illness presents an experience that is inexplicable to the person as their fundamental assumption that they can rely on the reality of their thoughts and perceptions is challenged (NCCMH 2014). The experience of hallucinations, perceptions of the world that are no longer reliable, difficulties in thinking and making themselves understood by others, have a significant effect. For some people with schizophrenia, self-esteem and self-perception are eroded over the long term as a result of depressive symptoms accompanying schizophrenia (Davidson 2020). Helplessness and hopelessness are associated with depression and are also the outcomes of self-concepts that are negative, expectations of poor outcome of the illness and a locus of control that is external to the person. Thus the person has low self-esteem and self-efficacy, feels that the outcome of the illness is beyond their control and thinks that they can do nothing to influence the course of the illness.

Stigma has a particularly toxic effect on people with schizophrenia who lack a clear and stable positive sense of self to act as a protective buffer (Davidson 2020; Parnas & Henriksen 2014), and self-stigmatisation, or internalised stigma, is central to negative impacts on self-image (SANE 2019). Self-stigmatisation occurs when a person agrees with the negative prejudices held by others (Oliveira et al 2015) and internalises such stereotypical assumptions. Holubova and colleagues (2016) found a positive association between negative coping strategies and self-stigma in people with schizophrenia. The authors identified that people with schizophrenia who used coping strategies associated with escape tendencies, resignation and self-accusation, tended to stigmatise themselves more than those with low levels of self-stigma. Self-stigmatisation affects the person's sense of self-efficacy, confidence and empowerment, is associated with poorer social and occupational functioning and lower income, increased levels of depression and demoralisation, less willingness to engage with treatment, and is indicative of poorer quality of life and poorer treatment outcomes (Holubova et al 2016; Oliveira et al 2015; Yilmaz & Okanh 2015).

The person with schizophrenia can be seen as in a dilemma. Do they reject the idea of having a mental illness, called lacking insight, or accept that they have a mental illness with the resultant stigmatisation and self-stigmatisation that occurs? Keen and colleagues (2017) suggest that significant emotional adjustment is associated with the meaning individuals attach to being diagnosed with schizophrenia, and that such a diagnosis can leave people experiencing intense internal and external shame. Internal shame is associated with negative self-evaluation and external shame is linked to the expected appraisals of others as shaming and stigmatising, which in turn is associated with depression (Keen et al 2017). This is also a dilemma for mental health service providers. How can service providers encourage acceptance of mental illness when we know that the consequence of such acceptance is likely to be self-stigmatisation? Research identifies that accepting a schizophrenia label is not necessarily helpful for individuals in terms of reducing distress and may have negative consequences for help-seeking and therapeutic alliances (Keen et al 2017). In the process of encouraging insight into the illness, services need to consider ways to promote an individual's mental health literacy in order to increase a person's understanding of their disorder and treatment, enhance their knowledge of resources to manage the illness (Crowe et al 2018), and offset the potential impacts of self-stigma. Crowe and colleagues (2018) found there was an inverse relationship between self-stigma and mental health literacy, indicating the importance of mental health knowledge in reducing stigma. Kao and colleagues (2017) identified that people with schizophrenia have the capacity to counteract the stigma of mental illness through stigma resistance. Stigma resistance is associated with self-esteem, self-reflection and adaptive coping.

QUALITY OF LIFE

People with schizophrenia have a significantly lower quality of life than those without (Dong et al 2019). Many people with schizophrenia have lives marked by impoverishment and loneliness. Housing options may be sub-standard or they may have drifted into a life of homelessness, accessing shelter where they can. Some live in boarding houses of varying comfort and quality; others may live in group homes, hostels or supported independent accommodation. While many families provide support, which affects quality of life, this may not be the chosen option for the person with schizophrenia or their family.

In Dong and colleagues' (2019) meta-analysis comparing quality of life in people with schizophrenia and healthy controls, people with schizophrenia had low quality of life in physical, psychological, social and environmental domains. The authors proposed several potential issues related to schizophrenia that can lead to poor life satisfaction, high psychological stress and low quality of life: adverse impacts of psychotic symptoms and co-morbidities; poor nutrition and reduced physical activity; social isolation and lack of access to environmental resources; limited employment opportunities; and stigma and discrimination. Oliveira and colleagues (2015) identified that people with schizophrenia tended to have an expectation of being stigmatised and rejected, and that this led to a reduction in self-efficacy, eroded empowerment and reduced quality of life. The quality of life of a person living with schizophrenia is multifactorial and that challenges mental health services to consider beyond the biological illness model how to provide services that increase quality of life and satisfaction with life.

RECOVERY

Understandings of recovery have evolved over the past few decades. The traditional view of recovery from illness has been dominated by a biomedical conceptualisation of rehabilitation concerned with the amelioration of symptoms, and the use of medication and perhaps some psychosocial education to achieve this. This has been described as 'clinical recovery' (Cavelti et al 2016, p. 93; Galletly et al 2016, p. 424), and in the case of schizophrenia, necessitates the remission of positive and negative symptoms (Chan et al 2018). However, 'personal recovery' has been identified by people who have experienced mental illness and have used mental health services (Cavelti et al 2016, p. 93; Galletly et al 2016, p. 424). From a subjective perspective, personal recovery relates to the development of ways to manage the threat to the person's sense of self and meaning of their place in the world. It incorporates having a personally meaningful and productive life and identity, reclaiming autonomy, having a positive sense of self and achieving self-determination with or despite the limitations of the illness (Chan et al 2018; Harris & Panozzo 2019). Thus recovery as a concept involves not only the provision of high-quality evidence-based treatment, but also the active involvement of clients and their families in a process that supports people to live satisfying lives, despite the enduring illness. To embrace the concept of recovery in relation to schizophrenia means to challenge services that provide messages of hopelessness and accuse clients of not being motivated, or being too 'chronic' to be able to have goals and aspirations. The mental health consumer movement has been active in the process of bringing to awareness of mental health services the importance of understanding the subjective experience of mental illness.

Patricia Deegan, who has undertaken her own recovery process from mental illness, and whose seminal writings have informed mental health recovery understandings, describes recovery as '… a journey of the heart' (Deegan 1996). Deegan argues that recovery is based on the awareness that people who have been diagnosed with mental illness are firstly human beings who can act, change their situation, speak for themselves and become the experts in their own recovery process. Recovery is an intra- and interpersonal journey concerned with 'hope, social connection, relationships, personal responsibility, empowerment, meaningful life activities, a positive identity, full life beyond illness and personal growth' (Jacob et al 2017; Price-Robertson et al 2017; Slade et al 2014).

In stories of consumers' perspectives of recovery, there is a strong emphasis on hope. The reflection to consumers with schizophrenia that it is an inevitably deteriorating illness, that they will need to take medication for the rest of their lives and that their dreams and aspirations are highly unlikely to be achieved, causes them to believe that all their efforts will be futile (Deegan 1996). Deegan suggests that 'apathy, withdrawal, isolation and lack of motivation' are more than negative symptoms of schizophrenia, but represent a 'hardening of the heart' by the person as a way of surviving. To care about the loss of hopes and dreams is to lay oneself open to possibility, and to despair and hopelessness if those possibilities do not eventuate. The greatest danger is if those people who are there to provide support and care embody that hopelessness and despair, and give up on hope of recovery because the person is seen as unmotivated to change or simply too low functioning (Deegan 1996). People describe the important aspects of recovery from mental illness as being hope, wellbeing, self-identity, self-responsibility and empowerment, meaning in life, social inclusion, education, self-advocacy and peer support (Jose et al 2015; Slade 2013).

People with schizophrenia have also identified the incremental and non-linear nature of the recovery process, which is often learned over time through trial and error. Davidson's (2020) extensive research on recovery and people experiencing severe mental illness has identified that improvements are gradual for many people, possibly interspersed with setbacks, and the markers of improvement are often not dramatic but occur indirectly, in small ways in everyday life. The modest and indirect events of recovery in action may be experienced as making decisions and choices about mundane, everyday activities such as selecting a radio station, or feeling small moments of intense pleasure through listening to music, or having a receptive interaction and being confirmed by another person, or experiencing subtle shifts in self-worth. The seemingly trivial nature of these actions and experiences are in fact the building blocks of recovery, in the form of self- and social-acceptance, reclaiming agency, and being self-aware in the present (Davidson 2020). However, healthcare practitioners and others in the person's network may fail to recognise these actions. People with mental illness also emphasise the importance of a sense of self in relation to the illness that is not related to the illness. A key initial step in recovery appears to be possible when the person is able to separate the illness and its effects from their sense of self; in other words, developing a 'normal' identity, rather than an illness-dominated identity (Davidson 2020; Jacob et al 2017).

Studies of the impact of hopelessness on outcomes for people with schizophrenia indicate that a sense of hopelessness predicts a poor rehabilitation outcome. Hopelessness has been linked to self-concepts that are negative, low expectations of self and the future and a sense of being under the control of external forces. However, individuals who believe in themselves and possess a positive sense of self, are more hopeful and optimistic about life and have good levels of wellbeing (Chan et al 2018). The acceptance of the negative messages of society, including healthcare professionals, clearly affects the rehabilitation possibilities for the individual. Conversely, services that are recovery-oriented are marked by optimism, focus on choice and interpersonal support, assist people to pursue hopes and aspirations, and pay attention to vocational rehabilitation (Chan et al 2018; Slade 2013).

The recovery process is fundamentally relational (Price-Robertson et al 2017) and the therapeutic relationship has been identified as an essential component of treatment of schizophrenia (Galletly et al 2016). In order to develop therapeutic relationships that are recovery-focused, nurses and other clinicians need a clear understanding of those assumptions that underpin the way they view consumers (Harris & Panozzo 2019). Hope-inspiring therapeutic relationships have been shown to predict positive change in social and vocational activity in young people with psychotic illness (Berry & Greenwood 2015). Confronting the assumptions of hopelessness, of the consumer as the passive recipient of treatment with which they must comply, of the consumer as unmotivated, apathetic and inevitably deteriorating into chronicity, requires the clinician to examine the foundations of their beliefs and practice. It requires a level of critical analysis of the services offered and the treatment philosophies that underpin that service.

A fruitful recovery journey from schizophrenia often needs the collaboration of the person, the family, health professionals and the support of other survivors from mental illness. Exacerbation of psychotic symptoms is not uncommon and can interrupt the recovery journey. Programs informed by recovery concepts have been developed and introduced in Australia, the United States and Britain, and the concept of recovery has been adopted as the framework for mental health services. Most recovery-informed programs involve education of both clients and their families. The Illness Management and Recovery Program (Slade et al 2014), piloted in the United States and Australia, teaches illness self-management strategies to people with severe mental illness. It includes five strategies – psychosocial education about mental illness and treatments, cognitive behaviour approaches to medication adherence, a relapse prevention plan, social skills training and coping skills training. The structured program commences with and focuses on self-directed problem definition, problem-solving, pursuit of meaningful goals and an exploration of what recovery means for the individual. Measures of recovery include personal confidence and hope; willingness to ask for help; goal and success orientation; positive reliance on others; and not being dominated by symptoms. Importantly, none of the factors used to measure recovery include the absence of symptoms or an emphasis on independence. Rather, measures reflect a belief that the important issues in recovery are learning to live with and manage the illness.

PRINCIPLES OF CARE

While models of care for people with schizophrenia usually include a pharmacological approach to treat psychotic symptoms, it is increasingly understood that an integrated approach to care that includes medication, and psychosocial and educational interventions tailored to a person's needs, will lead to improvement in the course and outcomes of schizophrenia (Vita & Barlati 2018; Zizolfi et al 2019). Comprehensive models of care that have been evaluated as effective include attention to medication needs, psychosocial education for the person and their family and a range of options in relation to social and vocational skills. The relationship between the key health professional and the person may be one of the most potent factors in success of treatment.

Medication

Medication is often seen as the mainstay of treatment for schizophrenia, and for many people medication has proven to be valuable. The newer antipsychotics have been shown to be effective and to have a lower side-effect profile than the older anti-psychotics. However, for many people antipsychotic medication is associated with adverse effects, including neurological, metabolic, sexual, endocrine, sedative and cardiovascular side effects (Galletly et al 2016). For some people medication may be life-saving and even the reduction of some psychotic symptoms can make a difference to their quality of life. Young people, especially those experiencing a first episode of psychosis, are particularly sensitive to the side effects of antipsychotic medication, and a cautionary approach of 'starting low and going slow' is used when prescribing psychotropic medication for this group (Early Psychosis Guidelines Writing Group 2016). Finding the right medication in the optimal dose is a collaborative effort between the treating team and the person with schizophrenia (for comprehensive information on psychotropic drugs see Australian Medicines Handbook 2020; Galletly et al 2016).

There are two major groups of antipsychotic drugs, both used in the treatment of schizophrenia: first-generation antipsychotics (FGAs) and second-generation antipsychotics (SGAs). The choice of medication is usually related to the likelihood of adverse side effects. Both FGAs and SGAs have demonstrated efficacy for many people with psychotic illness in reducing psychotic symptoms, and are recommended treatment of both acute and longer term psychotic illnesses (Galletly et al 2016). However, response to FGAs is not universal and for some people the response may be partial or not at all. Additionally, medication may have very limited impact on the negative symptoms or cognitive dysfunction discussed earlier in the chapter, which are more strongly associated with decreased functioning than positive symptoms (Charzyńska et al 2015; Owen et al 2016). However, while pharmacotherapy can contribute to a reduction in psychotic symptoms for some people, it does not have a considerable impact on improving social skills or cognitive deficits.

Examples of FGAs include chlorpromazine, fluphenazine, trifluoperazine and haloperidol. Examples of SGAs include amisulpride, aripiprazole, olanzapine, quetiapine and risperidone.

The major problem with the FGAs is debilitating extrapyramidal side effects, such as movement disorders

CASE STUDY 13.1

PART 1 LIVING WITH PSYCHOSIS

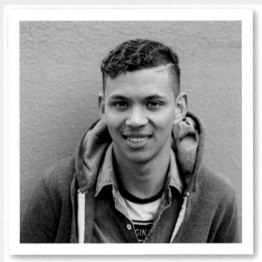

iStockphoto/Tassii.

Keiran is a 16-year-old who dropped out of high school 6 months ago. His plan was to complete his high school education and go to university to study physics; however, he found it increasingly difficult to concentrate over the previous 12 months and became increasingly withdrawn. Attempts by his family to talk to him about what was happening were met with hostility and further withdrawal. His family discussed their concerns at changes in him with their general practitioner, who suggested he attend the local youth mental health service for assessment; however, he refused to go. His father felt the changes may have been related to the stress of the exams, a break-up with his girlfriend and the death of his grandfather. Keiran became increasingly withdrawn, would not attend social occasions, and tended to spend much more time alone in his room. Six weeks ago he was admitted to the local mental health adolescent inpatient unit following a serious attempt to take his own life. He was found to have symptoms of a psychotic illness. He believed he was being followed, that thoughts were being removed from his brain and that his life and the lives of his family members were in danger. He could not identify the source of the danger or the identity of his followers. His attempt on his own life was because he believed that his family would be spared if he was sacrificed. He has been discharged from hospital on medication and referred to the early psychosis mental health team.

CASE STUDY QUESTIONS

1. Identify the vulnerability, stress and protective factors that Keiran might have.
2. As Keiran's community nurse, what do you think are the important principles of care at this time?
3. You attempt to educate Keiran about psychosis, but he is clearly distressed about the information and he does not keep his next appointment. What might be the reason for this and what might you do?

(muscle spasms, motor restlessness and abnormal involuntary movements). Some of these can be managed with medication. The major problem with SGAs is their link with sedation, increased appetite, weight gain and the development of metabolic syndrome marked by diabetes and heart disease. Olanzapine, clozapine and quetiapine are particularly noted for their link with metabolic effects (Australian Medicines Handbook 2020).

The evidence for medication treatment remains strong, with an impetus for early treatment with antipsychotic medication to reduce psychotic symptoms. However, many people show no, or at best only partial response in positive symptoms, with existing antipsychotic medications (Owen et al 2016). Additionally, antipsychotic medications are associated with a range of side effects, so choice of medication is a process based on identifying and titrating medication to achieve the least side effects with the greatest desired outcome for the individual (Owen et al 2016).

The argument has been made by some mental health service users that while medications are a choice for reducing symptoms, they are not the only choice and medication compliance should not be seen as the only way symptoms can be managed. Medication can go a considerable way to improving the recovery journey for some people. However, antipsychotics are associated with a substantial variation in effect and tolerability between individuals (Galletly et al 2016), and a significant proportion of people with schizophrenia will continue to have ongoing psychotic symptoms at some level (National Collaborating Centre for Mental Health [NCCMH] 2014). While many people identify medication as important to their recovery, many others stress that medication does not provide all the necessary ingredients for recovery. There is evidence that while antipsychotic treatment may be beneficial in the short term, some people with schizophrenia cope well in the long term without antipsychotic medication, and there is some suggestion that cognitive and social functioning may be improved without medication (Harrow et al 2012; NCCMH 2014).

In a 15-year follow-up study of people with schizophrenia, Harrow and Jobe (2007) found that there was a subgroup of people who did not immediately relapse when off medication and even showed signs of recovery. This group of people was characterised by good development prior to the illness, positive personality and attitude, a lower level of vulnerability, greater resilience and other favourable prognostic factors. A 20-year prospective study of people with schizophrenia by Harrow and colleagues (2012) identified a subgroup of participants who had ceased antipsychotic medication at their two-year follow-up, and subsequently remained medication-free for the next 18 years. These participants experienced periods of recovery and significantly better post-hospital course and outcome than those on antipsychotics throughout the time period, and this was linked to greater resiliency. These studies indicate that not all people who develop a schizophrenic illness need to use antipsychotic medication on an ongoing basis for the foreseeable future. However, many people with schizophrenia will be on medication and benefit from it and it is important that mental health services are developed in a way that ensures collaboration about medication.

PSYCHOSOCIAL EDUCATION

It is a fundamental right of patients to receive a comprehensive explanation of their illness and to be given the chance of an informed involvement in the drafting of their treatment (Bauml et al 2006).

Programs that emphasise psychosocial education have been shown to positively affect the course of the illness, and the life of the person with the illness. People who participate in psychoeducational programs such as the Illness Management and Recovery Program report high satisfaction with the program, finding it helpful for increasing knowledge and insight about illness, managing symptoms and for progressing towards personal goals (McGuire et al

2014; Tan et al 2016). Participants in Tan and colleagues' (2016) study experienced a reduced number of admissions and length of stay, reduced symptoms and improved social functioning. This program is delivered in modules using a combination of motivation-based, educational and cognitive behavioural strategies over multiple sessions. The following topics are addressed:

- Recovery strategies
- Practical facts about mental illness
- Stress-vulnerability model and treatment strategies
- Building social support
- Using medications effectively
- Drug and alcohol use
- Reducing relapses
- Coping with stress
- Coping with persistent symptoms
- Getting your needs met in the mental health system
- Living a healthy lifestyle (McGuire et al 2014).

The topics of the Illness Management and Recovery Program are consistent with the essential elements of psychosocial education groups outlined by Bauml and colleagues (2006), as therapeutic interaction, clarification and enhancement of coping competence through 'briefing patients about their illness, problem-solving training, communication training and self-assertiveness training' (p. S3). Therapeutic interaction is the approach adopted by the clinician as a 'therapist orientation guide' (p. S6), who explains the process of the illness with empathic understanding of the impact it has on the individuals in the group. The group process encourages sharing of experiences, modelling problem-solving behaviours and conveying respect and esteem for the opinions and struggles of group members. The clarification process reflected in the psychosocial educational model encourages a process of mutual respect for knowledge – both knowledge of self-experience and professional knowledge about the illness. This process allows for mutual understanding to develop between and among therapists and group members. The element of enhancing coping competence recognises the importance of acknowledging loss and grief in the process of coming to terms with the illness and what it may mean. This process emphasises strengths and not limitations, explores how medication can best work for the group members and identifies crisis management plans. It also emphasises the members of the group as the experts in their own illness (Bauml et al 2006).

CASE STUDY 13.1

PART 2

Keiran had a second admission 2 years later. He was diagnosed with schizophrenia with paranoid features. He had become increasingly withdrawn, agitated and distressed. Police had been called to a disturbance in a local shopping centre where Keiran was in severe distress and warning shoppers that the food was contaminated. He became more distressed when one of the store managers and security staff tried to remove him from the shopping centre. On admission he claimed that his bedroom had been bugged, and that he was getting special messages from his computer that there was a threat of contaminated food in his local area. He claimed that there was a conspiracy to kill him because of what he knew. The police recognised that he was either mentally ill or affected by drugs, and took him to the hospital.

After his first episode he had enrolled in computer courses at a local college, had joined a local church group and had started bushwalking and cycling to get fit. He was feeling well and decided to stop taking his medication as he did not like the side effects. Keiran had continued to live with his parents, who were supportive. However, recent stressors included his siblings moving out of home, his parents going on holiday, and he had contracted a flu-like virus that caused him to take time off from college.

Unfortunately, during the time Keiran was relapsing into a psychotic illness he had frightened his neighbours and fellow students by talking about the computers relaying warnings. He had been behaving strangely in church, looking agitated and frightened. Keiran was deeply embarrassed about having a mental illness and had not told his friends at college or his social or church group, as he feared the consequences.

Since his discharge following his second admission, Keiran has been increasingly depressed and isolated. He has not returned to college, avoids contact with his neighbours and friends, and has not resumed social activity.

CASE STUDY QUESTIONS

4. As Keiran's community nurse, what approach would you take?
5. Review the information on stigma, self-stigmatisation and stigma resistance and consider what support Keiran might need to approach the problem of what to tell people about his previous behaviour.
6. Review the information on peer support. What might be the value in Keiran engaging with a peer-support worker?

FAMILY AND CARERS

The families of people with schizophrenia are clearly very important to the way the illness progresses. Many early studies of families explored the negative impact of families (Warner 2004), seeking causal relationships between the family communication, particularly from mothers, and the generation or the course of the illness. Some studies identified high-expressed emotion (the number of negative, critical comments directed at the person with schizophrenia) as having a negative effect on the course of the illness. More recent studies have identified the positive effects of communication between family members, particularly mothers and their adult children with schizophrenia. Essentially the social context of family is central to an individual's experiences of severe mental illness, and family members' emotions, behaviours and attitudes towards mental illness are strong predictors of both relapse and recovery (Price-Robertson et al 2017). Greenberg and colleagues (2006) found that people with schizophrenia reported higher quality of life when their mothers were demonstrably warm and made positive comments about them. The mothers who were warm and

positive (described by the authors as pro-social) displayed three types of behaviour: they encouraged activities that emphasised the abilities of their adult child with schizophrenia, they made acknowledgement of small positive steps and they were less reactive to residual symptoms such as lack of energy and detachment (Greenberg et al 2006).

When the person with schizophrenia is also a parent, consideration needs to be given to the needs of all family members, including the children. When there are children in the household, mental health services need to make specific consideration for their need for age-appropriate education, support and care (Foster et al 2012; Grove et al 2017; O'Brien et al 2011). The issue of stigmatisation of people with mental illness affects the children of parents with schizophrenia as well as their parents. People with schizophrenia who are also parents may need additional support to continue in their role. Family-focused practice is the provision of psychosocial support to the whole family unit, which can reduce subjective and objective burden for family members, improve mental health literacy, and support family relationships and children's wellbeing (Foster et al 2019).

Many people with schizophrenia live with or have regular contact with their families, and their families may be their major source of support and social communication. Family psycho-education about mental illness has a strong evidence base and has been demonstrated to provide positive outcomes, including the reduction of relapse rates, enhanced recovery from symptoms and improved family wellbeing (Harvey & O'Hanlon 2013; Psychiatric Times 2012). A range of models of family psycho-education programs have been developed, with interventions involving 12 or more sessions over 6–12 months with single or groups of families, or brief workshops. However, they all share common elements of a non-blaming attitude, involving family as partners in care, information sharing, coping skills and problem-solving (Harvey & O'Hanlon 2013; Pollio et al 2006). The aims of psycho-education programs are to provide people with schizophrenia and their families with information about mental illness, including symptoms, treatments and services, early intervention and prevention of relapse, coping and management strategies; to give families the opportunity to ask questions; to encourage support from a group of peers; to reduce stigmatisation; and to increase communication between health services and families.

PEER SUPPORT

Peer support programs have been demonstrated as valuable for people with mental illness who are struggling to manage their illness. These programs are based on a belief in the value of peer and mutual help, a levelling of power relationships, community engagement and self-determination, and include key principles of respect, shared responsibility and mutual agreement on what is helpful (Fortuna et al 2019). Peer-support programs are led by people who have experienced mental illness and use their lived experience to support others in their recovery (Slade et al 2014). Peer workers usually focus on providing information, teaching recovery skills, providing support and encouraging self-advocacy. Peer-led programs and peer-support workers have demonstrated benefits on subjective outcomes, including hopefulness, empowerment, control and agency, clinical outcomes encompassing self-care, symptom reduction and lowered admission rates, and social outcomes, including friendships and community connection (Chan et al 2014; Fortuna et al 2019; Slade et al 2014) and adherence to medication (Boardman 2014). A qualitative study of the role of shared experience in a peer-support program included normalising

the experience of illness, providing comfort and personal connection, and inspiring hope (Gidugu et al 2015).

IMPLICATIONS FOR NURSING

Nursing plays an integral role in the healthcare of people recovering from schizophrenia. Nurses need to have a knowledge base that includes understanding about schizophrenia and its course and treatment, knowledge of human responses to psychotic experiences and knowledge of those interventions that will ameliorate distress in the person and their family. Nursing skills need to include the ability to form therapeutic relationships that are based on collaboration (McCloughen et al 2011), and to maintain and engender hope in people with severe mental illness.

Nursing care needs to be informed by recovery principles of attention to the subjective experiences, and choice, optimism, empowerment and interpersonal support (Harris & Panozzo 2019). The most important role that nurses can undertake is the establishment of a collaborative therapeutic alliance with both the person and their family. This relationship can underpin all subsequent treatments. The establishment of such a relationship may take time, but persistent, consistent interactions that seek to understand the person and their situation in a respectful way are powerful in reducing anxiety and instilling hope (Harris & Panozzo 2019).

Assessment is an important part of the therapeutic process and is comprehensive and ongoing. In addition to assessment of mental state, including substance use assessment and risk assessment, nurses need to assess physical health, response to medication and psychosocial status.

People with severe mental illness like schizophrenia have a high rate of physical illness that is not well detected by mental health clinicians (Happell et al 2016). People with schizophrenia have particular vulnerabilities to their health status related to the side effects of medication, and social factors such as difficulty with engaging in physical activity. Nurses are in an ideal position to encourage regular health checks, to promote contact between a general practitioner and the person and to promote a healthy lifestyle (Happell et al 2014; McCloughen et al 2016).

Nurses need to advocate for services that are consumer-centred. There are many barriers within traditional mental health services to the development of consumer-centred services (Carroll et al 2006). For mental health services to be focused on recovery, they also need to be focused on the strengths and resources

CASE STUDY 13.2

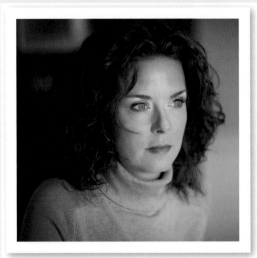

iStockphoto/NADOFOTOS.

Audrey is a 35-year-old woman who has had five admissions to an acute psychiatric unit in the last 10 years. On her first admission she was diagnosed with depression following a suicide attempt. She has been subsequently diagnosed with a schizoaffective disorder and finally with schizophrenia. The exacerbations of her illnesses usually follow increased stress and are marked by an acute onset and delusions with strong religious content. Audrey has managed to complete a university degree in business management and to gain experience as an office manager in a small business. She enjoys her work and her employer is aware of her mental illness and has been supportive.

Audrey has no family history of schizophrenia; however, several family members have been treated for depression. She describes a fairly happy childhood until her adolescence when her father died suddenly and she, her two brothers and her mother had to move into her grandparents' home. She experienced disruption to her schooling and has recently disclosed that she endured ongoing sexual assault by an uncle who visited the house. Threats from her uncle that the family would be thrown out if she told anyone prevented her from disclosing the assaults to anyone. The assaults continued until she left home after her first admission to hospital. Audrey has had no counselling for childhood sexual assault. She complains of flashbacks to the assaults that intrude on her thinking and disrupt her sleep.

Audrey lives on her own in a small unit. She volunteers with a bush-care group who meet monthly, and she belongs to a book club. She has one friend whom she met in hospital, but has not kept contact with other friends as she does not want to tell them about her illness.

She takes medication to treat her depression and psychosis. She is currently on an atypical (second-generation) antipsychotic and an antidepressant, although she admits she does not always take these medications in the way her psychiatrist prescribed them, as she finds the side effects of weight gain and tiredness limiting. She admits to adjusting her medication dosage at weekends as she feels she is brighter and more sociable when she does. She also admits that when she does this in a context of increased stress she is more likely to relapse.

CASE STUDY QUESTIONS

1. As Audrey's community nurse, how would you approach discussion about the management of her medication? What principles would you use to frame the discussion?

2. Audrey asks about what might have caused her illness. What issues are important to discuss? What resources might you refer her to?

3. What stressors may have contributed to her illness?

of people with mental illness rather than deficit and pathology-focused (Xie 2013). The inclusion of peer-support programs within mental health services requires nurses to question their attitudes to and the roles that they assign to people who have had or have a mental illness. Working alongside consumer peers requires a shift in thinking from the health professional as expert to one of mutual respect, exploration and learning. Nurses are in a position to drive change in the way mental health services are delivered.

In both inpatient and community mental health settings, nurses are in an ideal position to provide and advocate for a range of psychotherapeutic interventions, including education about the illness and the treatment, for the person and their family, either in formal groups or in informal discussions; problem-solving approaches to psychosocial problems; development of relapse recognition plans; encouragement to use medication constructively; provision of assertive community treatment; and identification of a range of resources that may be useful in maintaining and sustaining community tenure (Beebe 2007).

Nurses are also in an ideal position to advocate for the provision of a range of vocational and living skills support services that are in turn appropriately supported by mental health services.

CONCLUSION

Schizophrenia is a serious mental illness; however, the stereotypes of deterioration, alienation from society and paternalistic care are not inevitable. Some people recover; some people have periods of good functioning between episodes of being unwell. Recovery-focused services are person-centred, peer supported and strengths-based. Recovery-focused services do not give up hope that a person, even when they have symptoms that do not respond well to medication, can live a satisfying and productive life.

Reflective Questions

Please refer to the multimedia resources listed for this chapter on the Evolve website when responding to these questions.

1. When, and in what way, might each of these resources be useful to you in clinical practice?
2. When would you consider referring a person who has experienced a psychotic illness, or their family, to one of these resources?
3. In what way might it be helpful for a person with schizophrenia to hear about the experiences of other people with mental health conditions?

RECOMMENDED READING

Davidson L 2020. Recovering a sense of self in schizophrenia. Journal of Personality 88, 122–132.

Fossey E, Harvey C, McDermott F 2020. Housing and support narratives of people experiencing mental health issues: making my place, my home. Frontiers in Psychiatry 10, Article 939, 1–14.

Hancock N, Smith-Merry J, Jessup G et al 2018. Understanding the ups and downs of living well: the voices of people experiencing mental health recovery. BMC Psychiatry 18, 121.

Reflection on Recommended Readings

Critically evaluate what factors support recovery from mental illness and what factors impede recovery. Consider internal factors such as nature of illness, education and skills, self-stigmatisation and personality. Also consider external factors such as family structure, social relationships, stigmatisation, employment/education opportunity, housing, poverty and the accessibility of mental health services.

REFERENCES

American Psychiatric Association 2013. Diagnostic and statistical manual of mental disorders: fifth edition (DSM-V). American Psychiatric Association, Arlington, VA.

Australian Medicines Handbook Pty Ltd 2020. Australian medicines handbook 2020.

Barabassy A, Szatmári B, Laszlovszky I et al 2018. Negative symptoms of schizophrenia: constructs, burden, and management. In: F. Durbano (ed.), Psychotic disorders. An update, pp. 43–62. Intechopen http://dx.doi.org/10.5772/intechopen.73300

Bauml J, Frobose T, Kraemer S et al 2006. Psychoeducation: a basic psychotherapeutic intervention for patients with schizophrenia and their families. Schizophrenia Bulletin 32, 1–9.

Beebe LH 2007. Beyond the prescription pad. Psychosocial treatments for individuals with schizophrenia. Journal of Psychosocial Nursing and Mental Health Services 45(3), 35–43.

Bennett C, Sundram S, Farhall J et al 2012. Schizophrenia and related disorders. In: G Meadows, J Farhall, E Fossey et al. (eds), Mental health in Australia: collaborative community practice, 3rd ed. OUP, Melbourne.

Berry C, Greenwood K 2015. Hope-inspiring therapeutic relationships, professional expectations and social inclusion for young people with psychosis. Schizophrenia Research 168, 153–160.

Boardman G, McCann T, Kerr D 2014. A peer support programme for enhancing adherence to oral antipsychotic medication in consumers with schizophrenia. Journal of Advanced Nursing 70(10), 2293–2302.

Bögle S, Boden Z 2019. 'It was like a lightning bolt hitting my world': feeling shattered in a first crisis in psychosis. Qualitative Research in Psychology, 1–28.

Carroll CD, Manderscheid RW, Daniels AS et al 2006. Convergence of service, policy, and science toward consumer-driven mental health care. The Journal of Mental Health Policy and Economics 9(4), 185–192.

Cavelti M, Homan P, Vauth R 2016. The impact of thought disorder on therapeutic alliance and personal recovery in schizophrenia and schizoaffective disorder: an exploratory study. Psychiatry Research 239, 92–98.

Chan RCH, Mak WWS, Chio FHN et al 2018. Flourishing with psychosis: a prospective examination on the interactions between clinical, functional, and personal recovery processes on well-being among individuals with schizophrenia spectrum disorders. Schizophrenia Bulletin 44(4), 778–786.

Chan SWC, Ziqiang L, Klainin-Yobas P et al 2014. Effectiveness of a peer-led self-management programme for people with schizophrenia: protocol for a randomized controlled trial. Journal of Advanced Nursing 70(6), 1425–1435.

Charzyńska K, Kucharska K, Mortimer A 2015. Does employment promote the process of recovery from schizophrenia? A review of the existing evidence. International Journal of Occupational Medicine and Environmental Health 28(3), 407–418.

Cheng SC, Walsh E, Schepp KG 2016. Vulnerability, stress, and support in the disease trajectory from prodrome to diagnosed schizophrenia: diathesis-stress-support model. Archives of Psychiatric Nursing 30, 810–817.

Chong HI, Teoh SL, Bin-Chia Wu et al 2016. Global economic burden of schizophrenia: a systematic review. Neuropsychiatric Disease and Treatment 12, 357–373.

Cooke A (ed.) 2014. Understanding psychosis and schizophrenia. British Psychological Society, Leicester UK.

Crowe A, Mullen PR, Littlewood K 2018. Self-stigma, mental health literacy, and health outcomes in integrated care. Journal of Counseling and Development 96, 267–277.

Cunningham C, Peters K 2014. Aetiology of schizophrenia and implications for nursing practice: a literature review. Issues in Mental Health Nursing 35, 732–738.

Davidson L 2020. Recovering a sense of self in schizophrenia. Journal of Personality 88, 122–132.

Davis J, Eyre H, Kacka FN et al 2016. A review of vulnerability and risks for schizophrenia: beyond the two hit hypothesis. Neuroscience and Biobehavioral Reviews 65, 185–194.

Deegan PE 1996. Recovery as a journey of the heart. Psychiatric Rehabilitation Journal 19(3), 91–97.

Department of Health and Ageing 2013. National mental health report 2013: tracking progress of mental health reform in Australia 1993–2011. Commonwealth of Australia, Canberra.

Dong M, Lu L, Zhang L et al 2019. Quality of life in schizophrenia: a meta-analysis of comparative studies. Psychiatric Quarterly 90, 519–532.

Early Psychosis Guidelines Writing Group & EPPIC National Support Program 2016. Australian clinical guidelines for early psychosis, 2nd edn. Orygen The National Centre of Excellence in Youth Mental Health, Melbourne.

Espinosa R, Valiente C, Rigabert A et al 2016. Recovery style and stigma in psychosis: the healing power of integrating. Cognitive Neuropsychiatry, 1–10.

Fortuna KL, Brooks JM, Umucu E et al 2019. Peer support: a human factor to enhance engagement in digital health behavior change interventions. Journal of Technology in Behavioural Science 4, 152–161.

Foster K, Goodyear M, Grant A et al 2019. Family-focused practice with EASE: a practice framework for strengthening recovery when mental health consumers are parents. International Journal of Mental Health Nursing 28, 351–360.

Foster K, O'Brien L, Korhonen T 2012. Developing resilient children and families when parents have mental illness: a family-focused approach. International Journal of Mental Health Nursing 21(1), 3–11.

Fusar-Poli P, Tantardini M, DeSimone S et al 2017. Deconstructing vulnerability for psychosis: meta-analysis of environmental risk factors for psychosis in subjects at ultra high-risk. European Psychiatry 40, 65–75.

Galletly C, Castle D, Dark F et al 2016. Royal Australian and New Zealand College of Psychiatrists clinical practice guidelines for the management of schizophrenia and related disorders. The Australian and New Zealand Journal of Psychiatry 50(5), 1–117.

Gammelgaard I, Christensen TN, Eplov LF et al 2017. 'I have potential': experiences of recovery in the individual placement and support intervention. International Journal of Social Psychiatry 63(5), 400–406.

Gidugu V, Rogers ES, Harrington S et al 2015. Individual peer support: a qualitative study of mechanisms of its effectiveness. Community Mental Health Journal 51, 445–452.

Giusti L, Ussorio D, Tosone A et al 2015. Is personal recovery in schizophrenia predicted by low cognitive insight? Community Mental Health Journal 51, 31–37.

Glynn SM 2014. Bridging psychiatric rehabilitation and recovery in schizophrenia: a life's work. American Journal of Psychiatric Rehabilitation 17, 214–224.

Greenberg JS, Knudsen KJ, Aschbrenner KA 2006. Prosocial family processes and the quality of life of persons with schizophrenia. Psychiatric Services 57(12), 1771–1777.

Grove C, Riebschleger J, Bosch A et al 2017. Expert views of children's knowledge needs regarding parental mental illness. Children and Youth Services Review 79, 249–255.

Happell B, Gaskin CJ, Stanton R 2016. Addressing the physical health of people with serious mental illness: a potential solution for an enduring problem. International Journal of Social Psychiatry 62(2) 201–202.

Happell B, Stanton R, Platania Phung C et al 2014. The cardiometabolic health nurse: physical health behaviour outcomes from a randomised controlled trial. Issues in Mental Health Nursing 35, 768–775.

Harris B, Panozzo G 2019. Barriers to recovery-focused care within therapeutic relationships in nursing: attitudes and perceptions. International Journal of Mental Health Nursing 28, 1220–1227.

Harrow M, Jobe TH 2007. Factors involved in outcome and recovery in schizophrenia patients not on antipsychotic medications: a 15-year multifollow-up study. The Journal of Nervous and Mental Disease 195(5), 406–414.

Harrow M, Jobe TH, Faull RN 2012. Do all schizophrenia patients need antipsychotic treatment continuously throughout their lifetime? A 20-year longitudinal study. Psychological Medicine 42, 2145–2155.

Harvey C, O'Hanlon B 2013. Family psycho-education for people with schizophrenia and other psychotic disorders and their families. Australian and New Zealand Journal of Psychiatry 47(6), 516–520.

Hilker R, Helenius D, Fagerlund B et al 2018. Heritability of schizophrenia and schizophrenia spectrum based on the nationwide Danish twin register. Biological Psychiatry 83, 492–498.

Holubova M, Prasko J, Hruby R et al 2016. Coping strategies and self-stigma in patients with schizophrenia-spectrum disorders. Patient Preference and Adherence 10, 1151–1158.

Jacob S, Munro I, Taylor BJ et al 2017. Mental health recovery: a review of the peer-reviewed published literature. Collegian 24, 53–61.

Jose D, Ramachandra LK, Ghandi S et al 2015. Consumer perspectives on the concept of recovery in schizophrenia: a systematic review. Asian Journal of Psychiatry 14, 13–18.

Kao Y-C, Lien Y-J, Chang H-A et al 2017. Stigma resistance in stable schizophrenia: the relative contributions of stereotype endorsement, self-reflection, self-esteem, and coping styles. The Canadian Journal of Psychiatry 62(10), 735–744.

Keen N, George D, Scragg P et al 2017. The role of shame in people with a diagnosis of schizophrenia. British Journal of Clinical Psychology 56, 115–129.

Madaan V, Bestha DP, Kolli V 2014. Prodrome: an optimal approach. Early identification and monitoring of at-risk patients has the potential to improve outcomes. Current Psychiatry 13(3), 17–20, 29–30.

McCloughen A, Foster K, Kerley D et al 2016. Physical health and wellbeing: experiences and perspectives of young adult mental health consumers. International Journal of Mental Health Nursing 25, 299–307.

McCloughen A, Gillies D, O'Brien L 2011. Collaboration between mental health consumers and nurses: shared understandings, dissimilar experiences. International Journal of Mental Health Nursing 20, 47–55.

McGuire AB, Kukla M, Green A et al 2014. Illness management and recovery: a review of the literature. Psychiatric Services 65, 171–179.

Mueser K, Drake RE, Bond GR 2016. Recent advance in supported employment for people with serious mental illness. Current Opinion in Psychiatry 29(3), 196–201.

National Collaborating Centre for Mental Health (NCCMH) 2014. Psychosis and schizophrenia in adults. The NICE guideline on treatment and management. Updated edition 2014. Clinical guideline No. 178. National Institute for Health and Care Excellence.

O'Brien L, Anand M, Brady P et al 2011. Children visiting parents in inpatient psychiatric facilities: perspectives of parents, carers and children. International Journal of Mental Health Nursing 20(2), 137–143.

Oliveira SEH, Esteves F, Carvalho H 2015. Clinical profiles of stigma experiences, self-esteem and social relationships among people with schizophrenia, depressive and bi-polar disorders. Psychiatry Research 229, 167–173.

Owen MJ, Sawa A, Moretensen PB 2016. Schizophrenia. Lancet 388, 86–97.

Parnas J, Henriksen MG 2014. Disordered self in the schizophrenia spectrum: a clinical and research perspective. Harvard Review of Psychiatry 22(5), 251–265.

Peters E, Ward T, Jackson M et al 2016. Clinical, sociodemographic and psychological characteristics in individuals with persistent psychotic experiences with and without a 'need for care'. World Psychiatry 15, 41–52.

Pollio DE, North CS, Reid DL et al. 2006. Living with severe mental illness – what families and friends must know: evaluation of a one day psychoeducation workshop. Social Work 51(1), 31–38.

Price-Robertson R, Obradovic A, Morgan B 2017. Relational recovery: beyond individualism in the recovery approach. Advances in Mental Health 15(2), 108–120.

Psychiatric Times 2012. An evidence-based practice of psychoeducation for schizophrenia 29(2), 1–4. Online. Available: www.psychiatrictimes.com/evidence-based-practice-psychoeducation-schizophrenia

Pugliese V, Bruni A, Carbone EA et al 2019. Maternal stress, prenatal medical illnesses and obstetric complications: risk factors for schizophrenia spectrum disorder, bipolar disorder and major depressive disorder. Psychiatry Research 271, 23–30.

SANE Australia 2019. Reducing stigma. Online. Available: www.sane.org/information-stories/facts-and-guides/reducing-stigma#what-is-stigma

Sickel AE, Seacat JD, Nabors NA 2014. Mental health stigma update: a review of consequences. Advances in Mental Health 12(3), 202–215.

Slade M 2013. 100 ways to support recovery: a guide for mental health professionals, 2nd edn. Rethink, London.

Slade M, Amering M, Farkas M et al 2014. Uses and abuses of recovery: implementing recovery-oriented practices in mental health systems. World Psychiatry 13, 12–20.

Tan CHS, Ishak RB, Lim TXG et al 2016. Illness management and recovery program for mental health problems: reducing symptoms and increasing social functioning. Journal of Clinical Nursing 26, 3471–3485.

Thornicroft G, Mehta N, Clement S et al 2016. Evidence for effective interventions to reduce mental-health-related stigma and discrimination. Lancet 387, 1123–1132.

van Nierop M, Viechtbauer W, Gunther N et al 2015. Childhood trauma is associated with a specific admixture of affective, anxiety, and psychosis symptoms cutting across traditional diagnostic boundaries. Psychological Medicine 45(6), 1277–1288.

Vita A, Barlati S 2018. Recovery from schizophrenia: is it possible? Current Opinion in Psychiatry 31, 246–255.

Warner R 2004. Recovery from schizophrenia, 3rd ed. Brunner Routledge, New York.

Xie H 2013. Strengths-based approach for mental health recovery. Iranian Journal of Psychiatry Behavioural Science 7(2), 5–10.

Yilmaz E, Okanh A 2015. The effect of internalized stigma on the adherence to treatment in patients with schizophrenia. Archives of Psychiatric Nursing 29, 297–301.

Zipursky RB, Agid O 2015. Recovery, not progressive deterioration, should be the expectation in schizophrenia. World Psychiatry 14, 94–96.

Zizolfi D, Poloni N, Caselli I et al 2019. Resilience and recovery style: a retrospective study on associations among personal resources, symptoms, neurocognition, quality of life and psychosocial functioning in psychotic patients. Psychology Research and Behaviour Management 12, 385–395.

CHAPTER 14

Principles for Nursing Practice: Depression

ROBERT BATTERBEE

LEARNING OBJECTIVES

When you have completed this chapter, you will be able to:

* identify the epidemiology, clinical features and assessment of depression
* understand potential pharmacological and psychotherapeutic treatment approaches
* identify nursing assessment and management implications of depression
* understand the potential disability impacts of depression
* apply knowledge to a clinical case study.

KEY WORDS

antidepressant	epidemiology of depression
depression	major depression
dysthymic disorder	

INTRODUCTION

In the course of life, there is sadness and pain and sorrow, all of which, in their right time and season are normal – unpleasant, but normal. Depression is an altogether different zone because it involves a complete absence: absence of affect, absence of feeling, absence of interest. The pain you feel in the course of major clinical depression is an attempt on nature's part (nature after all abhors a vacuum) to fill up an empty space. But for all intents and purposes, the deeply depressed are just the walking, waking dead (Wurtzel 1994, p. 19).

Depression is a public health issue of global proportions. It is estimated that some 300 million people worldwide suffer from depression (World Health Organization [WHO] 2018). Depression is associated with significant distress for individual sufferers and their families, and can lead to impairment in educational, social, family and employment functioning and outcomes. As would be expected for a common and serious illness, a significant proportion of health expenditure in

Australia is devoted to the treatment of depression. Approximately 12% of the Australian adult population will seek help for a mental health problem each year, with 58.6% of those people seeking help with depressive disorders (Burgess et al 2009). The direct cost of treating depression each year is estimated to be in excess of $600 million. The true cost of depression for the community, which includes the indirect costs associated with the reduced productivity that accrues from a disabling condition, defies quantification. In Australia, depression has been identified as a National Health Priority Area in an attempt to elevate depression to the same level of community consciousness and coordinated health policy response – in the form of prevention, assessment and treatment – as heart disease, diabetes and cancer (Department of Health and Ageing 2013).

Nurses working in a variety of settings are well placed to be able to play a role in the identification, assessment and management of depression. The fact that depression is disconcertingly prevalent means that nurses working in acute hospital, community, primary and aged care contexts will encounter individuals with clinically significant depression, and they may be the first clinicians to directly explore the likelihood of depression. Early identification and timely, effective treatment is the single-most likely means by which the burden of depression for individuals, their families and carers, and the community can be reduced. Evidence-based treatments for depression are highly effective in reducing the impact of depression on the person and on occupational, social, family and relationship functioning.

Suicide is a significant problem that is related to depression. There is evidence of a worldwide reduction in suicide rates during 2000–16, which is reflected in the rates in most industrialised countries (excepting the United States) (WHO 2019). Despite advances in evidence-based treatments, suicide-related deaths in the Australian context have remained stable over the last century (Bastiampillai et al 2019; Jorm 2019). It remains a reality that each year over 3000 Australians choose to end their lives by suicide, many or most of whom have been depressed or were suffering from another mental disorder at the time of their death, with over three-quarters of suicide deaths occurring among men (Australian Bureau of Statistics [ABS] 2018). This is a statistic that underscores the importance and potential of nurses and clinicians from varying disciplines to understand the epidemiology, clinical features, assessment, treatment and management of the depressive disorders.

THE SCOPE OF THE PROBLEM: THE EPIDEMIOLOGY OF DEPRESSION

Over the past two to three decades there has been significant research interest in identifying and understanding the epidemiology of depression (and mood disorders). This activity has, in large part, been driven by improved methodological approaches (e.g. the use of standardised diagnostic interviews) for undertaking large-scale community surveys to assess incidence and prevalence at a population level. In Australia, the 2007 National Survey of Mental Health and Wellbeing initiative identified prevalence rates of mental disorders. This survey used the same methodology as the WHO *World Mental Health Survey*, allowing comparison across countries (Slade et al 2009). In the 2007 Australian National Survey, a sample of approximately 8841 people living in the community and aged between 16 and 85 years were interviewed using the World Health Survey Initiative diagnostic instrument (the Composite

International Diagnostic Interview), which identified that in the 12-month period prior to interview 6.2% of the adult population had experienced an identifiable and clinically significant depressive disorder (major depressive episode) (Slade et al 2009).

A consistent finding across studies of the epidemiology of depression is a strong female preponderance, with women having a higher rate of prevalence than males. Recent figures show that 11.6% of Australian women reported depression or feelings of depression in 2017–18 compared with 9.1% of men (ABS 2019).

The causes of this apparent gender difference have been the focus of significant research interest. It has been proposed that the gender 'difference' may be an artefactual finding, as women are more likely to seek help, that women are more likely to recall episodes of depression over their lifetime than men, or that women might be more likely to reflect on or amplify their mood states than men, who employ distraction or denial as means of coping with dysphoria. However, these explanations have not been substantiated and a complex interplay of biological vulnerability, social roles and stress events may play a part (Parker 2019). Other studies have also linked this increased risk of depression to hormonal and biochemical effects across the lifespan; during puberty, antenatally and postnatally, and during menopause (Stickel et al 2018). Childhood sexual abuse has been linked to the risk of postnatal depression (Hutchens et al 2017), and extensive research has confirmed the links between childhood trauma and mental illness (Bellis et al 2019).

IDENTIFYING THE DISABILITY IMPACTS OF DEPRESSION

In 2010, the WHO and the World Bank commissioned the Global Burden of Diseases, Injuries and Risk Factors study (Whiteford et al 2013). The study, first conducted in 1996, represented the most comprehensive attempt to quantify and explicate the mortality and disability impacts (burden of disease) of all diseases, injuries and risk factors using robust methodological approaches. Disability was estimated by using the Disability Adjusted Life Year (DALY) measure, which expresses the years of life lost (YLL) due to premature death and years lived with a disabling illness of specified duration and severity (Whiteford et al 2013). Mental illness contributed a significant proportion of DALY-measured disability, with the burden attributable to depressive disorders having the 'highest proportion of total burden across all regions' (Ferrari et al 2013; Whiteford et al 2013).

In the Australian context, mental and substance use disorders are estimated to account for approximately 14.6% of the total burden of disease, measured using DALYs. Depression is the third leading cause of burden in Australia, behind lower back pain and ischaemic heart disease (AIHW 2019).

Disability related to depression is due to the continuing behavioural, biological, psychomotor and psychological depressive symptoms that can affect every facet of life experience. The symptoms of depression are presented on page 238 of this chapter. The continuation of these symptoms over time results in a reduced capacity to enjoy and engage with pleasurable activities in a personal, family and social context. There is some evidence that men may experience more disability impacts associated with depressive and anxiety disorders. It is possible that this difference may be attributable to men being less likely to disclose and/or seek help in respect of mental health disorders, limiting their access to effective treatments and supports (Rice et al 2017).

DEPRESSION, THE WORKPLACE AND DISABILITY

In recent years there has been recognition that depression in the workplace is a significant issue. Work forms an important part of the life of most people. There is good evidence to suggest that work can be beneficial to a person's mental health (Modini et al 2016). Paid work obviously provides an income that allows at least the potential for individuals to live as healthy a life as possible; work, whether paid or otherwise, also provides meaning and purpose in the lives of many people.

A stable and rewarding workplace can impact in a positive way on a person's mental health. The opposite of this also holds true; a workplace that is unrewarding or involves stress and job strain can be detrimental to an individual's mental health. Job strain is particularly associated with jobs that place high physical and psychological workload demands on employees, accompanied by few decision-making responsibilities.

A recent study has reported that those experiencing high job strain are more likely to develop mental illness by the age of 50, regardless of gender or occupation. Furthermore, the study estimates that common mental health problems, such as depression and anxiety, could be reduced by 14%, if job strain were eliminated (Harvey et al 2018).

Employers increasingly understand that workplace depression is a major issue. There are examples of workplace programs designed to identify and refer employees who are depressed and/or strategies aimed at making workplaces mental-health-promoting by changing aspects of job demands and employee dynamics.

DEPRESSION AND MEDICAL ILLNESS

There is a complex relationship between depression and physical illnesses. Having a serious or chronic physical health condition, such as cardiovascular disease or diabetes, is in itself a risk factor for developing a depressive disorder (Read et al 2017). There is also evidence that depression is a risk factor for developing a physical illness and early mortality. Epidemiological studies have identified a higher prevalence of depression in people with a number of physical illnesses, including coronary heart disease, cerebrovascular accident, diabetes, cancer, Parkinson's disease, HIV/AIDS, hepatitis C, epilepsy, arthritis and osteoporosis, compared with the general population (American Psychiatric Association 2010; Bica et al 2017; Clarke & Currie 2009).

The relationship between heart disease and depression is complex. There is evidence that major depression is an independent risk factor for the development of heart disease. A recent meta-analysis of 30 published studies of the relationship between depression and cardiovascular disease concluded that depression is associated with a significant increased risk of coronary heart disease and myocardial infarction (Gan et al 2014). A number of potential psychosocial (increased prevalence of lifestyle and traditional cardiac risk factors; medication adherence) and biological (effects of stress on the autonomic nervous system, endocrine, platelet and inflammatory systems) explanations for the association between depression and the onset of heart disease have been identified (Dhar & Barton 2016). The risk of mortality increased among those who experience depression following a myocardial infarction (Meijer et al 2011).

It is hardly surprising that medical illnesses that are chronic, debilitating or painful can cause stress and predispose an individual to depression. While a low mood in the course of chronic illness and disability may be understandable, symptoms of depression should always indicate the need for correct identification, assessment and management where necessary (National Institute for Health and Care Excellence [NICE] 2016).

CLINICAL FEATURES OF DEPRESSION AND ASSESSMENT APPROACHES

Depressed, sad or dysphoric mood is a common and normal response to life's challenges and uncertainties. There would be few people who could not relate to the experience of having felt sad in response to a loss of some kind; this level of normal range of emotion and emotional reactivity does not in and of itself constitute 'clinical' depression. Distinguishing circumstances, where depressed mood is indicative of a depressive disorder requiring definitive treatment, as against an understandable and transient feeling state, is a key challenge for clinicians working in a variety of clinical settings.

Major (clinical) depression is distinguished from what might be understood to be 'normal' depression on the basis of the presence of certain symptoms and the severity, duration and persistence of these symptoms. There is no single or pathognomonic symptom that is necessary or sufficient for the diagnosis of major depression. Although pervasive feelings of lowered mood or sadness are frequent features of major depression, it is not clear that depressed mood per se is the core pathological change. It has been suggested that mood disturbance may be an epiphenomenon of a syndrome of core deficits in relation to energy, motivation and activation. This possibility is suggested by the fact that some individuals who report depressive symptoms of reduced energy and motivation, poor concentration, inability to feel pleasure, reduced appetite and sleep problems do not report feeling sad or depressed in their mood (Joyce 2004). A concept analysis of depression in women from a nursing perspective found that the principal attribute observed in depression in women was not lower mood, but 'inhibition or delay in motor function' (Armendariz-Garcia et al 2013, p. 274).

There are two widely used international diagnostic classification systems for mental disorders: The Diagnostic and Statistical Manual of Mental Disorders (DSM-V) (5th edn), published by the American Psychiatric Association (2013), and the International Statistical Classification of Diseases and Related Health Problems: Classification of mental and behavioural disorders (ICD 10 rev. 2016), originally published by the WHO (1992). Both systems identify operationalised diagnostic criteria for each of the mental disorders, including depression and other disorders of mood.

For a diagnosis of major depressive disorder to be made, DSM-V requires the presence of at least a 2-week period of depressed mood or loss of interest or pleasure in most activities. The depressed mood or loss of interest and pleasure must be present for much of nearly every day, on the basis of an individual's self-report or the observation of others. In children, the predominant mood state can be one of irritability. In addition, at least four of the following behavioural, biological, psychomotor or psychological symptoms must be present:

- significant increase or decrease in weight when not dieting (e.g. a change of more than 5% of body weight in a 1-month period), or decrease in appetite nearly every day. In children, failure to reach expected weight gains is also relevant
- insomnia or hypersomnia nearly every day
- psychomotor agitation or retardation nearly every day
- fatigue or loss of energy nearly every day
- loss of enjoyment of previously pleasurable activities (anhedonia)
- feelings of worthlessness or excessive or inappropriate feelings of guilt (which may reach delusional intensity) nearly every day (not merely self-reproach or guilt about being ill)
- diminished ability to concentrate, or indecisiveness, nearly every day (based on subjective account or the report of others)
- recurrent thoughts of death (not just fear of dying), recurrent suicidal ideation without a specific plan, or a suicide attempt, or a specific plan for committing suicide (adapted from American Psychiatric Association 2013; Malhi et al 2015).

The average age of onset of a first episode of depression is in the late 20s. Depression can, however, occur at any age. Both childhood and late-life depression are relatively common, and are sometimes under-recognised and treated (Charles & Fazeli 2017).

In children, depression can sometimes present quite differently from adults. Depressed children may display behavioural symptoms such as apathy, withdrawal, irritability, regression, crying or complain of somatic symptoms such as headache or stomach aches (Charles & Fazeli 2017).

Depression in older people has been estimated to occur at a rate of approximately 2–5%, while in residential aged care settings, such as hostels or nursing homes, the rate is estimated to be much higher, at 6–18%. In older people one of the key challenges from an assessment point of view is disentangling and distinguishing symptoms of depression from conditions commonly associated with poor physical health, or the effects of prescribed medication (ABS 2008; Hazell et al 2019).

Depression: Chronicity and Recurrence

The duration of an episode of major depression is variable, lasting from weeks to years in some cases. Left untreated, and assuming that a person has been kept safe, major depression can remit of its own accord in 6 to 9 months (American Psychiatric Association 2010). The likelihood of recurrence after an episode of treated depression is approximately 40% within 1 year and 80% of people will have a recurrence during their lifetime (Malhi et al 2015). Worldwide, depression is the dominant cause of disability, and a significant contributor to the burden of disease (WHO 2017).

Taken together, these findings underscore the potential level of disability that can accrue from recurrent episodes of major depression (major depressive disorder). Depression can contribute to chronicity and disability in other circumstances: where a dysthymic disorder (a low-grade and chronic form of depression) is present; where full remission of symptoms in response to adequate treatment is elusive (treatment resistance); or where symptoms are persistent in nature (chronic depression).

Persistent Depressive Disorder

Persistent depressive disorder (PDD), also often referred to as dysthymia, is a diagnostic category within the DSM-V that refers to a chronic low-grade depression of at least 2 years (American Psychiatric Association 2013). It is possible for individuals with dysthymic disorder to have periods of acute exacerbation (where diagnostic criteria for a major depressive episode is met); this is often known as 'double depression', due to the combination of an acute severe depression being overlaid on a background of chronic depression of mild to moderate severity (Mann et al 2013).

Treatment Resistance

Approximately 30% of people with major depression will not respond to adequate antidepressant therapy within an expected time period, such as showing signs of improvement within the first 4 weeks of treatment. Switching antidepressant agents and/or the addition of an augmentation agent are common means by which treatment resistance is managed. Augmentation agents are those that when added to the antidepressant are thought to have a potentiating effect. Various augmentation strategies have been applied in practice, including lithium, triiodothyronine (T3), buspirone, pindolol, antipsychotic agents (first generation and atypical agents), anticonvulsants, folates, oestrogens and psychostimulants. In several randomly controlled trials, a combination of cognitive behavioural therapy (CBT) and pharmacotherapy has been reported as an effective treatment strategy for treatment-resistant depression (Li et al 2018; McKnight & Geddes 2013; Wiles et al 2014).

Chronic Depression

Approximately 10% of individuals who are treated for a major depressive episode will remain depressed in 12 months, despite appropriate treatment, and another 10–20% will experience only a partial remission in their symptoms. Clinical approaches to the treatment of chronic depression include making changes in antidepressant regimens (dose adjustment or switching agents), considering the use of ECT or adding a psychotherapeutic approach to the package of treatment (American Psychiatric Association 2010; Leuzinger-Bohleber et al 2019).

RECURRENCE AND INTER-EPISODE FUNCTIONING

About half of those who experience a first episode of major depression will go on to experience at least one other episode. The course of recurrent major depressive disorder is highly variable in terms of both episode duration and the interval of time between episodes. Some people have recurrent episodes separated by periods of years, while others experience clusters of episodes. There is evidence that some people have increased frequency of episodes as they age.

While most people who have recurrent depression experience a return to their normal level of functioning between episodes, approximately 25–35% of people have persistent residual symptoms, or social and occupational impairment. Persisting inter-episode symptoms and impairment increase the risk of a subsequent episode of major depression. For this reason biopsychosocial treatments aimed at promoting a full return to baseline levels of function are an important aspect of the treatment of depression (American Psychiatric Association 2010; Rush & Thase 2018).

CASE STUDY 14.1

PART 1

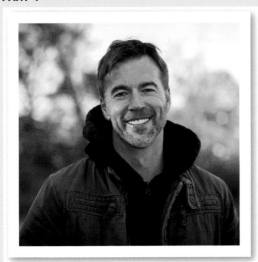

iStockphoto/NADOFOTOS.

Tom is a 35-year-old married man who works as a computer software developer. He specialises in educational programs. Tom lives with his wife, Collette and their children, Carly who is 6 years old, a son Connor, who has just turned 4, and a new baby, Samantha, just 6 months old.

Collette has been concerned about Tom since prior to the birth of the latest baby. The youngest child was very much wanted by both of them; however, since around the time of the birth Collette has noticed that Tom has been distant and preoccupied. Since the birth he has not been sleeping well and seems to have lost his appetite. He has become increasingly withdrawn and irritable at home, spending his evenings and weekends working in his study. He has always taken his work very seriously and worked long hours; however, he has also previously prioritised spending time with Collette and the children, especially on weekends. Lately, Tom has shown less interest in the children, often appearing visibly irritated when the older children ask him to spend time with them. When Collette most recently raised Tom's withdrawn behaviour with him, reminding him that they both had a strong commitment to ensuring a rich family life, with time spent together as a family, he replied, 'I cannot do everything – I have to work to keep us. Don't put any more pressure on me.'

Tom himself has noticed that he hasn't been himself, although his coping style has always been one of 'soldiering on', and he hasn't felt comfortable discussing his own concerns with Collette. Collette suggests that he talk to their general practitioner about what has been happening; however, Tom does not have a strong relationship with the GP and feels reticent about discussing personal issues and feelings.

Tom has been experiencing trouble concentrating and completing tasks at work, requiring him to work longer hours to get through his work. His work performance was raised with him at a recent performance review. His supervisor was sympathetic and assumed that his sliding performance was related to the new baby, and tiredness from broken sleep. His supervisor had noted that Tom was sometimes irritable with his colleagues and had been heard to be quite snappy and unhelpful to a client on the phone. The supervisor suggested that he would have expected that things would have settled by now and that Tom would again be contributing at work. The supervisor suggested that Tom consider seeking medical assessment and set another date for follow-up of this discussion.

Tom feels upset by the performance review. He is aware of his work difficulties and he finds himself thinking about the supervisor's comments frequently, feels guilty about not contributing at home and guilty about his work performance. He feels he has failed himself by not meeting his own expectations.

In fact, the baby is an excellent sleeper and has been for months. A wakeful baby is not the problem. For the past 5 months Tom has had trouble sleeping. He falls asleep easily enough, but wakes at approximately 2 am each morning and is then unable to return to sleep.

Tom has lost weight; approximately 9 kgs in the 6 months. He has had to buy new clothes for work. Tom can't explain his weight loss. He has stopped participating in the between-firm sporting activities, running at lunchtime, and had expected to gain weight.

Tom has noticed that he now takes the lift at work because he becomes breathless if he takes the stairs. He also has regular headaches that are not always relieved by simple analgesia.

Tom feels that his relationship with Collette is under strain. He's aware of tension associated with him having lost interest in sex in recent months.

One morning on his way to work Tom notices a Beyond Blue advertisement on the side of a government bus. Tom recalls that Beyond Blue, Australia's national depression initiative, was mentioned at a continuing professional development seminar on workplace stress that he attended some months ago. When Tom arrives at his office he uses the internet to search the Beyond Blue website; he reads that some of the things that he has been experiencing in recent months could be symptoms of depression.

CASE STUDY QUESTIONS

1. What are some of the symptoms that Tom has been experiencing that suggest he may have a depressive disorder?

2. What other aspects of Tom's presentation and recent history should a nurse be concerned about?

MAPPING THE TERRAIN: SOME ISSUES IN SUBTYPING AND CLASSIFYING DEPRESSIVE DISORDERS

Depression is a term used to describe states of mood that are part and parcel of human experience, being felt by nearly everyone at times of, say, grief, loss or life stress. Depression is also understood to refer to a serious and, in some cases, life-threatening illness that requires clinical assessment and treatment. At face value it is tempting to assume a link between feeling states that are commonplace but generally transient and what is understood to be 'clinical' depression – an essentially single phenomenon that is distinguished by severity and persistence.

The extent to which depression represents a single dimensional phenomenon, as against a range of discrete disorders with differing symptoms and, by extension, treatment characteristics, has been the focus of close to a century of debate. The identification of meaningful subtypes of depression – either clinically or in research – is a profitable exercise if subtypes are associated with differential response to treatment. In a clinical setting, for example, being able to identify the circumstances under which a psychological versus a biological treatment approach would be most appropriate, or being able to decide with some confidence which of a range of treatments would be most suitable, would have significant utility.

DSM-V describes a number of subtypes of depression: Major Depressive Disorder (MDD); Persistent Depressive Disorder (PDD); Disruptive Mood Dysregulation Disorder (DMDD); Pre Menstrual Dysphoric Disorder (PMDD); substance/medication induced depressive disorder; and depressive disorder due to another medical condition (American Psychiatric Association 2013). All subtypes are marked by changes in mood, which can be depressed, irritable, angry or can fluctuate. However, the extent of the presence of other symptoms varies across subtypes (American Psychiatric Association 2013; Malhi et al 2015).

THE COMPLEX AND MULTI-STRANDED CAUSES OF DEPRESSION

Depression is a complex disorder, or set of disorders, for which the underlying causes are not fully understood. Current thinking in relation to the pathophysiology of many mental disorders, including depression, involves the likely interaction of biological, psychological psychosocial and environmental factors (Jesulola et al 2018).

Biological Factors

The possibility of biological factors playing a role in the aetiology of depression has been proposed since antiquity. Hippocrates postulated that 'melancholy' was caused by an excess of 'black bile' (Thomas & Grey 2016). Interest in attempting to identify biological foundations of depression gained momentum from the 1950s, when it was observed that iproniazid (an anti-tuberculin) led to a noticeable improvement in the mood of those undergoing treatment for tuberculosis. More or less contemporaneous observations were also made that reserpine (initially used as an anti-hypertensive agent) and chlorpromazine (initially developed as an anti-histamine) reduced symptoms of psychosis. Taken together, these findings encouraged research into identifying biological aspects of mood and psychotic disorders, and drove what has become the modern era of psychopharmacology. Since the 1960s, research directed at identifying biological substrates of and treatments for mental disorders has continued apace (O'Brien & Fanker 2006).

Genetics: The Role of Heredity in Depression

Depression tends to run in families, raising the possibility of there being a genetic contribution to the aetiology of depressive disorders. This tendency has been demonstrated in a number of well-designed family studies. The odds ratio of an immediate relative of a person with a history of major depression also being affected has been calculated to be 2.84 (95% CI; 2.31–3.49); in other words, an almost threefold increase in risk (Sullivan et al 2000). Two of the three adoption studies published to date provide support for a genetic role, where there is increased risk of being affected by depression even when offspring of those with major depression have been raised in adoptive families. Twin studies have shown that the rate at which monozygotic twins are concordant (both affected) for depression is approximately 50%, whereas for dizygotic twins concordance is between 10% and 25% (Sullivan 2004). Genetic factors have been linked to the development of post-partum depression, along with psychosocial factors (El-Ibiary et al 2013).

Research has shown that the interaction between predisposed genetic and environmental factors influences depression. Individuals with a genetic predisposition, who then encounter stressful life events, are considerably more likely to become depressed than those with only one of these factors present (Lohoff 2010; Wong et al 2011).

Neurotransmission

Serotonin – a neurotransmitter that plays a role in the regulation of a number of biological functions, including sleep, appetite and libido – has been the focus of significant research interest in relation to its potential role in the pathophysiology of depressive disorders. Data from a number of studies have found an association between low serotonin levels and depression, and artificial drug-induced depletion of serotonin (e.g. by reserpine) has been observed to precipitate depression. A number of antidepressant agents (e.g. the selective serotonin reuptake inhibitors [SSRIs]) increase levels of serotonin in the central nervous system (CNS), implying that reduced levels of CNS serotonin play a role in the pathogenesis of depression.

There are interrelationships between the serotonergic and noradrenergic neurotransmitter systems, and noradrenaline has also been a focus of interest for its potential role in depression. Noradrenaline has a role in regulating autonomic nervous system responses and in the regulation of arousal, and a number of processes involved in depression, including mood and sleep. Studies investigating noradrenergic function have yielded equivocal findings, but remain a focus of interest due to some antidepressant agents having upregulation effects on noradrenaline (O'Brien & Fanker 2006; Schweitzer & Tuckwell 2004).

Psychological and Psychosocial Factors

Psychosocial stress and life events

Three psychosocial threads have been examined in relation to their potential role in precipitating depression: persistent stress (e.g. enduring environmental and life stressors); life events (dramatic and sudden stressors, such as grief and loss); and the availability of social support (the protective nature of having supportive social networks). There appears to be a relationship between life events and the development (or relapse) of depression (Paykel 2004).

CASE STUDY 14.1

PART 2

Tom doesn't want to consult the family GP, Dr Martin. He doesn't feel comfortable discussing his situation with Dr Martin, who has treated Collette and the children for many years. Tom approaches Ben, the in-house nurse employed by the company where he works. Tom has always had a friendly relationship with Ben because Ben plays in the between-firm soccer tournament.

Tom meets with Ben and describes his concerns and the contents of material from the Beyond Blue website that he has printed out. Tom has highlighted some of the contents of this material, made handwritten notes on the paperwork and made a list of questions for Ben.

Ben asks Tom if he has ever experienced an episode with similar experiences in the past. Tom tells Ben that he took a semester off university due to 'not coping' with the demands of the course. However, with gentle probing about anything else that might have been happening at that time, Tom becomes tearful and says that his father died that year. He then notes that he did not think it was such an issue as his father had left the family when Tom was very young and he had little to do with him during his childhood. Ben learns that this episode was associated with weight loss, poor concentration, loss of energy, ruminations of guilt and failure and insomnia. Tom tells Ben that he went travelling, but didn't seek any formal treatment at the time. Tom did not discuss his symptoms with anyone at the time, not even his best friend from childhood. Tom tells Ben that his view at the time was that 'I just had to pull myself together'.

Tom states that his mother, Lucy, has had treatment for 'bad nerves' on and off throughout her adulthood. Tom is unsure of the exact nature of Lucy's diagnosis, but he believes that she has 'seen counsellors' and 'taken pills'. He tells Ben that he believes that his mother's problems had impacted on her ability to be as good a mother as she could have.

Ben asks Tom if this episode feels the same or different to the one he experienced while at university. Tom states that he believes that his current symptoms are 'ten times worse' than the previous episode. He states that 'nothing or no one' gives him any pleasure anymore. He describes his mood as 'dead' and he states that his mood has been 'stuck' at this point for all of the past 7 months. Tom describes feeling that his whole body is slowed down. He tells Ben that he knows it might sound silly, but his limbs feel heavier than they once did, making everything he does an effort.

CASE STUDY QUESTIONS

3. What factors may have contributed to Tom's development of a depressive disorder?
4. Is Tom experiencing any symptoms suggestive of a depressive subtype? If so, which subtype?
5. What other questions should Ben ask Tom in relation to his recent experiences and symptoms as part of his initial assessment?

Personality factors

Personality style has also been considered as a factor that may increase an individual's vulnerability for the development of depression. It is possible that people with certain personality types may use internalising defence mechanisms (e.g. self-blame), and that these patterns of coping may increase vulnerability to psychological disturbances such as depression (O'Brien & Fanker 2006). Conversely, resilience — the ability to cope with stress and to recover from adversity — may provide protection against the severity of depression (Malhi et al 2015).

APPROACHES TO THE TREATMENT AND MANAGEMENT OF DEPRESSION

The overall approach to the assessment and management of depression aims to relieve symptoms, reduce negative sequelae (morbidity) and limit disability (Malhi et al 2015).

The following principles have been identified:

1. Comprehensive (diagnostic) assessment
2. Assess and ensure safety
3. Provide education to the person who is affected, and their family and carers
4. Establish a therapeutic relationship
5. Provide support and care
6. Provide advice and recommendations for treatment (e.g. evidence-based biological and/or psychotherapeutic interventions)
7. Ongoing assessment of treatment response
8. Promote treatment adherence (e.g. through active assessment and management of treatment-emergent adverse effects)
9. Evaluate and respond to associated impairments
10. Preventing relapse.

Choice of treatment is usually driven by factors such as severity, depressive subtype, previous history of successful treatment and patient preference (Joyce 2004; Malhi et al 2015).

Mild to moderate depression may be treated with psychological therapy, along with moderation to environmental factors that perpetuate depressed mood. Consideration should be given to psychoeducation, physical health, sleep hygiene, exercise, and review of lifestyle, including stressors, alcohol and other drug consumption and diet.

Psychotherapeutic Approaches

A variety of psychotherapeutic (talking therapy) approaches to the treatment and management of depression have been proposed and used. Psychotherapy

was the dominant approach until the 1950s, when effective antidepressant drugs first came into widespread use. Two approaches – CBT and interpersonal therapy – have been widely used and have empirical support for their effectiveness in depression (American Psychiatric Association 2010; Hacker et al 2016; Malhi et al 2015; McKenzie et al 2004). Two other forms of cognitive therapy – mindfulness-based cognitive therapy, and acceptance and commitment therapy – have been introduced and it is suggested that they both are effective in moderating depressive symptoms and may be helpful in averting recurrence of depressive episodes (Hacker et al 2016; Malhi et al 2015; Maxwell & Duff 2016). In mild depression, supportive counselling, problem-solving and education may be sufficient and effective in the first instance (Health and Social Care Information Centre 2015; Royal Australian and New Zealand Clinical Practice Guidelines for the Treatment of Depression 2004).

Cognitive behavioural therapy

Extensive literature indicates that CBT is extremely effective in the treatment of depression (Cuijpers et al 2013; Zhang et al 2019). CBT is often used as an umbrella term to describe a range of cognitive and behavioural therapies, strategies and techniques that are used to help the person identify and challenge and restructure unhelpful thinking. In relation to depression, this often includes the collaborative formulation of thoughts, emotions, behaviour and physical symptoms using a conceptual model. This is illustrated in a model adapted from Greenberger & Padesky (2015), shown in Figure 14.1.

The model helps the person to make sense of the relationship between their negative thoughts and other components affecting their wellbeing. An example of this is shown in Figure 14.2, where a person believes that they are different from others.

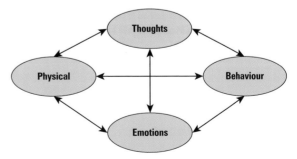

FIG. 14.1 **A Basic Cognitive Behavioural Conceptual Model.** Adapted from: Greenberger & Padesky 2015.

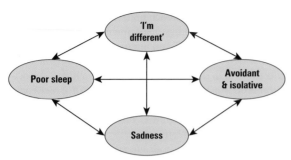

FIG. 14.2 A Cognitive Behavioural Conceptualisation of Depression. Adapted from: Greenberger & Padesky 2015.

Techniques and therapeutic interventions are then used to help restructure or calibrate unhelpful cognitions and thus positively impact wellbeing, as demonstrated in Figure 14.3.

Interpersonal therapy

Interpersonal therapy (IPT) is a psychotherapy technique that focuses on losses, life transitions, social and other interpersonal skill-related aspects of the person. Therapy is directed towards addressing these issues through promoting mourning, understanding the link between experience and feeling states and the development of skills that promote supportive and functional interpersonal relationships. While there is some evidence from controlled studies supporting the superiority of IPT over placebo for the treatment of depression, further studies are required to fully establish efficacy (McKenzie et al 2004). Again, IPT may not be effective in severe depression (Parker & Fletcher 2007).

'Biological' Approaches
Medication

The pharmacological treatment of depression has been a fertile area of research and practice since the late

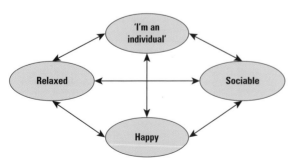

FIG. 14.3 An Example of a Positive Cognitive Behavioural Conceptualisation. Adapted from: Greenberger & Padesky 2015.

1950s with the introduction of imipramine (a tri-cyclic antidepressant). Its clinical usage is now widespread. The efficacy of imipramine impelled what David Healy has termed the 'anti-depressant era', a period of significant activity in relation to identifying, trialling and introducing into clinical practice an array of antidepressant agents (Healy 1997).

An antidepressant agent is usually indicated in circumstances where a major depressive episode has been established. Antidepressants would almost always be indicated in circumstances where melancholic or psychotic subtypes of depression are present (Bauer et al 2002). Selection of an antidepressant agent would usually be determined on the basis of the following factors:

- the likelihood that the agent will work (efficacy)
- the likelihood that a person will be able to tolerate any adverse effects
- aspects of the person's symptoms (e.g. choosing a sedating antidepressant if insomnia is an issue)
- avoiding certain agents if they are likely to affect medical issues (agents that may affect blood pressure).

Mann (2005) has provided a useful summary of the clinical use of antidepressant agents in the treatment of depressive disorders. Table 14.1 provides a summary of commonly used antidepressants, therapeutic dose ranges, relative safety in overdose and adverse effect profile.

Electroconvulsive therapy

First used clinically in 1938, electroconvulsive therapy (ECT) retains a role as a particularly useful treatment for severe depression (Moxham et al 2017). The availability of a range of effective antidepressant agents has tended to relegate the use of ECT to situations where rapid resolution of symptoms is required (e.g. the presence of a very severe low mood, high suicide risk, dehydration and/or nutritional compromise). ECT is also used in circumstances where treatment resistance, failure to respond to adequate trials of antidepressant agents or an inability to tolerate pharmacological approaches is an issue. ECT involves the induction of a generalised tonic-clonic seizure in an anaesthetised patient via electrical stimulation. The basis for the therapeutic efficacy of ECT is poorly understood, but is believed to relate to the action of the seizure rather than the electrical stimulus (American Psychiatric Association 2010; UK ECT Review Group 2003).

St John's Wort

The herb St John's Wort (*Hypericum perforatum*) has been the focus of interest in the past decade in both the popular media and the scientific literature on the basis

TABLE 14.1
Commonly Used Antidepressants: Doses, Safety and Adverse Effect Profile

Agent and Class/ Mechanism of Action	Starting Dose	Standard Dose[a]	Lethality in Overdose	Adverse Effects		Anti-Cholinergic Effects[b]	Nausea or GI Effects	Sexual Dysfunction	Weight Gain	
	Mg/Day	Insomnia or Agitation		Sedation	Hypo-Tension					
Selective Serotonin Reuptake Inhibitors Ssris										
Fluoxetine	20	20–40	Low	Moderate	None or mild	None or mild	None or mild	Moderate	Moderate	Mild or infrequent
Paroxetine	20	20–40	Low	Moderate	None or mild	None or mild	Mild	Moderate	Moderate	Mild or infrequent
Sertraline	50	50–150	Low	Moderate	None or mild	None or mild	None or mild	Moderate	Moderate	Mild or infrequent
Fluvoxamine	50	100–250	Low	Moderate	Mild	None or mild	None or mild	Moderate	Moderate	Mild or infrequent
Citalopram	20	20–40	Low	Moderate	None or mild	None or mild	None or mild	Moderate	Moderate	Mild or infrequent
Escitalopram	20	20–40	Low	Variable	Moderate	None or mild	None or mild	Moderate	Moderate	Mild or infrequent
Tricyclic Agents										
Amitriptyline	25–50	100–300	High	None or mild	Moderate	Moderate	Severe	None or mild	Mild	Moderate
Dothiepin	25–50	100–300	High	None of mild	Moderate	Moderate	Moderate	None or mild	Mild	Moderate
Imipramine	25–50	100–300	High	Moderate	Mild	Moderate	Moderate	None or mild	Mild	Moderate
Nortriptyline	25–50	75–200	High	Mild	Mild	Mild	Mild	None or mild	Mild	Mild
Clomipramine	25–50	100–250	High	Mild	Moderate	Moderate	Moderate	Mild	Mild	Moderate

Continued

TABLE 14.1
Commonly Used Antidepressants: Doses, Safety and Adverse Effect Profile – cont'd

Agent and Class/Mechanism of Action	Starting Dose Mg/Day	Standard Dose[a]	Insomnia or Agitation	Lethality in Overdose	Adverse Effects Sedation	Hypo-Tension	Anti-Cholinergic Effects[b]	Nausea or GI Effects	Sexual Dysfunction	Weight Gain
Desipramine	25–50	100–300		High	Mild	None or mild	Moderate	Mild	None or mild	Mild
Mono-Amine Oxidase Inhibitors										
Phenelzine non-reversible	15	30–90		High	Moderate	Mild	Moderate	Mild	Mild	Moderate
Moclobemide reversible	150	150–300		Low	Mild	None or mild	None or mild	Mild	Mild	None or mild
Other Agents										
Mianserin	30	60–120		Low	None or mild	Moderate	Mild	Mild	Never or mild	Mild
Mirtazapine	30	30–60		Low	None or mild	Severe	Mild	None or mild	Mild	Severe
Ventafaxine	37–75	75–225		Moderate	Moderate	None or mild	None or mild	None or mild	Moderate	Moderate
Duloxetine	30	30–60		Low	Variable	Moderate	Low	None or mild	Frequent	None or mild
Reboxetine	8	8–12		Low	Frequent	Low	Low	None or mild	Mild	Low
Desvenlafaxine	50	50–200		Low	Low	Low	Low	Low	Low	Low

a These doses reflect usual practice, and may vary depending on clinical circumstances.
b Anti-cholinergic side effects include dry mouth, constipation, sweating, blurred vision and urinary retention.

of its purported antidepressant properties. There is some evidence that St John's Wort is superior to placebo in trials of its efficacy in the treatment of depression (Seifritz et al 2016), although its comparative efficacy against conventional antidepressants has not been fully established. Until data emerges from well-designed randomised controlled studies of the efficacy of St John's Wort, its use as a stand-alone treatment for depression cannot be recommended. Having said this, there is evidence from community-based studies that St John's Wort is commonly used as a means of gaining relief from depression, and patients should be asked if they are taking any herbal or non-prescribed preparations in the assessment process (Jorm et al 2004; Kessler et al 2001). There is evidence that St John's Wort possesses enzyme-inducing properties, which means that it can interfere with the metabolism of a number of prescribed drugs and cause significant drug interactions (American Psychiatric Association 2010).

Omega-3 fatty acids

The brain is a lipid-rich organ, and lipids are involved in the structure and function of all cell membranes in the brain, raising the possibility that omega-3 fatty acid supplementation could have a therapeutic effect and role. There is significant current interest in the potential role of omega-3 fatty acids in the treatment of a range of disorders, including cardiovascular and mental disorders. To date, studies of the use of omega-3 fatty acids in the treatment of depression have involved omega-3 fatty acids being given as an adjunctive therapy; for example, combined with a conventional antidepressant. The evidence of efficacy is currently difficult to interpret due to the small nature of the studies and methodological differences between studies, but the potential role of omega-3 fatty acids in the treatment of depression is interesting and warrants further consideration (American Psychiatric Association 2010; Malhi et al 2015).

Vitamin D

Vitamin D insufficiency and deficiency has been questioned as one of the factors that may lead to depression. Vitamin D is provided from diet, from supplements and from exposure to sunlight, and deficiency of the vitamin can result from insufficient exposure to sunlight, or decreased ability of the skin to synthesise the vitamin. A review of vitamin D and depression research by Parker and colleagues (2017) suggests that there is some evidence that vitamin D deficiency is linked to depression. However, the authors caution against assuming causality. Vitamin D supplements

may be helpful, particularly for patients with depression whose daily activity is limited to indoors.

COMBINATION OF TREATMENTS: PHARMACOTHERAPY AND PSYCHOTHERAPY

Antidepressants of different types (tricyclic antidepressants, SSRIs and others) and evidence-based psychological therapies (particularly CBT and IPT) have been demonstrated to be reasonably effective for a range of depressive illnesses (Cuijpers et al 2015). However, a meta-analysis of combined treatments suggested that treatment of depression that included both pharmacological treatment and psychological therapy was more effective than either treatment alone or a placebo, or a placebo combined with a psychological therapy (Cuijpers et al 2015; Karyotaki et al 2016). Psychological therapy alone was demonstrated to be as effective as a combined psychological therapy and medication in the long term (Karyotaki et al 2016).

PRINCIPLES OF NURSING CARE
Providing a Supportive Therapeutic Relationship

Given the high prevalence of depression across all age groups and all social backgrounds, and the very high prevalence in people who have medical illnesses, it is inevitable that nurses in all areas of medical services will encounter people who have depressive symptoms and/or illnesses. For some nurses working in community mental health services, encounters with people with depression will occur because of self-referral, or secondary referral from GPs or other nursing services. Other nurses working in inpatient mental health services will care for people already diagnosed with a depressive illness of such severity that the person requires 24-hour nursing care. For nurses working in other specialties, whether inpatient or community-based, the people they encounter with depression may have a comorbid illness; be children or adolescents, older people, or relatives who are also carers of people with chronic illness. Whatever the setting for nursing care, there are a number of factors that need to be considered. These include the establishment of trust and rapport through a supportive therapeutic relationship; the fostering of optimism and hope; education about depression and its treatments; ongoing assessment of depressive symptoms and suicidality; the use of specific cognitive interventions; and communication with colleagues.

Elizabeth Wurtzel's (1994) description of depression being akin to a state of 'walking, waking dead' gives a sense of how distressing and unpleasant the experience of being depressed can be. The establishment of a therapeutic relationship in which rapport and trust are established is a cornerstone of effective nursing care. The quality of the therapeutic relationship is associated with outcome and an important nursing role when caring for people with depression (Zugai et al 2015). It is important that the nurse provides time and space to talk, listening without judgement. Empathic responses to expressions of distress and gentle exploration of thoughts and feelings acknowledge the validity of the person's distress and can allow the person to elaborate (Berman et al 2018).

Assessment of Depression

Nurses play an important role in the initial and ongoing assessment of depression. A nurse may be the first clinician to identify depression as a problem because a nurse cares for people in a range of settings with a range of disabilities and illness, across the lifespan.

Nurses are often well positioned to provide assessment on a 24-hour basis in the case of hospital settings, or over a significant ongoing time period in the case of community-based settings. If patients are expressing thoughts of hopelessness, loss of interest, loss of energy, feeling agitated and upset, are not enjoying food or company, further exploration is useful. While distress in patients is not unusual, it should not be accepted that this distress is not related to depression without further assessment. Assessment should include consideration of changes (increases or decreases) in domains such as nutrition and hydration, interactiveness, mood, energy, sleep, motivation, concentration, ability to experience pleasure, suicide risk and patterns of depressive thinking.

Part of the assessment role is the knowledge about what to do if you identify that depression may be part of the health picture you are seeing. Knowledge about appropriate referral pathways is important.

Providing Education

One of the key roles that nurses can play in the treatment and management of depression is the provision of education to the person who is depressed and their family and carers. Education can explore issues around the nature of depression (e.g. that it is a common and treatable disorder), and strategies for coping with the experience of depression and treatment. Education about medication is important and should include managing initial side effects, and giving medication an adequate trial.

Depressed Thinking

Strategies for dealing with the negative thinking patterns that some depressed people have can involve helping the person to identify and evaluate alternative viewpoints about particular thoughts, feelings or actions. For example, it can be helpful to challenge a statement such as, 'I am not getting any better; I will never be rid of this depression' with responses such as, 'You have been able to sit with me today and talk about how you are feeling for longer than previous days; this is a sign of improvement'. It is helpful to respond in ways that acknowledge an individual's experience, while at the same time encouraging a more positive outlook; for example: 'I understand that you are still feeling depressed and that it is taking some time for you to feel improvement, but you have been able to spend more time out of your room today, you have eaten and have interacted with me. These are signs of improvement' (O'Brien & Fanker 2006).

Promoting Sleep

Sleep disturbance is a frequent feature of mood disorder, including depression, and includes problems getting to sleep at night (initial insomnia), overnight wakefulness and inability to resume sleep (middle insomnia), or early morning wakening. Disrupted sleep can make navigating the daily tasks of living significantly more difficult and compound feelings of tiredness and fatigue, both of which can then have the effect of making the subjective experience of being depressed more unendurable. Some antidepressant agents, especially the SSRIs and selective serotonin noradrenaline reuptake inhibitors (SSNRIs) can also either induce or increase insomnia, especially during the first few weeks of treatment (Wichniak et al 2017).

Strategies to promote adequate sleep are important foci of nursing care of the depressed person. Nursing advice and intervention can assist with promoting adequate sleep (Berman et al 2018; O'Brien & Fanker 2006). For example, the nurse can:

- assist the person to establish a regular sleep routine, such as listening to relaxing music or having a warm bath prior to going to bed, and going to bed at the same time every night
- provide advice about the potential value of avoiding alcohol, caffeine and nicotine, especially in the late afternoon or evening, due to their stimulant effects
- encourage the introduction of regular exercise in the late afternoon

- assist the person to establish a comfortable environment that is conducive to sleeping; for example, controlling the intrusion of noise and light
- provide advice about avoiding daytime napping, wherever possible, to increase the likelihood of feeling sleepy at night
- assist with teaching relaxation techniques, such as progressive muscle relaxation
- suggest that the person get up at night and undertake an activity in another room (e.g. reading) rather than lying in bed tossing, turning and ruminating about their inability to sleep
- encourage the avoidance of stimulating activities while in bed, such as reading or watching television
- suggest the potential value of using soothing and relaxing stimuli, such as burning essential oils, massage or listening to meditative music.

Promoting Activity and Exercise

There has been significant research interest in recent years in relation to the potential antidepressant effect of exercise. A number of studies have demonstrated that exercise has been associated with decreased severity of depressive symptoms among people 'prescribed' exercise versus no-exercise control groups. It is possible that there are biological and psychosocial factors at play, as exercise can promote the release of neurotransmitters such as serotonin; there are also potentially positive psychosocial reinforcers that can be derived from exercise (e.g. social interaction, sense of achievement and mastery, promotion of sleep). Exercise can potentially distract people from negative thinking and reduce the feelings of tiredness and fatigue that can accompany depression. The effect sizes, or the size of the relationship between the variables of exercise and reduced depression scores in reported studies, to date have been relatively modest, with exercise perhaps best regarded as an adjunctive component of treatment rather than a treatment in and of itself (Stanton et al 2015). Research reviews into exercise in the treatment of depression indicate positive effect across age groups and severity of depression (McDowell et al 2018; Rhyner & Watts 2016; Schuch et al 2018). The introduction of any exercise program needs to consider issues around a person's baseline level of fitness and exercise tolerance, and any concurrent medical problems that might have an influence on the appropriateness of introducing exercise.

Diet

Appetite may be severely affected by acute depressive episodes, and both food and fluid intake need careful monitoring during this phase. Recent research has focused on the role of diet in the onset and recurrence of depression and indications are that healthy diet patterns are associated with a reduced risk of depression and that poorer diet patterns are linked to mental health problems generally and depression specifically, particularly in childhood and adolescence. This evidence would indicate that the role of diet is important not only to physical health maintenance but to mental health maintenance (Malhi et al 2015).

Withdrawn Behaviour

Withdrawn behaviour is common among people who are experiencing depression. Retreating into a withdrawn state is to some extent understandable given that depression often causes reduced energy, reduced motivation and fatigue. Depression also affects a person's willingness (or capacity) to interact with others, and the subjectively distressing and alienating experience of being depressed can promote a desire for aloneness. Crowe and O'Malley have described withdrawn behaviour as potentially reflecting a depressed person's '… desire for refuge, confinement, protection and escape' (2004, p. 272).

Nurses can use a range of strategies to assist patients who experience withdrawn behaviour during the course of an episode of depression. Identifying and understanding a person's subjective experience of the need to withdraw is an important starting point in determining helpful interventions, including the following.

- Acknowledge the person's need for aloneness, but reformulate activity and social interaction as important antidepressant strategies in and of themselves.
- Identify time to interact with a person on a one-to-one basis to encourage communication.
- Encourage the person to feel comfortable to be around other people, even if they feel initially unable to interact for any length of time.
- Use positive reinforcement or encouragement in response to a person's efforts to interact.
- Encourage a graded approach to activity and interaction with others; for example, starting with as little as 15 minutes of social contact and building up gradually as mood improves.
- Encourage the use of passive stimulants (e.g. a radio), especially while a person might be experiencing the nadir of their depressed mood (Crowe & O'Malley 2004; Schultz & Videbeck 2013).

Suicidality

Assessing and responding to potential risk of suicide is a key component of the management of depression.

Nurses who work with people who are suspected or known to be depressed should canvass the issues of suicide candidly during initial and ongoing assessments. Received notions that asking directly about suicide risk can 'put the idea in people's minds' and/or increase the likelihood of suicidal behaviour are myths; many people who are suicidal are relieved to be able to divulge their thoughts or plans in a supportive environment. Nursing strategies for managing suicidal risk and behaviour include:

- Assess risk openly and on an ongoing basis, by asking questions related to thoughts, intentions or plans directed towards self-harm or suicide.
- Consider information from families, carers or friends, who might have knowledge about risk not divulged by the person who is depressed or at risk.
- Give consideration to whether assessment by a specialist mental health clinician is warranted, in order to assess whether definitive treatment or a change in care environment (one-on-one nursing, admission to a mental health unit, detention under mental health legislation) is necessary.
- Frame suicidal behaviour as a symptom of overwhelming stress and/or an illness, and encourage the view that suicidal thinking can pass with support, safe care and the initiation of treatment.
- Employ strategies, such as encouraging the person to focus on 'reasons for living', and encourage use of self-soothing and distracting techniques (Antai-Otong 2016; Chu et al 2015).

Self-soothing and Pleasant Events

Nurses can assist people to adopt self-soothing strategies that are designed to bring comfort or respite from depression, including relaxation, distracting strategies, identifying and facilitating pleasant events and the use of aromatherapy or other complementary interventions.

CONCLUSION

Depression is a common, disabling and potentially life-threatening illness. Over the past three decades there have been steady improvements in the body of knowledge in relation to the effective treatment of depressive disorders. Nurses working in a variety of clinical settings have potential roles in the assessment, identification and management of depression. Early identification and management is the single best means by which the disabling effects of depression can be prevented, at both individual and community levels.

CASE STUDY 14.1

PART 3

Ben asks Tom a direct question in relation to whether he has had any thoughts of suicide. Tom avoids eye contact with Ben and appears to become visibly anxious and agitated. After a significant pause Tom states that he sometimes thinks that Collette and his children would be 'better off without him'. He goes on to state that he has investigated if his life insurance policy would pay a benefit to Collette in the event that he 'took the coward's way out'. When Ben explores this further with Tom, Tom admits to having had thoughts of suicide involving jumping from a height or driving his vehicle into a stationary object at speed.

CASE STUDY QUESTIONS

6. What immediate steps should Ben take in relation to the disclosures that Tom has made to him?
7. What types of treatments, interventions or supports are likely to be appropriate for Tom, given the symptoms that he has reported? Consider the range of psychotherapeutic and pharmacological interventions, as well as interventions involving family.

Reflective Questions

1. In what settings should nurses consider asking their patients about depression and suicidality?
2. Depression is a significant public health issue. What are some of the potential public health responses that could be used to increase the recognition and treatment of depression?
3. What are some of the ways that workplaces can respond to the issue of workplace depression?

RECOMMENDED READING

Antai-Otong D 2016. What every ED nurse should know about suicide risk assessment. Journal of Emergency Nursing 42, 31–36.

Hawley LL, Padesky CA, Hollon SD et al 2017. Cognitive-behavioral therapy for depression using mind over mood: CBT skill use and differential symptom alleviation. Behavior Therapy 48(1), 29–44.

Polacsek M, Boardman GH, McCann TV 2019. Help-seeking experiences of older adults with a diagnosis of moderate depression. International Journal of Mental Health Nursing 28(1), 278–287.

REFERENCES

American Psychiatric Association 2013. Diagnostic and statistical manual of mental disorders (DSM-V), 5th edn. APA, Arlington VA.

American Psychiatric Association 2010. Practice guideline for the treatment of patients with major depressive disorder, 3rd edn. APA, Arlington VA.

Antai-Otong D 2016. What every ED nurse should know about suicide risk assessment. Journal of Emergency Nursing 42, 31–36.

Armendariz-Garcia NA, Alonso-Castillo MM, Lopez-Garcia KS et al 2013. Depression in women: concept analysis from the nursing perspective. Investigacion y Educacion en Enfermeria 312, 270–276.

Australian Bureau of Statistics (ABS) 2019. Mental and behavioural conditions. Online. Available: www.abs.gov.au/ausstats/abs@.nsf/Lookup/by%20Subject/4364.0.55.001~2017-18~Main%20Features~Mental%20and%20behavioural%20conditions~70

Australian Bureau of Statistics (ABS) 2018. Causes of death, Australia. Online. Available: www.abs.gov.au/ausstats/abs@.nsf/Lookup/by%20Subject/3303.0~2017~Main%20Features~Intentional%20self-harm,%20key%20characteristics~3

Australian Bureau of Statistics (ABS) 2008. National Survey of Mental Health and Wellbeing. ABS, Catalogue No 4326.0. Canberra.

Australian Institute of Health and Welfare (AIHW) 2019. Australian Burden of Disease Study: impact and causes of illness and death in Australia 2015. AIHW, Canberra. Online. Available: www.aihw.gov.au/reports/burden-of-disease/burden-disease-study-illness-death-2015/contents/table-of-contents

Bastiampillai T, Allison S, Looi JC et al 2019. Why are Australia's suicide rates returning to the hundred-year average, despite suicide prevention initiatives? Reframing the problem from the perspective of Durkheim. Australian and New Zealand Journal of Psychiatry 54(1), 2–14.

Bauer M, Whybrow P, Angst J et al 2002. WFSBP Taskforce on Treatment Guidelines for Unipolar Depressive Disorders. World Federation of Societies of Biological Psychiatry. Guidelines for biological treatment of unipolar depressive disorders Part 1: acute and continuation treatment of major depressive disorder. World Journal of Biological Psychiatry 31, 35–43.

Bellis MA, Hughes K, Ford K et al 2019. Life course health consequences and associated annual costs of adverse childhood experiences across Europe and North America: a systematic review and meta-analysis, The Lancet Public Health 4(10), e517–528.

Berman A, Snyder SJ, Levett-Jones T et al 2018. Kozier and Erb's fundamentals of nursing [4th Australian edition], Pearson Australia, Melbourne.

Bica T, Castelló R, Toussaint LL et al 2017. Depression as a risk factor of organic diseases: an international integrative review. Journal of Nursing Scholarship 49(4), 389–399.

Burgess PM, Pirkis JE, Slade TN et al 2009. Service use for mental health problems: findings from the 2007 National Survey of Mental Health and Wellbeing. Australian and New Zealand Journal of Psychiatry 43, 615–623.

Charles J, Fazeli M 2017. Depression in children. Australian Family Physician 46(12), 901.

Chu C, Klein KM, Buchman-Schmitt JM 2015. Routinized assessment of suicide risk in clinical practice: an empirically informed update. Journal of Clinical Psychology 7112, 1186–1200.

Clarke D, Currie K 2009. Depression, anxiety and their relationship with chronic diseases: a review of the epidemiology, risk and treatment evidence. Medical Journal of Australia 1906, s54–s60.

Crowe M, O'Malley J 2004. Mental health nursing care for individuals experiencing mood disorders. In: P Joyce, P Mitchell (eds), Mood disorders: recognition and treatment. University of NSW Press, Sydney.

Cuijpers P, Berking M, Andersson G et al 2013. A meta-analysis of cognitive-behavioural therapy for adult depression, alone and in comparison with other treatments. The Canadian Journal of Psychiatry 58(7), 376–385.

Cuijpers P, De Wit L, Weitz E et al 2015. The combination of psychotherapy and pharmacotherapy in the treatment of adult depression: a comprehensive meta-analysis. Journal of Evidence-Based Psychotherapies 152, 147–168.

Department of Health and Ageing 2013. National mental health report: tracking progress of national mental health reform in Australia 1993–2011. Commonwealth of Australia, Canberra.

Dhar AK, Barton DA 2016. Depression and the link with cardiovascular disease. Frontiers in Psychiatry, 7, 33.

El-Ibiary SY, Hamilton SP, Abel R 2013. A pilot study evaluating genetic and environmental factors for post-partum depression. Innovations in Clinical Neuroscience 109–10, 15–22.

Ferrari AJ, Charlson FJ, Norman RE et al 2013. Burden of depressive disorders by country, sex, age, and year: findings from the Global Burden of Disease Study, 2010. PLoS Medicine 1011, e1001547.

Gan Y, Gong Y, Tong X et al 2014. Depression and the risk of coronary heart disease: a meta-analysis of prospective cohort studies. BMC Psychiatry 14(1), 371.

Greenberger D, Padesky CA 2015. Mind over mood: a cognitive therapy treatment manual for clients: Guilford Press.

Hacker T, Stone P, MacBeth A 2016. Acceptance and commitment therapy – do we know enough? Cumulative and sequential meta-analyses of randomized controlled trials. Journal of Affective Disorders 190, 551–565.

Harvey SB, Sellahewa DA, Wang MJ et al 2018. The role of job strain in understanding midlife common mental disorder: a national birth cohort study. The Lancet Psychiatry 5(6), 498–506.

Hazell CM, Smith HE, Jones CJ 2019. The blurred line between physical ageing and mental health in older adults: implications for the measurement of depression. Clinical

Medicine Insights: Psychiatry 10. https://doi.org/10.1177/1179557319885634

Health and Social Care Information Centre (HSCIC) 2015. Improving access to psychological therapies report. Online. Available: www.hscic.gov.uk/catalogue

Healy D 1997. The antidepressant era. Harvard University Press, Cambridge MA.

Hutchens BF, Kearney J, Kennedy HP 2017. Survivors of child maltreatment and postpartum depression: an integrative review. Journal of Midwifery & Women's Health 62(6), 706–722.

Jesulola E, Micalos P, Baguley IJ 2018. Understanding the pathophysiology of depression: from monoamines to the neurogenesis hypothesis model – are we there yet? Behavioural Brain Research 341, 79–90.

Jorm, AF 2019. Lack of impact of past efforts to prevent suicide in Australia: please explain. Australian and New Zealand Journal of Psychiatry 53, 379–380.

Jorm AF, Griffiths KM, Christensen H et al 2004. Actions taken to cope with depression at different levels of severity: a community survey. Psychological Medicine 34, 293–299.

Joyce P 2004. The assessment and classification of depression. In: P Joyce, P Mitchell (eds), Mood disorders: recognition and treatment. University of NSW Press, Sydney.

Karyotaki E, Smit Y, Henningsen KH et al 2016. Combining pharmacotherapy and psychotherapy or monotherapy for major depression? A meta-analysis on the long-term effects. Journal of Affective Disorders 194, 144–152.

Kessler R, Soukup J, Davis R et al 2001. The use of complementary and alternative therapies to treat anxiety and depression in the United States. American Journal of Psychiatry 158, 289–294.

Leuzinger-Bohleber M, Hautzinger M, Fiedler G et al 2019. Outcome of psychoanalytic and cognitive-behavioural long-term therapy with chronically depressed patients: a controlled trial with preferential and randomized allocation: Résultat d'une thérapie psychanalytique et cognitivo-comportementale à long terme chez des patients souffrant de dépression chronique : un essai contrôlé avec allocation préférentielle et randomisée. Canadian Journal of Psychiatry 64(1), 47–58.

Li JM, Zhang Y, Su WJ et al 2018. Cognitive behavioral therapy for treatment-resistant depression: a systematic review and meta-analysis. Psychiatry Research 268, 243–250.

Lohoff FW 2010. Overview of the genetics of major depressive disorder. Current Psychiatry Reports 12(6), 539–546.

Malhi GS, Bassett D, Boyce P et al 2015. Royal Australian and New Zealand College of Psychiatrists clinical practice guidelines for mood disorders. Australian and New Zealand Journal of Psychiatry 4912, 1087–1206.

Mann J 2005. The medical management of depression. New England Journal of Medicine 353, 1819–1834.

Mann JJ, McGrath PJ, Roose SP (eds) 2013. Clinical handbook for the management of mood disorders. Cambridge University Press, New York.

Maxwell L, Duff E 2016. Mindfulness: an effective prescription for depression and anxiety. The Journal for Nurse Practitioners 126, 403–409.

McDowell CP, Dishman RK, Hallgren M et al 2018. Associations of physical activity and depression: results from the Irish Longitudinal Study on Ageing. Experimental Gerontology 112, 68–75.

McKenzie J, Carter J, Luty S 2004. Psychological therapies for depression. In: P Joyce, P Mitchell (eds), Mood disorders: recognition and treatment. University of NSW Press, Sydney.

McKnight R, Geddes J 2013. Cognitive–behavioral therapy improved response and remission at 6 and 12 months in treatment-resistant depression. Annals of Internal Medicine 158(8), JC7–JC7.

Meijer A, Conradi HJ, Bos EH et al 2011. Prognostic association of depression following myocardial infarction with mortality and cardiovascular events: a meta-analysis of 25 years of research. General Hospital Psychiatry 33(3), 203.

Modini M, Joyce S, Mykletun A et al 2016. The mental health benefits of employment: Results of a systematic meta-review. Australasian Psychiatry, 24(4), 331–336.

Moxham, L, Robson P, Pegg S 2017. Mental healthcare in the Australian context. In: P Lemone, T Dwyer, T Levett-Jones et al (eds), Medical–surgical nursing: critical thinking for person-centred care. Pearson Australia, Frenchs Forest NSW.

National Institute for Health and Care Excellence (NICE) 2016. Multimorbidity: clinical assessment and management. NG56 (NICE, London). Online. Available: www.nice.org.uk/guidance/ng56/resources/multimorbidity-clinical-assessment-and-management-pdf-1837516654789

O'Brien L, Fanker S 2006. Mental health breakdown. In: E Chang, J Daly, D Elliott (eds), Pathophysiology applied to nursing. Elsevier, Sydney.

Parker G 2019. The role of environmental and psychosocial factors in depression. In: J Quevedo, AF Carvalho, CA Zarate (eds), Neurobiology of depression. Academic Press, Elsevier, London.

Parker GB, Brotchie H, Graham RK 2017. Vitamin D and depression. Journal of Affective Disorders 208, 56–61.

Parker G, Fletcher K 2007. Treating depression with the evidence-based psychotherapies: a critique of the evidence. Acta Psychiatrica Scandinavica 1155, 352–359.

Paykel E 2004. Psychosocial stress and depression. In: P Joyce, P Mitchell (eds), Mood disorders: recognition and treatment. University of NSW Press, Sydney.

Read JR, Sharpe L, Modini M et al 2017. Multimorbidity and depression: a systematic review and meta-analysis. Journal of Affective Disorders 221, 36–46.

Rhyner KT, Watts A 2016. Exercise and depressive symptoms in older adults: a systematic meta-analytic review. Journal of Aging and Physical Activity 24, 234–246.

Rice SM, Aucote HM, Parker AG et al 2017. Men's perceived barriers to help seeking for depression: longitudinal findings relative to symptom onset and duration. Journal of Health Psychology 22(5), 529–536.

Royal Australian and New Zealand College of Psychiatrists Clinical Practice Guidelines Team for Depression 2004. Australian and New Zealand clinical practice guidelines for the treatment of depression. Australian and New Zealand Journal of Psychiatry 38, 389–407.

Rush AJ, Thase ME 2018. Improving depression outcome by patient-centered medical management. American Journal of Psychiatry 175(12), 1187–1198.

Schuch FB, Vancampfort D, Firth J et al 2018. Physical activity and incident depression: a meta-analysis of prospective cohort studies. American Journal of Psychiatry 175(7), 631–648.

Schultz JM, Videbeck SL 2013. Lippincott's manual of psychiatric nursing care plans (9th ed.). Wolters Kluwer/Lippincott Williams & Wilkins Health, Philadelphia.

Schweitzer I, Tuckwell V 2004. The neurobiology of depression. In: P Joyce, P Mitchell (eds), Mood disorders: recognition and treatment. University of NSW Press, Sydney.

Seifritz E, Hatzinger M, Holsboer-Trachsler E 2016. Efficacy of Hypericum extract WS 5570 compared with paroxetine in patients with a moderate major depressive episode – a subgroup analysis. International Journal of Psychiatry in Clinical Practice 20(3), 126–132.

Slade T, Johnston A, Browne MA et al 2009. 2007 National Survey of Mental Health and Wellbeing: methods and key findings. Australian and New Zealand Journal of Psychiatry 43, 594–605.

Stanton R, Franck C, Reaburn P et al 2015. A pilot study of the views of general practitioners regarding exercise for the treatment of depression. Perspectives in Psychiatric Care 51(4), 253–259.

Stickel S, Wagels L, Wudarczyk O et al 2018. Neural correlates of depression in women across the reproductive lifespan – an fMRI review. Journal of Affective Disorders 1(246), 556–570.

Sullivan P 2004. The genetic epidemiology of major depression. In: P Joyce, P Mitchell (eds), Mood disorders: recognition and treatment. University of NSW Press, Sydney.

Sullivan P, Neale M, Kendler R 2000. Genetic epidemiology of major depression: review and meta-analysis. American Journal of Psychiatry 157, 1552–1562.

Thomas J, Grey I 2016. From black bile to the bipolar spectrum: a historical review of the bipolar affective disorder concept. Archives of Depression and Anxiety 2(1), 10–15.

UK ECT Review Group 2003. Efficacy and safety of electroconvulsive therapy in depressive disorders: a systematic review and meta-analysis. Lancet 361, 799–808.

Whiteford HA, Degenhardt L, Rehm J et al 2013. Global burden of disease attributable to mental and substance use disorders: findings from the Global Burden of Disease Study 2010. The Lancet 382, 1575–1586.

Wichniak A, Wierzbicka A, Walęcka M et al 2017. Effects of antidepressants on sleep. Current Psychiatry Reports 19(9), 63.

Wiles N, Thomas, L, Abel A et al 2014. Clinical effectiveness and cost-effectiveness of cognitive behavioural therapy as an adjunct to pharmacotherapy for treatment-resistant depression in primary care: the CoBalT randomised controlled trial. Health Technology Assessment (Winchester, England) 18(31), 1.

Wong CCY, Caspi A, Williams B et al 2011. A longitudinal twin study of skewed X chromosome-inactivation. PloS One 6(3), e17873.

World Health Organization (WHO) 2019. World health statistics 2019: monitoring health for the SDGs sustainable development goals. World Health Organization. Online. Available: https://apps.who.int/iris/bitstream/handle/10665/324835/9789241565707-eng.pdf.

World Health Organization (WHO) 2018. Depression. Online. Available: www.who.int/news-room/fact-sheets/detail/depression.

World Health Organization (WHO) 2017. Depression and other common mental disorders: global health estimates. Online. Available: http://hesp-news.org/2017/02/23/depression-and-other-common-mental-disorders-global-health-estimates/

World Health Organization (WHO) 1992. Classification of mental and behavioural disorders. ICD-10 revision 2016. WHO, Geneva.

Wurtzel E 1994. Prozac nation. Young and depressed in America. A Memoir. Quartet Books, London.

Zhang A, Borhneimer LA, Weaver A et al 2019. Cognitive behavioral therapy for primary care depression and anxiety: a secondary meta-analytic review using robust variance estimation in meta-regression. Journal of Behavioral Medicine 42(6), 1117–1141.

Zugai JS, Stein-Parbury J, Roche M 2015. Therapeutic alliance in mental health nursing: an evolutionary concept analysis. Issues in Mental Health Nursing 36(4), 249–257.

CHAPTER 15

Principles for Nursing Practice: Advanced Dementia

ESTHER CHANG • AMANDA JOHNSON

LEARNING OBJECTIVES

When you have completed this chapter, you will be able to:
- comprehend the pathophysiology of a person who has dementia
- adopt a holistic approach in managing the symptoms and behaviours of a person with advanced dementia, especially in pain management
- identify the potential challenges and implications for nursing a person with advanced dementia
- recognise that communication skills are essential in the provision of nursing care to a person with advanced dementia and their family
- appreciate the importance of family carers as an integral feature in planning care for the person with advanced dementia.

KEY WORDS

advanced dementia	communication
Alzheimer's	family
carers	pain management

INTRODUCTION

Worldwide there is much evidence to suggest that recognising dementia as a chronic disease through awareness, early diagnosis, good management and research, is paramount to providing effective care (Alzheimer's Disease International 2015; Snowden et al 2017). Dementia is becoming an increasingly burdensome health issue in both Australia and New Zealand, and is currently the second leading cause of death in Australia (Dementia Australia 2021). This burden is felt even more so by specific Australians, such as those from Aboriginal and Torres Strait Islander backgrounds (ATSI), with three to five times as many ATSI people experiencing dementia as within the general population (Flicker & Holdsworth 2014). The rates of dementia among rural and urban Aboriginal people in New South Wales and the Northern Territory are three times higher than the non-Indigenous population (Lindeman et al 2017).

Dementia dramatically changes the lives of people who live with it, including their families (Dixon 2017). An ATSI summit held by Alzheimer's Australia and the National Aboriginal and Torres Strait Islander Dementia Advisory Group (NATSIDAG) (2015) identified that there are few services located within communities, and mainstream service delivery does not identify cultural connection as key to service delivery. This places people with dementia from ATSI communities at an increased risk of further social isolation. Furthermore, a very low level of culturally appropriate residential care is available for ATSI communities, with mainstream services ill equipped to provide culturally appropriate care (Alzheimer's Australia and NATSIDAG 2015).

The National Cross-Cultural Dementia Network was established in Australia in 2003 to address the broad range of needs specific to people from CALD backgrounds and to ensure their needs are met. A similar situation exists in New Zealand with dementia care for Māori people, and given that the number of people aged over 65 is predicted to be seven times that of non-Māori people from 2011 to 2026, and that they are more likely to experience chronic health conditions than non-Māori people, dementia care specific to the Māori is imperative (Dyall 2014).

Dementia is associated with several diseases characterised by impairment of brain function, inclusive of memory, understanding and reasoning (Alzheimer's Association 2021). This group of diseases leads to a progressive, incurable decline in cognitive abilities and normal daily functioning which severely limits quality of life (Alzheimer's Association 2021). Dementia is also acknowledged as the leading cause of disability in older Australians (Australian Institute of Health and Welfare [AIHW] 2020). In 2020 it was estimated that between 400 000 and 459 000 people currently have dementia in Australia (AIHW 2020), while figures for New Zealand were 62 287 in 2016 – 1.3% of the population (Alzheimer's New Zealand & Deloitte 2017).

Projections in Australia for 2030 estimate an increase in people affected by dementia to 550 000 and 900 000 by 2050 (AIHW 2020; Dementia Australia 2020). Similarly, diagnoses of dementia are forecast to triple to 170 212 by 2050 in New Zealand (Alzheimer's New Zealand & Deloitte 2017). Dementia is frequently linked to advancing age, affecting less than 1% of the population under 65 years of age and one in four people aged 85 years or older (AIHW 2012).

Alzheimer's disease is the most common form of dementia and may contribute to 60–70% of cases (World Health Organization [WHO] 2016). Although research continues to identify the causes, there are typical changes seen in the brain – shrinkage and a build-up of abnormal proteins. Vascular dementia is the second-most common form of dementia. This group of conditions is caused by poor blood supply to the brain because of a stroke or several mini-strokes, or by the slow build-up of blood vessel disease in the brain. Lewy Body dementia is less common, characterised by the presence of 'Lewy Bodies', which are abnormal clumps of protein in the brain. These cause changes in movement, thinking, behaviour and alertness. People with Lewy Body disease can fluctuate between almost normal functioning and severe confusion within short periods and may also hallucinate, seeing things that aren't really there.

Fronto-temporal dementia is another less common group of conditions, affecting the frontal and/or temporal lobes of the brain. If a person has affected frontal lobes, they will have increasing difficulty with motivation, planning and organising, controlling emotions and maintaining socially appropriate behaviour. If temporal lobes are affected, the person will have difficulty with speaking and/or understanding language. The boundaries between each form of dementia are difficult to distinguish, and some people might have a combination of dementias (e.g. vascular dementia and Alzheimer's disease).

While there is no cure or treatment to stop the underlying decline and death of brain cells, various treatments are used to improve memory, thinking and reasoning problems (e.g. drugs to boost performance of chemicals in the brain that carry information from one brain cell to another). Various new treatments aimed at stopping or significantly delaying the progression of Alzheimer's are being investigated in clinical trials. Examples include treatments targeting plaques (e.g. via recruiting the immune system, preventing destruction or production blockers) and keeping a protein called 'tau' from tangling or reducing inflammation (Gandy & Sano 2015; Small & Greenfield 2015). Other avenues being researched include insulin resistance, heart and blood vessel health and hormones (e.g. oestrogen) (Morris et al 2012; Small & Greenfield 2015). There has also been considerable progress in identifying genetic risk factors in healthy young adults, with the aim to develop gene therapy, as well as to implement future preventative treatments as early as possible (Mormino et al 2016).

The Australian projections support the prediction that within two decades health and residential aged care spending will constitute the third highest source of spending (Access Economics 2009). Further, by 2023 dementia will be one of the fastest growing sources of major disease burden, overtaking coronary heart disease (Access Economics 2009). In acknowledging these projections, the Australian Government has recognised dementia as a National Health Priority and increased the budget to $16 billion for aged care, as well as implementing various initiatives to tackle the challenges for individuals with dementia, carers, the community and care professionals (Australian Government Department of Health 2016).

In New Zealand, in 2007 there were over 32 000 people with dementia. By 2011, 48 182 New Zealanders had dementia – 1.1% of the New Zealand population. This represented an increase of over 18% in 3 years, from 40 746 people in 2008 (Alzheimer's New Zealand 2013). As a disease, dementia is now ranked as the second leading cause of death in Australia (Australian Bureau of Statistics [ABS] 2020) and the fourth leading cause of death among the population aged 65 years and over in New Zealand (Alzheimer's New Zealand 2013). The number of deaths directly attributed to dementia in 2010 represented 6.3% of all Australian deaths overall, demonstrating a 3.4% increase since 2001, almost doubling during this time period and expected to continue to rise with the projections previously detailed (ABS 2010). It is highly probable that a similar pattern of increase will be reflected in the New Zealand population in worldwide trends (WHO 2012). Symptoms of advanced dementia frequently resemble those of a person dying from advanced cancer (Cartwright 2011; Chang et al 2009). This scenario suggests people with dementia would significantly benefit from the interventions traditionally directed to cancer-related end-of-life care (Mitchell et al 2009; van der Steen 2010); however, palliative care interventions are infrequently accorded to this group of people, so their needs are likely to be unmet (Chang et al 2009; Chang & Walter 2010). Further exacerbation of this lack of palliative care intervention may also be attributed to the person with advanced dementia possessing impaired communication (Johnson et al 2009). As a result of this and the disease itself, the symptoms of dementia, such as pain, are likely to present as a challenge for family and professional carers.

ADOPTING A HOLISTIC APPROACH

The pathology of dementia means that many challenges and disruptions occur along the illness trajectory, manifesting as a multitude of symptoms across cognitive, functional, behavioural and psychological areas (Grand et al 2011; Montine et al 2019). Because of the extensive needs of individuals with dementia, they often require care beyond traditional medical practice (Grand et al 2011). The person becomes increasingly reliant on caregivers to provide their entire essential physical, psychological and social needs (Long 2009). The challenge faced by nurses is to provide high-quality care that addresses all these facets. Hughes (2013) reported that people with dementia are less likely to have their pain and spiritual and religious needs addressed than those without dementia. Dementia can rob a person of their personhood (Hughes 2013). It is important to treat the person as an individual (Grand et al 2011), with care for the whole person as the main goal. A holistic approach to practice also encourages nurses to integrate care, self-responsibility, spirituality, and reflection in their lives (Klebanoff 2013). The nurse's practice in caring for a client with advanced dementia is complex and multi-layered, as a direct consequence of dementia pathology. The

basic principle of care is to meet the needs of the person by managing their total symptom experience rather than responding to discrete segments; for example, attending to a person's emotional status while also assessing their pain (Hughes 2013).

The illness trajectory of dementia is frequently slow and insidious, with family often acting as the primary caregivers for substantial periods of time. Ultimately, for most people with dementia, a move to institutional care in a residential aged care facility (RACF) is required (WHO 2012). The long involvement of family carers is unique to this client group; nurses, as part of their holistic approach and principle of care, must include the family in their caregiving. Recognising how family are feeling has a direct impact on the person with dementia (Nugent 2005), and may further contribute to their anxiety, depression, wandering and other displays of behaviour. It is through the relationships the nurse has with the person and their family and the actions the nurse demonstrates in providing holistic care that healing occurs. Healing in this context means seeing the person as a whole, attending to all dimensions of care, giving meaning to their life, offering hope to the family and showing compassion, respect and patience. It is from this understanding that nurses can make a difference to the life of the person affected by dementia and their family. Holistic nursing therefore delivers nursing care that addresses the person's physical, intellectual, emotional and spiritual dimensions. Holistic nursing refers to a kind of nursing practice which focuses on the patient as a whole as opposed to merely treating the symptoms of their present condition (RegisteredNursing.org 2020). The person and their family's needs are also considered as an inter-related entity of these dimensions (Taylor 2009). If holistic nursing is not undertaken, significant levels of distress and suffering may be experienced by the person and their family (Maher & Hemming 2005).

When nurses believe and demonstrate through their actions that they view a person as a whole human being, embracing the interconnectedness of mind, body and spirit, evidence of a holistic approach to the delivery of nursing care is present (Klebanoff 2013). Erickson sees a person's wholeness as the dynamic interaction of the mind, body and spirit components within the person, between and among others and with the universe (2007, p. 140). For a healthy state to exist, balance and harmony must be present in all aspects of the person's life – physical, social, emotional, cognitive and spiritual – irrespective of the presence or absence of physical disease (Erickson 2007). This implies that in the presence of disease, a person has the potential to achieve a state of wellbeing if their needs are addressed holistically and the person remains in a relational context with other people (Erickson 2007). In these circumstances, the person seeks, in partnership with the nurse, to ameliorate the imbalance and disharmony present through the alleviation of suffering, promotion of comfort, finding inner peace, assisting with healing and preventing illness and injury (Erickson 2007; Mariano 2007). Practising in this way demonstrates a shift in care from being disease-oriented to embracing the needs of the person and their family (Erickson 2007; O'Brien-King & Gates 2007).

The following principles underpin holistic nursing: understanding the person as a unique human being who possesses a connectedness with everyone and everything; recognising the need for healing in states of illness where cure is not possible, but where management of symptoms will lead to the alleviation of suffering; promoting comfort and restoration of balance and harmony; engaging in care practices that embrace both the science and the art of nursing; performing nursing care in relationship with the person and their family based on the values of compassion, respect, trust and authenticity; and participating in self-care activities to promote healing and personal development of self (Mariano 2007; Nugent 2005).

When a holistic approach to care is adopted, the journey taken by both the nurse and the patient is of a healing nature. This journey is predicated on the notion that healing is reflective of the following: having a presence; intent; unconditional acceptance; love and compassion (Erickson 2007, pp. 154–9). Healing leads to the attainment of wellbeing in the presence of disease for the patient and, for the nurse, provides an energy source derived from the balance and harmony achieved that nurtures the nurse to continue caregiving. Understanding where the person and their family are at is the beginning point of the journey for the nurse, the person with dementia and their family members (Mariano 2007). Holistic nurses are those that recognise, treat, and care for each individual differently (Practical Nursing Organisation 2020).

Assessment of the person and their family's needs, at this point, offers the opportunity to identify and discuss care options across the illness trajectory in the context of the person's preferences (Mariano 2007). Understanding the personal characteristics of the individual allows for the tailoring of interventions to support the person's deficits, to maximise their strengths and to identify the coping mechanisms of the person and their family (Kolanowski & Whall 2000, p. 74) in the management of end-of-life issues.

Holistic nursing therefore offers nurses a means of practice that responds to the whole person by addressing their physical, psychological, social, spiritual and cultural needs as a collective entity rather than directing care to discrete segments of a disease (Erickson 2007; Maher & Hemming 2005; Klebanoff 2013). For example, a person with dementia may scream or lash out as a result of feelings of anxiety, fear or depression due to their incapacity to express themselves and not as a consequence of dementia pathology (Kolanowski & Whall 2000, p. 69). Alternatively, in the presence of non-assessed or misdiagnosed fatigue, thirst, hunger and/or pain, a person with dementia may respond by wandering, physical aggression and disruptive vocalisations (Kolanowski & Whall 2000, p. 70), or exacerbations of these behaviours in response to an unmet physiological need.

Nurses who engage in a holistic nursing approach use a repertoire of actions that demonstrate their commitment to the concept of holism, including touch, massage, eye contact, moderated and empathic voice, comfort measures, aromatherapies, exercise, music, active listening, creation of trusting relationships, an approach that is non-confrontational and calm and the sensitive eliciting of information (Erickson 2007; Kolanowski & Whall 2000; Maher & Hemming 2005; Nugent 2005).

The case studies in this chapter show how holistic nursing care can be considered in practice. They show the interrelationship that exists between a person's mind, body and spirit and their care needs.

In Case Study 15.2 James doesn't recognise his children anymore. In this situation the nurse can use holistic nursing care to support both the individual and their family in their experiences of loss.

These two case studies highlight the complexity of providing holistic care and involving the family in the care of the person, viewing the person as a whole and understanding the significance of the interconnectedness between the components of mind, body and spirit, in order to meet the needs of the person and their family.

Understanding the pain experience in the case of advanced dementia is a subjective experience, as illustrated in the definition by McCaffrey (1968), which is still commonly used today: 'Pain is whatever the experiencing person says it is, existing whenever he or she says it does'. The challenge for the nurse, then, is how to assess and manage pain in people with advanced dementia, who cannot usually communicate verbally how they feel due to the disease processes involved. It is commonly believed that people with dementia have a

CASE STUDY 15.1

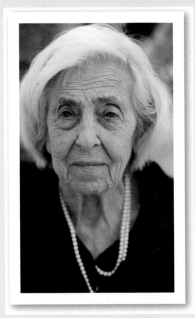

iStockphoto/francesco_de_napoli.

Rebecca is a 75-year-old woman who was diagnosed with vascular dementia 12 months ago. She had been living with her husband, who is also her caregiver. They have no children. Five months ago, Rebecca was admitted to the residential aged care facility (RACF) because of her behavioural problems. Her husband was increasingly concerned about her wandering, aggressive manner and the potential risk of harm. Other co-morbidities included heart disease, diabetes, anxiety and depression and a history of cholecystectomy 10 years ago.

The staff in the RACF identified that Rebecca was in the advanced stage of dementia. She had a Mini-Mental State Examination (MMSE) score of 14; she walked with the assistance of one nurse and was at a high risk of falling if she tried to ambulate independently. Rebecca has recently displayed frequent episodes of extreme agitation. She regularly calls out loudly, bangs things like plates against the wall, is resistant to care and often becomes more physically aggressive to staff when they provide care. She previously attended resident activities run by the diversional therapist, but this has stopped because the other residents complained that she was too disruptive and noisy.

Rebecca is receiving regular antipsychotic medication and 6-hourly paracetamol for pain. When Rebecca appears to have pain, the care staff initiates non-pharmacological pain interventions known to settle her, such as spending some time with her, distracting her to reduce her distress and agitation. She will sometimes settle without medication. Rebecca's husband Jim, a retired businessman, comes to visit her every day. She is less agitated when he is there.

From a holistic nursing perspective, the nurse would communicate with Rebecca's husband in the planning of care and decision-making to manage Rebecca's symptoms.

CASE STUDY QUESTIONS

1. What are the key elements of care for Rebecca?
2. What are the key elements of building a trusting relationship with Rebecca and her husband so that they feel valued?
3. How do you provide holistic care for Rebecca?

---

decreased ability to experience pain; however, this conviction may be due to the pain tools used that rely on verbal report (Smigorski & Leszek 2010). Pain is under-recognised and under-treated in advanced dementia (Abbey 2013; Jansen et al 2017; Jordan et al 2011). A paper on bioethical issues in dementia by the Nuffield Council on Bioethics (2009) reported research that people with dementia receive poor end-of-life care, in particular poor pain control. It also found that older hospitalised people with dementia were less likely to receive palliative care than those who did not have dementia. Corbett and colleagues (2016), in their study, clearly articulated a need for an evidence-based pain management program for people with dementia. This is

consistent with the Alzheimer's Australia (2014a) survey of care professionals and family carers' findings, in which 22% of former family carers felt that pain was not managed well at end of life for the person with dementia, 41% of care professionals had received no training on assessment of pain in people with dementia, and 7% of care professionals indicated they were uncomfortable with their ability to assess and manage pain for people with dementia. Consistent with previous reports, 27% of care professionals did not think adequate pain control (if it might also hasten death) was a legal choice for people in Australia or were unsure. This topic is discussed further below in advance care planning.

CASE STUDY 15.2

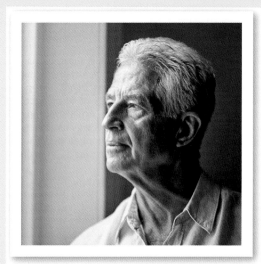

iStockphoto/PeopleImages.

James is a 65-year-old man. He was diagnosed with Alzheimer's dementia 4 years ago and has a history of hypertension and cardiovascular disease. James was admitted to an RACF a year ago because his wife could no longer care for him at home. He required assistance to transfer from bed to chair, and assistance with all his activities of daily living. His wife was unable to lift him without assistance.

James's notes reveal that he is confined to a chair, requiring two nurses to transfer him using a Pelican belt or similar equipment. He is now incontinent of both urine and faeces if not taken to the toilet regularly and incontinent overnight. He can communicate a little, but his vocabulary is very restricted. He requires staff assistance to feed him a normal diet. James was unable to complete any of the MMSE questions; his MMSE was therefore assessed as being zero.

Staff members have identified that James's condition is deteriorating. He has lost weight and is becoming increasingly frail. James is taking regular Celestone, Clamoxyl Duo, Chlorvescent and analgesics intermittently (prn), if staff note that he appears to be in pain on movement. He no longer recognises his wife or children during their visits. This distresses his children a great deal, as they want him to share their lives, and those of their small children. He has no advance care directive, no evidence that any discussion about prognosis or end-of-life care has been undertaken, nor goals of care stated.

From a holistic nursing perspective, the nurse would communicate with his wife in the planning of care and decision-making of advance care directives for James.

CASE STUDY QUESTIONS

1. What are the key elements of advance care planning for James?
2. How do you involve the family in the care of James?
3. What are some of the topics that might be discussed at a meeting with the family?

Impairment in communicative ability, self-report, has been recognised as the primary reason for inadequate pain management in this group (Sheu et al 2011). Another challenge is that people with dementia do not follow a linear trajectory towards death, and as a result, pain management can be variable (Aupperle et al 2004). In addition, an observable behaviour symptom (e.g. agitation) may be symptomatic of conditions other than pain, highlighting the complexities in symptom management in people with advanced dementia. There is also a common belief that being a neurological disorder, central nervous system experience of pain in dementia is reduced (Reynolds et al 2008). However, significant pain is a common experience in advanced dementia (Aminoff & Adunsky 2004; Black et al 2006; Corbett et al 2016; Feldt, Warne et al 1998; Ferrell 1995; Gove et al 2010; Jansen et al 2017; Kupper & Hughes 2011; McClean 2000; Parmelee 1996; Smigorski & Leszek 2010; Won et al 2004; Young 2001).

As stated in the *Australian guidelines for a palliative approach in residential aged care* (Australian Government Department of Health and Ageing 2006, p. 62), 'One of the most difficult aspects for the aged care team who is caring for the resident with advanced dementia is assessing whether they are experiencing pain'. Clinical experience of the authors supports this finding, with many Australian aged care nursing clinicians stating that the ability to not only assess but also address pain issues for the cognitively impaired resident remains a constant issue of concern as clinicians struggle to function within a system not designed or educated to cope with this challenge. Therefore, the emphasis of pain management is discussed in this chapter.

The literature indicates that people with dementia are at high risk for unrecognised, untreated or under-treated pain (Black et al 2006; Evans 2002; Jansen et al 2017; Reynolds et al 2008; Shega et al 2006; Snow & Shuster 2006). Apart from the challenges in assessment described above, this situation may be partly due to a common perception among many in our community, as well as trained health professionals, that individuals with dementia do not experience pain because of their impaired cognitive state (Boller et al 2002; Malotte & McPherson 2016) and their inability to verbalise and self-report their pain. This is not a logical assumption, because although communication deficits and motivational and complex thinking impairments may blunt pain behaviour, they do not necessarily alter pain perception (Shuster 2000). Even towards the end of life such individuals continue to interact with their environment and are not in a vegetative state (Boller et al 2002; Volicer & Hurley 1998).

Most people with advanced dementia are over the age of 65 (WHO 2012), and as such are likely to have underlying medical conditions that can cause pain (McClean 2000). In advanced dementia, pain is frequently the result of constipation or diarrhoea, lodged food particles, contractures, decubitus ulcers or urosepsis (Smith 1998). Other possible causes of pain include sore gums, broken teeth and cavities, headaches, back pain, osteoarthritis, hip fractures, skin rash, sore throat and cold (Rabins et al 2006). A US study on nursing homes found that there was a lack of good quality palliative care, with distressing symptoms and burdensome interventions being more common in people at the end stage of dementia, unless their relatives were well informed (Cervo et al 2009). For people with advanced dementia, pain may be expressed in terms of irritability, increased confusion or resistance to care. Nursing staff are in an ideal position to be able to notice changes in function or behaviour that may be signs of pain, as they are so closely involved in the care of the person that only they may be able to interpret the meaning of the symptoms. They also have an ethical and legal obligation to make all attempts to ensure the comfort and pain management of their patients, especially for those who are unable to express their pain verbally (Burns & McIlafrick 2015; Kerr & Chenoweth 2003).

ASSESSING PAIN IN PEOPLE WITH ADVANCED DEMENTIA

An expert-based consensus statement of pain assessment in older adults recommended that adequate assessment is vital in providing a basis for clinical decision-making and optimal care (Hadjistravropoulos et al 2007; Herr et al 2011; Jansen et al 2017; Malotte & McPherson 2016). One of the main reasons that pain management in patients who are older and cognitively impaired is inadequate is that there is a lack of or inappropriate assessment (Hadjistravropoulos et al 2007; Malotte & McPherson 2016; Smigorski & Leszek 2010). A systematic approach is required, using all members of the caring team within the facility, including family members.

Experts recommend that best practice for this population is to utilise behavioural observation-based assessment, due to difficulties with recall, interpretation of sensations and verbal expression in dementia (AGS Panel on Persistent Pain in Older Persons 2002; American Medical Directors Association 2005; Australian Government Department of Health and Ageing 2006). Thus, nursing staff base their decisions on an objective assessment of pain relief needs rather than simply relying on subjective impressions. An attempt should always be made to obtain a self-report of pain from the person with advanced dementia before changing to behavioural observation (Snow & Shuster 2006), because 'any reports of pain from the cognitively impaired resident should be accepted as just as valid and reliable as those of residents who can communicate' (Australian Pain Society 2005). Kerr and Chenoweth (2003) recommend the following interviewing skills when assessing pain in people with cognitive impairment: ask simple and specific questions about how the person is feeling (e.g. 'Do you have an ache?'); speak calmly and at a pace the person can comprehend; adopt a caring and patient manner; maintain eye contact and keep checking that the person understands the question; and use a safe, quiet environment. However, the nurse should also remember that, if the person's self-report of pain is negative, and pain discomfort behaviours are present, pain is likely (Snow & Shuster 2006). A family carer report is also recommended if one is available, as they are familiar with the person's usual demeanour (Kerr & Chenoweth 2003). A study by Corbett and colleagues (2016) found communication to be central on their landscape of pain management in people with dementia living in care homes. Thematic analysis revealed the need for pain awareness in staff, miscommunication among staff and carers, lack of confidence and responsibility, inconsistency of care and the need for staff training. They found that, despite examples of good practice, there were deficiencies in these areas which were consistent with similar work in this field (Petriwskyj et al 2015), with the need for formal structure and support for staff. Other components of pain assessment, apart from behavioural observation, include physical assessment and a comprehensive review of the history of the person with dementia. Physical touch appears to be lacking when reviewing how pain is assessed in the resident with dementia. Health professionals and carers tend to base their decisions on verbal response rather than physical examination of the body and the reactions of the person with advanced dementia. Clinical examination of the individual, using a simple physical assessment that includes movement of the limbs while observing the person with dementia, will provide evidence of pain even in a person at the end stage of dementia, who may grimace, moan or resist being moved. The findings, when taken together with the results from using a pain assessment tool, the nurse's clinical judgement and the opinions of other care staff and family members, will provide evidence on which to base pain interventions.

The medical history should also be reviewed, especially in relation to factors and conditions known to be associated with pain. Additionally, it is useful to know the history of the pain being experienced itself. Useful questions include: 'When did the pain start?'; 'What aggravates the pain?'; 'What relieves the pain?' and 'Is there a certain time of the day when the pain is present?' While a resident with advanced dementia may not be able to recall and respond to these questions, family members and other members of the care team may be able to assist.

Potential Behavioural Indicators of Pain

The American Geriatrics Society identified six main types of pain behaviours and indicators, based on a literature review (AGS Panel on Persistent Pain in Older Persons 2002). These are listed in Table 15.1 with specific examples of observable behaviours. However, it is important to consider the influence of culture on the expression of pain, so not all cues listed will apply (Kerr & Chenoweth 2003).

Tools for Assessment of Pain for Advanced Dementia

People with advanced dementia unable to self-report their pain are particularly at risk for under-recognised or under-treated pain, and the symptoms of dementia can be exacerbated by the pain experience. For example, the person may be more irritable, aggressive, depressed or withdrawn, with changed appetite or sleep. Recognition of these non-verbal behaviours as a potential sign of discomfort needs to be systematically addressed, with the use of appropriate pain assessment tools. Herr and colleagues (2006) conducted a critical review of existing tools issued for pain assessment in non-verbal older adults with dementia. The tools they identified as meeting criteria are listed in Table 15.2. All the tools require the rater to observe the person and

TABLE 15.1
Pain Behaviours/indicators

Pain Behaviour/ indicator	Example
Facial expressions	Slight frown, sad, frightened face, grimacing, wrinkled forehead, closed or tightened eyes, any distorted expression, rapid blinking
Verbalisations, vocalisations	Sighing, moaning, groaning, grunting, chanting, calling out, noisy breathing, asking for help
Body movements	Rigid, tense body posture, guarding, fidgeting, increased pacing, rocking, restricted movement, gait or mobility changes
Changes in interpersonal interactions	Aggressive, combative, resisting care, decreased social interactions, socially inappropriate, disruptive, withdrawn, verbally abusive
Changes in activity patterns or routines	Refusing food, appetite change, increase in rest periods or sleep, changes in rest pattern, sudden cessation of common routines, increased wandering
Mental status changes	Crying or tears, increased confusion, irritability or distress

AGS Panel on Persistent Pain in Older Persons 2002.

rate the behaviours in terms of their presence, intensity, or frequency (Snow & Shuster 2006). Although existing tools are still in the early stages of development and testing, particularly in terms of established validity (Herr et al 2011), the advantage of these tools is that their use raises the nurse's awareness of the need to assess the patient for pain, and they provide an objective assessment that can augment the nurse's subjective judgement. One must always remember that a tool is only as good as the assessor and cannot take away the clinical judgement of the health professional or carer. Bearing this in mind, how then does the nurse ensure that all residents with possible pain are assessed? Adopting a systematic approach to pain assessment and management is the best practice (Kovach, Cashin & Sauer 2006; Kovach, Logan et al 2006; Kovach, Noonan et al 2006; Malotte & McPherson 2016; Snow & Shuster 2006).

TABLE 15.2 Pain Assessment	
Pain Assessment Tool	**Authors**
Abbey Pain Scale (Abbey)	Abbey et al (2004)
Assessment of Discomfort in Dementia (ADD) protocol*	Kovach et al (1999)
Checklist of non-verbal pain indicators (CNPI)	Feldt, Warne et al (1998)
Certified Nursing Assistant Pain Assessment Tool (CPAT)	Cervo et al (2009)
Discomfort of Dementia of the Alzheimer's Type (DS-DAT)	Hurley et al (1992)
The Doloplus 2	Lefebvre-Chapiro & the Doloplus Group (2001)
The Face, Legs, Activity, Cry, and Consolability Pain Assessment Tool (the FLACC)	Merkel et al (1997)
Mahoney Pain Scale	Mahoney & Peters (2008)
Noncommunicative Patient's Pain Assessment Instrument (NOPPAIN)	Snow, Weber, O'Malley et al (2004)
Pain Assessment Checklist for Seniors with Limited Ability to Communicate (PACSLAC)	Fuchs-Lacelle & Hadjistravropoulos (2004)
Pain Assessment for the Dementing Elderly (PADE)	Villanueva et al (2003)
Pain Assessment in Advanced Dementia (PAINAD)	Warden et al (2003)
Pain Assessment In Noncommunicative Elderly (PAINE)	Cohen-Mansfield & Lipson (2008)

*Since this review the authors of the ADD have refined the protocol to develop the Serial Trial Intervention, which has been positively evaluated using a randomised controlled trial
Kovach, Logan et al 2006.

Systematic Approach to Assessment of Pain

One example of a systematic approach for this population is the Serial Trial Intervention (STI) developed by nurses (Kovach, Noonan et al 2006) to systematically assess and treat the unmet needs of people with dementia. This approach is a refinement of the Assessment of Discomfort in Dementia (ADD) protocol that has previously been found to be effective in improving pain assessment and management in nursing home residents with dementia (Pieper et al 2011; Corbett et al 2016; Malotte & McPherson 2016). The STI identifies the cause of discomfort behaviours and then treats the causes, such as pain, that lead to discomfort behaviours, and has been evaluated in a randomised controlled trial. The study of 114 nursing home residents with moderate or severe dementia found that those who received the STI had significantly lower levels of discomfort, were more likely to return to their baseline levels, received a broader scope of physical affective assessment and received more pharmacological comfort treatments, than those in the control group (Kovach, Logan et al 2006). An application of this approach to the cases in this chapter will be given below.

APPLYING A SYSTEMATIC APPROACH TO THE ASSESSMENT OF PAIN

Current best practice guidelines set out by the Australian Government are that pain management should be conducted using a comprehensive assessment of the resident's pain and evidence-based analgesic decision-making (Guideline Adaptation Committee 2016).

Table 15.2 shows behavioural measures of pain assessment tools derived from a review (Herr et al 2006). Measures satisfied the criteria of being:

- based on behavioural indicators of pain
- developed for assessment of pain in non-verbal older adults with severe dementia or evaluated for use with non-verbal older adults
- available in English
- psychometrically evaluated.

A position statement with clinical practice recommendations set out by Herr and colleagues (2006) poses the following hierarchy of pain assessment techniques for dementia, based on findings by Pasero and McCaffery (2011) and Hadjistravropoulos and colleagues (2007):

1. Obtain self-report. Self-report of pain is often possible in mild-to-moderate cognitive impairment,

but ability to self-report decreases as dementia progresses.

2. Search for potential causes of pain. Consider common chronic pain aetiologies: musculoskeletal and neurological disorders are the most common causes of pain in adults.

3. Observe patient behaviour. Observe facial expressions, verbalisations/vocalisations, body movements, changes in interactions, changes in activity patterns or routines and mental status. Behavioural observation should occur during activity whenever possible.

In the cases of Rebecca and James, any one of the behaviours listed in Table 15.1 could alert the nurse to the possibility that they may be experiencing pain. Rebecca is reportedly agitated, and is frequently resistive to care and physically aggressive. Both of them have heart disease, disabling conditions known to cause pain and lower quality of life (Cunningham 2006; Frondini et al 2007). People with cognitive impairment who behave aggressively are significantly more likely than those with non-aggressive behaviours to have two or more pain-related diagnoses, including strokes, contractures and decubitus ulcers (Bradford et al 2012). However, Rebecca's disruptive behaviours could also reflect other problems, such as depression, boredom or over- or under-stimulation (Snow & Shuster 2006).

Using a systematic approach to managing the symptoms of Rebecca and James, the nurse would respond to the behavioural symptoms by implementing multiple levels of assessment and treatment, tailored to the individual person (Kovach, Cashin & Sauer 2006; Mathys 2018). Detailed explanation of this approach can be found in Kovach, Cashin and Sauer (2006) and Snow and Shuster (2006).

1. Conduct a physical need assessment, focusing on conditions associated with discomfort. In the cases of Rebecca and James, there could be behavioural indications of specific locations of discomfort, so the nurse could physically move Rebecca's and James's limbs and watch for verbal and non-verbal cues that might indicate pain, such as grimacing; or when Rebecca is taken for a walk while assessing her movement.

2. Examine environment and activity pacing (alternating in excessive periods of stimulation and rest) to identify potential causes of behaviour and treat accordingly if assessment is positive. For Rebecca and James, this would involve checking that sources of environmental stress, such as the chair used by James, are eliminated, or reduced to a minimum. Rebecca and James both require combinations of meaningful human interaction and rest, even if they appear not to be responding. This is an important step to help identify whether a particular symptom (e.g. agitation) is due to pain or other reasons, such as lack of meaningful human interaction or stimulation.

3. Initiate an analgesic regimen trial when indicated by physical examination. This would also be started if no clear potential cause of discomfort can be identified and non-pharmacological interventions to increase comfort have been unsuccessful. This should be carefully monitored and regularly reassessed. In Rebecca's case, paracetamol was ineffective in controlling the pain. Although the pain was reduced after staff spent considerable time distracting her, this form of management is time-consuming, increases environmental stress and adds to the strain of caring (Kovach, Noonan et al 2006). It does not assist with the underlying cause of the pain. Regular analgesic regimens will assist here. James is also only being given analgesia 'as required'. With his history of diabetes and cardiovascular disease, he should be commenced on an 'around the clock' treatment regimen, starting with paracetamol. The fact that Rebecca was not given a stronger pain reliever than paracetamol is reflective of common under-treatment of pain that occurs in this population (Black et al 2006; Evans 2002; Shega et al 2006; Snow & Shuster 2006). However, the situation does appear to be improving, with a Swedish study (Haasum et al 2011) finding that people with dementia were more likely than those without dementia in a residential setting to receive analgesia. Perhaps awareness is increasing in medical and allied health staff on pain management in dementia. Adopting a palliative approach to the care of people with dementia (Guideline Adaptation Committee 2016) in the case of Rebecca means that a strong analgesic may be appropriate in the absence of effective pain relief following simple analgesia. Although nurses do not have a prescribing role, they play a crucial role in decisions about assessment, medication regimens and management procedures, as well as reviewing practice and outcomes (Cunningham 2006).

4. Non-pharmacological intervention trial: this occurs when indicated by Step 2 (examination of environment and activity pacing). Examples that could be applied to Rebecca and James include reduced or increased environmental/sensory stimulation, soothing and supportive verbal communication and/or touch, physical exercise/movement/massage,

and music therapy (Snow & Shuster 2006). Best practice guidelines recommend that these treatments be used to complement analgesia and may decrease the amount of analgesia required (AGS Panel on Persistent Pain in Older Persons 2002; American Medical Directors Association 2005). Review the use of complementary therapies such as aromatherapy and relaxation techniques.

5. If behaviour continues, consult with other disciplines or practitioners.
6. Using this approach requires persistence in terms of regular assessment, management and reassessment.

PRINCIPLES OF COMMUNICATION WITH FAMILY IMPACT ON THE COMMUNITY

When planning care for a person with advanced dementia, the health and wellbeing of family members who act as primary carers (family carers) need to be assessed, monitored and referral made for interventions, if indicated. Family carers provide physical care and emotional support to the person with dementia throughout the illness trajectory, frequently undertaking this responsibility even before a diagnosis is made (Brooks et al 2015). The care they provide is time-consuming, sometimes unpleasant, emotionally and physically stressful, and falls outside the bounds of normal family relationships (Yap et al 2005). For these reasons, the health and quality of life of the family carer may be adversely affected by their caring role. Dementia family carers may also be required to initiate, supervise and sometimes evaluate the effectiveness of medications (Brodaty & Green 2002) and act as the substitute decision-maker, providing consent for complex healthcare decisions for the person with dementia who no longer has the capacity to either consent to, or refuse, treatment (Brooks et al 2015).

Potential Impact on Family Carers and the Community

Family carers can experience negative health outcomes because of their caring role. While some carers report positive impacts and great satisfaction in their role, many experience deleterious effects on their emotional, psychological and physical health, social activities and support networks, ability to work and finances (Abbey 2013; Brooks et al 2015). Carers of people with dementia have poorer physical and psychological health, life expectancy, quality of life and economic security (Books et al 2015; WHO 2012). The social, economic and health impact of dementia not only on the family but the community as a whole is vast.

Brooks and colleagues (2015) reported on the impact of the caring role on informal carers who are providing support for someone with dementia living in the Australian community, and the evidence base for effective supports for carers. Most people with dementia living in the community (91%) are dependent on family members to care for them, usually the spouse or adult child of the person with dementia. Support can range from helping the person with dementia with activities of daily living, personal care, and managing behavioural and psychological symptoms of dementia, as well as making difficult decisions about treatment options, use of services, finances, and long-term care (Brooks et al 2015). Additional responsibilities for some carers include paid work, children and other family commitments. Almost one-quarter of community dwelling people with dementia do not access any formal services, with approximately 200 000 Australians providing unpaid care to a person with dementia (Brooks et al 2015).

Factors influencing poorer consequences for the carer include carer age (approximately half are over age 65), co-residency, previous health, personality, coping style, the severity and type of dementia, and the availability of social support (Brooks et al 2015). Although a range of supports and services are available for carers in Australia, including information, education and training, psychosocial therapies, case management approaches, social support groups, respite care and multicomponent programs that combine these, many carers find difficulty in accessing the supports when and where they need them (Brooks et al 2015). Access Economics projects that by 2029 there will be a shortage of 94 266 full-time equivalent (FTE) family carers (Access Economics 2009). Enabling people with dementia to live in the community for as long as possible requires an increased policy focus on enabling carers to access the support services they need in order to sustain their role. Attention to carer demographics and preferences will enable increased social policy responsiveness to the needs of carers and care recipients (Deloitte Access Economics 2015).

Impact of Transition to Residential Aged Care on the Person With Dementia and their Families

While both the family carer(s) and the person with dementia usually both desire that the person remain living at home for as long as possible, a large number ultimately require transition to an RACF due to the increasing complexities of their care. The decision to place a person with dementia into an RACF can often be characterised by stress, emotional upheaval and feelings of relief, loss, grief and guilt (Alzheimer's Australia NSW 2012). For the person with dementia, moving into a RACF or a hospital can also be disorienting, disempowering and emotional (Abbey 2013; Alzheimer's Australia 2012). In addition, the progression of dementia is also occurring, which can exacerbate the problem. More commonly, the move from home is a speedy one, and carers and the individual with dementia encounter a lack of choice and decision-making (Alzheimer's Australia NSW 2012). This occurs due to a desire of families for their loved ones to stay at home for as long as possible (Alzheimer's Australia NSW 2012). Policy and practice changes are needed to improve the quality and seamlessness of the transition from home to residential aged care.

Many families utilise home care packages to enable the person with dementia to live at home for as long as practical (Abbey 2013). One Australian Government aged care reform, *Living Longer. Living Better* (Australian Government Department of Health 2016) has been implemented in response to the recognition that the current cost of replacing family carers with paid carers is $5.5 billion per year (Access Economics 2009), as well as the social and health impacts on carers.

LIVING WITH DEMENTIA: PERCEPTIONS OF PEOPLE WITH DEMENTIA AND CARERS

While there is a growing literature on the lived experience of carers of people with dementia (e.g. Kindell et al 2014), most research has focused on people with early-stage dementia (Johnson 2016). Johnson (2016) explored the lived experience of people with moderate-stage dementia using an interpretive phenomenological analysis. Themes that emerged from semi-structured interviews of six participants were awareness and understanding of dementia, clarity and confusion, social support and relationships, living with dementia and life lived. In contrast to common perceptions that dementia is a kind of 'living death', there were descriptions of a continuing humanity. All participants were aware of their cognitive impairments, of others treating them differently, and that they needed support from others. However, they took it on themselves as being responsible to lower the burden on others by adapting to their difficulties (e.g. making others feel less anxious around them or trying hard to communicate clearly). Although the author recognised the bias in her sample, in that she recruited participants who were happy to discuss their dementia, this study does encourage more inclusion of people with moderate dementia as

participants in research, in that very meaningful discussions can be had with a great deal to be learned from such individuals.

Research has shown an increasing shift towards gaining perspectives on people with dementia from the findings of the first Australian survey of people with dementia conducted in 2014 (Alzheimer's Australia 2014b). Results of 188 respondents indicated that the social consequences of dementia can be devastating, and in support of Johnson's (2016) findings, participants were aware of a negative change in how people responded to them, including friends and family (e.g. avoiding spending time with them, less social contact in the community, difficulty communicating in shops, a perception that people felt uneasy around them). The survey results also identified priorities recommended by participants, including the need to change our communities to make them more dementia-friendly, particularly through better communication (e.g. better signage, increased community awareness, better access to health services and transport) to support people with dementia in participating in the community (Alzheimer's Australia 2014a).

ASSESSMENT OF FAMILY CARERS

Assessment of role strain potentially affecting the health of the family carer is an important dimension of nursing work. Validated tools are available to assist the assessment, such as the Caregiver Strain Index (Robinson 1983), widely utilised in Australia (Australian Government Department of Veterans' Affairs). In New Zealand, the Caregiver Assessment Tools (Guberman et al 2000) are recommended, although they require being adapted for use with Māori and Pacific Islander people (New Zealand Guidelines Group 2003). Assessment for depression is also necessary. One simple way for a nurse to screen a family carer for depression (Arrolls et al 2005) is to ask the family carer to answer 'yes' or 'no' to two questions: 'During the past month have you often been bothered by feeling down, depressed or hopeless?' and 'During the past month have you been bothered by little interest or pleasure in doing things?' These questions assess whether two core symptoms of depression are present. A 'yes' response to these questions may indicate the family carer is depressed. One further question, 'Is this something with which you would like help?', with three possible responses – 'yes', 'no' or 'yes, but not today' – will assist the nurse to determine whether the family carer wants assistance. If indicated, the family carer can be referred to their usual medical practitioner for further investigation and treatment.

Consideration must also be given to the assessment of the family carer's previous grief and loss experiences to provide appropriate support. Less-educated family carers with lower incomes who are experiencing more depressive symptoms are more likely to experience complicated grief reactions after the death of the person with dementia (Hebert et al 2006). Family carers therefore may require referral to a counsellor, social worker, pastoral care worker or other spiritual adviser for additional support. Many family carers adjust rapidly following the death of the person with dementia. This adjustment has been attributed to remarkable resilience, possibly due to the prolonged period of caring before death, giving rise to a sense of relief following their loved one's demise (Schulz et al 2003).

During the assessment process it is necessary to establish which family carer is the legal substitute decision-maker for the person with dementia, able to give consent for medical and dental treatments. Legal requirements vary within Australia, and differ also from New Zealand, so the nurse needs to inquire locally about the legal standard for consent. Failure to identify the correct person may result in medico–legal difficulties and family conflict when the person with dementia is unable to make their own decisions (Peisah et al 2006). Disputes about treatment, or the absence of a legal substitute decision-maker, require intervention from a legal authority, such as a guardianship board or similar, to make decisions in the best interests of the person with dementia. Rebecca's husband (Case Study 15.1) appears to be the substitute decision-maker for his wife. If he does not have legal authority to consent to treatments being given or withheld, then his decisions about his wife's care can be challenged.

Interventions to Assist Family Carers

James's wife (Case Study 15.2) was exhausted by her caring role, and as James's medical condition deteriorated, her quality of life and wellbeing were also being eroded, to the point that her children implored her to admit James to a RACF, which she did. What could be done to assist James's wife and other family carers? Effective interventions across the dementia trajectory that have been shown to help family carers, and may delay admission of the person with dementia to a RACF, include giving the family carers information about the course of dementia and what to expect; giving them long-term social support, in the form of counselling and support groups; and improving their problem-solving skills so they can handle new situations as they arise (Mittelman 2005; WHO 2012). Teaching them to

think in a more clinical manner about their role – that is, more objectively – may also help (Hepburn et al 2005). Interventions for family carers are more successful if the person with dementia is also involved (Brodaty et al 2005). A home care program in India (Dias et al 2008) found that providing information to carers on dementia, guidance on behaviour management, a single psychiatric assessment and psychotropic medication if needed, effectively reduced caregiver strain and improved their mental health.

Encouraging the family carer to take a break from their caregiving duties is also beneficial, by providing respite care, which may be available on a daily basis in the home, or a daycare centre; or for longer periods of a few weeks to months at a time, in a RACF, depending on the area in which the person with dementia is living (Guideline Adaptation Committee 2016). While James (Case Study 15.2) lived at home, his wife may have required encouragement to use her respite time to undertake some physical activity, such as a walk, to relieve stress and maintain her own physical health and to attend her own medical and dental appointments as necessary. Now that he has been admitted to a RACF, the staff should encourage her to continue with these activities, as well as encouraging her to eat a healthy diet, get as much sleep as possible and maintain contact with her social circle whenever she can, to reduce social isolation. Not all family carers use available support services, either because they don't think they need them or because they are not aware of their availability. Nurses in all care sites can assist family carers by making sure the family carer receives information and referral to available support services in their area (Brodaty et al 2005).

In terms of caregiver interventions, it is important to conduct a comprehensive assessment of the needs, strengths, weaknesses and available resources to guide the selection of the intervention (WHO 2012).

THE FAMILY CARER ROLE IN PLANNING CARE FOR THE PERSON WITH DEMENTIA

An advance care directive (also called 'advance health-care directive' or 'living will') may be either a document or an oral statement that gives instructions in advance of a health-related event, either consenting to, or refusing, certain treatments if the affected person does not have the capacity to make their own decisions. The legal requirements for making an advance care directive differ in each state and territory of Australia, and in New Zealand, so nurses need to inquire about their local laws in relation to directives.

In both Australia and New Zealand the making of an advance care directive is relatively uncommon, with only 14% of Australians making one (White et al 2014). Findings of the survey of carers (Alzheimer's Australia 2014b) found that 60% reported that the person with dementia they cared for did not have an advance care plan or they were unsure if they did. Nurses working with people with advanced dementia may find that there is no formal advance care directive available when caring for people with dementia and decisions fall to the family carer or other appointed guardian legally responsible for that person. For many carers of people with dementia, not knowing the right decision and being afraid of doing the wrong thing is a major source of stress (Hughes 2013). Having an advance care directive can help ease this stress.

The solution to the lack of a directive is to engage the family carer in a series of conversations about the likely future healthcare needs of the person with dementia, and together reach consensus about a future plan of care that optimises the quality of life and wellbeing of the person with dementia, and utilises a palliative approach to treat symptoms as they arise (Abbey 2013). Family carers may feel unprepared to make difficult end-of-life decisions and lack adequate information about the dementia trajectory (Sampson et al 2010), which is why the focus should be on giving them accurate, honest information during a number of encounters (Abbey 2013). Research evidence remains scant. One study (Koopmans et al 2007) revealed that the majority (85%) of people with dementia die before the very end stage of dementia is reached; and death, regardless of when it occurs, is most commonly associated with cachexia/dehydration (35.2%), cardiovascular disorders (20.9%) and acute pulmonary diseases such as pneumonia (20.1%), so decisions about future treatment or palliation of the symptoms associated with these causes of death need to form part of the plan of care. In the study by Koopmans and colleagues (2007), approximately 9% of people with dementia died of an unknown, acute cause. Nurses therefore also need to help family carers understand that death may occur due to other conditions that may be unpredictable.

An Australian study found that families of dementia patients who had died and who had advance care directives demonstrated less stress, anxiety and depression than those who did not (Detering et al 2010). Thus, despite the reluctance of carers to write plans (Sampson et al 2010), advance care planning appears to be effective in ensuring quality patient care, as well as the wellbeing of carers. Cartwright (2011) developed a publication and a seminar series for Alzheimer's Australia to provide a guide to people with dementia and their families and carers about the legal options that people have available to them to plan their end-of-life care. Such initiatives may help to dispel myths and encourage greater utilisation of advance care plans.

Some evidence that advance care directives have a positive impact on outcome is from the findings of carers and care professionals surveyed on their perceptions of end-of-life care that people with dementia received (Alzheimer's Australia 2014b). In most cases, both family carers and care professionals indicated that the wishes of people with dementia were adhered to. However, 20% of family carers were dissatisfied with adherence to the wishes of the person with dementia, and nearly one-third (31%) of care professionals experienced a situation where they were unable to follow the end-of-life care wishes of a person with dementia. Perceived barriers to providing quality end-of-life care by family carers and care professionals included a lack of documented wishes, legal issues, difficulties with communication, and the culture of the organisation.

CONCLUSION

Advanced dementia brings numerous somatic, affective and behavioural symptoms, impairments and co-morbidities. Diagnosing and managing pain and other symptoms in people with advanced dementia is often made difficult by the communicative difficulties of the person with dementia. Pain and other symptoms may exacerbate the behavioural symptoms of dementia and the uncertain illness trajectory of advanced dementia. Nursing staff, because they are closely involved in the care of the person with dementia, often detect and interpret changes in behaviour that may signal pain. Furthermore, they play a pivotal role in managing the medication regimen of such patients. Adopting a systematic and holistic approach to assessment and management of pain and other symptoms in advanced dementia means that patients are more likely to receive appropriate treatment. These challenges can also point to the need for professional development and training needs for carers. Advance care directives expressing the aged care resident's prospective care preferences would give clinicians clearer guidelines for responding to the patient and would assist in negotiating care decisions with family members.

Acknowledgement

Dr Karen Hancock in all the previous editions. Sally Easterbrook, Megan Luhr and Kathleen Harrison in the first edition.

RECOMMENDED READING

Bjørkløf G, Helvik A, Ibsen T et al 2019. Balancing the struggle to live with dementia: a systematic meta-synthesis of coping. BMC Geriatrics, 19:295 https://doi.org/10.1186/s12877-019-1306-9.

Brooks D, Ross C, Beattie E 2015. Caring for someone with dementia: the economic, social, and health impacts of caring and evidence-based supports for carers. Paper 42 prepared for Alzheimer's Australia. Online. Available: www.dementia.org.au/sites/default/files/NATIONAL/documents/Alzheimers-Australia-Numbered-Publication-42.pdf.

Garrido S, Dunne L, Stevens C et al 2020. Music playlists for people with dementia: trialing a guide for caregivers. Journal of Alzheimer's Disease 77(1) 219–226.

REFERENCES

Abbey J 2013. Wrestling with dementia and death. A report for Alzheimer's Australia. Paper 34 prepared for Alzheimer's Australia. Online. Available: www.dementia.org.au/sites/default/files/NATIONAL/documents/Alzheimers-Australia-Numbered-Publication-34.pdf.

Abbey J, Piller N, Bellis, DE et al 2004. The Abbey Pain Scale: a 1-minute numerical indicator for people with end-stage dementia. International Journal of Palliative Nursing 10(1), 6–13.

Access Economics 2009. Keeping dementia front of mind: Incidence and prevalence 2009–2050. Online. Available: www.dementia.org.au/sites/default/files/20090800_Nat__AE_FullKeepDemFrontMind.pdf.

AGS Panel on Persistent Pain in Older Persons 2002. The management of persistent pain in older persons. Journal of the American Geriatrics Society 50, S205–S224.

Alzheimer's Association 2021. Types of dementia. Online. Available: www.alz.org/dementia/types-of-dementia.asp.

Alzheimer's Australia and the National Aboriginal and Torres Strait Islander Dementia Advisory Group (NATSIDAG) 2015. Continuing the conversation: addressing dementia in Aboriginal and Torres Strait Islander Communities. 2015 National Communique. Online. Available: www.dementia.org.au/sites/default/files/NATIONAL/documents/ATSI-summit-communique.pdf.

Alzheimer's Australia 2014a. End-of-life-care for people with dementia: survey report. Online. Available: www.dementia.org.au/sites/default/files/EOI_ExecSummary_Web_Version.pdf

Alzheimer's Australia 2014b. Living with dementia in the community: challenges and opportunities: a report of national survey findings. September 2014. Online. Available: www.dementia.org.au/sites/default/files/DementiaFriendlySurvey_Final_web.pdf

Alzheimer's Australia NSW 2012. The most difficult decision: dementia and the move into residential aged care. Discussion paper number 5. Online. Available: www.dementia.org.au/sites/default/files/20121016-NSW-PUB-Moving_To_Res_Care.pdf

Alzheimer's Disease International (ADI) 2015. World Alzheimer report 2015. The global impact of dementia an analysis of prevalence, incidence, cost and trends. ADI, London. Online. Available: www.alzint.org/resource/world-alzheimer-report-2015/.

Alzheimer's New Zealand 2013. Reports and statistics. Online. Available: www.alzheimers.org.nz/information/reports-statistics.

Alzheimer's New Zealand & Deloitte 2017. Dementia Economic Impact Report 2016. Deloitte. Online. Available: www.alzheimers.org.nz/getmedia/79f7fd09-93fe-43b0-a837-771027bb23c0/Economic-Impacts-of-Dementia-2017.pdf/.

American Medical Directors Association 2005. Clinical practice guideline: pain management in the long-term care setting. AMA, Columbia, MD.

Aminoff B, Adunsky A 2004. Dying dementia patients: too much suffering, too little palliation. American Journal of Alzheimer's Disease and Other Dementias 19(4), 243–247.

Arroll B, Goodyear-Smith F, Kerse N et al 2005. Effect of the addition of a 'help' question to two screening questions on specificity for diagnosis of depression in general practice: diagnostic validity study. British Medical Journal 331, 884–886A.

Aupperle PM, MacPhee ER, Strozeski JE 2004. Hospice use for the patient with advanced Alzheimer's disease: the role of the geriatric psychiatrist. American Journal of Alzheimer's Disease and Other Dementias 19, 94–104.

Australian Bureau of Statistics (ABS) 2020. Causes of death, Australia 2019: Cat no. 3303.0. Online. Available: www.abs.gov.au/ausstats.

Australian Government Department of Health 2016. Ageing and aged care programs. Online. Available: https://agedcare.health.gov.au/programs.

Australian Government Department of Health and Ageing (DHA) 2006. Guidelines for a palliative approach in residential aged care enhanced version. DHA, Canberra.

Australian Institute of Health and Welfare (AIHW) 2020. Dementia snapshot. Online. Available: https://www.aihw.gov.au/reports/australias-health/dementia

Australian Institute of Health and Welfare (AIHW) 2012. Dementia in Australia. Online. Available: www.aihw.gov.au/getmedia/199796bc-34bf-4c49-a046-7e83c24968f1/13995.pdf.aspx?inline=true

Australian Pain Society 2005. Pain in residential aged care facilities. Management strategies. Online. Available: www.apsoc.org.au/Pain-in-RACF2-Resources

Black BS, Finucane T, Baker A et al 2006. Health problems and correlates of pain in nursing home residents with advanced dementia. Alzheimer Disease and Associated Disorders 20(4), 283–290.

Boller F, Verny M, Hugonot-Diener L et al 2002. Clinical features and assessment of severe dementia. A review. European Journal of Neurology 9(2), 125–136.

Bradford A, Shrestha S, Snow AL et al 2012. Managing pain to prevent aggression in people with dementia: a non-pharmacologic intervention. American Journal of Alzheimer's Disease and Other Dementias 27(1), 41–47.

Brodaty H, Green A 2002. Defining the role of the caregiver in Alzheimer's s disease treatment. Drugs and Aging 19(12), 891–898.

Brodaty H, Thomson C, Thompson C et al 2005. Why caregivers of people with dementia and memory loss don't use services. International Journal of Geriatric Psychiatry 20(6), 537–546.

Brooks D, Ross C, Beattie E 2015. Caring for someone with dementia: the economic, social, and health impacts of caring and evidence based supports for carers. Paper 42. Prepared for Alzheimer's Australia. Online. Available: www.dementia.org.au/sites/default/files/NATIONAL/documents/Alzheimers-Australia-Numbered-Publication-42.pdf.

Burns M, McIlfatrick S 2015. Nurses' knowledge and attitudes towards pain assessment for people with dementia in a nursing home setting. International Journal of Palliative Nursing 21(10), 479–487.

Cartwright C 2011. Planning for the end of life for people with dementia: a report for Alzheimer's Australia. Alzheimer's Australia. Online. Available: www.dementia.org.au/sites/default/files/start2talk/5.0.4.10%20Cartwright_Planning%20for%20the%20end%20of%20life_%20Part%20one.pdf.

Cervo F, Bruckenthal P, Chen J et al 2009. Pain assessment in nursing home residents with dementia: psychometric properties and clinical utility of the CNA pain assessment tool CPAT. Journal of the American Medical Directors Association 10(7), 505–510.

Chang A, Walter LC 2010. Recognizing dementia as a terminal illness in nursing home residents. Archives of Internal Medicine 170(13), 1107–1109.

Chang EM, Daly J, Johnson A et al 2009. Challenges for professional care of advanced dementia. International Journal of Nursing Practice 15(1), 41–47.

Cohen-Mansfield J, Lipson S 2008. The utility of pain assessment for analgesic use in persons with dementia. Pain 134(1–2), 16–23.

Corbett A, Nunez K, Smeaton E et al 2016. The landscape of pain management in people with dementia living in care homes: a mixed methods study. International Journal of Geriatric Psychiatry Online 31(12), 1354–1370.

Cunningham C 2006. Managing pain in patients with dementia in hospital. Nursing Standard 46, 54–58.

Deloitte Access Economics 2015. The economic value of informal care in Australia in 2015. Carers Australia.

Dementia Australia 2020. Media release: No longer a statistic. Online. Available: https://www.dementia.org.au/about-us/news-and-stories/news/no-longer-statistic-0

Detering K, Hancock A, Reade MC et al 2010. The impact of advance care planning on the end of life care in elderly patients: randomized controlled trial. British Medical Journal 340, 847.

Dias A, Dewey ME, D'Souza J et al 2008. The effectiveness of a home care program for supporting caregivers of persons with dementia in developing countries: a randomised controlled trial from Goa, India. PLoS ONE 3(6), e2333. Online. Available: www.plosone.org/article/info%3Adoi%2F10.1371%2Fjournal.pone.0002333.

Dixon N 2017 Dementia Economic Impact Report. Deloitte Access Economics 2016 published in March 2017.

Dyall L 2014. Dementia: continuation of health and ethnic inequalities in New Zealand. The New Zealand Medical Journal 27(1389), 68–80.

Erickson HL 2007. Philosophy and theory of holism. Nursing Clinics of North America 42, 139–163.

Evans BD 2002. Improving palliative care in the nursing home: from a dementia perspective. Journal of Hospice and Palliative Nursing 4(2), 91–102.

Feldt KS, Warne MA, Ryden MB 1998. Examining pain in aggressive cognitively impaired older adults. Journal of Gerontological Nursing 24(11), 14–22.

Ferrell BA 1995. Pain evaluation and management in the nursing home. Annals of Internal Medicine 123, 681–687.

Flicker L, Holdsworth K 2014. Aboriginal and Torres Strait Islander people and dementia: a review of the research. A report for Alzheimers Australia. Paper 41, October 2014.

Frondini C, LanFranchi G, Minardi M et al 2007. Affective, behavior and cognitive disorders in the elderly with chronic musculoskeletal pain: the impact on an aging population. Archives of Gerontology and Geriatrics 44 (Suppl. 1), 167–171.

Fuchs-Lacelle S, Hadjistravropoulos T 2004. Development and preliminary validation of the pain assessment checklist for seniors with limited ability to communicate PASLAC. Pain Management in Nursing 5, 37–49.

Gandy S, Sano M 2015. Solanezumab – prospects for meaningful interventions in AD? Nature Reviews. Neurology 11(12), 669–670.

Gove D, Sparr S, Dos Santos Bernardo A et al 2010. Recommendations on end-of-life care for people with dementia. The Journal of Nutrition, Health and Aging 14(2), 136–139.

Grand J, Caspar S, MacDonald S 2011. Clinical features and multidisciplinary approaches to dementia care. Journal of Multidisciplinary Healthcare 4, 125–147.

Guberman N, Keefe J, Fancey P et al 2000. CARE tool and caregiver risk screen. University Institute of Social Gerontology, Centre de recherché sur les services communautaires CLSC René Cassin. Online. Available: www.msvu.ca.

Guideline Adaptation Committee 2016. Clinical practice guidelines and principles of care for people with dementia. Sydney.

Haasum Y, Fastbom J, Fratiglioni L et al 2011. Pain treatment in elderly persons with and without dementia: a population-based study of institutionalized and home-dwelling elderly. Drugs and Aging 28(4), 283–293.

Hadjistravropoulos T, Herr K, Turk D et al 2007. An interdisciplinary expert consensus statement on assessment of pain in older persons. The Clinical Journal of Pain 23(1), S1–S43.

Hebert R, Dang Q, Schulz R 2006. Preparedness for the death of a loved one and mental health in bereaved caregivers of patients with dementia: findings from the REACH study. Journal of Palliative Medicine 9(3), 683–693.

Hepburn KW, Lewis M, Narayan S et al 2005. Partners in caregiving: a psychoeducation program affecting dementia family caregivers' distress and caregiving outlook. Clinical Gerontologist 29(1), 53–69.

Herr K, Bjoro K, Decker S 2006. Tools for assessment of pain in nonverbal older adults with dementia: a state-of-the-science review. Journal of Pain and Symptom Management 31(2), 170–192.

Herr K, Coyne P, McCaffery M et al 2011. Pain assessment in the patient unable to self-report: position statement with clinical practice recommendations. Pain Management Nursing 12(4), 230–250.

Hughes J 2013. Models of dementia care: person-centred, palliative and supportive. A discussion paper for Alzheimer's Australia on death and dementia. Paper 35 June 2013. Online. Available: www.dementia.org.au/sites/default/files/NATIONAL/documents/Alzheimers-Australia-Numbered-Publication-35.pdf

Hurley AC, Volicer BJ, Hanrahan PA et al 1992. Assessment of discomfort in advanced Alzheimer patients. Research in Nursing and Health 15, 369–377.

Jansen B, Brazil K, Passmore P et al 2017. Exploring healthcare assistants' role and experience in pain assessment and management for people with advanced dementia towards the end of life: a qualitative study. BMC Palliative Care 16(6). Online. Available: https://doi.org/10.1186/s12904-017-0184-1

Johnson A, Chang E, Daly J et al 2009. The communication challenges faced in adopting a palliative care approach in advance dementia. International Journal of Nursing Practice 15(5), 467–474.

Johnson F 2016. Exploring the lived experience of people with dementia through interpretive phenomenological analysis. The Qualitative Report 21(4), 695–711.

Jordan A, Hughes J, Pakresi M et al 2011. The utility of PAINAID in assessing pain in a UK population with severe dementia. International Journal of Geriatric Psychiatry 26(2), 118–263.

Kerr S, Chenoweth L 2003. Pain management. In: R Hudson (ed.), Dementia nursing: a guide to practice. Ausmed Publications, Melbourne.

Kindell J, Sage K, Wilkinson R et al 2014. Living with semantic dementia: a case study of one's family experience. Qualitative Health Research 24(3), 401–411.

Klebanoff N 2013. Holistic nursing: focusing on the whole person. American Nurse Today 8(10).

Kolanowski AM, Whall AL 2000. Toward holistic-theory based intervention for dementia behavior. Holistic Nursing Practice 14(2), 67–76.

Koopmans RT, van der Sterren KJ, van der Steen JT 2007. The 'natural' endpoint of dementia: death from cachexia or dehydration following palliative care? International Journal of Geriatric Psychiatry 22, 350–355.

Kovach C, Weissman D, Griffie J et al 1999. Assessment and treatment of discomfort for people with late-stage dementia. Journal of Pain and Symptom Management 18, 412–419.

Kovach CR, Cashin JR, Sauer L 2006. Deconstruction of a complex tailored intervention to assess and treat discomfort of people with advanced dementia. Journal of Advanced Nursing 55(6), 678–688.

Kovach CR, Logan B, Noonan PE et al 2006. Effects of the serial trial intervention on discomfort and behavior in demented nursing home residents. American Journal of Alzheimer's Disease and Other Dementias 21(3), 147–155.

Kovach CR, Noonan PE, Schildt AM et al 2006. The serial trial intervention: an innovative approach of meeting needs of individuals with dementia. Journal of Gerontological Nursing 32(4), 18–26.

Kupper AL, Hughes J 2011. The challenges of providing palliative care for older people with dementia. Current Oncology Reports 13, 295–301.

Lefebvre-Chapiro S, The Doloplus Group 2001. The Doloplus–2 scale – evaluating pain in the elderly. European Journal of Palliative Care 8, 191–194.

Lindeman M, Smith K, LoGiudice D et al 2017. Community care of Indigenous people: an update. Australasian Journal of Ageing 36(2), 124–127.

Long C 2009. Palliative care for advanced dementia. Approaches that work. Journal of Gerontological Nursing 35(11), 19–24.

Maher D, Hemming L 2005. Understanding patient and family: holistic assessment in palliative care. British Journal of Community Nursing 10(7), 318–322.

Mahoney A, Peters L 2008. The Mahoney pain scale: examining pain and agitation in advanced dementia. American Journal of Alzheimer's Disease and Other Dementias 23, 250–261.

Malotte K, McPherson M 2016. Identification, assessment, and management of pain in patients with advanced dementia. Mental Health Clinician 6(2), 89–94. https://doi.org/10.9740/mhc.2016.03.89.

Mariano C 2007. Holistic nursing as a specialty: holistic nursing – scope and standards for practice. The Nursing Clinics of North America 42(2), 165–188.

Mathys M 2018. Pharmacologic management of behavioral and psychological symptoms of major neurocognitive disorder. Mental Health Clinician 8(6), 284–293. Doi: https://doi.org/10.9740/mhc.2018.11.284.

McCaffrey M 1968. Nursing practice theories related to cognition, bodily pain, and man-environment interactions. UCLA Students Store, Los Angeles.

McClean W 2000. Practice guide for pain management for people with dementia in institutional care. The Dementia Services Development Centre, University of Stirling, Stirling.

Merkel SI, Voepel-Lewis T, Shayevitz JR et al 1997. Practice applications of research The FLACC: a behavioural scale for postoperative pain in young children. Pediatric Nursing 23, 293–297.

Mitchell SL, Teno JM, Kiely DK 2009. The clinical course of advanced dementia. New England Journal of Medicine 361(16), 1529–1538.

Mittelman M 2005. Taking care of the caregivers. Current Opinion in Psychiatry 18(6), 633–639.

Mittelman MS, Haley WE, Clay OJ et al 2006. Improving caregiver well-being delays nursing home placement of patients with Alzheimer disease. Neurology 14,67(9), 1592–1599.

Montine T, Adesina A, Sonnen J 2019. Dementia pathology. Online. Available: https://emedicine.medscape.com/article/2003174overview.

Mormino E, Sperling R, Holmes A et al 2016. Polygenic risk of Alzheimer disease is associated with early- and late-life processes. Neurology 87(5), 481–488.

Morris JK, Burns JM 2012. Insulin: an emerging treatment for Alzheimer's disease dementia? Current Neurology and Neuroscience Reports 12, 520–527.

New Zealand Guidelines Group 2003. Assessment processes for older people. Online. Available: www.health.govt.nz/publication/assessment-processes-older-people

Nuffield Council on Bioethics 2009. Dementia: ethical issues. Nuffield Council on Ethics. Online. Available: www.nuffieldbioethics.org/wp-content/uploads/2014/07/Dementia-report-Oct-09.pdf.

Nugent J 2005. A passion for caring: applying holistic skills in dementia care. NurseLink Australia, Adelaide.

O'Brien-King M, Gates MF 2007. Teaching holistic nursing: the legacy of Nightingale. Nursing Clinics of North America 42(2), 309–333.

Parmelee PA 1996. Pain in cognitively impaired older persons. Clinical Geriatric Medicine 12, 473–487.

Pasero C, McCaffery M 2011. Pain assessment and pharmacological management. Mosby, St Louis.

Peisah C, Brodaty H, Quadrio C 2006. Family conflict in dementia: prodigal sons and black sheep. International Journal of Geriatric Psychiatry 21(5), 485–492.

Petriwskyj A, Gibson A, Webby G 2015. Staff members' negotiation of power in client engagement: analysis of practice within an Australian aged care service. Journal of Aging Studies 33, 37–46.

Pieper M, Achterberg W, Francke A et al 2011. The implementation of the serial trial intervention for pain and challenging behavior in advanced dementia patients (STA OP!) a cluster randomized trial. BMC Geriatrics. Online. Available: https://bmcgeriatr.biomedcentral.com/articles/10.1186/1471-2318-11-12

Practical Nursing Organisation 2020. The importance of holistic nursing care: how to completely care for your patients. Online. Available: https://.practicalnursing.org/importance-holistic-care-how-completely-care-patients.

Rabins PV, Lyketsos CG, Steele CD 2006. Practical dementia care, 2nd ed. Oxford University Press, New York.

RegisteredNursing.org 2020. Holistic nurse. Online. Available: www.registerednursing.org/specialty/holistic-nurse/

Reynolds KS, Hanson LC, DeVellis RF et al 2008. Disparities in pain management between cognitively intact and cognitively impaired nursing home residents. Journal of Pain Symptom Management 35, 388–396.

Robinson BC 1983. Validation of a caregiver strain index. Journal of Gerontology 38(3), 344–348.

Sampson E, Jones L, Thune-Boyle I 2010. Palliative assessment and advance care planning in severe dementia: an exploratory randomized controlled trial of a complex intervention. Palliative Medicine 25(3), 197–209.

Schulz R, Mendelsohn AB, Haley WE et al 2003. End-of-life care and the effects of bereavement on family caregivers of persons with dementia. The New England Journal of Medicine 349(20), 1936–1942.

Shega JW, Hougham GW, Stocking CB et al 2006. Management of non-cancer pain in community-dwelling persons with dementia. Journal of the American Geriatrics Society 54(12), 1892–1897.

Sheu E, Versloot J, Nader R et al 2011. Pain in the elderly: validity of facial expression components of observational measures. The Clinical Journal of Pain 27(7), 593–601.

Shuster J 2000. Palliative care for advanced dementia. Clinics in Geriatric Medicine 16(2), 373–386.

Small GW, Greenfield S 2015. Current and future treatments for Alzheimer disease. The American Journal of Geriatric Psychiatry 23, 1101–1105.

Smigorski K, Leszek J 2010. Pain experience and expression in patients with dementia, health management. Online. Available: www.intechopen.com/books/health-management/the-experience-and-expression-of-pain-in-patients-with-dementia.

Smith SJ 1998. Providing palliative care for the terminal Alzheimer patient. In: L Volicer, A Hurley (eds), Hospice care for patients with advanced progressive dementia. Springer Publishing, New York.

Snow AL, Shuster JL Jr 2006. Assessment and treatment of persistent pain in persons with cognitive and communicative impairment. Journal of Clinical Psychology 62(11), 1379–1387.

Snow AL, Weber JB, O'Malley KJ et al 2004. NOPAIN: a nursing assistant-administered pain assessment instrument for use in dementia. Dementia and Geriatric Cognitive Disorders 17, 240–244.

Snowden M, Steinman L, Lesley E et al 2017. Dementia and co-occurring chronic conditions: a systematic literature review to identify what is known and where the gaps in the evidence? International Journal Geriatric Psychiatry 2017, Vol 34(4), 357–371.

Taylor D 2009. Living with medicines for dementia – patient and carer perspectives. Pharmacy Practice Research Trust, University of Bath, UK.

van der Steen J 2010. Dying with dementia: what we know after more than a decade of research. Journal of Alzheimer's Disease 22, 37–55.

Villanueva MR, Smith TL, Erickson JS et al 2003. Pain assessment for the dementing elderly: reliability and validity of a new measure. Journal of the American Medical Directors Association 1–8.

Volicer L, Hurley A 1998. Hospice care for patients with advanced progressive dementia. Springer Publishing, New York.

Warden V, Hurley AC, Volicer L 2003. Development and psychometric evaluation of the pain assessment in advanced dementia scale. Journal of the American Medical Directors Association 4(1), 9–15.

White B, Tilse C, Wilson J et al 2014. Prevalence and predictors of advance directives in Australia. Internal Medicine Journal 44(10), 975–980.

Won AB, Lapane KL, Vallow S et al 2004. Persistent non-malignant pain and analgesic prescribing patterns in elderly nursing home residents. Journal of the American Geriatrics Society 52, 867–874.

World Health Organization (WHO) 2016. Dementia fact sheet. Online. Available: www.who.int/news-room/fact-sheets/detail/dementia

World Health Organization (WHO) 2012. Dementia: a public health priority. WHO, Geneva.

Yap LKP, Seow CCD, Henderson LM et al 2005. Family caregivers and caregiving in dementia. Reviews in Clinical Gerontology 15(3–4), 263–271.

Young DM 2001. Pain in institutionalised elders with chronic dementia. PhD dissertation. University of Iowa, Iowa City.

CHAPTER 16

Principles for Nursing Practice: Stroke

CALEB FERGUSON

LEARNING OBJECTIVES

When you have completed this chapter you will be able to:
- identify established modifiable and non-modifiable stroke risk factors
- understand the underlying pathophysiological mechanisms of stroke
- understand the difference in etiology and treatment between ischaemic and haemorrhagic stroke
- understand primary and secondary stroke prevention strategies
- identify rehabilitation goals in light of cognitive or functional deficits related to stroke.

KEY WORDS

acute stroke care	stroke rehabilitation
haemorrhagic stroke	stroke support
ischaemic stroke	patient education
stroke risk factors	

INTRODUCTION

Stroke is Australia's third largest cause of death and a major contributor to disability (Australian Institute of Health and Welfare [AIHW] 2020). Stroke is a debilitating condition and a huge personal and economic burden, not only for the survivor and their loved ones but for society as a whole. Stroke is often sudden in onset, leaving long-lasting effects from which the individual may never fully recover to their prior level of functioning. Despite the burden of stroke, its modifiable risk factors are well established and so too are its long-term impacts. However, there have been many innovations in stroke care over the last decade. These include innovative models of pre-hospital care (such as stroke ambulances), the advent of multidisciplinary acute stroke units, nursing protocols, thrombolysis and endovascular clot retrieval for acute ischaemic stroke.

This chapter discusses stroke incidence, signs and symptoms, hospital care, diagnosis, types, acute care and rehabilitation issues that may arise during the care trajectory. Two case studies are presented to demonstrate care priorities for two different types of stroke.

STROKE

Stroke is one of the most common causes of death and adulthood disability. The estimated global lifetime risk of stroke is one in four. Those living in East Asia, Central Europe and Eastern Europe are at greatest risk (GBD Lifetime Risk of Stroke Collaborators 2018). However, one in every six people will be impacted by stroke in Australia (Stroke Foundation 2020). Most recent data (2017) shows that in Australia there were 56,000 new and recurrent strokes (Stroke Foundation 2017), which equates to one stroke every nine minutes. In 2017, there were estimated to be 475,000 Australians living with stroke, yet this is predicted to increase to over one million by 2050 (Stroke Foundation 2017). The economic impact of stroke in Australia is estimated to be $5 billion each year. While advanced age is a key risk factor for stroke, stroke does not just affect older adults. The Stroke Foundation (2020) estimates in Australia, one-third of all stroke survivors are of working age (under the age of 65 years). Further, stroke is estimated to kill more women than breast cancer and more men than prostate cancer.

As a consequence, stroke prevention is a health priority, as there are many identified risk factors that can be modified or targeted to save countless lives, as well as lifelong expense. It is estimated approximately 80% of all strokes are preventable (O'Donnell 2016).

Stroke can occur in two main ways, either through a sudden blockage of cerebral arterial blood flow, such as found in ischaemic stroke (80% of cases), or through the rupturing of cerebral arteries in haemorrhagic stroke, such as intracerebral haemorrhage (15%), or subarachnoid haemorrhage (5%) (see Fig. 16.1) (Donnan et al 2008).

Stroke is a condition characterised by the gradual or rapid non-convulsive onset of neurological deficits that fit a known vascular territory and persist beyond 24 hours. This abrupt cessation or alteration in cerebral arterial blood flow directly affects the part of the brain supplied by the artery; consequently there is loss of function which is directly related to the signs and symptoms exhibited by the patient. The physical manifestation of stroke (signs and symptoms) can be transient or permanent, depending on the extent of brain cell death, the patient's existing co-morbidities, how early it is diagnosed, the type of stroke, the area of brain affected, treatment options available, preventing potentially avoidable complications from the stroke and rehabilitation options available.

RISK FACTORS AND PRIMARY PREVENTION

Risk factors for stroke have shared risk factors with common chronic diseases, particularly those involving the cardiovascular system. These can include physiological, social and behavioural determinants. These factors can influence one another, further compounding the devastating effects of stroke. Understanding the following risk factors and actively preventing them (if possible) is considered as primary prevention.

Social Factors

Potential risk factors or vulnerability towards conditions can be avoidable, but due to personal circumstances may be extremely difficult to overcome and can be seen as (personally) unmodifiable. Social determinants have been and will continue to be used to determine an individual's predisposition to conditions such as stroke. Factors associated with social disadvantage, such as level of education, informed health decisions and access to healthcare, all contribute to overall risk (Scanlon & Lee 2007).

Advanced Age

With advancing age also comes the increased risk of stroke (Iadecola et al 2009). The incidence of mortality

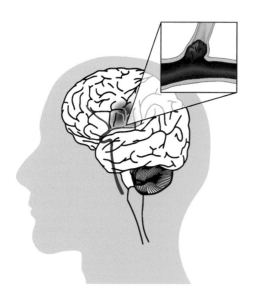 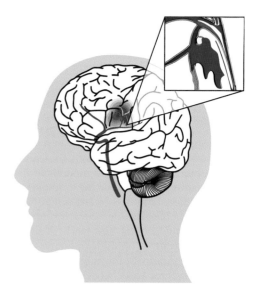

Artery blocked by blood clot
Ischaemic stroke
(embolic and thrombotic)

Artery bursts causing a bleed
Haemorrhagic stroke
(subarachnoid and intracerebral)

FIG. 16.1 **Two Main Types of Stroke 1) Ischaemic and 2) Haemorrhagic.** © National Stroke Foundation.

and ongoing severity morbidity associated with stroke also increases with age (Lloyd-Jones et al 2010).

The National Health and Hospitals Reform Commission commissioned the AIHW to undertake projections of Australian healthcare expenditure. The resulting publication, released in 2008, was to determine health expenditure from 2003 to 2033. In relation to stroke, it projected that although the number of strokes was going to rise over time due to an ageing and growing population to 55.9%, the age-standardised incidence rate of stroke would decline (40.4% and 40.6% for males and females, respectively) (Goss 2008).

Ethnicity

There is evidence that ethnic background is associated with biological predisposition and/or social determinants towards developing certain conditions. In the United States, those of African–American or Hispanic descent (Lloyd-Jones et al 2010) are more likely to experience a stroke than the general population. In Australia, Aboriginal and Torres Strait Islander peoples are up to three times more likely to have a stroke and twice as likely to die from stroke than non-Indigenous Australians (Thrift & Hayman 2007). This may also be related to modifiable determinants of health compounding these risks. In the New Zealand population, Māori/Pacific Islander and Asian/other people are at higher risk of ischaemic stroke, but there are similar rates of subarachnoid haemorrhage across all ethnic groups (Feigin et al 2006).

Family History

Positive family history of conditions has been well established as an indicator for risk. Through ongoing genetic research, numerous genes have been identified as known risk factors for both ischaemic and haemorrhagic stroke (Nahed et al 2007). Unfortunately, the availability of genetic testing and awareness of this particular risk are not widespread. Education is required about the positive outcomes of pre-emptive screening and possible modifiable risk factors.

Sex

Sex differences are commonly seen in most cardiovascular conditions. Men are more likely than women to have a stroke below the age of 65, but after the age of 75 women are at higher risk (Towfighi et al 2007). The reason for this may be related to the failure of many men to have regular check-ups or act on early warning signs and symptoms of conditions such as stroke (Scanlon & Lee 2007). In the age group above

75, women have a tendency to experience more strokes and have worse outcomes (quality of life, depression, disability) than men; the exact reason behind this is not well understood, yet this may be due to differences in clinical presentation or treatment bias, including clinician bias (Gargano & Reeves 2007).

Transient Ischaemic Attack (TIA)

A transient ischaemic attack (TIA) mimics stroke symptoms and is sometimes referred to as a 'mini stroke'. The symptoms last less than 24 hours and spontaneously resolve. The causes of TIAs are predominantly embolisms that can originate from atherosclerotic plaque or thrombosis from elsewhere in the body (such as from atrial fibrillation). TIAs must be comprehensively investigated because of the increased risk of stroke (Lloyd-Jones et al 2010). The risk of stroke after TIA is approximately 5% at 7 days and 10–15% at 90 days (Giles & Rothwell 2007, 2009).

Hypertension

There are numerous clinical consequences of hypertension, none more serious than the associated vascular changes, such as loss of smooth motor function (Iadecola 2009). These changes can weaken (thus rupture) or degrade (through constant vasoconstriction to maintain the hypertensive state) the cerebral vasculature to such an extent that stroke is inevitable. Lowering blood pressure is an effective method for reducing the risk of stroke and subsequent stroke (Lakhan & Sapko 2009).

Hypercholesterolemia

Hypercholesterolemia is of concern due to changes of the vascular system, particularly changes that occur in the cerebral vascular system. However, its direct effects on the cerebral vascular system and stroke are currently widely debated. Regardless of this, the indirect effects can be attributed to the damage caused to the arteries supplying the heart, causing cardiac dysfunction, which may in turn lead to ischaemic stroke through embolisation (Prinz & Endres 2011).

Carotid Stenosis

The increased incidence of clot formation (and thus thrombosis and embolism) associated with stenosis of the carotid arteries also increases the potential for stroke (Altaf et al 2007). This stenosis may also be attributed to the atherosclerotic changes associated with hypercholesterolaemia, as mentioned previously, leading to emboli lodging in (usually) the middle cerebral artery (MCA).

Atrial Fibrillation

Atrial fibrillation (AF) is the most common cardiac arrhythmia, which primarily affects older people and has a tendency to produce emboli secondary to turbulent blood flow in the atria. These in turn are 'flicked off' towards the path of least resistance (aorta – carotid arteries – cerebral arterial circulation) until they can travel no further, lodging in an arterial vessel and causing an embolic stroke. People living with AF have an increased risk of more severe stroke with greater levels of disability (Gattellari et al 2011; Wang et al 2003). It is recommended that patients with AF be treated with anticoagulation to decrease the risk of stroke (Brieger et al 2018; Ferguson et al 2014).

Diabetes

Apart from the well-established effects that diabetes has on all vital functions of the body, its effects on the vascular system in particular not only substantially increase the risk of stroke, but also lead to worse patient outcomes (Giorda et al 2007; Yakubovich & Gerstein 2011). If untreated, hyperglycaemia can further complicate recovery, as it is linked to associated brain oedema, as well as infarct expansion within 24 hours of initial stroke (Baird et al 2003). Oedema related to the infarcted brain tissue expands within the limited space of the cranial vault and causes adjacent brain cells to also be damaged and potentially temporarily or permanently cease functioning.

Tobacco Smoking

Tobacco smoking is a well-established risk factor for all cardiovascular disease (CVD), including stroke (Scanlon 2006). Nicotine, apart from being highly addictive, is also a known carcinogen. The effects of smoking tobacco cause hypertension, tachycardia and vasoconstriction of all arteries. Each of these on its own could cause stroke; together the likelihood is increased. Smokers' risk for stroke is approximately double that of non-smokers (Lloyd-Jones et al 2010).

Excessive Alcohol Consumption

Evidence for the relationship between alcohol use and stroke can be seen as conflicting, as the effects of alcohol can be both beneficial and detrimental. The anticoagulation effect of moderate alcohol use is beneficial for ischaemic stroke, lessening the potential for clot or thrombosis formation (Goldstein & Hankey 2006). However, the overall risk increases exponentially with heavy alcohol use (Reynolds et al 2003), as the increased anticoagulation effect of alcohol use also increases the risk of haemorrhagic stroke.

Overweight and Obesity

There are clear links between obesity and any number of chronic conditions, and stroke is no different. The risk of ischaemic stroke – in particular, stroke caused by atherosclerosis – is increased by 10% to 20% with obesity (Chen et al 2006). Obesity puts the individual at risk of hypertension and diabetes, both known risk factors for stroke, and further increases their potential. Studies have also demonstrated that regular exercise can also reduce the risk of stroke (Gallanagh et al 2011). The current Stroke Foundation recommendation is an hour of exercise on most days of the week.

Other Factors

Hormone replacement therapy (HRT) and the contraceptive pill are associated with an increase of stroke incidence. However, they are not seen as priorities in assessing and preventing stroke (Lloyd-Jones et al 2010).

NURSE-LED CLINICS FOR STROKE

Advanced practice and nurse-practitioner stroke and TIA clinics are becoming common as an innovative model of care. These nurse-coordinated models are evidenced to be cost effective, are favoured by patients and contribute to improved patient outcomes (O'Brien et al 2016). Nurse-led multidisciplinary models of care have demonstrated improved patient outcomes for other chronic cardiovascular disease conditions, including atrial fibrillation, chronic heart failure, diabetes, hypertension and hypercholesterolemia (Hendriks et al 2012; Rich et al 1995; Shaw et al 2014). There is scope to expand such models into stroke prevention and follow-up, through taking an integrated care approach to stroke care.

PRE-HOSPITAL CARE

Of critical importance for stroke survival is appropriate and timely hyperacute and pre-hospital care. International guidelines support this rapid response to presenting symptoms in order to optimise patient outcomes (Hachinski et al 2010; Stroke Foundation 2018). Symptoms associated with stroke should never be ignored, as any delay in diagnosis and treatment can further exacerbate the individual's condition and lead to preventable complications, including death. Mobile stroke unit (MSUs) models for pre-hospital care are becoming more readily available. One of these is the Melbourne Mobile Stroke Unit. This service has reduced time to thrombolysis therapy and provided earlier access to endovascular clot retrieval services.

While relatively innovative and not widely available, these models of care have the potential to revolutionise pre-hospital care, and contribute to reduced stroke disability and improved patient outcomes when scaled nationally (Zhao et al 2020).

Signs and Symptoms of Stroke

Alteration in blood flow is directly attributed to a sudden loss of function, demonstrated by common signs and symptoms. These can include:

- weakness, numbness or paralysis of the face, arm or leg on either or both sides of the body
- difficulty speaking or understanding (expressive and receptive aphasia)
- dizziness, loss of balance or an unexplained fall
- loss of vision, or sudden blurred or decreased vision in one or both eyes
- headache, usually severe and sudden in onset, or unexplained change in the pattern of headaches
- difficulty swallowing (dysphagia) (Stroke Foundation 2020).

Stroke symptoms typically last more than 24 hours or result in death (not to be confused with TIAs, which last less than 24 hours). The Stroke Foundation has developed a public media campaign to increase awareness around stroke and what to do. The campaign (which started in 2006) is aimed at presenting the symptoms of stroke simply, allowing for assessment that could be performed by anyone, thus increasing the likelihood of rapid assessment and appropriate treatment (Stroke Foundation 2020). The campaign is based on the acronym FAST:

- Facial weakness – can the person smile? Has their mouth or eye drooped?
- Arm weakness – can the person raise both arms?
- Speech difficulty – can the person speak clearly and understand what you say?
- Time to act fast – seek medical attention immediately (Stroke Foundation 2020).

This process allows the assessor to decide on the appropriate action for their patient or loved one as quickly as possible, as there is a very small window of opportunity in which to seek treatment to reverse or lessen the potentially devastating and fatal side effects of stroke.

DIAGNOSIS

Once clinical signs and symptoms of stroke are present the individual has a very limited amount of time to receive time-critical treatment to obtain maximum benefit. This time frame has been conservatively estimated at 2 hours (Adams et al 2007). On presenting to the emergency department (ED), rapid assessment and diagnosis should be performed to exclude all other possibilities. Signs and symptoms of stroke do mimic other possible life-threatening conditions, and differential diagnosis to stroke can include, but is not limited to, traumatic brain injury, migraine, hypoglycaemia, seizure, brain tumour and systemic infection. The first and most definitive diagnostic test is the computed tomography (CT) scan. A CT scan can at least differentiate very quickly between ischaemic and haemorrhagic stroke, as well as other possible diagnoses such as brain tumour or trauma. Haemorrhagic strokes often have telltale signs of acute blood characterised by a white appearance, or hyperdense regions anywhere within the cerebrospinal fluid pathways (the ventricles, gyri and sulci, etc.), whereas ischaemic stroke areas of infarction may appear dark or hypodense within normal structures of the brain (Wardlaw et al 2004). Sometimes, however, ischaemic stroke may not be evident on a CT scan for up to 48 hours after initial symptoms are present (Frizzell 2005). At this point treatment for stroke diverges. If a CT scan excludes haemorrhagic stroke or other differential diagnosis, then appropriate treatment is commenced. If it confirms haemorrhagic stroke then further investigation is necessary to determine the source of the bleed. This is usually performed by angiography, which can be done by CT scan or magnetic resonance imaging (MRI) scans, but most commonly is done with fluoroscopy digital subtraction. Angiography of the cerebral arteries allows visualisation of abnormalities such as aneurysms or arteriovenous malformations.

TYPES OF STROKE

Ischaemic Stroke

Ischaemic strokes account for the vast majority of all strokes – between 80 and 85% (Therapeutic Guidelines Limited 2011). Its presentation is similar to haemorrhagic, but its treatment is very different due to the nature of the cerebral blood flow disruption. The three main types of ischaemic stroke are thrombotic, lacunar and embolic.

- *Thrombotic stroke* is usually a result of atherosclerosis weakening the cerebral artery wall to such an extent that a thrombus forms and eventually blocks the artery. This type of stroke accounts for roughly 30% of all strokes and predominantly affects large vessels of the brain (Therapeutic Guidelines Limited 2011).
- *Lacunar stroke* accounts for about 15% of all strokes and is regarded as a subtype of the thrombotic

stroke (Therapeutic Guidelines Limited 2011). The reason for this is that it develops in a similar way to thrombotic stroke, but on smaller vessels usually in and around the brain stem.

- *Embolic stroke* occurs as a result of an embolism travelling into the cerebral circulation and eventually becoming lodged in the capillary bed, leading to loss of blood flow and cell death. These emboli frequently come from the heart due to atrial fibrillation, artificial heart valves or myocardial infarction. They can also occur due to other cardiovascular disorders such as deep vein thrombosis or through surgery or trauma that frees particles of adipose tissue or air bubbles. This type of stroke accounts for approximately 20% of all strokes (Therapeutic Guidelines Limited 2011).

There are also strokes that can occur from rare conditions such as dissection, venous infarction and vasculopathies, accounting for approximately 5% of all strokes. There are also strokes that develop from unknown causes, which make up about 15% of all strokes (Therapeutic Guidelines Limited 2011).

Haemorrhagic Stroke

Haemorrhagic stroke accounts for approximately 15–20% of all strokes and over 50% of the mortality related to all strokes (Therapeutic Guidelines Limited 2011). Its devastating effects require at times both medical and neurosurgical intervention. This type of stroke includes both intracerebral haemorrhage (10% of all strokes) and subarachnoid haemorrhage (SAH) (5% of all strokes) (Therapeutic Guidelines Limited 2011). Both types of haemorrhagic stroke occur due to ruptured blood vessels. This can be attributed to trauma, but more commonly it is weakened cerebral vessels as a result of atherosclerotic changes, hypertension, congenital malformations and a mixture of previous causes, or can also be idiopathic.

SAH affects approximately 6.5 people per 100 000 throughout Australia and New Zealand every year (Brophy et al 2000) with devastating effects. Usually SAH is caused by a weakened blood vessel, which may be berry-like in shape, have an appearance of a general weakening of one particular area (fusiform) or by arteriovenous malformation (AVM). An AVM affects cerebral vasculature in such a way that it is both arterial and venous in nature. This 'mixed' circulation causes the vessels to develop into multiple fistula-like formations that also drastically weaken them, particularly to increases of pressure. Once ruptured, there is an increased risk of re-bleed shortly after the initial event, as well as cerebral vasospasm (which can induce an

ischaemic stroke up to 28 days post initial SAH), hydrocephalus and hyponatraemia associated with the initial and any subsequent bleeds (Diringer 2009).

ACUTE STROKE CARE

Once the stroke has been defined as being ischaemic or haemorrhagic, ongoing treatment is determined. The two types of stroke require very different approaches to care as there are contraindications for some treatment modalities in both. Despite the differences in approach, however, there is clear evidence in both cases for the need for specialist stroke care, usually in the form of a dedicated stroke unit within a large public hospital. These units are characterised by a focus on rapid, comprehensive assessment and early management, utilising a multidisciplinary team (Adams et al 2007; Hachinski et al 2010; Stroke Foundation 2018). High-level evidence supports the existence of these highly specialised units, which have been shown to improve overall patient outcomes (Lakhan & Sapko 2009) by reducing associated mortality by approximately 20%. In comparison with less organised services, these specialised units also have reduced rates of morbidity (Lakhan & Sapko 2009; Therapeutic Guidelines Limited 2011).

Ischaemic Stroke Care

The principles of ischaemic stroke care are to reduce and try to re-establish cerebral health; prevent any further formation of clots, cerebral oedema, increase cerebral perfusion, control for pain and protect from further damage the area of the body that now has the resultant neurological deficit.

Acute treatment for ischaemic stroke requires initial dissolving of the clot (thrombosis or embolism) in the acute stage, commonly referred to as thrombolytic or 'clot buster' therapy, but this must be administered within a very short period after onset of symptoms. Intravenous alteplase (t-PA) has been shown to improve long-term outcomes in both morbidity and mortality for selected patients (van der Worp & van Gijn 2007). The criteria for determining who is eligible for t-PA are as follows:

- ischaemic stroke confirmed (by CT or MRI scan)
- onset of symptoms is within the previous 4.5 hours
- no major changes of early ischaemia (on CT or MRI scan)
- no other contraindication for thrombolytic therapy:
  - bleeding disorder
  - recent peptic ulceration
  - serious medical condition
  - recent surgery

- the availability of a specialised stroke unit or high dependency unit care
- aggressive treatment of hypertension
- frequent monitoring of blood pressure
- neurological assessment (including Glasgow Coma Scale)
- close monitoring for at least 24 hours post-infusion (Stroke Foundation 2018; Therapeutic Guidelines Limited 2011).

Clot retrieval or embolectomy is another novel treatment for acute ischaemic stroke. This therapy is very much in its infancy, and is available for a select group of eligible patients only. At present, this therapy is only available in some metropolitan hospitals in capital cities within Australia; however, due to improvements in systems such as ambulance directs and telehealth, hopefully we will see greater use of such innovative therapies.

The use of aspirin within 48 hours of ischaemic stroke has been shown to reduce mortality/morbidity to approximately one death or recurrent stroke per 100 people in the first few weeks (Therapeutic Guidelines Limited 2011). Aspirin works by inhibiting thromboxanes, which are substances that influence platelet aggregation and thus clot formation. However, aspirin cannot be used in conjunction with thrombolytic therapies.

Evidence-Based, Nurse-Managed Acute Stroke Protocols

A study by Middleton and colleagues (2011) identified the importance of managing fever, hyperglycaemia and swallowing function in the acute stroke setting. Their study demonstrated that multidisciplinary evidence-based protocols commenced by nurses for managing fever, hyperglycaemia and swallowing dysfunction led to improved patient outcomes, including reduced mortality and improved function outcomes. This underscores the importance of nurses regulating normal temperature and adequately managing fever, conducting a simple swallow screen and referral to a speech pathologist on admission, and managing blood sugar levels in patients with acute ischaemic stroke.

PREVENTION OF SECONDARY COMPLICATIONS

Graduated Compression Stockings

The prevention of secondary complications, such as respiratory complications, pneumonia and venous thromboembolism, is of primary importance in the acute setting. There are a few evidence-based strategies that reduce the risk of venous thromboembolism (e.g. deep vein thrombosis (DVT), and pulmonary embolism (PE)). These include the application of graduate compression stockings, intermittent calf compression and subcutaneous anticoagulation with heparin or enoxaparin. The efficacy of graduate compression stockings for DVT prophylaxis remains a controversial practice given the recent results of CLOTS Trial 1, which did not support the use of thigh-length stockings in patients admitted to hospital with acute stroke. Further, CLOTS Trial 2 did not provide evidence of overall benefit or harm of the use of graduated compression stockings after stroke (CLOTS Trial Collaboration 2013). The current Stroke Foundation Guidelines (2018) offer limited recommendations on the application of graduated compression stockings; however, advise against thigh-length stocking application. Early mobilisation and adequate hydration are highlighted as key recommendations in the prevention of DVT and PE.

Oral Health

Maintaining oral health immediately post-stroke and during rehabilitation is critical. Two-thirds of stroke survivors will have a level of cognitive or functional disability after their stroke event and may require support and assistance to achieve optimal oral care, where self-care is not able or optimal. Informal caregivers and family members should be educated and trained to support stroke survivors undertake this important personal care.

Secondary Prevention

Follow-up therapy has been shown to decrease the likelihood of future strokes. It is termed secondary prevention, while primary prevention is used to prevent initial stroke.

Secondary prevention usually involves (Davis & Donnan 2012; Therapeutic Guidelines Limited 2011):
- anti-platelet therapy
- aspirin or clopidogrel
- anti-hypertension therapy, if hypertension is evident
- anticoagulation, if atrial fibrillation is diagnosed
- smoking cessation
- treatment of hypercholesterolaemia
- carotid endarterectomy, for carotid stenosis.

HAEMORRHAGIC STROKE CARE

The principles of haemorrhagic stroke care are to correct the site of rupture (if possible), reduce any associated intracranial pressure and cerebral oedema, manage the unconscious patient, maintain airways and breathing, and reduce pain from headache.

Once the stroke is identified as haemorrhagic, consultation is sought by the patient's parent unit (usually a medical or dedicated stroke unit) for neurosurgical services for intervention. If a clearly defined cause is apparent through diagnosis investigation, be it an aneurysm or AVM, then corrective surgery, such as clipping on endovascular coiling of the damaged vessel, is an option. If there is no clear reason for the haemorrhage, further investigation is warranted. Regardless of the outcome of the investigations, aggressive blood pressure lowering must be initiated to reduce haematoma expansion (Bederson et al 2009; Therapeutic Guidelines Limited 2011). However, if the bleed is large, a craniectomy and evacuation of the clot, or drainage of bloodstained cerebrospinal fluid (which may cause hydrocephalus) through the insertion of an external ventricular drain, may need to be performed to relieve pressure on the already damaged brain. Those suffering from an SAH of aneurysmal origin are at an increased risk of cerebral vasospasm, which may cause further stroke. Cerebral vasospasm should be aggressively treated and once an aneurysm is stabilised, hypertensive and hypervolemic therapy should be commenced to improve perfusion and dilation of cerebral vessels (Therapeutic Guidelines Limited 2011).

IMPACT OF STROKE

Stroke impacts individuals in many different ways. It may affect a person's mobility, ability to undertake activities of daily living (ADLs), their relationships and family, their emotions and psychological functioning and wellbeing (see Fig. 16.2).

REHABILITATION

Approximately 25–30% of stroke patients are candidates for comprehensive rehabilitation (Good et al 2011). Stroke rehabilitation is individual to each patient and is dependent on a number of factors, including the type of stroke (ischaemic or haemorrhagic), the area of brain affected, size of stroke, pre-existing co-morbidities and/or risk factors and initiation of appropriate treatment and complications immediately after the stroke. However, there are some common problems that are universal to stroke rehabilitation.

- Movement:
  - limb spasticity or contracture
  - loss of motor strength or sensation
  - loss of balance

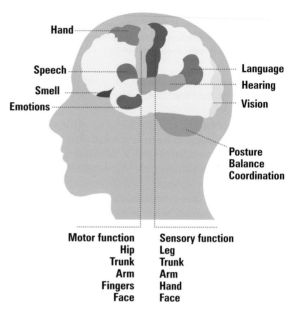

Different function areas of the brain

Hand

Speech

Smell

Emotions

Language

Hearing

Vision

Posture
Balance
Coordination

Motor function	Sensory function
Hip	Leg
Trunk	Trunk
Arm	Arm
Fingers	Hand
Face	Face

FIG. 16.2 **The Impact of Stroke.** © National Stroke Foundation.

- dysphagia
- VTE and DVT prevention
- pressure injury prevention.
- Cognition:
  - changes in attention span or memory
  - fatigue
  - agnosia or apraxia
  - aphasia
  - alterations in mood
  - fear, anxiety and depression
  - incontinence.

Therefore, rehabilitation and effective discharge planning should be directed at achieving the maximum level of function to undertake ADLs, drive, return to work, pursue leisure activities and enjoy a sexual life (Stroke Foundation 2018). It may be that maximal recovery will not be achieved because of a lack of provision of services available in some areas of Australia and internationally (Hachinski et al 2010), and so the nurse has a responsibility to ensure that the patient is appropriately referred to services prior to discharge from hospital.

Apart from ongoing physical therapy, the patient will also need ongoing services in relation to respite care, outpatient visits to speech and occupational therapy or psychology services, and perhaps assistance with home duties, transport or cooking (Good 2011). The nurse discharging the patient will have a critical role in facilitating the forging of these links to ensure ongoing care is delivered and so make the transition to home effective.

Brain repair and recovery after stroke involves a process of axonal sprouting in connected cortical neurons and, in basic terms, occurs when neural connections take over lost functions secondary to stroke (Benowitz & Carmichael 2010; Carmichael 2010). As a result, a reorganisation of motor, sensory, language and other cognitive operations within the brain can occur (Benowitz & Carmichael 2010). This is possibly further facilitated by skill learning through rehabilitation exercises.

Physical repair and functional recovery commonly occur in the weeks and months after stroke (Benowitz & Carmichael 2010). The extent of this recovery will initially be determined by the resolution of the ischaemic area surrounding the infarction and the ability of the brain to reorganise itself in such a way that new areas of the brain can perform functions originally performed by the now damaged area.

Better results seem to correlate with early and frequent practices of simple skills that stimulate the use of the affected muscle groups (Krakauer 2006). Indeed, Krakauer referred to research that demonstrates recovery is maximised when the skills that are designed to be practised can be varied in some way (e.g. reaching for a glass and reaching for a toothbrush), and so enabling memory about more general applications of the skill, which then can be applied to ADLs. Further, success may be achieved if the practice sessions are punctuated with rest periods that are more frequent and longer as time goes on, allowing motor memory of these activities to be formed.

The recovery phase is characterised by a reduction in cerebral oedema and an increased activation of the neuronal network (Rijntjes 2006). There is an initial increased neuronal activity of the unaffected side, which, when this level of activity has peaked, is then followed by increased neuronal activity of the affected side (Rijntjes 2006). This activity seems to be at the basis of reorganisation. Reorganisation of the brain involves areas of the brain performing functions they did not previously perform (Krakauer 2006).

Thus recovery is the result of several factors: spontaneous recovery of areas that were previously swollen but not damaged; focused rehabilitation interventions to facilitate motor learning; and compensation, which is the use of alternative muscle groups to achieve the same end; for example, using the right hand instead of the left to pick something up. For motor recovery, for example, the stroke sufferer needs to learn the sequence of movements, along with velocity, which is achieved by using visual and proprioceptive cues (Krakauer 2006).

The result is to reduce the level of physical impairment through the minimisation of cerebral damage. In addition, the rehabilitation process assists the sufferer to overcome the consequences of any residual physical impairment through reorganisation or motor learning.

The nurse's role in rehabilitation comprises numerous functions and brings a distinctive holistic perspective to the patient care process (Miller et al 2010). As the Nursing and Midwifery Board of Australia (NMBA) Registered Nurse Standards for Practice (2018) describes, a registered nurse:

- thinks critically and analyses nursing practice, engages in therapeutic and professional relationships and maintains the capability for practice
- comprehensively conducts patient assessments, develops and actions a plan for care
- provides safe, appropriate and quality nursing care and evaluates outcomes.

As members of the interdisciplinary stroke rehabilitation team, RNs are responsible for identifying, developing and then implementing treatment plans to address therapy goals for stroke survivors. This is in addition to their role in the management of co-morbid existing conditions (that were present) prior to, complicated by, or directly attributed to the stroke (Miller et al 2010).

PATIENT AND CAREGIVER EDUCATION

Stroke survivor and informal caregivers' educational needs are diverse and complex. They need to know many aspects of care, including information on secondary stroke prevention, treatment and recovery. The most common reported caregiver needs include information regarding manual handling, rehabilitation exercises and activity abilities, psychosocial and behavioural changes, nutritional advice, as well as managing impairments in the long term (Hafsteindottir et al 2011). Stroke survivors and their caregivers have many unmet educational needs. It is important that nurses consider the optimal timing and delivery of education. This must be patient-centred and tailored to meet the needs of the individual, as patients often prefer individualised information as opposed to generic risk-based information. Providing support via a post-stroke follow-up clinic, stroke survivor peer support groups, or by phone or internet platforms, are contemporary approaches to after-discharge care and follow-up to meet educational needs.

Access to Quality Information

The Stroke Foundation's EnableMe platform, My Stroke Journey and StrokeLine are good examples of high-quality resources and support platforms that patients and their caregivers may find helpful. EnableMe allows users to interact with other stroke survivors, their families and friends and have access to high-quality, credible stroke information. Stories, insights and tips can also be shared as part of rehabilitation and recovery processes. The platform hosts information, including videos, blogs and podcasts from other stroke survivors, their families and healthcare professionals.

CASE STUDY 16.1

ISCHAEMIC STROKE

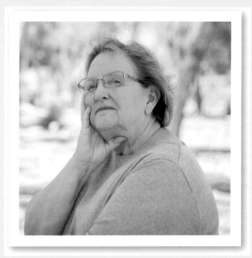

iStockphoto/Feverpitched.

Barbara presented with left-sided weakness involving her face and upper and lower limbs, and dysarthria after going to the toilet to use her bowels. Barbara is a 68-year-old female with a past history of hypertension, hypercholesterolaemia, paroxysmal atrial fibrillation and type 2 diabetes mellitus.

Non-contrast scans of the brain, followed by a CT perfusion of the brain demonstrate no evidence of acute intracranial haemorrhage, but a chronic lacunar infarct is seen, as well as a possible left posterior cerebral artery infarct. As she met all the criteria for thrombolysis therapy (rt-PA), she was administered therapy within 2 hours of onset of stroke signs and symptoms.

Barbara's dysarthria improved within 2 hours of receiving thrombolysis; however, she had residual deficits with balance and coordination, but not strength. She was admitted to inpatient rehabilitation and was discharged after 14 days. She had outpatient follow-up organised for the nurse-practitioner stroke follow-up clinic to implement secondary prevention strategies.

CASE STUDY 16.2

STROKE REHABILITATION

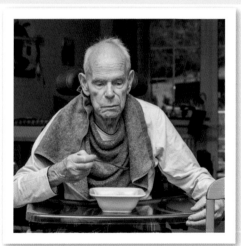

iStockphoto/Jan-Schneckenhaus.

James is an 81-year-old gentleman admitted to the acute stroke unit with rapid atrial fibrillation, pain on the right side of his face and neck, dizziness, nausea and a productive cough. Previous medical history included AF, hypertension, ischaemic heart disease, type 2 diabetes and a previous PE. A CT head scan revealed a right cerebellar infarct. A carotid duplex scan identified that James has no flow in his left internal carotid artery.

He was commenced on dabigatran this admission, and was discharged with a transitional aged care package of home support. He was provided with the Stroke Foundation 'My Stroke Journey' resource on discharge from hospital.

CONCLUSION

The global burden of stroke and its associated mortality and morbidity are concerning. Stroke prevention strategies, early diagnosis and appropriate pre-hospital, hyper-acute care and rehabilitation are key national health priorities. As nurses, it is our duty to provide evidence-based, patient-centred care to patients, as well as ongoing education about their condition to patients and their informal caregivers, along with information about interventions to reduce potentially avoidable complications.

Reflective Questions

Refer to Case Studies 16.1 and 16.2 and consider the following questions.

1. Describe five non-modifiable and five modifiable stroke risk factors. What health behaviour change strategies could you apply to assist individuals at high risk of stroke?
2. In what ways can stroke impact an individual? What are some of the factors that might influence a patient's outcome after stroke?
3. What are the core components of quality nursing care in acute stroke management?
4. Describe three innovations in Australian stroke care in the last decade.

Acknowledgement

Thanks to James Kevin, Bronwyn Coulton and Andrew Scanlon for their contributions to previous editions of this chapter.

RECOMMENDED RESOURCES

Collaboration Stroke Unit Trialists 2013. Organised inpatients (stroke unit) care for stroke. The Cochrane Database of Systematic Reviews (9), CD000197.

Ferguson C 2016. How to recognize a stroke and what you should know about their treatment. The Conversation. Online. Available: theconversation.com/how-to-recognise-a-stroke-and-what-you-should-know-about-their-treatment-63651

Ferguson C, Hickman LD, Lal S et al 2016. Addressing the stroke evidence-treatment gap. Contemporary Nurse 1–5.

Stroke Foundation 2018. Clinical guidelines for stroke management. Online. Available: strokefoundation.org.au/What-we-do/Treatment-programs/Clinical-guidelines

REFERENCES

Adams HP Jr, del Zoppo G, Alberts MJ et al 2007. Guidelines for the early management of adults with ischemic stroke: a guideline from the American Heart Association/American Stroke Association , Stroke Council, Clinical Cardiology Council, Cardiovascular Radiology and Intervention Council, and the Atherosclerotic Peripheral Vascular Disease and Quality of Care Outcomes in Research Interdisciplinary Working Groups. Stroke; a Journal of Cerebral Circulation 38(5), 1655–1711.

Altaf N, MacSweeney ST, Gladman J et al 2007. Carotid intra-plaque hemorrhage predicts recurrent symptoms in patients with high-grade carotid stenosis. Stroke; a Journal of Cerebral Circulation 38(5), 1633–1635.

Australian Institute of Health and Welfare (AIHW) 2020. Deaths in Australia. Online. Available: www.aihw.gov.au/reports/life-expectancy-death/deaths-in-australia/contents/leading-causes-of-death

Baird TA, Parsons MW, Phanh T et al 2003. Persistent post-stroke hyperglycemia is independently associated with infarct expansion and worse clinical outcome. Stroke; a Journal of Cerebral Circulation 34(9), 2208–2214.

Bederson JB, Connolly ES Jr, Batjer HH et al 2009. Guidelines for the management of aneurysmal subarachnoid hemorrhage: a statement for healthcare professionals from a special writing group of the Stroke Council, American Heart Association. Stroke; a Journal of Cerebral Circulation 40(3), 994–1025.

Benowitz LI, Carmichael ST 2010. Promoting axonal rewiring to improve outcome after stroke. JAMA: The Journal of the American Medical Association 290(8), 1049–1056.

Brieger D, Amerena J, Attia J et al 2018. National Heart Foundation of Australia and Cardiac Society of Australia and New Zealand: Australian clinical guidelines for the diagnosis and management of atrial fibrillation 2018. Medical Journal of Australia 209(8), 356–362.

Brophy BP, Riddell J, Mee E et al 2000. Epidemiology of aneurysmal subarachnoid hemorrhage in Australia and New Zealand: incidence and case fatality from the Australasian Cooperative Research on Subarachnoid Hemorrhage Study (ACROSS). Stroke; a Journal of Cerebral Circulation 31, 1843–1850.

Carmichael ST 2010. Targets for neural repair therapies after stroke. Stroke; a Journal of Cerebral Circulation 41(10 Suppl.), S124–S126.

Chen HJ, Bai CH, Yeh WT et al 2006. Influence of metabolic syndrome and general obesity on the risk of ischemic stroke. Stroke; a Journal of Cerebral Circulation 37(4), 1060–1064.

CLOTS trials collaboration, Dennis M, Sandercock P et al 2013. The effect of graduated compression stockings on long-term outcomes after stroke: the CLOTS trials 1 and 2. Stroke; a Journal of Cerebral Circulation 44(4), 1075–1079.

Davis SM, Donnan GA 2012. Clinical practice. Secondary prevention after ischemic stroke or transient ischemic attack. The New England Journal of Medicine 366(20), 1914–1922.

Diringer MN 2009. Management of aneurysmal subarachnoid hemorrhage. Critical Care Medicine 37(2), 432.

Donnan GA, Fisher M, Macleod M et al 2008. Stroke. Lancet 371(9624), 1612–1623.

Feigin V, Carter K, Hackett M et al 2006. Ethnic disparities in incidence of stroke subtypes: Auckland Regional Community Stroke Study 2002–2003. Lancet Neurology 5(2), 130–139.

Ferguson C, Inglis SC, Newton PJ et al 2014. Atrial fibrillation: stroke prevention in focus. Australian Critical Care: Official Journal of the Confederation of Australian Critical Care Nurses 27(2), 92–98.

Frizzell JP 2005. Acute stroke: pathophysiology, diagnosis, and treatment. AACN Clinical Issues 16(4), 421–440, quiz 597–598.

Gallanagh S, Quinn TJ, Alexander J et al 2011. Physical activity in the prevention and treatment of stroke. ISRN Neurology 2011, 953818.

Gargano JW, Reeves MJ 2007. Sex differences in stroke recovery and stroke-specific quality of life: results from a statewide stroke registry. Stroke; a Journal of Cerebral Circulation 38(9), 2541–2548.

Gattellari M, Goumas C, Aitken R et al 2011. Outcomes for patients with ischaemic stroke and atrial fibrillation: the PRIMS Study (A Program of Research Informing Stroke Management). Cerebrovascular Diseases 32, 370–382.

GBD 2016 Lifetime Risk of Stroke Collaborators 2018. Global, regional, and country-specific lifetime risks of stroke, 1990 and 2016. New England Journal of Medicine 379(25), 2429–2437.

Giles MF, Rothwell PM 2009. Transient ischaemic attack: clinical relevance, risk prediction and urgency of secondary prevention. Current Opinion in Neurology 22(1), 46–53.

Giles MF, Rothwell PM 2007. Risk of stroke early after transient ischaemic attack: a systematic review and meta-analysis. The Lancet. Neurology 6(12), 1063–1072.

Giorda CB, Avogaro A, Maggini M et al 2007. Incidence and risk factors for stroke in type 2 diabetic patients: the DAI study. Stroke; a Journal of Cerebral Circulation 38(4), 1154–1160.

Goldstein LB, Hankey GJ 2006. Advances in primary stroke prevention. Stroke; a Journal of Cerebral Circulation 37(2), 317–319.

Good DC, Bettermann K, Reichwein RK 2011. Stroke rehabilitation. CONTINUUM: Lifelong Learning in Neurology 17(3 Neurorehabilitation), 545–567.

Goss J 2008. Projection of Australian health care expenditure by disease 2003 to 2033. Health and Welfare Expenditure Series, N. 36.

Hachinski V, Donnan GA, Gorelick PB et al 2010. Stroke: working toward a prioritized world agenda. [Review.] Stroke; a Journal of Cerebral Circulation 41(6), 1084–1099.

Hafsteindottir TB, Vurgunst M, Lindeman E et al 2011. Educational needs for patients with a stroke and their caregivers: a systematic review. Patient Education Counselling 85(1), 14–25.

Hendriks JML, deWit R, Crijns HJGM et al 2012. Nurse-led care vs usual care for patients with atrial fibrillation. European Heart Journal 33, 2692–2699.

Iadecola C, Park L, Capone C 2009. Threats to the mind: aging, amyloid, and hypertension. Stroke; a Journal of Cerebral Circulation 40(Suppl. 3), S40–S44.

Krakauer JW 2006. Motor learning: its relevance to stroke recovery and neurorehabilitation. Current Opinion in Neurology 19(1), 84–90.

Lakhan SE, Sapko MT 2009. Blood pressure lowering treatment for preventing stroke recurrence: a systematic review and meta-analysis. International Archives of Medicine 2(1), 30.

Lloyd-Jones D, Adams RJ, Brown TM et al 2010. Heart disease and stroke statistics – 2010 update. Circulation 121(7), e46–e215.

Middleton S, McElduff P, Ward J et al 2011. Implementation of evidence-based treatment protocols to manage fever, hyperglycaemia, and swallowing dysfunction in acute stroke (QASC): a cluster randomized controlled trial. The Lancet 378(9804), 1699–1706.

Miller EL, Murray L, Richards L et al 2010. Comprehensive overview of nursing and interdisciplinary rehabilitation care of the stroke patient. Stroke; a Journal of Cerebral Circulation 41(10), 2402–2448.

Nahed BV, Bydon M, Ozturk AK et al 2007. Genetics of intracranial aneurysms. Neurosurgery 60(2), 213–225, discussion 225–216.

Nursing and Midwifery Board of Australia (NMBA) 2018. Registered Nurse Standards for Practice. Online. Available: www.nursingmidwiferyboard.gov.au/codes-guidelines-statements/professional-standards.aspx

O'Brien E, Priglinger ML, Bertmar C et al 2016. Rapid access point of care clinic for transient ischemic attacks and minor strokes. Journal of Clinical Neuroscience 23, 106–110.

O'Donnell M, Chin SL, Rangarajan S et al 2016. Global and regional effects of potentially modifiable risk factors associated with acute stroke in 32 countries (INTERSTROKE): a case-control study. Lancet 388, 761–775.

Prinz V, Endres M 2011. Statins and stroke: prevention and beyond. [Research Support, Non-U.S. Gov't Review.] Current Opinion in Neurology 24(1), 75–80.

Reynolds K, Lewis B, Nolen JD et al 2003. Alcohol consumption and risk of stroke: a meta-analysis. JAMA: The Journal of the American Medical Association 289(5), 579–2588.

Rich MW, Beckham V, Wittenberg C et al 1995. A multidisciplinary intervention to prevent the readmission of elderly patients with congestive heart failure. New England Journal of Medicine 333(18), 1190–1195.

Rijntjes M 2006. Mechanisms of recovery in stroke patients with hemiparesis or aphasia: new insights, old questions and the meaning of therapies. Current Opinion in Neurology 19(1), 76–83.

Scanlon A 2006. Nursing and the 5As guideline to smoking cessation interventions. Australian Nursing Journal 14(5), 25–28.

Scanlon A, Lee G 2007. The use of the term 'vulnerability' in acute care. Why does it differ and what does it mean? Australian Journal of Advanced Nursing 24(3), 54–59.

Shaw RJ, McDuffie JR, Hendrix CC et al 2014. Effects of nurse-managed protocols in the outpatient management of adults with chronic conditions. Annals of Internal Medicine 161(2), 113–121.

Stroke Foundation 2020. Signs of stroke – FAST. FAST. Online. Available: http://strokefoundation.com.au/what-is-a-stroke/signs-of-stroke/.

Stroke Foundation 2018. Clinical guidelines for stroke management 2010. Online. Available: www.strokefoundation.com.au

Stroke Foundation 2017. No postcode untouched, stroke in Australia. Deloitte Access Economics. Online. Available: https://strokefoundation.org.au/-/media/5C7D7A2FE9E6488AB350DA6C2055F425.ashx?la=en

Therapeutic Guidelines Limited 2011. Stroke. Therapeutic Guidelines: Neurology, version 4 2011 (Vol. 2007). TGL, West Melbourne.

Thrift AG, Hayman N 2007. Aboriginal and Torres Strait Islander peoples and the burden of stroke. International Journal of Stroke 2(1), 57–59.

Towfighi A, Saver JL, Engelhardt R et al 2007. A midlife stroke surge among women in the United States. Neurology 69(20), 1898–1904.

van der Worp HB, van Gijn J 2007. Acute ischemic stroke. New England Journal of Medicine 357(21), 2203–2204.

Wang TJ, Massaro JM, Levy D et al 2003. A risk score for predicting stroke or death in individuals with new-onset atrial fibrillation in the community: the Framingham Heart Study. Neurobiology of Disease 37(2), 259–266.

Wardlaw JM, Keir SL, Seymour J et al 2004. What is the best imaging strategy for acute stroke? Health Technology Assessment (Winchester, England) 8(1), iii.

Yakubovich N, Gerstein HC 2011. Serious cardiovascular outcomes in diabetes: the role of hypoglycemia. Circulation 123(3), 342–348.

Zhao H, Coote S, Easton D et al 2020. Melbourne mobile stroke unit and reperfusion therapy. Stroke 51, 922–930.

CHAPTER 17

Principles for Nursing Practice: Parkinson's Disease, Multiple Sclerosis and Motor Neurone Disease

SONIA MATIUK

LEARNING OBJECTIVES

When you have completed this chapter you will be able to:

- describe the symptoms of Parkinson's disease (PD), multiple sclerosis (MS) and motor neurone disease (MND), and some of the treatments used to manage these disabling diseases
- discuss the possible impact each disease may have on the person living with PD, MS or MND
- discuss the possible challenges faced by family and/or friends in providing in-home care for people living with PD, MS or MND
- explain the importance of assessing the individual needs and providing an interdisciplinary, chronicity focused approach to supportive care
- discuss relevant strategies that would enable people and their caregivers to live well with neurodegeneration.

KEY WORDS

degenerative	neurological
interdisciplinary team	supportive care
mobility	

INTRODUCTION

While Parkinson's disease (PD), multiple sclerosis (MS) and motor neurone disease (MND) are distinct diseases in themselves, they have several characteristics in common, including the need for physical and supportive care as the disease progresses. All three diseases are neurodegenerative, progressive disorders of motor function accompanied by some non-motor symptoms, including some sensory function deficits in MS and PD. In all three, people may present with weakness and mobility-related symptoms, necessitating careful diagnostic testing and treatment of symptoms over time before a probable diagnosis can be made. Families report this time as a stressful and often frustrating period of indecision while they await a probable diagnosis.

Devastatingly for the person and their family, each disease is disabling and to some extent life limiting, with no known cause and no cure. While people diagnosed with some phenotypes of MS can expect to live for a relatively normal lifespan, their quality of life decreases over time. For people diagnosed with MND, the prognosis is far worse with 50% not expected to live 15–20 months from diagnosis (GBD 2016 Motor Neuron Disease Collaborators 2018). Life expectancy in PD has improved with new treatments; however, related complications may increase the number of disability-adjusted years of life (DALY), resulting in a median time from onset to death of 12.4 years (Deloitte Access Economics 2015a).

DALY is a statistical expression of the years of 'healthy' life lost to disability and death.

It is calculated as:

Years of life lost due to early death (YLL) + Years lost because of disability (YLD)

(Deloitte Access Economics 2015a)

As people with PD, MS or MND are largely cared for in the community, the chronic but progressive nature of these diseases presents unique lifestyle challenges for the person and their caregivers. Cognitive changes common to all three diseases create additional caregiver burden. Yet, every case is different and each person has their own cultural and social understanding of illness, its impact and the eventual end-of-life process. People with the disease and their caregivers become very knowledgeable about disease management. This expertise must be recognised and valued by members of the interdisciplinary healthcare team. In this chapter, case studies have been provided to develop your insight into the individual manner in which each disease may affect a person's life, their family and their relationships with the community.

Providing care for people with any of these neurological diseases requires careful management of complex and sometimes confronting symptomatology, as well as the variable presentation of motor and non-motor signs. An interdisciplinary approach is the preferred model of care, with nursing as a key discipline coordinating and providing care, facilitating advance care planning, giving advice, support and education and monitoring the effect of medication. Effective care will only occur if interdisciplinary team members are prepared to work together with patients and family caregivers to continually assess individual needs and collaboratively plan relevant supportive care, including careful advance care planning, timely access to community resources and end-of-life care (Dieplinger et al 2017).

PARKINSON'S DISEASE

Parkinson's disease (PD) was named for James Parkinson following the publication of his paper about 'shaking palsy'. PD is a chronic, degenerative neurological disorder, and is the fastest growing neurodegenerative condition in regards to prevalence, disability and death, with the number of people affected by PD more than doubling in the period 1990–2015 (GBD 2016 Parkinson's Disease Collaborators 2018). PD is characterised by the loss of dopamine-producing neurones in the substantia nigra and elsewhere in the brain. The depletion of dopaminergic neurons results in the characteristic triad of PD symptoms of tremor, rigidity and bradykinesia (You et al 2018). Dopamine is an important neurotransmitter in the basal ganglia, a collection of specialised brain cells in the brain stem that are responsible for the modulation of movement and coordination. Over time, PD spreads to the cerebral cortex affecting cognitive function, and in some cases cognitive deficit can appear early or even before motor deficits develop (Martini et al 2020), as evident in Nigel's story (Case Study 17.1). People with PD also lose facial expression (masked facies), which may be mistaken for indifference, an important feature for health professionals to recognise when providing care.

The cause of PD is unknown, but a range of endogenous and exogenous factors are thought to contribute to the risk of developing and progressing the development of PD. Although PD is seen in all age groups, a primary risk factor is increasing age with peak incident at 70–79 (Creed et al 2019). The growing incidence is reflective of the increasing percentage of the population in the older age groups and PD is slightly more prevalent in males than females (Deloitte Access Economics 2015b). It is estimated that 867 per 100 000 Australians over 50 years of age (Deloitte Access Economics 2015b), and 1% of New Zealanders over the age of 60 (Parkinson's New Zealand 2018) have PD. While PD is sporadic (idiopathic) in more than 90% of cases, genetic mutations – LRRK2, Parkin and PINK1 – have been linked with PD (Creed et al 2019). Exogenous factors that have been investigated include exposure to certain pesticides, physical activity, diet and drugs; however, the evidence is not conclusive (Belvisi et al 2019). There have also been studies made into factors that may provide some neuroprotective effects, including smoking and caffeine consumption, ibuprofen and β-adrenoceptor agonists; however, the evidence is not strong or consistent (Belvisi et al 2019).

PD is suspected when a person presents with bradykinesia and one of the following: muscular rigidity, resting tremor or postural instability. Exposure to toxins and other underlying causes need to be excluded and other supporting criteria met before a diagnosis can be established. An improvement in symptoms with L-dopa replacement medication confirms the diagnosis (Varadi 2020).

While PD has varied symptomatology, it usually presents asymmetrically. The signs of PD are divided into motor and non-motor (see Table 17.1).

CASE STUDY 17.1

NIGEL'S STORY

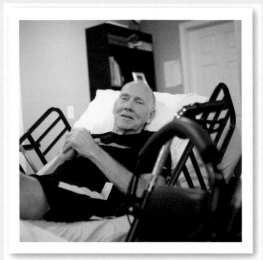

iStockphoto/LPETTET.

Looking back on my working life, it has been very fulfilling. I've had over 45 years as an architect, and have designed churches, shopping centres, schools and residences. When approaching retirement, our children had flown the coop and my wife and I were contemplating travel, sailing, music concerts, wood turning, gardening and reading all those books collected for when we had the time to relax and enjoy them. I noticed a tremor in my right hand and my gait had changed. As both my father and grandfather had Parkinson's disease, I suspected that it had come down to me too.

This diagnosis of Parkinson's disease was confirmed by our local GP, who prescribed Madopar, which helps to replace the dopamine lost in the brain. Madopar eased the hand tremor for a year or two, and I was able to continue to do wood turning and painting, but other deficits soon surfaced. I was now seeing a neurologist every 6 months. Slowed movement (bradykinesia), stooped posture which affected balance, and rigid muscles which caused pain, developed after the hand tremor. Then moving became more difficult with 'freezing' and 'sticky feet', and I found I had to count 'one, two, three, move' to get going again. When trying to relax at night, 'restless legs syndrome' kicked in and made it difficult to sleep. Sifrol was prescribed to treat stiffness, tremors, muscle spasms and poor muscle control, as well as restless legs syndrome which made it difficult to sleep at night, but while it helped for a while, it was not a cure. The active substance in Sifrol (pramipexole) is a dopamine agonist (a substance that imitates the action of dopamine).

Sifrol has some nasty side effects. A common one is hallucinations – I often saw people or furry animals that no one else saw and worried my wife by having conversations with invisible persons. These hallucinations didn't bother me, but seemed to worry others. Other side effects were bouts of suddenly falling asleep – by this time I had stopped driving as my motor deficits slowed my reactions. Behavioural changes began to happen. Some people take up gambling, or increased sexual desire or binge eating ... I became a compulsive shopper of books, tools and DVDs, and we now have a huge supply to store or clear. Elisabeth (my wife) wants them disposed of! Now with double vision, another effect of Sifrol and Parkinson's, I am unable to read or do the wood turning I looked forward to in retirement, and my writing has become very small and scratchy. Another problem is the 'Parkinson's face', where facial muscles become immobilised, leaving people with Parkinson's (PWP) with blank expressions. To those who aren't aware, we can appear disinterested, even bored. My speech also became very soft, often in a monotone, making it difficult to hold a conversation. A group of us from our support group did the intense Lee Silverman LSVT LOUD program and followed the voice exercises for some time – the main focus is to speak LOUD and it works, as long as one continues the exercises and remembers to speak loudly. The principles of LSVT LOUD were applied to limb movement in PWPs and an exercise program called LSVT BIG proved effective for some time. Unfortunately, as with many exercise programs, when you slip up and don't practise you lose the benefits gained. Our support group now includes a (compulsory) half-hour of exercises each month using DVDs from the 'Dance for Parkinson's' program developed by the Mark Morris Dance Studio in Brooklyn.

As the disease progresses, medications have to be modified or changed as they seem to wear off, and the 'ON' times become shorter and 'OFF' times become debilitating. Sifrol was stopped, Stalevo was introduced in combination with Madopar, and various additional medications were included to cope with panic attacks and difficulty in sleeping. Stalevo is a combination of carbidopa, levodopa and entacapone, and is taken five times a day with other Parkinson's medications, and it is crucial to administer them on time. Even 10 minutes late and I know it!

We now have neurologists in my city and I see them twice a year, but most of us feel that our treatment is best managed by our local GPs. We see them monthly, or more as required and they are aware of the daily challenges we have to face and modify medication as required. It's really difficult when nursing staff in hospitals aren't aware of the need to administer medications right on time, but fortunately this is much better now. Cognitive decline has progressed. While I'm still described as a gentle man, the dementia and hallucinations mean having a conversation is not possible. Until recently, I was cared for by Elisabeth and the family, but I am now in residential care. I enjoy all the activities, church services, entertainment groups, coffee hours, happy hours, doing word-searches and playing bingo.

TABLE 17.1
Motor and Non-Motor Symptoms of PD

Motor	Non-Motor
Classic triad of (resting) tremor, rigidity (inflexibility of limbs, neck or trunk) and bradykinesia to akinesia (slowness and difficulty in initiating movement)	Autonomic dysfunction: postural hypotension, abnormal sweating, gastrointestinal disturbances, sexual dysfunction
Postural instability, flexion on the trunk, gait difficulties with shuffling and freezing, reduced arm swing	Mood disturbances: depression, anxiety, apathy Psychotic symptoms: impulse control disorders, hallucinations
Akinesia presenting as difficulty turning in bed, small handwriting and a soft voice that is difficult to understand	Cognitive impairment: impaired judgement, identity confusion
	Sleep disturbances: restless leg syndrome, sleep apnoea
	Sensory phenomena: pain and paraesthesia, anosmia, ageusia

Varadi 2020.

When functional disability affects quality of life, medications such as levodopa are used to supplement the dopamine deficiency, with no effect on the degenerative course of this disease. However, clinical trials currently being conducted indicate the potential for antioxidants to slow the progression of PD (Angeles et al 2016). Research into neural implantation is also at the therapeutic trial stage (Kumar et al 2015).

As PD progresses, medication effects wear off between doses, signalling further degeneration. Since the 1980s, deep brain stimulation (DBS) has been used in selected cases to improve motor symptoms in advanced PD, but it has no benefit for non-motor symptoms such as cognitive decline. While studies indicate that DBS improves mobility, bradykinesia and time asleep, it does not stop disease progression (Liddle et al 2019). DBS has little effect on reducing hallucinations, speech or cognitive decline and in some cases can worsen these symptoms (Liddle et al 2019).

Altered Mobility and Fatigue

People with PD have different levels of motor function depending on whether they are in the 'off' or 'on' state. The 'off' state describes the patient when the disabling signs and symptoms of PD are most obvious, while the 'on' state describes the best the person can achieve with PD medications. The same patient who requires full care in feeding, showering and transferring may be able to manage their care independently or with assistance in the 'on' state, after their medications take effect. Conversational fluency, appropriateness, speech production and comprehension are negatively affected by low dopamine levels or an 'off' state (Straulino et al 2016). Although the impact of medication in speech

production remains unclear, it is vitally important that PD medications are taken at the prescribed time without delay, as they may be effective in improving other motor symptoms, such as stiff facial muscles.

Difficulty with gait, posture and balance compromises mobility. Showering, toileting and ambulating require careful assessment by a physiotherapist and an occupational therapist (OT) where available. Strategies can then be implemented for either prevention or management of priority or contributing problems related to mobility limitations, enabling the person to achieve a measure of independence within safety limits (Radder et al 2017). As the disease progresses, balance often deteriorates and falls are common. Walking aids may be required after review from the physiotherapist. Routines need to be planned around the 'on' time to enable the person to realise their daily goals.

Fatigue is a common, but not well recognised or understood, symptom of PD. Untreated fatigue can cause relationship stress, anxiety and poor quality of life. Sleep disturbances, depression and some PD medications can result in daytime tiredness. Therefore, it is important to monitor and treat, where possible, these contributing factors. When planning the daily routine, fatigue, as well as 'on' and 'off' states, need to be considered.

Dopamine replacement, in the form of levodopa, combined with a dopa decarboxylase inhibitor to prevent the peripheral side effects of levodopa, remains the first-line treatment for PD. In Case Study 17.1 Nigel takes Madopar, which is a combination of levodopa and benserazide. At the onset of PD this medication often returns the person close to a normal baseline, but with disease progression many people find that the 'on' time shortens, leading to motor fluctuations complicated by chorea-like involuntary movements called 'dyskinesias'. It is important to differentiate tremor from dyskinesia to ensure that correct treatment options such as radiofrequency thalamotomy, unilateral DBS and stereotactic radiosurgery are considered. An emerging treatment option for medication-refractory essential tremor is focused ultrasound thalamotomy, which has shown clinical efficacy, with rapid and lasting tremor relief and a higher safety profile than other available options (Langford et al 2018).

Other PD drug therapies include synthetic dopamine agonists (rotigotine patch, ropinirole, pramipexole and apomorphine), which act on the dopamine receptor sites with a similar but weaker action, except for apomorphine (Torti et al 2019). Apomorphine, a by-product of morphine without opiate activity, is an injectable dopamine agonist that has a comparable effect to levodopa. It can be used as an injection to rescue the person from 'off' states or as an infusion for management of symptomatology. Postural hypotension is common with this group of medications and they are more likely to cause hallucinations in susceptible patients. Obsessional behaviours such as hyper-sexuality, excessive eating and excessive gambling are recognised as side effects of levodopa and dopamine agonist therapy in susceptible patients (see Case Study 17.1).

Entacapone prevents the rapid uptake of levodopa, creating a longer effect time. Anti-cholinergic drugs (benzhexol, benztropine) are rarely used in older people because they are poorly tolerated and of no benefit for motor symptoms. Amantidine is used to control dyskinesia, but is used in only approximately 10% of patients due to the common adverse side effects of hallucinations and confusion (Rascol et al 2020).

Dietary protein can interfere with the absorption of medications. Thus, medications should be given at least 30 minutes before food, wherever possible. Timing of the effect of medication is important and can be measured with PD diaries, where motor fluctuations and dyskinesias (which are side effects of long-term dopamine replacement), as well as 'on' and 'off' states, can be documented.

PD medications should be administered regularly as significant delay or omissions can lead to an exacerbation of PD symptoms and an increased risk of complications, such as falls, aspiration pneumonia and pressure injuries. PD medications should not be stopped abruptly to prevent the rare but life-threatening condition called neuroleptic malignant syndrome which manifests as high fever and extreme muscle rigidity, and without immediate intervention can lead to

renal failure, cardiac arrest and death (Alty et al 2016). Also many medications, including certain anti-emetics and phenothiazine medications, may cause acute and severe exacerbation of PD and should be avoided.

People with PD have difficulty in motor sequencing, highlighting the disabling nature of this condition. The use of external cues is very helpful to foster independence, especially with mobility, although swallowing or speech problems also respond to cues. Cues can be given by the nurse or caregiver, or, where possible, instigated by the person themselves. Some useful cues which initiate recovery from freezing of gait, include counting aloud (as Nigel describes in Case Study 17.1), stepping over a laser line, humming a marching tune, singing or pretending to climb a stair. Getting out of bed can be broken down into motor segments and cues can be used to get the patient through the entire sequence of movements.

Body Image

Many changes occur with PD that can lead to an altered body image. A stooped posture, slowness in movement and gait disturbance ages the person. Drooling, reduced facial expression, unblinking eyes, slowness in thought (bradyphrenia) and voice disturbances not only lead to a loss of personal dignity, but interfere with communication. The person may be perceived as having low intellect. Social isolation for both the person with PD and their caregiver can ensue. People with PD may resent their wishes, feelings and opinions being interpreted and reported by others and often feel shunned by previous friends as the condition progresses.

There are many complementary therapies available to treat non-motor symptoms and improve body image and quality of life. Natural therapies, herbs and over-the-counter medications have been used for constipation, urinary frequency and urgency, postural hypotension, sexual difficulties, depression, anxiety and dementia. However, preparations should be checked by the pharmacist to ensure they do not interfere with PD medications or aggravate PD symptoms.

Quality of Life

Quality of life (QOL) means different things to different individuals, but in PD, it is adversely affected for several reasons. Motor symptoms have an effect on areas such as role change, independence, working, driving and physical comfort. Yet, studies show non-motor symptoms such as pain and sexual limitations are more troublesome and have a negative impact on QOL (Gofton et al 2015). Depression is also a common feature of PD that impacts on QOL (Pontone et al 2016).

Psychosis in PD, which often manifests as visual hallucinations, affects up to 60% of people with PD and is associated with higher rates of carer distress, admission to nursing home placements and mortality rates (Lenka et al 2017). The causes of psychosis in PD are not well understood; however, risk factors include older age, longer duration of illness, higher severity of motor symptoms, the presence of sleep disturbances and cognitive impairment.

Social interaction diminishes as the disease progresses, not only because of body image changes, especially the Parkinson's face, but because of communication difficulties. Nigel's story describes the LSVT LOUD® program used to enhance voice production and facilitate communication. Health professionals should be aware that establishing an effective means of communication is paramount to developing a rapport with people with PD. When faced with people who have soft monotonic voices, rapid and/or slurred speech and reduced facial expression, it is important to listen to content rather than delivery of speech to gauge needs, mood and cognitive function. Ensuring a face-to-face position, making eye contact and using cues to encourage people to speak key words loudly, and the use of a pacing board if prescribed, are helpful and enable the personal expression of needs. For people unable to speak, communication boards paired with a pointing device are useful. Recent technological advances have brought many innovations, so that speech-generating devices can be individualised and operated via specialised switches like retinal scanners, even when fine hand motor control is severely impaired. The advent of smartphone and tablet devices has made sophisticated methods of communication affordable, portable and available to most people with PD. Regardless of how a person with PD communicates, it is essential to allow them ample time to express themselves and check that you have understood their intended message.

Family and Caregivers

As with the majority of chronic conditions, PD is a family affair. The dynamics, relationships and traditional roles in the family may change, and resentment, guilt and grieving can become major problems if changes are not addressed. Social support is important and counselling outside the family is often helpful to resolve these issues.

A well-informed family is more able to assist the person with PD to engage in advance care planning and make decisions about their care, as well as solving many of the day-to-day QOL issues. While direct caregiving may be exhausting in the later stages of PD, the family also carries the burden of the condition vicariously as observers of the toll that PD is taking on their loved one. Support for caregivers needs to include monitoring of health, particularly of older spousal caregivers, and opportunities for respite to avoid burn-out.

MULTIPLE SCLEROSIS

Multiple sclerosis (MS) is a chronic, autoimmune, demyelinating disease resulting in the development of lesions in the white matter of the brain and spinal cord (Kumar et al 2015). Myelin forms around the axon as an insulator that interprets and conducts the message along the fibre tract. In people with MS, acute inflammation causes demyelination of the axon, which if not resolved, leads to scarring. Following the inflammatory attack, remyelination may occur in some axons, enabling a return of function. Where myelin is lost, scarring or sclerosis occurs, slowing or impairing the transmission of the nerve impulse and increasing axon vulnerability to environmental influences. The size and distribution of the sclerotic plaques dictate the locations and types of symptoms experienced.

Geographical variations in incidence have led to several hypotheses about causal factors, such as environmental (including latitude) and genetic factors (Jelinek et al 2015). It is proposed that MS is activated in genetically predisposed people who have been exposed to a viral assault that precipitates an inflammatory reaction (Kular & Jagodic 2020). Environmental predictors include low levels of vitamin D, cigarette smoking and obesity in early life, as well as viral infections such as Epstein-Barr (Ascherio & Munger 2016).

MS is not a disease of old age, as most people are diagnosed between the ages of 20 and 50 years and some even younger (Rumrill Jr & Bishop 2019). The revised McDonald criteria indicates that two attacks typical of acute inflammatory demyelination in the central nervous system (observed or patient reported) in the absence of fever or infection, lasting more than 24 hours, with two or more lesions on the brain visible on magnetic resonance imaging (MRI), or objective clinical evidence of one lesion – for example, positive, unmatched cerebrospinal fluid oligoclonal bands – with associated history, confers probable MS (McNicholas et al 2019). This combination is required because abnormalities in one test – for example, the presence of lesions on an MRI – is inconclusive and could be the result of other disease processes. Accompanying symptoms may include unilateral visual impairment, ataxia, sensory impairment in trunk and limbs, difficulty in maintaining bladder control and spasticity (Rommer et al 2019).

TABLE 17.2
MS Phenotypes

Phenotype	Presentation
Relapsing remitting most common clinical course	Acute attacks (exacerbations) with neurological symptoms in one or more limbs Sensory disturbances
see Arona's story – Case Study 17.2	Optical, cerebellar and vestibular disturbances Pain, fatigue, sleep disturbances Partial or complete recovery between attacks
Secondary progressive progression from relapsing, remitting form Does not respond to MS medications Poor prognosis	Chronic neurodegeneration with no exacerbations Increased central fatigue, poor muscle activation resulting in eventual functional loss
Primary progressive More often in older people Does not respond to MS medications Poor prognosis	Continuous demyelination without remyelination No exacerbations Progressive gait difficulties leading to loss of mobility over time
Progressive relapsing	Continuous degeneration, with acute attacks occurring at intervals accompanied by minor recovery

Wolkorte et al 2016.

The course of MS differs among people, but there are four recognised phenotypes (see Table 17.2).

MS is the most common central nervous system disease in young adults worldwide, with approximately 10 Australians being diagnosed with MS every week (MS Research Australia 2018). Prevalence figures estimate that 25 600 Australians and 1 in 1000 New Zealanders live with MS, and three out of four of these are women (MS Research Australia 2020; Multiple Sclerosis Society of New Zealand [MSMZ] 2020). Interestingly, the incidence in the Māori population (without European contamination) is significantly smaller than for those of European descent (MSMZ 2020). Familial MS accounts for approximately 12.5% of cases (Steenhof et al 2018).

To prevent relapses, slow the progression of the disease and the accumulation of disabilities, disease modifying therapy with varying efficacy and safety profiles may be used, including interferon beta 1a and 1b and glatiramer acetate, natalizumab, alemtuzumab and fingolimod (Sanchirico et al 2019). Treatments for episodes of acute relapse or exacerbation of MS may include corticosteroids, plasmapheresis and in some cases immunosuppressants like methotrexate (Beh et al 2017).

Altered Mobility and Fatigue

Fatigue affects up to 80–90% of people with MS and is the chief complaint in approximately 60% of people with relapsing remitting MS (RRMS) (Wilting et al 2016). Its debilitating effects, not evident to others, are difficult to assess and quantify, making it hard to balance life, work, activity and rest. During the course of daily living, MS symptoms may be exacerbated by medication, intense periods of physical and/or emotional stress, such as work schedules or personal problems. Regular exercise is recommended to reduce fatigue, improve muscle tone, assist bladder and bowel function, and promote emotional wellbeing (see Arona's story in Case Study 17.2) (Razazian et al 2020).

Living with MS has physical and emotional implications for many aspects of daily life, including making provision for regular immunoregulatory antiviral injections. Work demands and life activities have to be programmed to include the management of side effects caused by immunoregulatory antiviral injection. Side effects can include influenza-like symptoms that affect approximately 75% of people with MS following injection and is more prevalent if given in the morning, but can disturb sleep quality when given at night and therefore cause fatigue during the day (Patti et al 2020).

Loss of sensation may induce numbness in the affected parts of the body, which can result in the person being unaware of injury. For example, loss of sensation in the face resembles the feeling generated by dental anaesthesia, causing the person to unknowingly bite their tongue or cheek without feeling pain. Likewise,

CASE STUDY 17.2

ARONA'S STORY

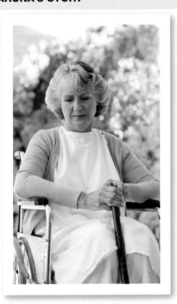

Shutterstock/wavebreakmedia.

I am now in my 35th year of living with MS. I was 26 years old, single and enjoying life as a secondary science teacher when I had my first attack of MS. This left me with reduced sensation in the skin across the entire left side of my body. My general practitioner referred me to a neurologist, who undertook a range of tests, including CAT (computed axial tomography, now referred to as CT) scans, visual evoke response tests to test optic nerve transmission and lumbar punctures. This was a stressful time of repeated testing before a diagnosis of relapsing remitting MS (RRMS) was finally made 18 months later.

When I was 27, I was told I should never work full-time, never get married or have children. In effect, I should just sit around and wait for all the bad things to happen! I felt that my social life had ceased, I was a lemon; no guy would want to know me! I decided to take some control of my destiny, so I changed my neurologist and began living life to the full. I taught for nearly 30 years, got married, had a son, and later divorced.

Over the years, MS has attacked my left side again and again, leaving a lasting left-sided weakness. During these attacks, I lost the sight in my left eye, the use of my left arm, and developed cerebellar ataxia, which upset my balance and coordination. It was like walking in thick mud and restricted my life activities. I was in my mid-40s when Betaferon became part of the pharmaceutical benefits scheme, making the antiviral, immunoregulatory drug affordable. I injected myself every second day, lessening the effects of MS attacks.

I was inspired by the work of an Australian doctor, Professor George Jelinek, who was also living with MS. He proposed that changing the fats in one's diet would rebuild the cell membrane phospholipid bi-layer and thus increase its resistance to MS. As a result, I became a fish-eating vegan and avoided chemical additives such as preservatives in food. My attacks became less severe, but I still had problems with balance and occasional vertigo. My movement is very affected by hot temperatures and humidity: I'm like a Raggedy Anne doll or someone who is drunk.

At about the young age of 49 years, I noticed a gradual deterioration in my cognitive capacity to process information and problem-solve, as well as increased fatigue. This affected my ability to continue school teaching and I retired for medical reasons 2 years later.

In 2005, I was hospitalised to treat a large fat cell necrosis on my thigh. As very few MS patients are hospitalised, the doctors and nursing staff knew very little about MS and its treatment. No one seemed to connect the lump in my leg with my injections, except for my GP. I had multiple intravenous drugs, went in with three allergies, and came out after 4 weeks with six allergies and a cannulation phobia! It was also very hard to manage my MS diet in hospital. I commenced a modified gym program to relax and tone (mostly done on machines).

Over the latter part of 2015 and into 2016, I had an exacerbation spread, bringing more mobility problems. I had a fall in a shop last year and fractured my left radius – 6 weeks in plaster, no gym, no driving! As a result, they changed my medication. I told my neurologist 'I'm sick of being a junkie'. His response was: 'I can give you a pill for that!' Aubagio and an anti-inflammatory. I'm certainly better! I saw him at the start of 2016, more mobility difficulties so into hospital for tests. Lumbar puncture, contrast CT scan, MRI, methylprednisolone infusion (4 days), nerve conduction test – the worst electric acupuncture, blood test and bone density scan – so relieved that it is non-invasive! I ran the gamut of another neurologist, haematologist, physiotherapy and endocrinologist. Nothing new, same old MS.

So I continue with an intensive exercise rehab program 5 days a week, 3 days at gym, 2 days on passive machines for body toning. This has helped me to be much steadier, although I have taken myself off the roster at church for now; I'm too slow and unsteady to be much help!

MS has seriously affected portions of my life, but there are worse things that could happen. I consider myself lucky. I live with and nurture MS rather than rejecting it. Information and education, strategies for dealing with situations, being able to help others cope with serious illness – there are many positives. My wonderful neurologist supports all my complementary approaches. I know more than most doctors about my condition, and they allow me to guide them. I respect this greatly.

hands or limbs may not detect heat from stoves or steam from a kettle, resulting in burns. People living with MS should be educated to avoid physical heat and stay cool in the summer. An increased body temperature brought on by hot baths, hot weather or infection slows nerve conduction and creates mobility and coordination problems (Gonzales et al 2017).

As well as being frustrating and socially challenging, tremors may reduce the person's ability to undertake tasks requiring fine motor skills. Neurological disturbances that alter the intent of voluntary movements, together with unpredictable loss of balance, can result in falls, bruising and ligament damage, as well as loss of confidence and self-esteem. Pain arising from muscle spasm is effectively treated with Baclofen. Unresolved spasms may result in contractures that restrict the range of movement of affected joints. Short-term use of walking aids may be appropriate, but use needs to be monitored by a physiotherapist to ensure other muscle groups, particularly the upper limbs, are not compromised. Likewise, physiotherapy may improve muscle strength, tone and posture, but fatigue must be avoided.

Body Image

Preserving positive body image is contingent on seeing the whole person who is living with MS and not the disabling condition. Listening to people's needs and encouraging them to make an effort with personal appearance diverts attention away from the disability focus and enhances self-esteem. However, MS-related changes affect body image and need to be addressed in a sensitive manner. For example, localised tissue reactions to drugs such as Betaferon often leave people with unsightly, persistent red blotches. Emphasising the role these medications play in staying well will encourage people to balance the blotchy image with the health benefit.

Maintaining hydration and muscle tone and avoiding infection are important keys to bladder control. Nevertheless, bladder control may be difficult to maintain during attacks, and as MS progresses, due to mobility factors impacting on ability to get to the toilet, undress, sit safely on the toilet etc. (Hentzen et al 2020). Frequency, urgency and the fear of incontinence threaten body image and QOL. Loss of bladder control may require a range of interventions from incontinence supports, medication to intermittent or continuous catheterisation. Progressive forms of MS may result in the need for long-term catheterisation, sometimes in the form of suprapubic catheterisation (Aharony et al 2017). Important body image issues may include the visibility

of a catheter, an impediment to sexual activity, and concern about the care needed to prevent infection. Effective management of the bowel, including treatment for constipation, managing the fear of incontinence and untimely flatus are also important for preserving body image. Neural disturbances may block the feeling of fullness in the bowel that signals the need for defecation. Recent studies suggest that electronic stimulation of the abdominal muscles may be effective in the management of chronic constipation (Singleton et al 2016).

Loss of sensation and motor function, drug therapy or psychological issues can affect the person's sex life. Sexual issues such as impotence, loss of libido, reduced lubrication and loss of sensation may result in slow arousal and decreased satisfaction. Patience together with medication and counselling can stimulate successful expressions of love.

Quality of Life

QOL is closely associated with personal empowerment. Being involved in care decision-making and setting their own priorities enables people living with MS to take control in chronic disease management (see Arona's example in Case Study 17.2).

The unpredictable nature of MS and the limitations on work, leisure and life roles can affect psychological and social functioning. Symptoms may change throughout the day and the timing of attacks cannot be predetermined. At some point in the course of the disease, 50% will experience depression and up to 90% of people with MS will experience fatigue (Greeke et al 2017). Therefore, staying positive and fighting depressive moods through involvement in a range of activities and modified exercise (as per Arona's example) are important for maintaining quality of life.

Variations in QOL can be correlated with the pattern, type and severity of symptoms being experienced and the context of the individual's demographic, socioeconomic, environmental and biopsychosocial circumstances (Bishop et al 2018). As effective communication is essential for social interaction, slurred speech (usually found in progressive forms of MS) makes communication difficult and may be mistaken by others for cognitive impairment or drunkenness, particularly when ataxia is also present. Difficulty with swallowing (dysphagia) is not considered a primary clinical feature of MS, but can have potentially life-threatening consequences and has been reported in 30–60% of people with MS, depending on the mode of assessment used (Solaro et al 2020). Assessment by a speech pathologist is recommended in cases where speech and swallowing difficulties persist.

Visual disturbances create reductions in visual acuity or double vision, making employment tasks and lifestyle activities, such as driving, difficult to perform. Cognitive function is affected in about 60% of people with MS, characterised by deficiencies in short-term memory, conceptual function and problem-solving. Recent studies into stimulating more effective cognitive function (termed cognitive rehabilitation) are promising, but outcomes vary with phenotype (D'Amico et al 2016). Compensatory strategies such as lists, diaries, visualisation techniques and avoiding detailed interactions in complex environments, are useful.

The community understanding of MS is limited. People with MS are often anxious about being labelled with the stigma of chronic illness or disability, and have been refused employment or 'forced' out of work as a productivity liability. Disclosure of MS might be avoided for fear of jeopardising relationships, the potential for employment or roles in community groups. Health professionals need to engage in community education and advocacy to enhance opportunities and acceptance of MS in the community.

Family and Caregivers

Living with the chronic, progressively disabling symptoms of MS affects family life in a number of ways, including roles, relationships, finances and general family organisation. The family caregiver's adaptive abilities will depend on family relationships prior to diagnosis, the attitudes to illness and rehabilitation, the effectiveness of their coping and stress management strategies and the availability of social support. Families have to accommodate the person's need for rest, symptom changes during an attack and adaptions to their life required to provide care when needed. Many people living with RRMS do not require intensive hands-on care. Instead they need love, understanding and support. In progressive forms of MS or during a severe attack, people need varying degrees of cognitive and physical assistance as well as psychological support.

Family members also have to contend with their own responses to physical and emotional losses, including lifestyle restrictions, relationship changes and communication challenges. Fear of future disease implications and end of life may also add to family stress. As with family caregivers in most situations, feelings of uselessness and guilt are common when family members are no longer able to provide care. Therefore, families are also people living with MS, who need supportive care at various times during the illness trajectory.

MOTOR NEURONE DISEASE

Motor neurone disease (MND) is a collective term that encompasses a number of neurodegenerative disorders, including amyotrophic lateral sclerosis (ALS), primary lateral sclerosis and progressive bulbar palsy. Degeneration occurs in the upper motor neurones of the cerebral cortex, the lower motor neurones in the spinal cord and the motor nuclei of the brain stem, resulting in multiple failures in nerve impulse transmission and denervation of muscles (Kumar et al 2015). The combination of upper and lower motor neurone involvement can be seen in muscle wasting (a lower motor neurone feature) and scarring of the corticospinal tract in the spinal cord (an upper motor neurone feature). While some sensory symptoms may present, the sensory system and intellect remain intact and the person is keenly aware of the degeneration of their body. Features of frontotemporal lobe dementia (FTD), such as changes in behaviour and language, disinhibition, apathy, compulsions and socially inappropriate actions, can also occur with ALS (Ahmed et al 2016). Like MS, MND is not a disease of old age. It mostly affects people aged between 40 and 60 years, with a mean age of onset at 55 years, an era of life when people are usually moving from direct parenting to living their own life, preparing for retirement and/or caring for elderly parents.

It is estimated that at any one time more than 2000 Australians and 400 New Zealanders are living with the disabling effects of MND (Deloitte 2015a; MND New Zealand 2020). These figures indicate that MND is not a common condition, yet it is the most common degenerative disorder of the motor-neuronal system in adults and the incidence of MND is rising.

While there is variation in the initial presentation of MND, progressive muscle weakness in one or more limbs, and/or speech and/or swallowing are typical signs. Problematically, the course of this disease is not consistent across cases and increasing muscle weakness, shrinkage and muscle fibre atrophy can occur at varying rates in different parts of the body. Several phenotypes are recognised as belonging to the MND syndrome, as detailed in Table 17.3.

Pain related to stress on joints associated with muscle decline, muscle spasm and cramping and pain on skin pressure are common to all phenotypes (Clarke 2016). On the other hand, regular fasciculations or twitching of a single muscle group are indicative of lower motor neurone dysfunction (Sleutjes et al 2015).

Extensive research is being undertaken to establish the cause of MND. Most cases are thought to be sporadic, but about 10% of cases are familial in origin,

TABLE 17.3
MND Phenotypes

Phenotype	Presentation
Amyotrophic lateral sclerosis (ALS) upper and lower motor neurone signs most common presentation	Brisk reflexes and local muscle wasting, particularly in the legs, feet, hands, arms, neck and head Visible fasciculations, emotional lability (atypical laughing or crying) with normal cognitive function Development of speech and swallowing dysfunction (in bulbar onset ALS, these appear first with tongue fasciculations, rapidly spreading to limbs with poor prognosis)
Progressive muscular atrophy mostly lower motor neurone involvement rare	Slow, progressive leg weakness and wasting that moves to arms and can involve the tongue, absence of reflexes, fasciculations, emotional lability Wasting and weakness often out of proportion
Flail arm more common in males	Upper girdle wasting, may include dropped head Bilateral increasing flaccidity of arms, limiting the person's ability to manipulate even the lightest of objects Slow spread to other parts of body
Lower limb onset	Gradual ascending distal weakness Increasing flaccidity in legs, quickly limiting the person's ability to mobilise
Primary lateral sclerosis upper motor neurone involvement longer life expectancy	Hyper reflexes and spasticity, preserved reflexes in wasted limbs More prone to emotional lability
Progressive bulbar palsy 1–2 year life expectancy	Often rapid degeneration of lower brain stem motor nuclei, speech, chewing and swallowing dysfunction, wasted tongue, drooling saliva

Huynh et al 2016; Kumar et al 2015.

attributed to more than 30 different genetic aberrations, with SOD1, C9orf72, FUS and TDP-43 being the more commonly mutated genes in MND (Mathis et al 2019). Genetic counselling in MND is complex, partly due to the strong influence ancestral origins have on the frequency of the genetic mutations. The most common genetic aberration in familial ALS (FALS) with European heritage is C9orf72 (see Gwen's story in Case Study 17.3), whereas for those with Asian backgrounds it's SOD1. RNA targeted therapies are being investigated as treatments for MND; however, as yet none has been found to be effective.

Although the mechanism of action of the drug Riluzole (called Rilutek in Gwen's story) is not entirely clear and its tablet format makes it increasingly difficult to swallow due to the development of dysphagia as the disease progresses, it is currently the only drug used in the treatment of MND and has been shown to extend life by a few months (Qureshi et al 2020). Life can also be extended through the use of assisted ventilation (Faull & Oliver 2016). While feeding via percutaneous endoscopic gastrostomy (PEG) improves nutritional status, it only corrects weight loss in the short term, has

no effect on function, but may contribute to survival advantage (Barone et al 2019). Thus, from diagnosis, an interdisciplinary palliative approach is the most effective way to provide care and promote QOL for people living with MND (Flemming et al 2020). Additionally, advance care planning needs to begin soon after diagnosis to facilitate conversations about symptom management and preparations for end-of-life care. Nurses and allied health professionals provide supportive care, including advance care planning, family education and equipment to sustain in-home care, institutional respite and acute care when patients need new treatments such as respiratory support, PEG placement or care related to co-morbidities.

Altered Mobility and Fatigue

Changes in mobility reflect the neural pathways affected by MND. Global symptoms may begin with disabling muscle cramps, stumbling or falling unexpectedly as the legs and/or feet muscles deteriorate. Loss of balance and difficulty holding objects or lifting anything impacts on the person's mobility and ability to undertake the activities of daily living (ADLs).

CASE STUDY 17.3

GWEN'S STORY (WRITTEN ON IPAD USING A MOUTH-HELD STYLUS)

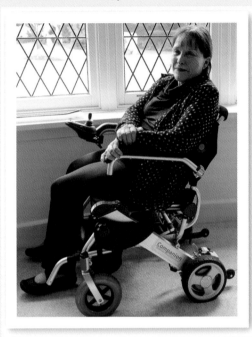

Fairfax Photos/Melissa Adams.

I was diagnosed with MND by a neurologist back in July 2012. For about a year prior to diagnosis, I was having problems with my hands. Things like doing up buttons or if I was writing for a long time my right hand would cramp up. I thought it was carpal tunnel, associated with my previous job as a horticulturalist and my current job as a Parks and Wildlife ranger, using machinery like chainsaws.

My father died 6 months after diagnosis with MND back in 1991 aged 50. He had lost muscle all over and had dementia symptoms. He would forget names and how to do simple tasks like dressing. His symptoms were picked up by a doctor from Scotland who was working at the local hospital. He had seen MND before in the UK. Dad's brother also died from MND that year. Back then we received no support, only a social worker who we saw a couple of times. Second time we saw a social worker was at the local agricultural show. She asked where Dad was. We said we had put Dad in hospital so we could have a break. By that stage Dad wandered around the house at night and Mum would stay up to watch him. The social worker thought this was ridiculous.

Back to me; during 2011 I saw my doctor about my hand. My doctor knew my dad had died from MND. The ultrasound report on both my hands attributed my symptoms to my job. My hands continued to get worse throughout 2011, so I was sent for CT scan of my neck that showed arthritis in my neck. I checked the internet and found that disc pressure on nerves in the spinal cord causes problems with hands, so I thought that was my problem. I was referred to a neurologist. While waiting for the appointment, I kept working and my partner Steve proposed to me.

When I finally got to see the neurologist, accompanied by Steve, he asked questions about my job and what my parents died of. He examined me, especially my muscle groups. He said, 'You're an intelligent person, so I am going to tell you straight that you have ALS'. He sent me for a lung function test and put me on Rilutek. Steve and I knew what MND meant because both our fathers had died from MND. I was dumbfounded by the diagnosis. It took me time to get my head round what that meant for me. The neurologist booked me into the local hospital for a few days for an MRI, blood tests, nerve conduct tests and a sleep study. My GP had suspected MND, but was surprised by the diagnosis.

Prior to my diagnosis, my older brother was seeing a neurogeneticist who was researching families with MND. They found the gene responsible for MND (C9orf72) in our family. My brother has the same symptoms as my dad.

Once I got my head round my diagnosis, I gave Steve the option of cancelling the wedding. He said he knew what he was in for and still wanted to marry me. We got married that October. Slowly over time I told family and friends about my diagnosis, trying to do it with humour. I contacted MND Queensland, who gave a name for a support group. I found the support group really handy for information and also its links to allied health, which improved access as I progressed. I was medically retired in early 2013. I had a small disability or death insurance which I accessed and allowed Steve to be my full-time carer. A wonderful friend who is a carpenter modified our house to make it easier for me to get around in my wheelchair. Steve, who is now my legs and arms, refers to the modifications as making the house 'Gwenable'.

I am determined to live my life to the fullest; my motto is here for a good time not a long time. I have a bucket list that we are working through. We went on a cruise for 72 days in 2014, halfway around the world visiting countries on my bucket list. Through the internet I was able to book disabled tours. In 2015 we went to Egypt and found disabled-friendly tours. Once travel overseas stopped my palliative care doctor asked if I was thinking about a PEG (percutaneous endoscopic gastrostomy). I know that MND will affect my ability to swallow and if my lung function gets worse, I won't be able to have a PEG. My only concern about the PEG was that I would be awake. As soon as they told me I would sleep during the procedure, I had the PEG. My PEG is really cool, one step towards being a cyborg.

I liken MND to Kinder Surprise chocolate; everyone has something different and something new every day.

Upper limb splinting may be useful and prolong capability, but caregivers quickly have to assume responsibility for tasks, such as doing up buttons, zips and shoe laces, turning pages, operating remote controls, showering, dressing, shaving, feeding and turning door knobs. In fact, anything that requires the hand to have strength and grip.

The early introduction of mobility aids is recommended to enhance independence and reduce the load on the degenerating muscles. Large pieces of equipment such as hoists and electric wheelchairs with high back support present particular problems because they are hard to manoeuvre and store in a family home. The presence of these mobility aids in the home indicates the extent of the disease progression to anyone who visits, preventing the ability to hide what might have been private knowledge into a more public arena. Health professionals need to be aware that mobility aids may threaten the person's self-image and compel them to confront the next stage of degeneration. Sensitivity to the emotional as well as the physical needs of the person and their family is important when discussing additional mobility supports. As entire muscle groups succumb to neuronal depletion, losses can seem to manifest overnight to the person and their family caregivers, threatening emotional wellbeing. OT and physiotherapy assessments need to be commenced soon after diagnosis and continue at regular intervals as new losses become evident.

People living with MND experience increasing chronic fatigue as their muscle tissue, including their intercostal muscles, diminishes. Fatigue increases throughout the day as fewer muscles are available to achieve the required workload. Exercise is important during the early stages of the disease, before significant atrophy leads to fatigue and reduced muscle strength (Zucchi et al 2019). Weakened respiratory muscles lead to chronic hypoventilation, making less oxygen available to the tissues. Non-invasive ventilation (NIV), usually delivered from a variable positive air pressure (VPAP) unit via a mask, improves oxygenation, relieves fatigue and increases life expectancy; however, it does not always improve QOL for the patient or caregivers in the later stages of the disease (Hazenberg et al 2016).

Body Image

With MND, body image is threatened by the relentless physical degeneration and increasing disability. Muscle wasting and weight loss are increasingly evident, particularly around the shoulders, trunk and sometimes the face. Losing the ability to participate in expected family routines and to undertake the personal ADLs not only alters personal roles and boundaries, but also threatens body image. Family members can do little more than watch their relative waste away and become more dependent. Body image is further jeopardised for people with bulbar symptoms. When swallowing becomes a problem, quantities of saliva that are normally swallowed may dribble uncontrollably from the mouth. Drooling and the need to be assisted with eating or PEG feeding are not consistent with social interaction. Children of people with MND may become embarrassed by the changed appearance and apparent loss of body control of their parent and cease having friends visit. This restricts opportunities to stay connected with social support systems and reduces quality of life for the person and their family.

Quality of Life

QOL for people living with MND is focused on effective symptom control and maintenance of personhood, including independence and social relationships. Early assessment, the establishment of a safe living environment and the well-timed introduction of functional devices that enable people to remain independent as long as possible, improve QOL for the person and family caregivers. The person with MND feels more in control of their life and the family caregiver is able to continue employment and other life activities for longer periods.

Symptom management in MND includes pain control, respiratory support, dysphagia management, drooling control, enhanced communication and, for some, management of emotional lability and cognitive changes. Pain resulting from strain on joints responds to anti-inflammatory medication; muscle relaxants such as Baclofen are useful for spasms from upper neurone damage; while skin pressure pain is relieved by repositioning, pressure-reducing aids, such as specialised seat and bed overlays and opioid medication (Everett et al 2020). Swallowing problems are managed initially by modified cups, postural changes, fluid thickening and food modification. Later, if the person agrees to active treatment, a gastrostomy is performed. Anticholinergic drugs, injecting the parotid glands with botulinum toxin or destruction of the salivary glands via radiotherapy can reduce saliva (Everett et al 2020). However, these treatments can also result in the development of tenacious saliva that is hard to swallow.

QOL through social relationships depends on effective communication. The loss of the ability to communicate limits social interactions to those who can socially engage without the need for verbal participation. This is especially important, as the majority of people with MND develop dysarthria and many will progress to anarthria during the course of the disease. There are a variety of communication solutions available, some electronic that can be accessed via specialised switches such as retinal scanners or neuromuscular switches, but often the simplicity of low-tech systems like laser pointers, picture and alphabet boards is preferred, especially within the older age group. Smartphone and tablet technology has increased accessibility and affordability for most people. However, their success is dependent on the rate of degenerative progression and the willingness of the person and others to adapt to that style of communication. For example, Lightwriters use synthesised voice that can sound unnatural, while Etran boards rely on eye movements and an attentive communication partner to spell out words. Despite these aids, communication can be hard work and social relationships decline.

Family and Caregivers
In Australia, most people with MND (as in Gwen's case) are cared for in the home by family members and many die at home. Access to community resources is sporadic, dependent on availability of services and eligibility criteria. If services are accessible, a pervasive issue for caregivers of people with MND plus frontotemporal lobe dementia, and the interdisciplinary team, is the impact of cognitive changes that can manifest as inflexibility when considering realistic solutions to challenges of daily care. This impacts on the uptake of in-home safety recommendations without consideration of the extra physical and emotional stress this may place on the caregiver, who may place their own wellbeing at risk while striving to fulfil the wishes of their person with MND. Advance care planning to encourage discussion and documentation of patient wishes before cognitive and behavioural decline and the initiation of life-sustaining treatments is therefore recommended (Murray et al 2016).

Care and support of a loved one with MND who is going to die has been described as relentless. As the person becomes less mobile and unable to carry out personal tasks the family members, usually a partner or child, have to provide care 24 hours each day of the week. Family caregivers experience many situations that cause them to redefine themselves and their relationship with the person living with MND (Dieplinger et al 2017). While family caregivers need and value the support of community resources, these resources should be integrated and structured so that family privacy and personal space in the family home are respected and preserved as much as possible. Providing time to support family caregivers rather than just meeting the physical needs of the person with MND is vital for the maintenance of effective in-home care.

The palliative care approach was until recently not offered to people with MND despite the progressive and terminal nature of the disease. There is, however, a growing recognition of the need to initiate palliative care services early to plan and regularly re-evaluate symptom management, and family support, rather than waiting until near the end of life (Flemming et al 2020).

EDUCATION FOR THE PERSON AND FAMILY LIVING WITH PD, MS OR MND
The management of PD, MS and MND is a shared function involving the person, their family or other caregivers and the interdisciplinary team. It is important that those who care for a person with PD, MS or MND understand the complexities of the condition, the motor and non-motor aspects and the relevant medications and treatment options. It is easier to understand the motor and sensory problems, but the non-motor problems, such as constipation, anxiety, depression, sexual difficulties and social withdrawal, can prove to be more insidious and chip away at QOL. Educational information needs to be incremental, relevant to achieving immediate care, address specific problems and be inclusive of planning for future care needs through advance care plan conversations. These conversations require advanced communication skills and sensitivity concerning the difficulty some may experience in confronting the reality of living with a chronic, degenerative illness. Therefore, health professionals need to be cognisant of the person or their family's existing knowledge, look for opportunities presented by changes in health status and recognise cues indicating readiness to engage in education and future planning. When disability from disease progression makes travelling to the clinic too difficult and for those in rural and remote locations, the emergence of telehealth is providing an effective tool to enhance support and promote communication between patients, family caregivers and health professionals (James et al 2019).

Discussions may include:
- effective ways to assist with ADLs and manage chronic care requirements to prevent injury
- repositioning techniques to relieve pressure and strain and to promote breathing
- communication techniques and devices, assisted coughing
- effective use of medications and complementary therapies to promote QOL
- use and maintenance of interventions such as PEG, NIV devices, mobility aids, suction units
- effective cueing strategies
- available community services and resources to support in-home care

- strategies for identifying and mobilising social support networks
- importance of talking about the impact of the disease on relationships, lifestyle, advance care planning and preparations for end of life
- strategies for managing the losses and emotional burden of caregiving
- caregiver health and wellbeing, including plans for personal time and resources for respite
- access to the resources of relevant associations:
  - The Parkinson's Society (www.parkinsons.org.au/) (www.parkinsons.org.nz/)
  - MS Society (www.msaustralia.org.au/) (www.msnz.org.nz/)
  - MND Association (www.mndaust.asn.au/) (www.mnd.org.nz/).

While members of the interdisciplinary team may initiate some of these topics, nurses are often required to revise, support and consolidate knowledge and skills, and facilitate advance care planning especially in rural and regional areas.

CONCLUSION

The degenerative, disabling and often chronic nature of PD, MS and MND create multiple physical, emotional and lifestyle challenges for people and their families. Changes in the level of mobility and capacity to self-care, as well as alterations in body image and self-concept, change the nature of roles and relationships and affect QOL. Support and encouragement that enables people to plan ahead and take control of disease management is integral to promoting a positive approach. Through understanding of the distinctive features of each disease and the available interventions, the interdisciplinary team will be equipped to provide focused support for people and their families living with PD, MS and MND.

Reflective Questions

1. Timely interventions are important for maintaining quality of life and enabling people to live at home. Describe the likely patient care needs and the corresponding interdisciplinary team members that could be involved in facilitating effective in-home care across each disease trajectory.
2. Discuss the place and importance of supportive care for family caregivers of people living with PD, MS and MND.
3. Describe the challenges and enablers for facilitating advance care planning among people living with PD, MS and MND.

Acknowledgement

The authors wish to thank the people living with PD, MS and MND for their willingness to share stories of their journey with each disease so that others may learn and improve their ability to provide supportive care.

RECOMMENDED READING

Harris DA, Jack K, Wibberley C 2018. The meaning of living with uncertainty for people with motor neurone disease. Journal of Clinical Nursing 27, 2062–2071.

Rommer PS, Eichstadt K, Ellenberger D et al 2019. Symptomatology and symptomatic treatment in multiple sclerosis: results from a nationwide MS registry. Multiple Sclerosis Journal 25(12), 1641–1652.

Tension E, Smink A, Redwood S et al 2020. Proactive and integrated management and empowerment in Parkinson's disease: designing a new model of care. Parkinson's Disease, DOI: 10.1155/2020/8673087

REFERENCES

Aharony SM, Lam O, Corcos J 2017. Treatment of lower urinary tract symptoms in multiple sclerosis patients: review of the literature and current guidelines. Canadian Urological Association Journal 11(3–4), E110–115.

Ahmed RM, Devenney EM, Irish M et al 2016. Neuronal network disintegration: common pathways linking neurodegenerative diseases. Journal of Neurology, Neurosurgery & Psychiatry 87(11), 1234–1241.

Alty J, Robson J, Duggan-Carter P et al 2016. What to do when people with Parkinson's disease cannot take their usual oral medications. Practical Neurology 16(2), 122–128.

Angeles DC, Ho P, Dymock BW et al 2016. Antioxidants inhibit neuronal toxicity in Parkinson's disease-linked LRRK2. Annals of Clinical and Translational Neurology 3(4), 288–294.

Ascherio A, Munger KL 2016. Epidemiology of multiple sclerosis: from risk factors to prevention: an update. Seminars in Neurology 36(2), 103–114.

Australian Bureau of Statistics 2019. 3303.0 – Causes of death, Australia, 2018 Australia's leading causes of death, 2018. Online. Available: www.abs.gov.au/ausstats/abs@.nsf/mf/3303.0

Barone M, Viggiani MT, Introna A et al 2019. Nutritional prognostic factors for survival in amyotrophic lateral sclerosis patients undergone percutaneous endoscopic gastrostomy placement. Amyotrophic Lateral Sclerosis and Frontotemporal Degeneration 20(7/8), 490–496.

Beh SC, Kildebeck E, Narayan R et al 2017. High-dose methotrexate with leucovorin rescue: for monumentally severe CNS inflammatory syndromes. Journal of the Neurological Sciences 372, 187–195.

Belvisi D, Pellicciari R, Fabbrini G et al 2019. Modifiable risk and protective factors in disease development, progression and clinical subtypes of Parkinson's disease: what do prospective studies suggest?, Neurobiology of Disease 134 (2020), 104671.

Bishop M, Fraser R, Li J et al 2018. Life domains that are important to quality of life for people with multiple sclerosis: a population-based qualitative analysis. Journal of Vocational Rehabilitation 51(1), 67–76.

Clarke J 2016. Pain in motor neurone disease. British Journal of Neuroscience Nursing 12(2), 85–87.

Creed RB, Menalled L, Casey B et al 2019. Basal and evoked neurotransmitter levels in Parkin, DJ-1, PINK1 and LRRK2 knockout rat striatum. Neuroscience 409, 169–179.

D'Amico E, Leone C, Hayrettin T et al 2016. Can we define a rehabilitation strategy for cognitive impairment in progressive multiple sclerosis? A critical appraisal. Multiple Sclerosis Journal 22(5), 581–589.

Deloitte Access Economics 2015. Economic analysis of motor neurone disease in Australia. Online. Available: www.mndaust.asn.au/Influencing-policy/Economic-analysis-of-MND-(1)/Economic-analysis-of-MND-in-Australia.aspx

Deloitte Access Economics 2015. Living with Parkinson's disease: an updated economic analysis 2014. Online. Available: https://d04df24a-57f9-43a8-8a9e-121c07e25be2.filesusr.com/ugd/d5412d_b84fd7411bc447b88136034e5cf4a077.pdf.

Dieplinger A, Kundt FS, Lorenzl S 2017. Palliative care nursing for patients with neurological diseases: what makes a difference? British Journal of Nursing 26(6), 356–359.

Everett EA, Pedowitz E, Maiser S et al 2020. Top ten tips palliative care clinicians should know about amyotrophic lateral sclerosis. Journal of Palliative Medicine 23(6), 842–847.

Faull C, Oliver D 2016. Withdrawal of ventilation at the request of a patient with motor neurone disease: guidance for professionals. BMJ Supportive & Palliative Care 6(2), 144–146.

Flemming K, Turner V, Bolsher S et al 2020. The experiences of, and need for, palliative care for people with motor neurone disease and their informal caregivers: a qualitative systematic review. Palliative Medicine 34(6), 708–730.

GBD 2016 Parkinson's Disease Collaborators 2018. Global, regional, and national burden of Parkinson's disease, 1990–2016: a systematic analysis for the Global Burden of Disease Study 2016. The Lancet Neurology 17(11), 939–953.

Gofton TE, Kumar H, Roberts-South A et al 2015. Validity, reliability, and insights from applying the McGill Quality of Life Questionnaire to people living with Parkinson's disease (MQoL-PD). Journal of Palliative Care 31(4), 213–220.

Gonzales B, Chopard G, Charry B et al 2017. Effects of a training program involving body cooling on physical and cognitive capacities and quality of life in multiple sclerosis patients: a pilot study European Neurology 78(1/2), 71–77.

Greeke EE, Chua AS, Healy BC et al 2017. Depression and fatigue in patients with multiple sclerosis. Journal of Neurological Sciences 380, 236–241.

Harris D, Jack K, Wibberley C 2019. Making her end of life her own: further reflections on supporting a loved one with motor neurone disease. International Journal of Palliative Nursing 25(6), 284–292.

Hazenberg A, Kerstjens HAM, Prins SCL et al 2016. Is chronic ventilatory support really effective in patients with amyotrophic lateral sclerosis? Journal of Neurology 263(12), 2456–2461.

Hentzen C, Villaume A, Turmel N et al 2020. Time to be ready to void: a new tool to assess the time needed to perform micturition for patients with multiple sclerosis. Annals of Physical and Rehabilitation Medicine 63(2), 99–105.

Huynh W, Simon NG, Grosskreutz J et al 2016. Assessment of the upper motor neuron in amyotrophic lateral sclerosis. Clinical Neurophysiology: Official Journal of the International Federation of Clinical Neurophysiology 127(7), 2643–2660.

James N, Power E, Hoden A et al 2019. Patients' perspectives of multidisciplinary home-based e-Health service delivery for motor neurone disease. Disability and Rehabilitation: Assistive Technology 14(7), 737–743.

Jelinek GA, Marck CH, Weiland TJ et al 2015. Latitude, sun exposure and vitamin D supplementation: associations with quality of life and disease outcomes in a large international cohort of people with multiple sclerosis. BMC Neurology 15(1), 1–6.

Kular L, Jagodic M 2020. Epigenetic insights into multiple sclerosis disease progression. Journal of Internal Medicine 288(1), 82–102.

Kumar V, Abbas AK, Aster JC 2015. Robbins and Coltran: pathologic basis of disease. Elsevier, Philadelphia.

Langford BE, Ridley CJA, Beale RC et al 2018. Focused ultrasound thalamotomy and other interventions for medication-refractory essential tremor: an indirect comparison of short-term impact on health-related quality of life. Value Health 21(10), 1168–1175.

Lenka A, Herath P, Christopher R et al 2017. Psychosis in Parkinson's disease: from the soft signs to the hard science. Journal of the Neurological Sciences 379, 169–176.

Liddle J, Beazley G, Gustafsson L et al 2019. Mapping the experiences and needs of deep brain stimulation for people with Parkinson's disease and their family members. Brain Impairment 20(3), 211–225.

Martini A, Weis L, Schifano R et al 2020. Differences in cognitive profiles between Lewy body and Parkinson's disease dementia. Journal of Neural Transmission (Vienna) 127(3), 323–330.

Mathis S, Goizet C, Soulages A et al 2019. Genetics of amyotrophic lateral sclerosis: a review. Journal of the Neurological Sciences 399, 217–226.

McNicholas N, Lockhart A, Yap SM et al 2019. New versus old: implications for evolving diagnostic criteria for relapsing-remitting multiple sclerosis. Multiple Sclerosis Journal 25(6), 867–870.

MND New Zealand 2020. Facts about MND. Online. Available: https://mnd.org.nz/about-mnd/

MS Research Australia 2018. MS on the rise in Australia but still flying under our radar. Online. Available: https://msra.org.au/news/ms-rise-australia-still-flying-radar/

MS Research Australia 2020. What is multiple sclerosis (MS)? Online. Available: https://msra.org.au/what-is-multiple-sclerosis-ms/

Multiple Sclerosis New Zealand (MSMZ) 2021. Who gets MS? Online. Available: www.msnz.org.nz/about/#WGM

Murray L, Butow PN, White K et al 2016. Advance care planning in motor neuron disease: a qualitative study of caregiver perspectives. Palliative Medicine 30(5), 471–478.

Parkinson's New Zealand 2021. What is Parkinson's? Online. Available: www.parkinsons.org.nz/understanding-parkinsons/what-parkinsons.

Patti F, Zimator GB, Morra VB et al 2020. Administration of subcutaneous interferon beta 1a in the evening: data from RELIEF study. Journal of Neurology 267(6), 1812–1823.

Pontone GM, Bakker CC, Chen S et al 2016. The longitudinal impact of depression on disability in Parkinson disease. International Journal of Geriatric Psychiatry 31(5), 458–465.

Qureshi I, Lovegren M, Wirtz V et al 2020. A pharmacokinetic bioequivalence study comparing sublingual Riluzole (BHV-0223) and oral tablet formulation of Riluzole in healthy volunteers. Clinical Pharmacology in Drug Development 9(4), 476–485.

Radder DLM, Sturkenboom LH, van Nimwegen M et al 2017. Physical therapy and occupational therapy in Parkinson's disease. International Journal of Neuroscience 127(10), 930–943.

Rascol O, Negre-Pages L, Damier P et al 2020. Utilization patterns of Amantadine in Parkinson's disease patients enrolled in the French COPARK Study. Drugs and Aging 37(3), 215–223.

Razazian N, Kazeminia M, Moayedi H et al 2020. The impact of physical exercise on the fatigue symptoms in patients with multiple sclerosis: a systematic review and meta-analysis. BMC Neurology 20(1), 1–11.

Rommer PS, Eichstädt K, Ellenberger D et al 2019. Symptomatology and symptomatic treatment in multiple sclerosis: results for a nationwide MS registry. Multiple Sclerosis Journal 25(12), 1641–1652.

Rumrill Jr, PD, Bishop M 2019. Multiple sclerosis: a high-incidence immune-mediated disease of the central nervous system. Journal of Vocational Rehabilitation 51(1), 1–9.

Sanchirico M, Caldwell-Tarr A, Mudumby P et al 2019. Treatment patterns, healthcare resource utilization, and costs among Medicare patients with multiple sclerosis in relation to disease-modifying therapy and corticosteroid treatment Neurology Theory 8(1), 121–133.

Singleton C, Bakheit AM, Peace C 2016. The efficacy of functional electrical stimulation of the abdominal muscles in the treatment of chronic constipation in patients with multiple sclerosis: a pilot study. Multiple Sclerosis International 2016, 4860315.

Sleutjes BT, Montfoort I, van Doorn PA et al 2015. Diagnostic accuracy of electrically elicited multiple discharges in patients with motor neuron disease. Journal of Neurology, Neurosurgery & Psychiatry 86(11), 1234–1239.

Solaro C, Cuccaro A, Gamberini G et al 2020. Prevalence of dysphagia in a consecutive cohort of subjects with MS using fibre-optic endoscopy. Neurological Sciences 41(5), 1075–1079.

Steenhof M, Nielsen NM, Stenager E et al 2018. Distribution of disease courses in familial vs sporadic multiple sclerosis. Acta Neurologica Scandinavica 139(3), 231–237.

Straulino E, Scaravilli T, Castiello U 2016. Dopamine depletion affects communicative intentionality in Parkinson's disease patients: evidence from action kinematics. Cortex; a Journal Devoted to the Study of the Nervous System and Behavior 77, 84–94.

Torti M, Bravi D, Vacca L et al 2019. Are all dopamine agonists essentially the same? Drugs 79(7), 693–703.

Varadi C 2020. Clinical features of Parkinson's disease: the evolution of critical symptoms. Biology 9(5), doi:10.3390/biology9050103

Wilting J, Rolfsnes HO, Zimmermann H et al 2016. Structural correlates for fatigue in early relapsing remitting multiple sclerosis. European Society of Radiology 26, 515–523.

Wolkorte R, Heersema DJ, Zijdewind I 2016. Reduced voluntary activation during brief and sustained contractions of a hand muscle in secondary-progressive multiple sclerosis patients. Neurorehabilitation and Neural Repair 30(4), 307–316.

You H, Mariani L-L, Mangone G et al 2018. Molecular basis of dopamine replacement therapy and its side effects in Parkinson's disease. Cell and Tissue Research 373(1), 111–135.

Zucchi E, Vinceti M, Malagoli C et al 2019. High-frequency motor rehabilitation in amyotrophic lateral sclerosis: a randomized clinical trial. Annals of Clinical and Translational Neurology 6(5), 893–901.

CHAPTER 18

Principles for Nursing Practice: Persistent Asthma

CHARLOTTE ALLEN

LEARNING OBJECTIVES

When you have completed this chapter you will be able to:

- describe the pathogenesis and diagnosis of persistent atopic asthma and the clinical features observed during exacerbation of the disease
- explain the triggers for exacerbation of persistent atopic asthma and steps that can be taken to avoid them
- describe the approaches to long-term management of this condition
- explain the principles underpinning the approaches to nursing practice in the treatment of persistent atopic asthma
- understand the psychological issues that can affect the care of patients with this chronic disorder.

KEY WORDS

airway hyper-responsiveness	exacerbation
asthma	peak expiratory flow
bronchodilation	

INTRODUCTION

Asthma is a term that describes a collection of clinical disorders, rather than a single disease, which have in common reversible airflow limitation to the lungs in response to certain triggers. The complex nature of the disease is highlighted by the distinction between the clinical manifestations of the disease in adults compared with children. Although the prevalence of wheezing is considered to be high in children under the age of 6 years, approximately half will cease wheezing by adolescence (Holt & Sly 2012). The incidence of the disease then tends to decline towards adulthood, with the most current figures indicating that asthma is one of Australia's most widespread chronic health problems, with 8.2–13.9% of children (up to 15 years of age) and 8.6–12.4% of adults reporting doctor-diagnosed asthma with treatment in the previous 12 months between the 2003–09 period (Australian Centre for Asthma Monitoring 2011). Additional information from a 2017–18 National Health Survey by the Australian Bureau of Statistics (ABS) showed that 2.7 million Australians have been diagnosed with asthma (ABS 2018). A further analysis by the Australian Institute of Health and Welfare (AIHW) revealed asthma to be in the top 15 causes of total disease burden in Australia in 2015, and the leading cause of disease burden in males aged between 5 and 14 years of age (AIHW 2020).

The key underlying disease process occurring in asthma is inflammation of the airway walls and lung parenchyma, the triggering of which induces bronchial hyperresponsiveness (BHR). The assessment of BHR by methacholine challenge testing is a mainstay of persistent or uncontrolled asthma diagnosis in adults and has a strong negative predictive power in excluding a diagnosis of asthma (Quaedvlieg et al 2009; Global Initiative for Asthma 2016a). One of the most common triggers of BHR in adults is inhaled allergens, which is the underlying basis of atopic or eosinophilic asthma. According to the National Asthma Council Australia, around 80% of people with asthma also have allergies (National Asthma Council Australia 2016a, 2016b), while data from the 2007–08 National Health Survey indicate that sinusitis and rhinitis are the most common respiratory co-morbid condition among people with asthma (Australian Centre for Asthma Monitoring 2011). Atopy is defined as the production of a particular isotype of antibody, termed immunoglobulin E (IgE) at low levels to a variety of environmental allergens; this is the underlying cause of allergic conditions such as rhinitis, atopic dermatitis (eczema) and allergic sensitisation to food allergens. Importantly, in terms of persistent allergic asthma, a diagnosis of atopy together with recurrent respiratory viral infections are strongly associated with the persistence of asthma into adolescence and adulthood (Holt & Sly 2012). Individuals with allergic rhinitis, atopic dermatitis or who are also sensitised to food or aero-allergens are considered to be at high risk for the development of persistent asthma (Guilbert et al 2016).

In addition to the atopic asthma 'phenotype', several other phenotypes representing asthma induced by non-atopic triggers represent a significant category of adult asthma sufferers; these include asthma exacerbations triggered by a variety of non-specific stimuli such as exercise, cold air, drugs (aspirin, NSAIDs),

occupational exposures and active or passive cigarette smoke exposure (Howrylak et al 2016). Respiratory infections, such as respiratory syncytial virus, rhinovirus and influenza viral infections, are also a common cause of asthma exacerbations in children, but cause a minority of exacerbations in adults (Johnston 1998; Rubner et al 2017). Clinically, additional subtypes (or 'endotypes') can be made based on the inflammatory phenotype, where 'eosinophilic' and 'non-eosinophilic' or 'neutrophilic' phenotypes can be diagnosed on the basis of the inflammatory cell types in induced sputum or bronchioalveolar lavage samples (Brooks et al 2013; Howrylak et al 2016). Although these inflammatory subtypes are not regularly identified in the day-to-day clinical management of the person with asthma, they may be useful in the design of new treatments for patients in which conventional anti-inflammatory therapies are not effective (Barnes 2012). In Case Study 18.1, Charlene's asthma exacerbation develops subsequent to an influenza infection, which may have heightened her responsiveness to other environmental triggers, including allergens.

The management of persistent asthma requires a comprehensive approach, the primary aim of which is to minimise the number and severity of asthma exacerbations. This will involve the identification and avoidance of triggers where possible, appropriate medications and education for patients, family and carers.

CASE STUDY 18.1

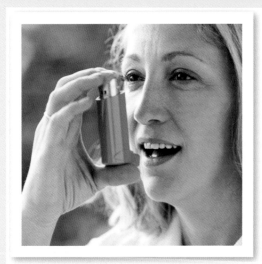

iStockphoto/vgajic.

Charlene is a 23-year-old female with a history of atopic asthma. She was first diagnosed with asthma by her family general practitioner (GP) when she was a child. During her childhood she has been hospitalised on several occasions for exacerbations of asthma. Charlene also has eczema and is allergic to nuts; however, she has no other relevant clinical history.

Charlene experiences symptoms of asthma on most days and seeks medical treatment several times each year to treat exacerbations of asthma, usually related to respiratory viral infections. Her usual asthma management includes the use of a rapid acting beta-2-agonist inhaler and a low-dose inhaled glucocorticosteroid.

Charlene has recently moved away from her family for the first time. She has just commenced studies at university and now shares a house with three other students. She has noticed that since moving into shared accommodation her asthma symptoms have worsened. The share house is in an older suburb, with poor heating and ventilation, and one of her housemates smokes cigarettes. She has recently had a respiratory bacterial infection following an influenza viral infection (treated with oral antibiotics and oral glucocor-ticosteroids); however, her asthma symptoms are slow to improve. She has not attended university on many occasions as she has been tired, kept awake at night due to coughing. She is worried about her approaching exams and is feeling fatigued, stressed and having trouble controlling her asthma symptoms (wheezing, breathlessness, night-time and early morning coughing).

At her mother's insistence, Charlene attends her GP again for treatment of her worsening symptoms and is subsequently referred to the practice asthma nurse for a review of her action plan and medications, including correct delivery device use.

Charlene and the practice asthma nurse meet at the medical clinic. During the consultation Charlene identifies her main concerns as anxiety regarding her worsening symptoms of asthma and about passing her approaching university exams. Charlene states that 'Sometimes I am really scared as I can't get my breath; it takes all my energy to relax so I can get air in and out of my lungs'. Charlene expresses how much she has enjoyed the independence of moving into a share house with other students, but feels that if her asthma remains out of control she will need to move back home – something she doesn't want to do. When the asthma nurse inquires about her medication regimen, Charlene discloses that she hasn't been taking the low-dose inhaled glucocorticosteroid over the past few months as she doesn't think it makes much difference to her asthma. In addition, when the asthma nurse asks Charlene to demonstrate her inhaler technique, she does not use a spacer, stating she is embarrassed to use a spacer as she feels this is only for children.

The asthma nurse identifies the following issues: poor understanding of medications and triggers, suboptimal use of medication devices, poor adherence to asthma action plan, anxiety related to asthma and reduced quality of life. Charlene and the asthma nurse work together to review her asthma action plan and to identify some realistic strategies that Charlene feels she could achieve over the following weeks. The asthma nurse involves Charlene in all decisions in order to respect her emerging independence and autonomy. The strategies focus primarily upon education regarding her medications, her technique of using inhalers and identification of triggers. In addition, Charlene expresses her desire to start yoga classes with some friends. A follow-up appointment is made for 6 weeks time.

At the follow-up meeting with the asthma nurse, Charlene discusses how she has been compliant with her medication use (rarely forgetting and using good technique), has had a reduction in symptoms, has had improved lung function and is attending yoga classes with friends. She remains in the share house and is still attending university.

BEHAVIOURS THAT CONTRIBUTE TO THE DEVELOPMENT OF THE CONDITION

Pathophysiology

Over 90% of adults and 80% of children with asthma are diagnosed as atopic and therefore management of this condition requires knowledge of the factors that trigger an allergic response. In the patient with persistent asthma, the key physiological feature underlying this condition is BHR, which in the context of allergic asthma manifests as a heightened or exaggerated bronchoconstrictor response to aeroallergens. The underlying basis for this condition is a persistent inflammatory response into the airways that ultimately results in airway remodelling, narrowing of the airways and heightened responsiveness to allergic and non-allergic triggers. How this condition develops over the life of a patient is still poorly understood. However, it seems probable that genetically susceptible individuals are primed at birth (or even in utero) to develop an atopic response to one or more environmental allergens. An understanding of the nature of the inflammatory response is important in order to guide correct diagnosis of the disease and choice of treatment approaches (Chung 2015).

It is interesting to note that the incidence of atopy and allergy in Western and developing nations, including Australia, is increasing. In the United States, for example, the number of people with asthma increased by 28% from 2001 to 2011 (Centers for Disease Control and Prevention 2013). Again, the reason for this is not fully understood, but its basis is likely to be in the early years of life and may perhaps relate to the increasing 'cleanliness' of urban home environments in these regions: the so-called 'hygiene hypothesis' (Strachan 1989). For example, there is evidence to suggest that early exposure to the high bacterial loads in some farm environments can prevent the development of atopy and asthma. A recent study in the United States comparing genetically similar Amish and Hutterite farming populations found a significant inverse relationship between household bacterial endotoxin levels and the incidence of asthma and allergic sensitisation in children, again supporting a role for bacterial exposure in preventing the development of atopy and asthma

(Stein et al 2016). Other environmental factors may also be at play, including increased levels of pollution in metropolitan regions and the likelihood of the increasing effects of global warming: increased atmospheric CO_2 levels are known to stimulate pollinosis, which can increase the levels of allergens in the atmosphere, while changing climates will alter the geographic spread of allergens and the types of allergens to which people are exposed (Liu 2015).

It is therefore important to identify allergen triggers where possible, so that avoidance strategies can be put in place for the patient. However, it may also be important to establish whether the environmental conditions of the patient have also changed. In the case of Charlene in Case Study 18.1, moving into an environment with high levels of passive smoke exposure represented a high-risk environment. The environment into which the patient is moving should be taken into account when considering discharge from hospital of the stabilised patient, and all other potential trigger factors should be considered (see below).

However, it should also be noted that a lack of diagnosis for atopy does not preclude a diagnosis of asthma – this is particularly the case for children – and asthma can develop in response to a variety of non-allergenic triggers. These include cold air, exercise, stress, oesophageal reflux and responses to medications, such as aspirin and non-steroidal anti-inflammatory drugs (NSAIDs). However, as Charlene has been diagnosed as atopic, it is likely that her exacerbation was triggered by an allergic response and we will therefore focus this discussion on the allergic triggers of asthma.

Allergen Triggers

For patients with allergic asthma, it is well established that exposure to allergens can trigger an asthmatic response. In Australia and other developed countries, one of the most common indoor allergic triggers is allergens of the house dust mite (HDM) *Dermatophagoides pteronyssinus* and *Dermatophagoides farinae*. HDM allergens usually take the form of small protein molecules that are part of the mite or are excreted as waste products (Holt & Thomas 2005). However, in addition to HDM, other common indoor allergens include animal dander from cats and dogs, cockroach allergens and, occasionally, moulds. Food allergens, such as peanuts and seafood, are also reported by some patients to induce asthma exacerbations, although this often occurs in conjunction with other more generalised food allergy reactions, such as skin rashes and gut symptoms that occur as part of a systemic anaphylactic response (National Asthma Council Australia 2016a, 2016b). Cat allergens are a particularly potent form of allergen: they are secreted by the sebaceous glands, salivary glands and uterus, stick to the hair and become airborne when hair is shed. About 50% of patients who are allergic to cats make IgE that binds to the cat allergen Fel d 1 – a uteroglobin (blastokinin) secreted by the uteruses of many mammals, the cat version of which is especially allergenic (Holt & Thomas 2005). The most important outdoor allergens are the pollens of grasses, weeds (especially ragweed), olive, birch and conifers. Patients may react to one or several of these allergens, but sensitisation will depend on geographical location.

Allergen Avoidance

The case for allergen avoidance in the prevention of asthma is complex. However, in some cases, allergen avoidance or reduced allergen exposure can be effective in reducing asthma symptoms and requirement for medications. For example, patients with a proven allergy to HDM can take measures to kill mites or restrict their breeding and remove the allergens they produce. However, in some individuals there may not be a direct relationship between allergen exposure and development of asthma symptoms. This may be the case because the individual is sensitised to more than one allergen or that allergen exposure is exacerbated by exposure to other triggers, such as influenza virus infection, cigarette smoke or medications. This is likely to be the case for Charlene, as several factors may be involved in triggering her exacerbation and contribute to the severity of symptoms – moving into a different environment, exposure to passive cigarette smoke and a recent influenza infection. Care should be taken to reduce allergen exposure and triggers in the home environment when the patient is stabilised.

THE IMPACT OF PERSISTENT ASTHMA ON THE QUALITY OF LIFE

The impact of living with asthma affects the quality of life. Box 18.1 illustrates key content areas and provides examples of personal experiences of how the lives of those with asthma are affected (Eberhart et al 2014). Exploring the personal experiences of people with asthma provides health professionals with the opportunity to see beyond the objective data of peak flows and respiratory rates and consider how living with a chronic process actually impacts on the quality of life. The case study of Charlene (Case Study 18.1) demonstrates many of the content areas identified by Eberhart and colleagues (2014) that impact on her life, including activities, school, affect/emotions, fear of a bad attack, stigma, lack of control and sleep.

> **BOX 18.1**
> **The Impact of Asthma on the Quality of Life**
>
> | Content Area | Operational Definition | Example of Personal Experience |
> | --- | --- | --- |
> | Impact on activities | Impact on valued activities or activities the person wants to do | I was unable to do all the things I wanted to do |
> | Impact on social relationships/physical intimacy | Impact of asthma on interpersonal relationships | Asthma placed stress on my relationships with family, friends, significant others, or co-workers |
> | Impact on work/school/home | Impact on ability to fulfil social roles and obligations, whether at work, school or home | I was kept from doing things I needed to do at work, school or home |
> | Affect/emotions | Impact on various kinds of negative affect (sad, angry, stressed, tired, worried, annoyed etc.) | I felt irritable |
> | Fear of death/bad attack | Fear of having a severe asthma attack and having one's life threatened | I worried about dying from an asthma attack |
> | Stigma/embarrassment | Feeling stigmatised by others due to asthma, or embarrassed by asthma and its treatment | I was embarrassed by using my inhaler in front of other people |
> | Worry about future health | Worry about the long-term effects of asthma on health | I worried about the long-term effects of asthma on my health |
> | Anticipation | Having to plan ahead to anticipate asthma triggers and avoid potentially problematic situations | It bothers me that I have to plan ahead |
> | Burden/always on mind | Having to constantly think about asthma; asthma as a burden that one carries around with them all the time | My asthma was on my mind |
> | Denial/minimisation | Denying or minimising the effect that asthma has on one's life | It was hard for me to admit I have asthma |
> | Lack of control/uncertainty | Being unable to control asthma, things that trigger asthma, or one's own life due to asthma | I felt frustrated that I can't control the things around me that trigger my asthma |
> | Financial impact | Financial/economic effect of asthma and its treatment | The cost of treating my asthma is a burden to me |
> | Dependence on medications | Burden associated with dependence on asthma medications | I found it annoying having to carry my inhaler with me |
> | Side effects of medication | Bothered by side effects of asthma medications on quality of life | I was bothered by side effects from asthma medication |
> | Impact on sleep | Impact of asthma on quality of sleep | It was hard to get a good night's sleep because of my asthma |
> | General impact on life goals/enjoyment of life | Impact of asthma on ability to achieve life goals or have an enjoyable and fulfilling life | I felt that asthma was preventing me from achieving what I want from life |

Adapted from Eberhart et al 2014.

CONTROL-BASED MANAGEMENT OF ASTHMA

For asthma, control refers to control of the manifestations of disease rather than prevention or cure; asthma can be treated but not cured. This should include control of the clinical features of the disease, including lung function abnormalities, as well as reducing the inflammation that underlies the disease.

Management of asthma to control symptoms and reduce the risk for exacerbations includes medications, identifying/treating risk factors and non-pharmacological therapies/strategies (Global Initiative for Asthma [GINA] 2016a, 2016b). In addition, each patient should receive training in asthma self-management through information on the disease, inhaler skills, adherence to therapy, a written asthma action plan, self-monitoring, and regular medication review (GINA 2016a, 2016b). In its revised 2016 version, the Global Initiative for Asthma proposes a circular control-based approach to manage asthma involving continuous assessment, treatment and review (Fig. 18.1) (GINA 2016a, 2016b).

Once asthma is diagnosed, the patient is initiated on a daily controller treatment based on inhaled corticosteroids (ICS), making sure that the patient has received proper instruction for the inhalant device utilisation (Fig. 18.2). The response to treatment is then reviewed

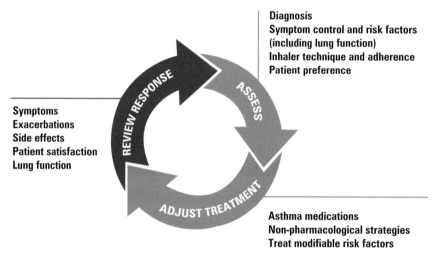

FIG. 18.1 **The Control-Based Asthma Management Cycle.** Global Initiative for Asthma (GINA) 2016.

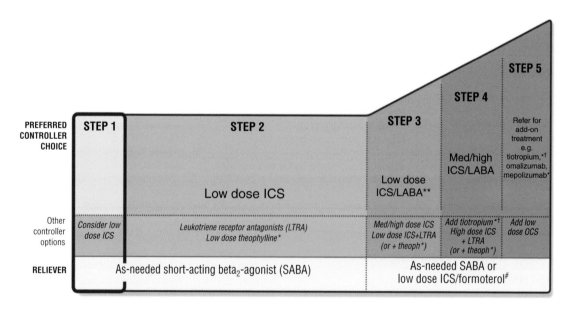

*Not for children <12 years.
**For children 6–11 years, the preferred Step 3 treatment is medium dose ICS
#For patients prescribed BDP/formoterol or BUD/formoterol maintenance and reliever therapy
†Tiotropium by mist inhaler is an add-on treatment for patients ≥12 years with a history of exacerbations

FIG. 18.2 **Stepwise Approach to Control Asthma Symptoms and Reduce Risk.** GINA 2016.

after about 3 months and the treatment adjusted in a step-wise manner (Fig.18.2). In general, initial step-up involves either increasing the dose of ICS, or adding a combination treatment with a long-acting beta-agonist (LABA). Further steps to intensify therapy may subsequently involve addition of a leukotriene receptor antagonist (LTRA) and/or a long-acting muscarinic antagonist (LAMA), such as tiotropium. If these measures do not improve asthma control, oral corticosteroids (OCS) and/or treatment with an anti-IgE antibody (omalizumab) is added. Asthma is a fluctuating disorder that necessitates regular review by a doctor and adjustment of controller treatment. Under guidance, skilled patients may also independently adapt their treatment, either stepping up maintenance and/or reliever therapy if symptoms worsen, or stepping down therapy when their asthma is well controlled. If symptoms and/or exacerbations persist under controller therapy, frequent issues should be assessed prior to escalating treatment any further, such as inhaler technique, adherence to therapy, risk factors (e.g. smoking) and co-morbidities (e.g. allergic rhinitis).

Inhaler Technique

The vast majority of patients (about 90%) fail to properly utilise their inhaler, contributing to inappropriate asthma control (National Asthma Council 2016c). The four 'Cs' may help to guarantee correct inhalant handling: (1) Choose the ideal device for the patient; (2) Check inhalant technique frequently; (3) Correct the errors in inhalant utilisation by demonstrating proper handling; (4) Confirm proper technique for each type of inhaler used (GINA 2016a, 2016b). Importantly, patients should avoid having two different types of inhalant devices, such as metered dose inhalers and dry powder inhalers as the techniques for their usage differ.

Adherence to Therapy

About half of the asthmatic patients fail to take controller medications as prescribed. Several reasons contribute to poor adherence, such as misunderstandings, forgetfulness, costs, fear of side effects, and not perceiving the necessity for treatment. In a first step, patients should be empathically queried about their medications and medication utilisation verified. If adherence is problematic, the patient should repeatedly be informed about their disorder, receive home visits by asthma nurses and benefit from a simplified medication regimen (e.g. once daily versus twice daily). Nursing staff should also regularly review best practice strategies for the delivery of medications and maintaining compliance to medication regimens.

Treating Modifiable Risk Factors and Co-Morbid Conditions

Smoking asthmatics should receive smoking cessation advice and allergies identified and treated if necessary. Frequent co-morbid conditions that affect asthma control are chronic rhinosinusitis and gastro-oesophageal reflux disease. Asthma control in obese patients is more difficult, necessitating careful dosage of medications. Usage of aspirin and NSAIDs may adversely affect asthma control and should generally be discouraged in asthmatics. With occupational asthma, patients describe workplace-related worsening of their symptoms and improvement during weekend or when on leave.

Other Treatments

Bronchial thermoplasty is a recently developed novel treatment that consists of bronchoscopic coagulation of the airway wall that reduces airway smooth muscle (Pretolani et al 2016). This treatment is reserved for highly selected patients with severe and refractory asthma that is not responsive to medical treatment. New generation biological treatments such as Omalizumab (anti-IgE antibody), and now also Mepolizumab (Anti-IL-5) and Benralizumab (Anti-IL-5R) may also be considered as additional treatment options in patients whose asthma is not controlled under GINA steps 4–5 (Fig. 18.2).

Asthma Action Plans

A written asthma action plan should be implemented in order to monitor the long-term use of medications and improve compliance. The plan should be reviewed regularly and adjusted according to progression of the disease. The individual plan must be fully explained to the patient and understood by them. The patient may be included in decisions on the action plan to take into consideration individual preferences; alternatively, patients may prefer their action plan to be decided by their doctor. An asthma action plan should include:
- guidance for identifying signs of worsening control
- clear instructions for how to respond to any given change in asthma control.

In adults, individualised asthma action plans have been shown to reduce absences from work, hospital admissions, emergency presentations to the GP, use of short-acting beta-2-agonists and to generally improve lung function.

An example of an asthma action plan as recommended by the National Asthma Council Australia can be seen in Fig. 18.3. This plan helps both the patient and the carer recognise and respond appropriately to worsening asthma (National Asthma Council Australia 2017).

ASTHMA ACTION PLAN

Take this **ASTHMA ACTION PLAN** with you when you visit your doctor

NAME	DOCTOR'S CONTACT DETAILS	EMERGENCY CONTACT DETAILS
DATE		Name
NEXT ASTHMA CHECK-UP DUE		Phone
		Relationship

😊 WHEN WELL *Asthma under control (almost no symptoms)*   ALWAYS CARRY YOUR RELIEVER WITH YOU

Peak flow* (if used) above:

Your preventer is:
                                    [NAME & STRENGTH]

Take .... puffs/tablets .... times every day
☐ Use a spacer with your inhaler

Your reliever is:
                                    [NAME]

Take .... puffs

When: You have symptoms like wheezing, coughing or shortness of breath
☐ Use a spacer with your inhaler

OTHER INSTRUCTIONS
[e.g. other medicines, trigger avoidance, what to do before exercise]

😐 WHEN NOT WELL *Asthma getting worse (needing more reliever e.g. more than 3 times per week, waking up with asthma, more symptoms than usual, asthma is interfering with usual activities)*

Peak flow* (if used) between .... and ....

Keep taking preventer:
                                    [NAME & STRENGTH]

Take .... puffs/tablets .... times every day

☐ Use a spacer with your inhaler

Your reliever is:
                                    [NAME]

Take .... puffs

☐ Use a spacer with your inhaler

OTHER INSTRUCTIONS   ☐ Contact your doctor
[e.g. other medicines, when to stop taking extra medicines]

😟 IF SYMPTOMS GET WORSE *Asthma is severe (needing reliever again within 3 hours, increasing difficulty breathing, waking often at night with asthma symptoms)*

Peak flow* (if used) between .... and ....

Keep taking preventer:
                                    [NAME & STRENGTH]

Take .... puffs/tablets .... times every day

☐ Use a spacer with your inhaler

Your reliever is:
                                    [NAME]

Take .... puffs

☐ Use a spacer with your inhaler

OTHER INSTRUCTIONS   ☑ Contact your doctor today
[e.g. other medicines, when to stop taking extra medicines]
Prednisolone/prednisone:

Take .... each morning for .... days

😫 DANGER SIGNS *Asthma emergency (severe breathing problems, symptoms get worse very quickly, reliever has little or no effect)*

Peak flow (if used) below:

DIAL 000 FOR AMBULANCE

Call an ambulance immediately
Say that this is an asthma emergency
Keep taking reliever as often as needed

NationalAsthma
CouncilAustralia
leading the attack against asthma

www.nationalasthma.org.au

* Peak flow not recommended for children under 12 years.

FIG. 18.3 **Asthma Action Plan.** © National Asthma Council Australia, www.nationalasthma.org.au.

ASTHMA ACTION PLAN
what to look out for

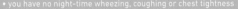

| WHEN WELL | **THIS MEANS:**
• you have no night-time wheezing, coughing or chest tightness
• you only occasionally have wheezing, coughing or chest tightness during the day
• you need reliever medication only occasionally or before exercise
• you can do your usual activities without getting asthma symptoms |

| WHEN NOT WELL | **THIS MEANS ANY ONE OF THESE:**
• you have night-time wheezing, coughing or chest tightness
• you have morning asthma symptoms when you wake up
• you need to take your reliever more than usual eg. more than 3 times per week
• your asthma is interfering with your usual activities |

| IF SYMPTOMS GET WORSE | **THIS MEANS:**
• you have increasing wheezing, cough, chest tightness or shortness of breath
• you are waking often at night with asthma symptoms
• you need to use your reliever again within 3 hours

THIS IS AN ASTHMA ATTACK |

| DANGER SIGNS | **THIS MEANS:**
• your symptoms get worse very quickly
• you have severe shortness of breath, can't speak comfortably or lips look blue
• you get little or no relief from your reliever inhaler
CALL AN AMBULANCE IMMEDIATELY: DIAL 000
SAY THIS IS AN ASTHMA EMERGENCY. | **DIAL 000 FOR AMBULANCE** |

| ASTHMA MEDICINES | **PREVENTERS**
Your preventer medicine reduces inflammation, swelling and mucus in the airways of your lungs. Preventers need to be taken **every day**, even when you are well.

Some preventer inhalers contain 2 medicines to help control your asthma (combination inhalers). | **RELIEVERS**
Your reliever medicine works quickly to make breathing easier by making the airways wider.
Always carry your reliever with you – it is essential for first aid. Do not use your preventer inhaler for quick relief of asthma symptoms unless your doctor has told you to do this. |

To order more Asthma Action Plans visit the National Asthma Council website. A range of action plans are available on the website – please use the one that best suits your patient.
www.nationalasthma.org.au

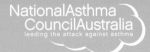
NationalAsthma
CouncilAustralia
leading the attack against asthma

Developed by the National Asthma Council Australia and supported by GlaxoSmithKline Australia.
National Asthma Council Australia retained editorial control.

FIG. 18.3, cont'd

Spirometry and Peak Expiratory Flow Measurements

Spirometry is a measurement of the time-dependent volume of air breathed into (inspiration) and out of (expiration) the lungs. The aim of spirometry is to detect the presence and variability of airflow obstruction, and to measure the degree of airflow limitation (referred to as obstruction) compared to either the predicted normal (reference value) or the individual's personal best value measured when their asthma is well controlled. Measurement of respiratory function is necessary in the diagnosis of asthma and to effectively manage treatment. Spirometry generates flow–volume loops that indicate the amount of air a person can breathe in and out (volume) and the speed or flow rate at which this can be achieved (flow) with the forced expiratory volume in 1 second (FEV_1) being a key parameter to diagnose airflow limitation (obstruction). For the GP, the shape of the flow–volume loops indicates the nature and severity of the patient's asthma and whether the patient responds to bronchodilation following inhalation of a short-acting beta-2-agonist bronchodilator (Fig. 18.4). A significant bronchodilator response occurs when either FEV_1 or FVC (forced vital capacity) increase by > 200 mL and $> 12\%$. In the correct clinical context this allows the diagnosis of asthma.

Peak flow, or peak expiratory flow (PEF), is the measurement of the peak rate, or maximum rate, at which an individual can expel air from the lungs. Peak flow measurements can be performed by the patient at home, providing an indication of airflow limitation (obstruction) and are usually scored as a percentage measurement of a person's 'best' result; that is, an average result recorded over a period of 1 or 2 weeks when their asthma is well controlled. The measurement can also be recorded as 'percentage predicted', the predicted value being a composite value of age, height, gender and ethnically matched non-asthmatic individuals. However, if a personal best value is known, this is generally a more reliable measure as it will take into account person–person variations. Peak flow measurements can be used for early detection of asthma worsening and help to intensify medical treatment, for example, when a PEF value falls below 80% of the predicted value, or personal best value, if known (see Fig. 18.5). PEF measurements can also be useful in monitoring responses to medications, such as inhaled corticosteroids, after a severe attack. In interpreting this type of monitoring, however, it is important that several readings are taken

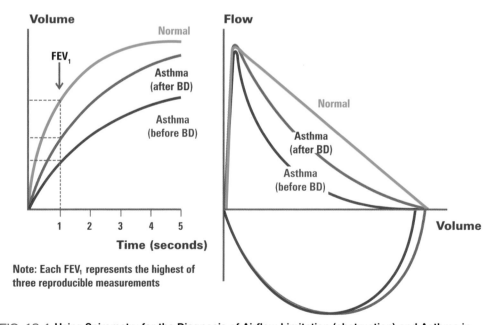

Note: Each FEV_1 represents the highest of three reproducible measurements

FIG. 18.4 Using Spirometry for the Diagnosis of Airflow Limitation (obstruction) and Asthma in Adults with the Bronchodilator (BD) Response Showing a Reversibility of Airflow Limitation. A significant bronchodilator response occurs when FEV_1 (or FVC: forced vital capacity) increase by > 200 mL and $> 12\%$. $FEV_1 =$ forced expiratory volume in 1 second. GINA 2016.

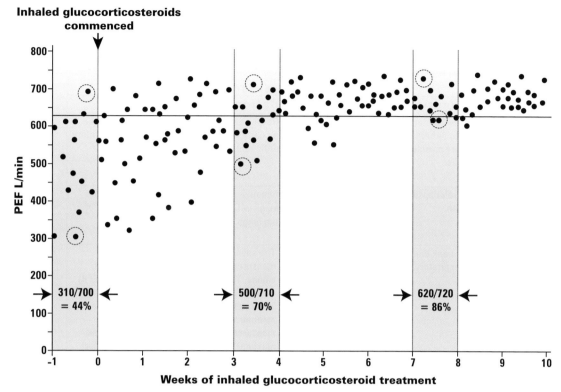

FIG. 18.5 **Measuring Variability of Peak Expiratory Flow.** GINA 2011.

over a prolonged period of time, as a variability between readings can occur (Fig. 18.5). Peak flow variability > 20% is consistent with either untreated or suboptimally treated asthma. Due to the wide range of 'normal' values and high degree of variability, peak flow readings only benefit a small proportion of people. Peak flow readings are effort-dependent and are not recommended for use in children under 12 years of age (GINA 2011). Predicted values of FEV_1, FVC and PEF based on age, sex and height have been obtained from population studies. These are being continually revised, and with the exception of PEF for which the range of predictive values is too wide, they are useful for judging whether a given value is abnormal or not. If precision is needed, for example, in the conduct of a clinical trial, use of a more rigorous definition (lower limit of normal [LLN]) should be considered. Careful instruction is required to reliably measure PEF because PEF measurements are effort-dependent. Use of spirometry and other measures recommended for older children and adults, such as airway responsiveness and markers of airway inflammation, is difficult and several require complex equipment, making them unsuitable for

routine use. However, children 4 to 5 years old can be taught to use a PEF meter, but to ensure reliability parental supervision is required.

Successive spirometry measurements before and after bronchodilator use allow diagnosis of airway obstruction, enable measurement of the degree of airway obstruction, monitor the effects of treatments, demonstrate the presence and reversibility of airway obstruction to the patient, provide objective feedback to the patient about the presence and severity of asthma and accurately back-titrate preventive medication to determine the minimum effective dose (National Asthma Council Australia 2016a).

FAMILY AND CARERS
Nursing Management
In planning the nursing management of the person with asthma, we have chosen to use the nursing process as the framework for nursing management. A detailed persistent asthma nursing care plan is shown in Fig. 18.6 (adapted from Gulanick & Myers 2013).

Nursing Diagnosis: Ineffective breathing pattern related to swelling and spasm of the bronchial tubes in response to allergies, drugs, stress, infection and inhaled irritants.

Expected Outcome: The patient to maintain optimal breathing patterns, as evidenced by regular respiratory rate or pattern.

Ongoing assessment	
Interventions	Rationale
Assess respiratory rate and depth, monitor breathing pattern. Assess for use of accessory muscles, retractions and flaring of nostrils.	Respiratory rate and rhythm changes can be an early warning sign to impending respiratory difficulties.
Assess relationship of inspiration to expiration.	Reactive airways allow air to move into the lungs with greater ease than to move out of the lungs.
Monitor peak expiratory flow rates and forced expiratory volumes.	The severity of the exacerbation can be measured objectively by monitoring these values. The peak expiratory flow rate (PEFR) is the maximum flow rate that can be generated during a forced expiratory manoeuvre with fully inflated lungs. It measures in litres per second and requires maximal effort. When done with good effort it correlates well with forced expiratory volume in 1 second (FEV_1) measured by spirometry and provides a simple reproducible measure of airway obstruction.
Assess vital signs every hour as needed if patient in distress.	
Assess fatigue.	Fatigue may indicate increasing distress leading to respiratory failure.

FIG. 18.6 **Persistent Asthma Nursing Care Plan.** Adapted from Gulanick & Myers 2013.

Monitor oxygen saturation by pulse oximetry, maintaining the oxygen saturation above 90% or higher, with oxygen as ordered by the physician.	
Assess breath sounds and note wheeze or other adventitious breath sounds.	Adventitious sounds may indicate a worsening condition or additional pathology such as pneumonia. Diminishing wheezing and inaudible breath sounds may indicate impending respiratory failure.
Assess level of anxiety.	Hypoxia and the sensation of 'not being able to breathe' is very frightening and may cause worsening hypoxia.

Therapeutic interventions	
Interventions	**Rationale**
Encourage the patient to sit upright, supported with pillows.	This position allows for adequate lung excursion and chest expansion.
Encourage slow deep breathing. Instruct patient to use pursed lip breathing for exhalation. Instruct to time breathing so that exhalation takes 2 to 3 times as long as inspiration.	Pursed lip exhalation facilitates expiratory airflow by helping to keep the bronchioles open. Prolonged expiration prevents air trapping.
Use B2-andrenergic agonist drugs by metered-dose inhaler (MDI) with spacer or nebuliser as prescribed.	B2-andrenergic agonist drugs relax airway smooth muscle.
Administer medications as prescribed.	Corticosteroids are the most effective anti-inflammatory drugs for the reversible airflow obstruction. During severe attacks, anticholinergics may be effective when used in combination with B2-andrenergic agonists.
Plan activity and rest to maximise patient's energy.	Fatigue is common with the increased work of breathing from the ineffective breathing pattern.

Nursing Diagnosis: Ineffective airway clearance related to bronchospasm, excessive mucus production and ineffective cough and fatigue.

Expected Outcome: Patient's airway is maintained free of secretions as evidenced by normal/improved breath sounds and normal ABGs or oxygen saturation if 90% or greater on pulse oximeter.

Ongoing assessment	
Interventions	**Rationale**
Auscultate lungs with each routine vital sign check.	This allows for early detection and correction of abnormalities.
Assess secretions noting colour, viscosity, odour and amount.	Thick tenacious secretions may indicate dehydration. Coloured or odourous secretions may indicate bleeding or infection.

FIG. 18.6, cont'd

Assess cough for effectiveness and productivity.	Consider possible causes of an ineffective cough, respiratory muscle fatigue, severe bronchospasm, thick tenacious sputum.
Assess patient's physical capabilities and activities of daily living (ADLs).	Fatigue can limit ADLs.
Monitor pulse oxygen saturation and ABGs.	Hypoxia can result from increased pulmonary secretions.

Therapeutic interventions	
Interventions	**Rationale**
Administer B2-andrenergic agonists (e.g. albuterol) by MDI or nebuliser, as prescribed.	B2-andrenergic agonist drugs relax airway smooth muscle.
Administer other medications as prescribed.	Corticosteroids are the most effective anti-inflammatory drugs for the reversible airflow obstruction. During severe attacks, anticholinergics may be effective when used in combination with B2-andrenergic agonists.
Encourage patient to cough and assist with effective coughing techniques:	
• Sit patient upright.	Promotes chest expansion.
• Splint chest.	
• Patient to use abdominal muscles.	Promotes comfort.
• Use cough techniques as appropriate.	Ability for a more forceful cough.
Assist in mobilising secretions to facilitate airway clearance:	
• Increase room humidification.	Humidity will help liquefy secretions.
• Perform chest physiotherapy; postural drainage, percussion and vibration.	
• Encourage 2 to 3 L fluid intake unless contraindicated.	To prevent dehydration and keep secretions thin.
• Encourage activity and position changes every 2 hours.	Activity helps mobilise secretions and prevents pooling in lungs.
• Perform nasotracheal suctioning as indicated if patient unable to effectively clear secretions.	
Anticipate intubation and mechanical ventilation, if required with a transfer to acute care setting.	

FIG. 18.6, cont'd

Nursing Diagnosis: Anxiety related to respiratory distress, change in health status, changes in environment and routines, and coping with chronic illness.

Expected Outcome: Patient's anxiety is reduced as evidenced by cooperative behaviour, demonstration of positive coping mechanisms and verbalised report of decreased anxiety.

Ongoing assessment	
Interventions	**Rationale**
Assess anxiety level, including vital signs, respiratory status, irritability, apprehension, and orientation.	Anxiety can affect respiratory rate and rhythm.
Assess oxygen saturation levels.	Anxiety increases with increasing hypoxia and may be an early warning sign of decreasing oxygen levels.
Assess theophylline level if patient is taking theophylline.	Theophylline increases anxiety.

Therapeutic interventions	
Interventions	**Interventions**
Stay with patient and encourage slow, deep breathing.	
Explain importance of remaining calm.	Maintaining calmness decreases oxygen consumption and work of breathing.
Keep significant other informed of patient's progress.	Information can help to relieve apprehension.
Avoid excessive reassurance.	Excessive reassurance may increase anxiety for many people.
Assist the patient with developing anxiety reducing skills (e.g. relaxation, deep breathing, progressive muscle relaxation positive visualisation, and reassuring self-statements).	Using anxiety-reduction strategies enhances the patient's sense of personal mastery and confidence.
Encourage patient to seek assistance from understanding significant other or healthcare provider if anxious feelings become difficult.	

Nursing Diagnosis: Deficit knowledge related to ineffective past teaching or learning, and unfamiliarity with resources.

Expected Outcome: Patient verbalises understanding of disease process and treatment.

Ongoing assessment	
Intervention	**Rationale**
Assess knowledge base of persistent asthma.	Asthma is a persistent disease and many new medications and treatments continue to be developed.
Assess educational, environmental, social and cultural factors that may influence teaching plan.	
Assess cognitive function and emotional readiness to learn.	

FIG. 18.6, cont'd

Therapeutic interventions	
Intervention	**Rationale**
Establish common goals with the patient.	
Actively include the patient in the decision process of the education and management.	
Instruct patient in anatomy and physiology of the respiratory system and provide information to appropriate level.	Information will assist the patient to understand the complexities of their airway problems.
Discuss the relation of the disease process of asthma related to signs and symptoms.	Information will assist the patient to understand the complexities of their airway problems.
Discuss the medications that the patient is taking, including: • Name of medication. • Action and role of each medication. • Dosage of medication. • Method of administration. • Care of the MDI or inhaler device • Side effects of medication. • Action on experiencing side effects. • Consequences of improper use. • Consideration of medication's influence with ADLs.	Return demonstrations on MDI or inhaler technique are necessary to ensure appropriate delivery of medications.
Discuss concept of energy conservation. Encourage resting as needed during activities, avoiding overexertion and fatigue, sitting as much as possible, and alternating heavy and light tasks.	Learning self-management skills may reduce dyspnoea from fatigue.
Discuss asthma action plan, including signs and symptoms of infection and worsening asthma and when to contact healthcare provider.	
Discuss triggers and factors that lead to exacerbations of asthma and how to avoid them.	
Discuss effect of smoking and refer patient or significant others to cessation of smoking program or support group.	

FIG. 18.6, cont'd

Discuss importance of specific therapeutic measures as listed:	
• **Breathing exercises** *Exercise 1* 　1. Lie supine, with one hand on chest and one on abdomen.	This exercise strengthens muscles of respiration.
2. Inhale slowly through mouth, raising abdomen against hand.	
3. Exhale slowly through pursed lips while contracting abdominal muscles and moving abdomen inwards.	
Exercise 2 　1. Walk; stop to take a deep breath. 　2. Exhale slowly while walking.	This exercise develops slowed, controlled breathing.
Exercise 3 　1. For pursed-lip breathing, inhale slowly through nose.	This exercise decreases air trapping and airway collapse.
2. Exhale twice as slowly as usual through pursed lips.	
• **Cough:** Lean forwards; take several deep breaths with pursed-lip method. Take last deep breath, cough through open mouth during expiration, and simultaneously contract abdominal muscles.	Effective method that prevents waste of energy.
• **Chest physiotherapy or pulmonary postural drainage.** Demonstrate correct methods of postural drainage: positioning, percussions, vibration.	Facilitates expectoration of secretions and prevents waste of energy.
• **Hydration:** Discuss importance of maintaining 1.5 to 2 L/day.	Decreases viscosity of secretions.
• **Humidity:** Discuss various forms of humidification.	Prevents drying of secretions.
Discuss the need for regular consultation by healthcare team for review of management, prescriptions, ongoing education.	

FIG. 18.6, cont'd

Discuss available resources:
  • **Asthma Australia.**
  • **National Asthma Council Australia.**	

Discuss the need for patient to obtain vaccines for pneumococcal pneumonia and yearly vaccine for influenza.	Vaccine decreases severity and occurrence of these diseases.
Discuss use of medical alert bracelet or other identification.	Alerts others to persistent asthma and severe allergies.
Include relevant others, including family members, in education to ensure patient has relevant knowledgeable help in time of crisis.	

FIG. 18.6, cont'd

Education for the Person and Family

Education for the person with persistent asthma is critical. Education can empower the person to effectively self-manage and take responsibility for their chronic illness. The education process should begin with the initial diagnosis of asthma and continue throughout all subsequent interactions between the patient, family and healthcare professionals. The aim of education is to empower the patient to effectively manage their asthma, in order to:

• achieve the optimum health (physical and psychological)
• reduce unplanned GP consultations, emergency department treatments and hospital admissions
• have the confidence to manage change in asthma conditions.

In adults, the use of asthma self-management education programs will involve:

• written information about asthma
• monitoring of asthma control, based on PEF and/or symptoms
• a written asthma action plan (see Fig. 18.3)
• regular review by a health professional (which may include a doctor, nurse or asthma educator). This will include review of medications, assessment in the correct use of inhalation device, recommendation of spacer device with MDI, assessment of asthma control, discussion of triggers, consideration of lifestyle choices and discussion and provision of feedback to the patient about their overall control of asthma.

In addition, the person, family and friends should also be educated about what to do in case of an emergency asthma attack. Asthma Australia has developed an asthma first aid plan that provides a useful summary of what to do in case of emergency (Table 18.1) (Asthma Australia 2016).

Self-Management Interventions

Self-management interventions (SMI) in persistent asthma involve more than providing information to the patient. The key feature of these interventions is to increase patients' involvement in and control of their treatment and its effect on their lives, in order to improve rates of adherence to medications and quality of life (Lawn & Schoo 2010). It is a process developed over time in partnership between the patient and health professionals, and enables the patient to actively participate in their asthma care with the doctor, nurse or asthma educator. It will include:

• understanding the nature of asthma (chronic inflammatory disease)

TABLE 18.1 Asthma First Aid Plan	
STEP 1	Sit the person upright and give them reassurance. Do not leave them alone.
STEP 2	Without delay, give 4 separate puffs of a blue inhaler (e.g. Ventolin). Give the medicine one puff at a time via a spacer device and ask the person to take 4 breaths from the spacer after each puff. If a spacer is not available, use the puffer on its own.
STEP 3	Wait 4 minutes. If there is no improvement, repeat steps 2 and 3.
STEP 4	If there is still little or no improvement call an ambulance.

Adapted from Asthma Australia 2016.

- being actively involved in planning care and the review process
- identifying activities that protect and promote health (including knowledge of medications and the correct use and care of inhaler devices)
- monitoring the signs and symptoms of asthma
- managing the psychosocial impact of chronic illness upon lifestyle.

CONCLUSION

Asthma is a complex condition that requires careful diagnosis and management. The underlying pathology of this condition is inflammation of the airways driven by a variety of allergic and non-allergic stimuli. However, a high proportion of people with asthma suffer from an allergic condition called atopy; therefore, a key step in the care of the allergic asthmatic patient is the identification of allergic triggers of the disorder and taking steps to avoid or minimise exposure to these. The key principle of nursing management of persistent asthmatic patients is to restore airway function to the optimal level for the individual and to instigate a treatment regimen to maintain optimal lung function. A key component in the management of the patient with persistent asthma is the development of an asthma management plan in conjunction with the patient and the doctor. This will aid in compliance with treatment in order to maintain optimal airway function, and help to identify signs and symptoms that will indicate when the condition is worsening and when treatment should be sought. Family and friends should also be educated as to the nature of this chronic condition, what to do in case of an acute exacerbation and ways that the patient's environment can be improved and maintained in order to minimise the risk of exacerbations occurring.

> ### Reflective Questions
>
> 1. Consider how you would explain the benefits of an asthma action plan to a patient with persistent asthma who has not previously had an action plan. What are the key aspects of the plan that the patient, family and carers should understand?
> 2. What are some of the key triggers for asthma exacerbations and what measures could be taken to avoid these triggers? What education could be provided to the patient by the practice nurse to improve the home or work environment?
> 3. How would you explain the benefits of a preventative inhaler to a teenager, and what strategies could you take to educate and improve patient compliance with inhaler use?

Acknowledgement

The editors and author would like to acknowledge the previous edition's authors Philip A. Stumbles, Prue Andrus and Christophe von Garnier.

RECOMMENDED READING

Eberhart NK, Sherbourne CD, Edelen MO et al 2014. Development of a measure of asthma-specific quality of life among adults. Quality of Life Research 23(3), 837–848.

Global Initiative for Asthma (GINA) 2016. Global strategy for asthma management and prevention. Online. Available: www.ginasthma.org.

National Asthma Council Australia 2016b. What is asthma? Online. Available: www.nationalasthma.org.au/understanding-asthma/what-is-asthma.

REFERENCES

Asthma Australia 2016. Asthma First Aid Plan. Online. Available: www.asthmaaustralia.org.au.

Australian Bureau of Statistics (ABS) 2018. National Health Survey 2017–18: First results. Online. Available: www.abs.gov.au/statistics/health/health-conditions-and-risks/national-health-survey-first-results/latest-release

Australian Centre for Asthma Monitoring 2011. Asthma in Australia 2011. AIHW, Canberra. Online. Available: www.aihw.gov.au/publication-detail/?id=10737420159.

Australian Institute of Health and Welfare (AIHW) 2020. Australian burden of disease study: impact and causes of illness and death in Australia 2015. Australian Burden of Disease Study series no. 19. BOD 22. AIHW, Canberra. Online. Available: www.aihw.gov.au/getmedia/c076f42f-61ea-4348-9c0a-d996353e838f/aihw-bod-22.pdf.aspx?inline=true

Barnes PJ 2012. Severe asthma: advances in current management and future therapy. The Journal of Allergy and Clinical Immunology 129, 48–59.

Brooks CR, van Dalen CJ, Hermans IF et al 2013. Identifying leucocyte populations in fresh and cryopreserved sputum using flow cytometry. Cytometry. Part B, Clinical Cytometry 84B(2), 104–113.

Centers for Disease Control and Prevention 2013. Asthma Facts – CDC's National Asthma Control Program Grantees. US Department of Health and Human Services, Centers for Disease Control and Prevention, Atlanta, GA.

Chung K 2015. Managing severe asthma in adults: lessons from the ERS/ATS guidelines. Current Opinion in Pulmonary Medicine 21, 8–15.

Eberhart NK, Sherbourne CD, Edelen MO et al 2014. Development of a measure of asthma-specific quality of life among adults. Quality of Life Research 23(3), 837–848.

Global Initiative for Asthma (GINA) 2016a. Global Strategy for Asthma Management and Prevention. Online. Available: www.ginasthma.org.

Global Initiative for Asthma (GINA) 2016b. Teaching slide set. Online. Available: http://ginasthma.org/gina-teaching-slide-set/.

Global Initiative for Asthma (GINA) 2011. At-a-glance asthma management pocket reference. Online. Available: www.ginasthma.org/guidelines-pocket-guide-for-asthma-management.html.

Guilbert TW, Mauger DT, Lemanske RF 2016. Childhood asthma-predictive phenotype. The Journal of Allergy and Clinical Immunology. In Practice 2, 664–670.

Gulanick M, Myers JL 2013. Nursing care plans: nursing diagnosis and interventions, 8th ed. Elsevier, St Louis.

Holt PG, Sly PD 2012. Viral infections and atopy in asthma pathogenesis: new rationales for asthma prevention and treatment. Nature Medicine 18(5), 726–735.

Holt PG, Thomas WR 2005. Sensitization to airborne environmental allergens: unresolved issues. Nature Immunology 6, 957–960.

Howrylak JA, Moll M, Weiss ST et al 2016. Gene expression profiling of asthma phenotypes demonstrates molecular signatures of atopy and asthma control. Journal of Allergy Clinical Immunology 137, 1390–1397.

Johnston SL 1998. Viruses and asthma. Allergy 53, 922–923.

Lawn S, Schoo A 2010. Supporting self-management of chronic health conditions: common approaches. Patient Education and Counseling 80(2), 205–211.

Liu A 2015. Revisiting the hygiene hypothesis for allergy and asthma. Journal of Allergy and Clinical Immunology 136, 860–865.

National Asthma Council Australia 2017. Asthma action plan. Online. Available: www.nationalasthma.org.au.

National Asthma Council Australia 2016a. Australian asthmahandbook. Online. Available: www.asthmahandbook.org.au/.

National Asthma Council Australia 2016b. What is asthma? Online. Available: www.nationalasthma.org.au/understanding-asthma/what-is-asthma?

National Asthma Council Australia 2016c. Media Release: Ninety percent of Australians with asthma use their inhalers incorrectly. Online. Available: www.nationalasthma.org.au/news/2016/ninety-per-cent-of-australians-with-asthma-use-their-inhalers-incorrectly

Pretolani M, Bergqvist A, Thabut G et al 2016. Effectiveness of bronchial thermoplasty in patients with severe refractory asthma: clinical and histopathological correlations. Journal of Allergy and Clinical Immunology. pii: S0091–6749(16), 30896-X.

Quaedvlieg V, Sele J, Henket M et al 2009. Association between asthma control and bronchial hyperresponsiveness and airways inflammation: a cross-sectional study in daily practice. Clinical and Experimental Allergy 39, 1822–1829.

Rubner FJ, Jackson DJ, Evans MD et al 2017. Early life rhinovirus wheezing, allergic sensitization, and asthma risk at adolescence. Journal of Allergy and Clinical Immunology 139(2), 501–507.

Stein MM, Hrusch CL, Gozdz J et al 2016. Innate immunity and asthma risk in Amish and Hutterite farm children. New England Journal of Medicine 375, 411–421.

Strachan DP 1989. Hay fever, hygiene, and household size. British Medical Journal 299, 1259–1260.

CHAPTER 19

Principles for Nursing Practice: Chronic Obstructive Pulmonary Disease

COLLEEN DOYLE • GAIL ROBERTS • SANDY WARD

LEARNING OBJECTIVES

When you have completed this chapter you will be able to:

- describe the main signs and symptoms of chronic obstructive pulmonary disease (COPD) and understand how common it is
- understand the mental health issues for the person with COPD
- describe the epidemiology of COPD
- understand the importance of self-management through attendance at pulmonary rehabilitation and patient education classes
- explain the main nursing principles relevant to the ongoing care of the person with COPD including palliation.

KEY WORDS

dyspnoea	mental health
exacerbation	pulmonary rehabilitation
hypoxaemia	

INTRODUCTION – WHAT IS COPD?

Chronic obstructive pulmonary disease (COPD), also known as chronic obstructive lung disease (COLD), is one of the most common diseases in the world, yet public awareness of the disease is much lower than for other lung diseases such as asthma (Australian Institute of Health and Welfare [AIHW] 2015; Dunt & Doyle 2012). One reason for this relates to the language used to describe the disease. COPD is not one single disease but an umbrella term for a group of diseases that are chronic irreversible disease processes which limit airflow to the lungs. In the past, COPD has also been referred to as chronic obstructive airway disease (COAD), chronic airflow limitation (CAL) and chronic obstructive respiratory disease. This differing terminology can lead to confusion and may impact on public understanding of the disease.

In practice, it may be difficult to differentiate between asthma, which is reversible airway limitation, and COPD, which is irreversible airway limitation. People with COPD experience breathlessness, coughing, wheezing, increased sputum production, sleep disturbance, fatigue and weight loss. Everyday activities, including bending over or walking short distances, become difficult due to breathlessness and the debilitating effects of the disease. Smoking is the main behavioural cause of COPD, but there is evidence that some individuals have a genetic susceptibility to developing COPD. Occupational or environmental exposures to dust and fumes also cause COPD (Global Initiative for Chronic Obstructive Lung Disease [GOLD] 2020). One of the most effective treatments for people with COPD is pulmonary rehabilitation, a program of exercise and education that can greatly improve quality of life. Influenza vaccinations are also effective in protecting against exacerbations. There is increasing evidence for the effectiveness of cognitive behaviour therapy (CBT) for managing depression and anxiety associated with the disease. Nurses should be aware that much can be done to improve the quality of life for their patients with COPD, by working collaboratively with them and their families to meet their individual needs at the various stages of the illness process. Distinguishing COPD from asthma can be difficult, especially in older adults and smokers. We no longer refer to Asthma COPD Overlap but recognise that features are shared between the two disorders of asthma and COPD (GOLD 2020).

The World Health Organization (WHO) provides the following definition of COPD:

> *Chronic obstructive pulmonary disease (COPD) is not one single disease but an umbrella term used to describe chronic lung diseases that cause limitations in lung airflow. The more familiar terms 'chronic bronchitis' and 'emphysema' are no longer used, but are now included within the COPD diagnosis.*
>
> *The most common symptoms of COPD are breathlessness, or a 'need for air', excessive sputum production, and a chronic cough. However, COPD is not just simply a 'smoker's cough', but an under-diagnosed, life threatening lung disease that may progressively lead to death (WHO 2016a).*

The Global Initiative for Chronic Obstructive Lung Disease defines COPD as:

> *a common, preventable and treatable disease (that) is characterized by persistent respiratory symptoms and airflow limitation that is due to airway and/or alveolar abnormalities usually caused by significant exposure to noxious particles or gases. COPD may be punctuated by periods of acute worsening of respiratory symptoms, called exacerbations (GOLD 2020).*

Therefore, COPD is a term for a collection of lung diseases that prevent the sufferer from breathing easily. In individuals with COPD, the lungs are damaged and the airways are partly obstructed, making it hard to breathe. Emphysema and chronic bronchitis have been described as types of COPD, but in fact, emphysema refers to the alveolar abnormalities featured in COPD, and chronic bronchitis refers to a physiological condition that can be present prior to or after a diagnosis of the airflow limitation that characterises COPD. The airflow limitation present with COPD is usually progressive and is associated with an abnormal inflammatory response of the lungs to noxious particles or gases (GOLD 2020).

HOW IS COPD RELATED TO ASTHMA AND OTHER LUNG FUNCTION DISEASES?

Lung function diseases are all characterised by limitations to airflow, which is measured via spirometry, a respiratory function test (RFT, also known as a lung function test). The separation of asthma and COPD aligns with the current treatment of the two lung conditions as separate although overlapping diseases (see Fig. 19.1). Currently accepted definitions emphasise the reversibility of asthma, which is highly responsive to treatment, while COPD is considered to be irreversible and characterised by progressive airway narrowing (GOLD 2020). Emphysema is a pathological diagnosis, and consists of alveolar dilation and destruction. Chronic bronchitis is defined as a daily cough with sputum production for at least 3 months for 2 or more consecutive years, although lungs normally produce about 30 millilitres of sputum daily, so sputum production on its own is not sufficient for a diagnosis. In practice, there may also be co-morbidity of lung disease in patients (GOLD 2020; Yang et al 2019).

People with COPD commonly refer to their condition by lay terms, such as 'asthma' or 'bronchitis' or 'emphysema'; however, they often have a combination of all three types of pathology in varying degrees. Chronic asthma stems from hyperactivity and thickening of airway walls over a prolonged period. The degree of reversibility on RFTs after bronchodilator administration distinguishes asthma (high degree of reversibility) from chronic asthma (low degree of reversibility). Emphysema involves the destruction of the peripheral airways including the alveoli, resulting in loss of lung elasticity, narrowing of the terminal airways and decreased surface area for gas exchange. During expiration, loss of elasticity may result in collapse of the terminal airways, which in turn increases the work of breathing. In comparison, chronic bronchitis exhibits a

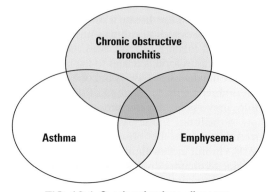

FIG. 19.1 **Overlapping lung diseases.**

persistent productive cough, due to hypertrophy and hyperplasia of the airway's mucus-producing cells. The upper airways are usually inflamed and swollen, resulting in debris and obstruction (GOLD 2020).

BURDEN OF DISEASE: COPD

Prevalence

The estimated prevalence of COPD worldwide is about 65 million people. This figure is expected to increase by 30% in the next 10 years, and COPD is likely to become the third largest cause of death worldwide by 2030 (WHO 2016a). In Australia, self-reported data indicate that about 4.8% of Australians, or 464,000 people, may have COPD (AIHW 2019). The Burden of Obstructive Lung Disease (BOLD) Study, also relying on self-reported data, estimated that the prevalence of COPD in Australia may be 7.5% for people aged over 40 years of age, and 29.2% for those aged 75 and over, although it remains under-diagnosed (Toelle et al 2013). Underestimation in self-reported data may be due to the fact that COPD is often not diagnosed until it begins to restrict a person's lifestyle and is moderately advanced.

Indigenous Australians have a higher burden of chronic disease than non-Indigenous Australians (AIHW 2020). In Australia in 2018–19, chronic respiratory disease accounted for 10% of the total burden of disease for Indigenous Australians over the age of 45, according to self-reported data (AIHW 2020). This represents about 2.3 times the prevalence among non-Indigenous Australians in the same age group (AIHW 2020). This figure is, however, likely to be an underestimate. In New Zealand the prevalence of COPD among the Indigenous Māori population is also estimated as about 2.5 times higher than the non-Indigenous New Zealand population.

The prevalence of COPD is generally the same in men and women, as the gender difference has reduced somewhat over time as more women in Western countries started smoking. It has been reported that there may be gender differences in the susceptibility to deleterious effects of smoking, with men showing greater susceptibility, possibly due to additive effects of exposure to pollutants and occupational dusts or chemicals (Watson et al 2006). While COPD appears more prevalent in men in later years, when smoking and occupational exposure are taken into account there is no gender difference (Watson et al 2006).

Mortality: COPD as a Cause of Death

Worldwide, COPD is the fourth leading cause of death, responsible for about 3.1 million deaths, or, approximately 5.6% of all deaths worldwide (GOLD 2020; WHO 2014). The lack of more precise prevalence figures is attributable to discrepancies in the definition of COPD, and to under-diagnosing of COPD worldwide (Buist et al 2007). In 2012 in Australia and New Zealand, deaths from COPD were calculated as 5.9% and 1.4% per 100,000 deaths respectively, and COPD accounted for 4% of all deaths in Australia and 5.1% of those in New Zealand (WHO 2015). In New Zealand, COPD is the third leading cause of death for men and the fourth for women, affecting over 200,000 adult New Zealanders over the age of 45 years (Health Navigator New Zealand 2016). In Australia in 2017, COPD was the fifth leading cause of death, after coronary heart disease, dementia and Alzheimer's disease, cardiovascular disease and lung cancer (AIHW 2019). It has been estimated that in New Zealand, the Māori population are up to five times more likely to die from COPD than the non-Māori population (Best Practice Advocacy Centre New Zealand [BPACNZ] 2015; Health Navigator New Zealand 2016; Ministry of Health NZ 2014, 2015).

Economic Burden of COPD

In 2008, the economic burden of COPD in Australia was estimated as $98.2 billion, $8.8 billion of which was estimated as direct financial costs, including employment or absentee-related costs; healthcare-related costs, including medications, community and acute care services, of about $900 million (of which $473 million is estimated as hospital costs); costs to wellbeing, and the cost to the community of premature death (Access Economics 2008; Lung Foundation Australia 2016a, 2016b). According to the AIHW, the most recent reliable available data show that in 2008–09, expenditure on COPD amounted to $929 million, which is 1.3% of all direct expenditure on diseases (AIHW 2016).

In 2013–14, an estimated 58,900 Australians aged 55 and over were hospitalised for COPD, representing 6% of hospitalisations in that period, and a rate of 1008 people with COPD per 100,000 population (AIHW 2016). The data also shows that hospitalisation rates for men reduced between 2004–05 and 2013–14, while rates for women remained fairly stable (AIHW 2016).

EPIDEMIOLOGY OF COPD

COPD Risk Factors

Perhaps contrary to common belief, a minority of cigarette smokers (10–20%) develop COPD, although tobacco smoking is the single highest behavioural determinant of COPD. Most people with COPD either smoke or have smoked in their past. About 20% of COPD occurs in people who have never smoked (GOLD 2020; Lamprecht et al for the BOLD Collaborative Research Group 2011). Among non-smokers, the prevalence of the disease has been determined by a large 25-year longitudinal Danish study as being between 4% to 9%, indicating the likely genetic, as well as environmental and behavioural factors that play a role in the development of COPD (GOLD 2020; Lokke et al 2006; WHO 2016b). It has also been identified that while smoking contributes about 15% of the variability in lung function, genetic factors may account for a further 40% (Wood & Stockley 2006). Observations of differences in the rate of decline in lung function, family aggregations of spirometry measures and higher rates of airflow obstructions among first-degree relatives of patients with COPD also suggest genetic influences (GOLD 2020).

Many determinants or risk factors are not 'behaviours' and, as such, are not easily avoided by the people with the disease. Dusty environments and smoking are both risk factors for developing COPD, but when combined, the risk of COPD increases greatly (Blanc & Toren 2007). Matheson and colleagues (2005) indicated that 15–19% of COPD in smokers and up to 31% of COPD in never-smokers can be attributed to occupational exposure to dust (Lamprecht et al 2011). Studies reviewed by Blanc and Toren indicated that exposures were to dust consisting of silica, coal, agricultural dusts, coke oven emissions and tunnelling dusts and fumes. Cement workers are also at high risk of developing chronic respiratory symptoms and COPD (Mwaiselage et al 2005).

In summary, risk factors may be associated with socioeconomic status and its relationship with the social determinants of health, which can link with lifestyle factors, cultural mores and occupational roles. The main risk factors have been identified as:

- tobacco smoking – including environmental tobacco smoke (passive smoking)
- indoor air pollution – including that created by fuel during cooking and heating
- occupational dust and chemicals – including exposure to cadmium, silica, asbestos or dusts
- outdoor air pollution – but current evidence suggests this may be less of a risk factor than other factors
- genetic predisposition, including alpha1-antitrypsin deficiency (GOLD 2020).

In recent years, the overall rate of smoking has continued to decline in Australian adults; in 2010 it was 15.9% and in 2013 it was 13.3% (AIHW 2015). However, some cultural groups continue to smoke more than others. People from Indigenous (Aboriginal and Torres Strait Islander, and Māori) backgrounds, some culturally and linguistically diverse (CALD) backgrounds, the lesbian, gay, bisexual, transgender and queer (LGBTQ) community, people with mental illness and substance use issues, and prisoners, all have higher smoking rates than in the general population, increasing the susceptibility of such groups to COPD (Baker et al 2006; Clarke & Coughlin 2012; Siru et al 2009). In addition, migrants now constitute about 25% of the Australian population, with approximately 14% having emigrated from countries of non-English-speaking backgrounds, some of which feature smoking as a more acceptable cultural practice (Baker et al 2006; Page et al 2007).

The GOLD Study has identified a clear link between social class and COPD, with greater prevalence among people of lower socioeconomic status (SES) (GOLD 2020; Rabe et al 2007). Low SES is associated with poorer health and higher mortality, and in Australia areas of low SES have higher rates of smoking, physical inactivity and obesity (AIHW 2019). Mortality from COPD tends to increase in Australia for both males and females with increased remoteness, although it is the effect of the social determinants of health on adults living in these areas, rather than the geographical remoteness per se, that contributes to this increase (AIHW 2019).

Diet and nutrition can affect most chronic diseases, and may also influence the presentation of COPD. Studies have shown that frequent consumption of cured meat is associated with increased risk for developing COPD (Jiang et al 2007; Varraso & Camargo 2015; Varraso et al 2015). Cured meats such as bacon, sausage, luncheon meats and cured hams are high in nitrites, which are used as a meat preservative. Nitrites may cause lung damage, producing structural changes similar to emphysema (tobacco smoke is another major source of nitrite in the body). Several studies have suggested that dietary antioxidants and foods rich in antioxidants (i.e. fruits and vegetables) may protect the airways against oxidant-mediated damage that leads to COPD (Varraso et al 2015).

EFFECTS OF COPD ON PHYSICAL HEALTH

People with COPD experience a broad spectrum of symptoms, depending on their particular lung pathology, the severity of their illness and their adaptation to it. Early symptoms of COPD may include breathlessness (dyspnoea), cough, wheeze, increased production of phlegm (sputum), sleep disturbance and fatigue (GOLD 2020). Fatigue also features in the latter symptoms of COPD and is often associated with escalating dyspnoea, increasingly frequent exacerbations, muscle wasting, loss of appetite and/or weight and cor pulmonale (right-sided heart failure).

Significant airflow obstruction may be present before the individual is aware of any symptoms. As such, it is no surprise that people are often diagnosed with COPD quite late in the disease trajectory. COPD has a 'relapse remitting' course, which Lynn (2001) and Murray and colleagues (2005) describe as one of illness over many months or years with occasional dramatic exacerbations; each episode may cause death, but the individual usually survives many such episodes before death. A trajectory model may assist in considering the course of the disease for individual patients (Corbin 1998; Rocker & Cook 2013). In the medium-to-later stages of COPD, increasingly frequent hospital admissions are not uncommon, reflecting deteriorating lung function and increasing susceptibility to infection. Exacerbations tend to be more common in people with moderate-to-severe COPD and of greater consequence in those with advanced disease (Sherwood Burge 2006).

PATHOPHYSIOLOGY OF BREATHLESSNESS

COPD severity is classified by the degree of obstruction during expiration on RFTs. However, evidence suggests that there is little correlation between the degree of obstruction on RFTs and the physical impairment or degree of dyspnoea endured by the individual (GOLD 2020; Wolkove et al 1989). Dyspnoea may vary from very mild breathlessness on exertion to rendering an individual housebound. A complex relationship of neural and biochemical factors control our respiratory rate, which is further modulated by emotional facets, such as tolerance of the individual to the sensation of dyspnoea, anxiety, previous experience and expectations. Intrapulmonary pathology (e.g. airway obstruction, impaired gas exchange, hyperinflation) together with extra-pulmonary factors (e.g. deconditioning, functional decline and muscle wasting) govern the biochemical factors that influence the central nervous system's control of respiration.

A fear of being dyspnoeic leads to heightened anxiety and discourages people with COPD from participating in activities that result in breathlessness, which in turn causes further deconditioning and activity avoidance. This vicious cycle of deconditioning, and

functional decline (see Fig. 19.2) is a common phenomenon and may be further precipitated by musculoskeletal problems (e.g. arthritis), inconvenience (e.g. driving is quicker than walking) or lack of enjoyment of exercise (e.g. colder climates). The principal intervention for people with COPD who are deconditioned is a course of pulmonary rehabilitation, which is discussed later in this chapter.

Respiratory assessment should consider the many alternative causes of dyspnoea (GOLD 2020). There is a plethora of non-COPD causes of dyspnoea, including heart disease, anaemia, pulmonary embolism, pleural effusion and pneumothorax. Those that relate to COPD include, but are not limited to, airway obstruction from sputum or foreign objects, bronchospasm, fatigue, and, in some cases, hypoxaemia. Worsening of dyspnoea may signify an exacerbation of COPD, which is often associated with increased sputum production and/or viscosity, wheeze, fever or pleuritic pain. Oxygen therapy is indicated in COPD during acute exacerbations where oxygen saturations (SpO_2) are decreased (e.g. < 92% on room air), or as a domiciliary therapy, where a person's partial pressure of oxygen (PaO_2) is < 55 mmHg on arterial blood gases. Unless there is evidence of hypoxaemia, supplementary oxygen will not usually relieve dyspnoea, although this is a common lay misconception. In administering oxygen therapy for people with COPD, the nurse must always consider the risk of oxygen toxicity and carbon dioxide retention, and observe closely for signs of respiratory system depression. It should also be noted that when delivering oxygen therapy to patients with COPD who have had an episode of hypercapnic respiratory failure, high oxygen concentrations may worsen their condition due to suppression of hypoxic ventilatory drive (Feller-Kopman & Schwartzstein 2012; Smith et al 2009). Although COPD patients with hypercapnic respiratory failure are not common (around 10% according to Plant and colleagues 2000), it is recommended that all

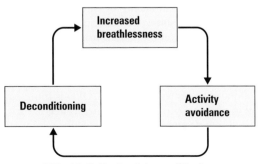

FIG. 19.2 **Cycle of deconditioning.**

patients with low oxygen saturation do receive oxygen therapy, and it is important to identify these patients as they particularly need continuous assessment while receiving oxygen therapy.

Altered Mobility and Fatigue

Regardless of the variation between individuals, dyspnoea is generally the most overt limitation on a person's activities of daily living (ADL). Around the time of diagnosis, people often report earlier limitation in usual activities of exertion (e.g. climbing stairs, playing with grandchildren), while in later stages household activities such as cleaning and cooking become increasingly difficult. Tasks that involve bending forwards, such as vacuuming, putting on shoes and making beds, are commonly reported as particularly challenging for people with COPD, perhaps due to the restriction of respiration in an already biomechanically-challenged thorax. Overhead chores, such as pegging out washing or storing groceries in an overhead cupboard, result in disproportionate dyspnoea, as does showering in a steamy, poorly ventilated bathroom. Tasks often need to be modified, or split into stages to avoid immediate limitation, due to dyspnoea or fatigue.

Secondary impairment may result when a physical inability to walk, drive or catch public transport to the shops leads to nutritional inadequacies. Weight loss associated with muscle wasting is common in the later stages of COPD and further impedes exercise tolerance and respiratory function. Low body mass index (BMI) is a well-documented risk factor for poor prognosis in COPD (Schols et al 1998), and, while the mechanisms for involuntary weight loss are not well understood (Ferreira et al 2001), impaired swallowing function in advanced COPD is one likely contributor (McGinley 2014). Increasing dyspnoea makes the 3- to 5-second breath hold required for swallowing difficult, and may increase the risk of aspiration and chest infection. Inhaled respiratory medications often result in a dry mouth, which further hampers safe swallowing function. These factors may lead to avoidance of particular foods or of eating altogether, resulting in nutritional deprivation.

While the physical limitations from COPD vary between individuals, they also vary greatly within individuals as the relapse and remitting course of exacerbations lessen a person's usual physical capabilities. It should also be remembered that COPD is more common in older people, thus age-related changes, such as reduced muscle strength and mass, fatigue, joint stiffness due to degenerative changes and bone loss, are commonplace, and may not be related to the individual's lung pathology.

Measurement of Physical Health

Many best practice interventions for COPD, while improving dyspnoea and quality of life (QOL), do not alter physiological lung function. Hence, assessment of the impact of interventions should focus on the initial goals of the intervention. That is, the use of tools that measure change in other outcomes, such as BMI, dyspnoea, functional capacity, the number of exacerbations and QOL, may be more appropriate than repeating RFTs. The goal of many COPD interventions is to decrease dyspnoea; however, dyspnoea is subjective and difficult to quantify. Scales such as the Borg Scale of Dyspnoea (Mahler et al 1987) and the Medical Research Council Scale of Dyspnoea (Bestall et al 1999) have been validated for use in this population. The measurement of functional capacity is often achieved using the 6 Minute Walk Test (American Thoracic Society 2002) or the Incremental Shuttle Walk Test (Singh et al 1992). These tests may also be used to assess for exertional desaturation or oxygen requirements, and are used by physiotherapists to prescribe exercise. It is worth remembering that physiological measurements of COPD (e.g. spirometry, 6 Minute Walk Test) do not necessarily correlate with the various symptoms of COPD. As such, quality-of-life tools and measures of dyspnoea may more accurately reflect a patient's perception of their disease severity or impairment, the impact of treatments and the fluctuations in symptoms (Yusen 2001).

Morbidity and Co-morbidity of COPD

Almost all people with COPD have at least one other chronic disorder, leading to the suggestion that the term 'co-morbidity' should be changed to 'multimorbidity' (Clini & Berghe 2013; Vanfleteren et al 2013). This change recognises that with diseases related to smoking often one disease does not dominate and cause the others; rather, there is a complex inter-relationship between a number of diseases. The clinical implication of this change is that patients with COPD should be investigated for concomitant chronic disorders, including osteoporosis, dyslipidaemia, hypertension, atherosclerosis and hyperglycemia.

EFFECTS OF COPD ON MENTAL HEALTH AND QUALITY OF LIFE

The effects of COPD on an individual's QOL and mental and physical health are not independent from each other. Symptoms such as breathlessness, insomnia, fatigue, poor appetite, reduced activity levels, feelings of guilt and anger, irritability, reduced self-esteem, just to mention a few, may all affect QOL and be related to COPD, to adjusting to COPD or to anxiety and/or depression.

Physical deconditioning may lead to social isolation as friends and hobbies become inaccessible, resulting in loneliness and its associated symptom of depression (Kara & Mirici 2004; Miravitlles & Rivera 2017). Similarly, the anxiety that a person feels in anticipation of dyspnoea may prevent them from being adequately motivated to attempt activity, resulting in further deconditioning and progressive dyspnoea. In addition, the presence of mental health conditions has been associated with longer hospitalisations, poorer survival rates, increased symptom burden and poorer physical and social functioning in COPD patients (Ng et al 2007).

Having a chronic illness such as COPD will inevitably impact on QOL. WHO defines QOL as an 'individual's perception of their position in life in the context of the culture and value systems in which they live and in relation to their goals, expectations, standards and concerns' (1997, p. 1). Thus defined, QOL is a broad concept that can be affected in a multitude of ways. In recognition of the breadth of this definition, along with the considerable impact health status and illness can have on QOL, investigations often focus on health-related quality of life (HRQOL) as a measure of QOL as it is affected specifically by health and healthcare (Kil et al 2010).

While HRQOL is an important factor in and of itself, it also has a significant impact on a range of other variables. It is a prognostic factor in COPD, with poor HRQOL associated with higher mortality and greater risk of hospitalisation (Balcells et al 2010). In a review, Tsiligianni and colleagues found the most significant factors associated with HRQOL to be dyspnoea, exercise tolerance and anxiety and depression (Tsiligianni et al 2011). A combination of depression and anxiety in a person with severe COPD has a more significant impact on HRQOL (Balcells et al 2010). Other factors found to be related to reduced HRQOL included being female, being under- or overweight, continuing to smoke, more severe COPD and the presence of comorbidities (Tsiligianni et al 2011).

Yusen (2001) describes HRQOL as a reflection of the health- and disease-related aspects, including the impact of disease, treatments and tests, of daily life and wellbeing. The goals of most interventions for COPD are, directly or indirectly, to improve QOL.

In choosing a tool to measure QOL, the nurse should consider whether a respiratory disease-specific QOL tool, such as the Guyatt Chronic Respiratory

Disease Questionnaire (Guyatt et al 1987) or the St George Respiratory Disease Questionnaire (Jones et al 1992), or a generic QOL tool, is more appropriate. The domains included in the choice of tool should reflect the intervention and its goals. For example, an exercise and education program of pulmonary rehabilitation may use a disease-specific QOL tool that covers domains such as physical, emotional, knowledge, mastery and fatigue. The tool's domains encompass the degree of dyspnoea on activities, the impact of disease on ADL and the frustration and feelings of hope or despair in living with COPD. The choice of tool should depend on the purpose – to measure overall impact of COPD at one point in time, or to test and retest QOL in response to an intervention. Whichever instrument is chosen, it should be reliable and valid in the population it is to be used for. For example, measuring QOL in a CALD population requires that the tool be either available in multiple languages, or validated when translated by an interpreter. Other considerations may include the literacy of the population, and whether the tool is designed to be administered by a healthcare professional or independently by the patients themselves.

Adjustment to Illness

Symptoms of COPD can present years after smoking has ceased and can occur in the absence of known risk factors. For many people, recurrent chest infections or insidious dyspnoea leads to a diagnosis some time after initial symptoms arise. Being diagnosed with a chronic disease such as COPD can be understandably confronting and distressing. COPD is irreversible, incurable and progressive, and the person diagnosed with COPD must make significant adjustments over multiple domains, including behavioural, emotional, psychological and social. The process of adjustment will be ongoing as the impact of the disease changes over time. In the behavioural domain, people with COPD may have to reduce their activity levels. The physical limitations from dyspnoea may require early retirement and a change of role in employment, social and family contexts. For people who have been active, independent and self-sufficient, the effect of COPD on their activities can be quite devastating (Ekici et al 2015; Falvo 2005). People with COPD must also endure significant lifestyle changes, with the acquisition of new habits (e.g. medications, exercise, modified activities) and the suppression of old habits (e.g. smoking, poor self-care).

Being diagnosed with COPD may result in altered self-perception, including body image. Social roles and relationships may change. An individual's loss of independence and restrictions on recreational activities may result in irritability, a sense of hopelessness (Burgel et al 2013; Yusen 2001), decreased confidence and lowered self-esteem. Frustration and powerlessness are also common in response to recurrent infections and the impossibility of predicting the timing or severity of exacerbations. There is evidence to demonstrate that acute exacerbations of COPD have a negative impact on health-related QOL and exercise capacity (Carr et al 2007) for the duration of the exacerbation and potentially for some time after, if the recovery is prolonged. Perhaps the most difficult adjustment people with COPD must face is adaptation to the sensation of shortness of breath and the associated fear of breathlessness and, at the extreme end, the fear of dying.

Impact on the Person and their Family

The sequelae of COPD and its treatments often bring sufferers embarrassment and can result in their avoidance of public situations. Breathlessness, a productive cough and the use of inhalers often lead to undue attention from the general public, so people with COPD may avoid enclosed spaces such as public transport. Some of the common visible physical symptoms that the patient and family must adjust to include portable oxygen or walking aids, clubbed fingers, Cushingoid features and bruising from steroid-based medications. Aside from dyspnoea, relinquishment of social activities with others may stem from more diverse causes, such as:

- stress incontinence as a side effect of pelvic floor pressure from frequent coughing
- travel restrictions, as persons with chronic hypoxaemia may not be able to fly due to atmospheric pressure changes at altitude
- a fear of 'holding up' the rest of the group due to low energy levels and fatigue.

Patients with COPD may also feel guilt, shame or anger about their illness and it is important to remember that COPD has a degree of stigma as a 'self-inflicted' illness (Sherwood Burge 2006), which health workers should avoid reinforcing.

Inevitably these symptoms and their impact on ADL and life role require support and understanding from family and caregivers. Relationships can be compromised and strained due to effects of the illness on family members. Partners may have to take on the role of carer, thereby sacrificing some of their own needs. There may be anger towards the person with COPD if the illness is seen as being caused by their own behaviour, such as smoking. This may be accompanied by guilt about feeling angry. There may also be anger

directed at others, such as employers, if the illness is seen to be a result of the occupational environment.

Family members may overestimate the impact of the disease and put their loved one in the sick role, reducing behavioural expectations, thereby reinforcing sickness behaviour and inadvertently contributing to deconditioning. Alternatively, some family members may not fully appreciate the impact of the disease on the activity levels of the person with COPD and hold unrealistic expectations of their capabilities (Falvo 2005; Gardiner et al 2010).

COPD may put considerable financial stress on a family if the person with the illness has ceased work and their partner has to alter their work arrangements in order to take on a caring role. There are also costs associated with medical treatment, hospitalisations and medication. A couple's intimate relationship may also be adversely affected. The person with COPD may feel anxiety about engaging in sexual activity due to the impact this has on their breathing (Falvo 2005).

Depression and Anxiety

Estimates of the prevalence of depression and anxiety in people with COPD vary widely, (depression: 8–80%; anxiety 6–74%), although the general consensus in the literature seems to be that the rates are high and that depression and anxiety are probably under-diagnosed and certainly under-treated (Doyle et al 2016; Yohannes et al 2010). It has been estimated that one in four people with COPD has significant depression, and 40% have clinical anxiety (Panagioti et al 2014). The variation in rates of depression and anxiety in people with COPD reported in the literature is in part related to the variety of measures used and whether they are diagnostic- or symptom-based.

In a large cohort study, Hanania and colleagues (2011) found that rates of depression in COPD are higher than in the general population and also higher than in the population of smokers. This suggests that COPD is at least a contributing factor to the depression experienced in this population. Within COPD populations, these researchers found that depression is more prevalent in women, in people with more serious COPD, in people who are over 60 years of age and in those who continue to smoke.

Depression in COPD leads to reduced functional capability, magnifies morbidity and worsens functional and health status of patients (Hanania et al 2011). Depression has been shown to have a negative impact on a range of health outcomes, including mortality, continued smoking, length of hospital stay and physical and social functioning, even when confounders such as chronicity of COPD and socioeconomic variables are controlled for (Ng et al 2007). An increased rate of exacerbations has also been associated with depression in COPD, resulting in higher levels of healthcare use. Hanania and colleagues (2011) estimated that only one-third of people with COPD and depression receive appropriate treatment and this is in spite of the observation that people with COPD and a depressive disorder are more likely to present with moderate to severe symptoms, which can have a significant negative impact on functioning.

Anxiety is particularly common in COPD as a result of dyspnoea (Gore et al 2000; Pulmar et al 2014) and may be exacerbated by the vicious cycle of deconditioning (see Fig. 19.2). A fear of becoming breathless leads to activity avoidance or fear of exercise, and results in further deconditioning. Anticipatory anxiety then results when the individual next attempts an activity that they perceive may result in breathlessness. Panic attacks and panic disorder are particularly prevalent in people with COPD, and rates are considerably higher than those found in the general population (Livermore et al 2010). Anxiety can be particularly difficult to identify in COPD patients due to the overlap of physiological symptoms in particular.

MANAGEMENT OF COPD

Among therapeutic options for managing COPD, smoking cessation is very important and the management option with the greatest impact on the individual's prospects. Drug treatments can reduce the frequency and severity of exacerbations, but no existing medications can modify the long-term reduction in lung function. Pulmonary rehabilitation has good evidence for improving symptoms and QOL. Surgical treatments, such as lung volume reduction and bronchoscopic lung volume reduction, are being studied (GOLD 2020).

Management of Psychological Symptoms

Given the high prevalence of symptoms of anxiety and depression in people with COPD, it is unfortunate that current national and international treatment guidelines devote little, if any, content to the treatment of psychological symptoms (Australian Physiotherapy Association [APA] & Australian Lung Foundation [ALF] 2009; GOLD 2020; Qaseem et al 2011). Current COPD-X guidelines include recognition of anxiety and depression as significant co-morbidities and recommend screening and referral to clinical psychologists for treatment (Yang et al 2019). One reason that treatment guidelines focus overwhelmingly on the physical characteristics of the disease may be due to the lack of

supporting evidence for effective treatments for the mental health component (Cafarella et al 2012). To date, there has not been sufficient investigation into treatments for anxiety and depression in people with COPD to warrant firm conclusions or evidence-based recommendations (Fritzsche et al 2011). Over the coming years this situation is likely to change as further research is undertaken and evidence begins to accumulate. In the meantime, it is possible to address the psychological aspects of COPD using what we already know.

First, given the prevalence rates and the impact of depression and anxiety on HRQOL, morbidity and mortality, the importance of monitoring patients with COPD for signs of depression or anxiety cannot be overstated. Deterioration in mood, increasing avoidance behaviour, high levels of fear and catastrophic or negative cognitions are all signs that suggest further assessment may be required. Screening instruments such as the Hospital Anxiety and Depression Scale (HADS) and the nine-item Patient Health Questionnaire (PHQ 9) are readily available and quick to administer. While these instruments are not intended to be diagnostic, they may indicate that a referral for more thorough assessment is warranted. Screening patients with COPD for depression and anxiety should be part of standard practice.

Pulmonary rehabilitation has been shown to improve HRQOL and depression levels in people with COPD (Bratas et al 2010), and is routinely recommended for people whose COPD has become functionally disabling in order to reduce fatigue, improve exercise tolerance, reduce the progression of the disease and prolong life expectancy (Addy 2007).

Unfortunately, depression and anxiety may impact on a person's capacity to engage with pulmonary rehabilitation, despite its effectiveness (Baraniak & Sheffield 2011). For example, Addy (2007) has argued that for people with anxiety about breathlessness, their fear that increased activity levels will exacerbate the condition results in a reluctance to engage in pulmonary rehabilitation. Such fear avoidance cycles can cause further disability through physical deconditioning. Addy recommends psychological treatment to address this problem using cognitive and behavioural interventions such as graded exposure.

Cognitive behaviour therapy (CBT) is an evidence-based psychological intervention that includes a wide range of behavioural and cognitive strategies targeting particular symptoms and disorders. Graded exposure is an example of one such behavioural technique. While the evidence for the effectiveness of psychological interventions, including CBT, for the treatment of depression and anxiety in COPD patients is mixed (Baraniak & Sheffield 2011), there is a strong evidence base for CBT in the treatment of anxiety and depression in the general population and CBT is also an effective treatment for anxiety and depression associated with chronic illness (Cafarella et al 2012).

Although the research into treatment for depression and anxiety in people with COPD is growing, there is an extensive body of research examining treatments for depression and anxiety in the general population, some of which have also been examined in people with co-morbid chronic diseases. Examples include pharmacological treatments, especially selective serotonin reuptake inhibitors (SSRIs), relaxation therapy, interpersonal psychotherapy (Cafarella et al 2012; Pulmar et al 2014) and mindfulness-based therapies, such as mindfulness-based cognitive therapy (MBCT) (Addy 2007). These all have the potential to ameliorate symptoms of depression and anxiety in people with COPD.

The treatment of depression and anxiety is the realm of the specialist, usually a psychologist, who will undertake a thorough psychological assessment and develop a targeted treatment plan with the patient. The role of the nurse may be to identify patients who are at possible risk of developing anxiety or depression, to identify signs and symptoms that may warrant further investigation and to make appropriate onward referrals. The nurse may also provide a pivotal role in encouraging the patient to seek further treatment and to provide reassurance that treatment for anxiety and depression is available.

Education for the Person with COPD and their Family – Pulmonary Rehabilitation

People with COPD are actively encouraged to participate in their care through education, shared decision-making, communication and information (NICE 2020). Pulmonary rehabilitation is a structured program of education and exercise for people with chronic lung diseases that aims to improve self-efficacy in relation to their condition, increase exercise tolerance, decrease dyspnoea and improve QOL. The structure of programs vary, although evidence-based guidelines recommend at least 6 weeks of attendance (APA & ALF 2009; Yang et al 2019).

Pulmonary rehabilitation is most commonly run by nurses and physiotherapists in a variety of healthcare settings, including acute care and community sites. While it is an ideal opportunity for multidisciplinary care of the individual, the role of the nurse may vary according to the diversity of other health professional disciplines that may be available and involved in the program. Historically, nurses with specialist skills have

played a primary role in patient education within these programs (APA & ALF 2009). Guidelines suggest that the education component of programs should be multidisciplinary and include information on self-management and the prevention and treatment of exacerbations (Ries et al 2007). According to Australian expert opinion (APA & ALF 2009), education topics should include knowledge of the respiratory system and what the lungs do, symptom recognition and management, the role of physical exercise, smoking cessation, correct use of medications, coping skills (including management of anxiety, depression and panic attacks), breathing techniques, airway clearance strategies, energy conservation and nutrition, among others. The exercise component of pulmonary rehabilitation programs should include endurance and strength training exercises for both upper and lower limbs (Ries et al 2007), as well as a home-based exercise program (APA & ALF 2009).

Trials of pulmonary rehabilitation programs have demonstrated clinically and statistically significant improvements in dyspnoea (Ries et al 2007) and QOL domains, including fatigue, mastery, emotional function and dyspnoea (Lacasse et al 2006; Ries et al 2007). Improvements in functional exercise capacity and maximal exercise capacity have been widely demonstrated, although results are not always statistically significant (Lacasse et al 2006). However, patients' perception of dyspnoea consistently improves (Lacasse et al 2006), suggesting that pulmonary rehabilitation results in improved perception and tolerance of dyspnoea regardless of objective change in exercise capacity. For patients with exercise-induced hypoxaemia, the use of supplementary oxygen during pulmonary rehabilitation is recommended (Ries et al 2007). There is evidence that functional improvements decline over 12–18 months if patients do not participate in a maintenance exercise program after completing a pulmonary rehabilitation course (Ries et al 2003; Ries et al 2007). However, the optimal format (e.g. frequency, duration) for maintaining benefits has not yet been established.

Other Issues to Consider: Palliative Care for COPD

Historically, people with COPD were not routinely referred to palliative care services for their end-of-life care. This may be because the timing of death in COPD is often uncertain until very late in the course of the disease (Gardiner et al 2010; GOLD 2020), unlike more typical palliative care diagnoses such as malignancy. However, recent literature has highlighted the relevance of palliative care in managing the end-of-life symptoms of COPD (Antoniu & Boiculese 2016; Buckingham et al 2015; Disler et al 2012; Gore et al 2000; Murray et al 2005; Seamark et al 2007; Vermylen et al 2015). Gore and colleagues (2000) describe COPD's course as a prolonged period of disabling dyspnoea, increasing hospital admissions and premature death. They further highlight that the experience of reduced QOL, psychological issues and unmet information requirements parallels that of lung cancer patients, who are more readily referred to palliative care services.

Features related to poor prognosis and possible consideration for palliative care include severe airflow obstruction ($FEV_1 < 30\%$ of predicted), severe dyspnoea at rest, hypoxaemia at rest on supplementary oxygen, hypercapnia ($PaCO_2 > 55$ mmHg), frequency of exacerbations, development of cor pulmonale, and unintentional and continuing weight loss or low BMI (Budweiser et al 2007; Lynn 2001; Seamark et al 2007).

In COPD there is often no clearly identifiable point at which management changes from active to palliative in focus (Murray et al 2005). Nursing care for end-of-life COPD should be specifically tailored to address symptoms, of which dyspnoea and anxiety are usually the most prominent. Unlike some other conditions, medications that would be considered part of active management, such as antibiotics, bronchodilators and steroids, may still play an important palliative role in the suppression of dyspnoea. Lynn (2001) describes the unique need for both disease-modifying and comfort-enhancing interventions simultaneously in end-stage COPD management. Constipation is also not unusual in the end-of-life phase (Seamark et al 2007), particularly if opioids are being used for dyspnoea management. While there is evidence to support oral and parenteral opioids to treat advanced dyspnoea (Jennings et al 2002), they should be used judiciously in COPD due to their depression of the respiratory system.

NURSING PRINCIPLES AND INTERVENTIONS

As the symptoms of COPD develop, the physical changes and their effects on a person's psychosocial wellbeing result in an increased need for both physical and emotional support. The nurse's role in COPD management varies across healthcare settings and the acuity of disease spectrum. Regardless of the setting, nurses should focus on working collaboratively with their patients to develop and continually appraise a care plan with interventions that minimise disease progression and maximise their QOL. For example:

- utilise interventions that encourage patient motivation. The relapse/remitting course of COPD means

that while symptoms are usually present in some form, the individual's care needs will fluctuate. The individual and/or their carers are responsible for their own care for a large proportion of the time and will benefit from enhanced self-efficacy skills to monitor and manage their condition. Patients should be encouraged to be involved in their care planning process to help empower them by promoting motivation, understanding and self-efficacy.
- assess for insomnia and encourage appropriate sleep hygiene habits. Insomnia in COPD is multi-factorial, and may be due to physiological COPD changes, age-related sleep pattern changes or medications, but is also a symptom of depression.
- changes in mental health status and ability to cope should be monitored and reported. Kara and Mirici (2004) suggest monitoring for signs of loneliness and depression. Nurse interventions may include referrals to strengthen social networks and relieve stress of family burdens. Referral to a psychologist for therapy to treat anxiety or depression should also be considered.
- encourage smoking cessation. Ironically, while smoking is often the causative factor of COPD, many patients with COPD who still smoke describe their continued habit as their last remaining pleasure in life, despite the knowledge that further harm will eventuate. Sensitively explore the role smoking has for the patient; careful timing of this discussion, and a gentle, non-judgemental approach is critical to effect change (Kilpatrick et al 2012). If the patient is amenable, encourage and educate regarding smoking cessation (GOLD 2020). Jointly consider referral to a smoking cessation specialist clinic, where available.
- provide support and education for family and caregivers as they too adjust to lifestyle and routine modifications.
- to help protect against possible exacerbations of COPD, encourage influenza vaccination and pneumococcal vaccination according to current evidence and guidelines (GOLD 2020; Poole et al 2007; Yang et al 2019).
- monitor functional capabilities. Encourage work simplification and activity modification where appropriate, and assess for increased care needs during exacerbations.
- during stable periods, encourage regular, graduated exercise to maintain functional capabilities. Consider referral to a pulmonary rehabilitation program if evidence of dyspnoea on exertion.
- monitor BMI and nutritional status. Consider referral to a dietitian if overweight or underweight.

- monitor airway clearance techniques. Consider referral to a respiratory physiotherapist if patient describes difficulty in clearing sputum.
- encourage self-monitoring of symptoms and the discussion of an action plan with their treating medical practitioner, including signs to seek medical attention when symptoms worsen.
- provide education on the prevention of exacerbations, including the avoidance of risk factors such as cold weather, pollution exposure or contact with people with a bacterial or viral infection (Sherwood Burge 2006).
- assess use of inhaled medication devices and provide education to the patient and carer to optimise drug administration. Misuse of inhaled devices may lead to inadequate drug dosing and suboptimal disease control (Rau 2006). Reassess capability to use usual inhaled devices during exacerbations as diminished respiratory reserve may impede optimal device use.
- titrate oxygen therapy as appropriate in the acute setting and monitor for side effects. Provide education regarding the use of domiciliary oxygen where prescribed, including safety considerations around the home.
- monitor for signs of aspiration whether obvious (e.g. changes in quality of voice, or coughing/choking on eating or drinking), or more subtle (pocketing of food/fluid around mouth, recurrent chest infections, difficulty managing some food consistencies). If evidence or suspicion of aspiration, consider referral to speech pathologist.

PRINCIPLES OF NURSING PRACTICE

The following principles of nursing practice apply to nursing patients with COPD:
- encourage medication compliance/optimise technique
- maximise functional ability/minimise further deconditioning
- recognise signs and symptoms of deterioration (and act promptly)
- educate patient/carer to recognise signs and symptoms
- support activity modification
- support symptom relief and comfort.

CONCLUSION

COPD is one of the most common diseases in the world. COPD is the umbrella term for some lung diseases, including emphysema and chronic bronchitis. The airflow limitation associated with COPD is usually progressive and is associated with abnormal inflammatory response of the lungs to noxious particles or gases. The nurse's role in COPD management, as discussed in this chapter, varies across the healthcare settings depending on the acuity of the disease. It is important that the nurse focuses on minimising disease progression, while at the same time working with the patient's family and significant others, to maximise their QOL (see Case Study 19.1 and 19.2).

CASE STUDY 19.1

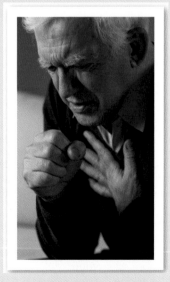

iStockphoto/KatarzynaBialasiewicz.

Mr A, a 78-year-old man, was admitted to RN Suresh's ward with an exacerbation of his COPD. His observations were initially stable and he was treated with intravenous antibiotics, oral corticosteroids and oxygen therapy via nasal prongs. He was breathless on minimal activity and required assistance with all his personal care and transfers.

During handover the following morning it was reported that Mr A's oxygen saturations had dropped overnight and his oxygen therapy was increased. When Suresh assessed Mr A he found that he was drowsier than on the previous day, although his oxygen saturations had improved. Suresh was concerned about possible carbon dioxide (CO_2) retention and reported his decreased conscious state to the treating doctor. Arterial blood gases (ABGs) confirmed a rising CO_2 and the doctor commenced Mr A on non-invasive ventilation (BiPAP) and decreased his fraction of inspired oxygen (FiO_2). His conscious state then required bed rest, full nursing care and frequent observations to monitor his respiratory and cardiovascular status while the BiPAP was in situ.

CASE STUDY 19.1 – cont'd

By the end of Suresh's shift, Mr A's ABGs were improving and his BiPAP had reduced from continuous to intermittent. By the next day, Mr A's pH and CO_2 were within normal range and the BiPAP was ceased. The ward nurses continued to observe Mr A closely for the remainder of his admission, administering only low flow oxygen (<3 litres per minute) and accepting oxygen saturations of 88–92% to avoid further CO_2 retention.

CASE STUDY 19.2

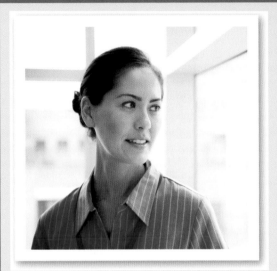

iStockphoto/JohnnyGreig.

Ana is a community health nurse working at a community health centre where an 8-week outpatient pulmonary rehabilitation program is run. Ana's role, together with a respiratory physiotherapist and an allied health assistant, includes pre- and post-program assessments in which comprehensive respiratory assessments are carried out and measures of exercise capacity are completed. During the assessments, Ana must not only assess the participants' respiratory system, but their overall health status, including their safety to exercise.

Ana encourages participants to set goals for themselves and monitors these each week. A team of allied health staff contribute to the program's education components including information, and if required, referral, for assistance in the management of anxiety and depression symptoms. The allied health team can also arrange a referral for an assessment of patients' homes by an occupational therapist to assess for any aids and modifications that may assist patients' QOL and promote their safety. Ana provides information on respiratory medications, the use of respiratory devices, smoking cessation and action plans for symptom monitoring and the management of exacerbations. Throughout the 8 weeks, Ana monitors each participant, taking regular observations and liaising closely with participants' GPs regarding symptoms and progress. At the conclusion, Ana assists participants to make a plan to maintain the physical benefits they have gained over the 8 weeks. Where appropriate, Ana includes family members in some of the planning process, if the patient wishes this, as it can support the patient and their carers.

Reflective Questions

1. Consider what information might be useful to a person with COPD who does not wish to undertake pulmonary rehabilitation.
2. A woman who is a long-term smoker and single parent to her three teenage children is admitted with pneumonia and diagnosed with COPD. How might this new diagnosis affect her emotional status?
3. Discuss the nursing education interventions that should be addressed and the most appropriate times for these to take place.
4. Participants of pulmonary rehabilitation programs frequently have co-morbidities, often related to smoking. What other systems should be assessed to ensure that a person is able to participate in a group exercise situation?

Acknowledgement

Rebecca Howard and Maree Daly contributed to writing earlier versions of this chapter.

RECOMMENDED READING

Yang I, Dabscheck E, George J et al on behalf of the Lung Foundation Australia and the Thoracic Society of Australia and New Zealand 2019. COPD-X guidelines: Australian and New Zealand guidelines for management of COPD. Lung Foundation Australia.

Global Initiative for Chronic Obstructive Lung Disease (GOLD) 2020. Global strategy for the diagnosis, management and prevention of COPD. Online. Available: http://goldcopd.org/.

National Institute of Clinical Excellence (NICE) 2020. NICE Pathways. Chronic obstructive pulmonary disease. Online. Available: https://pathways.nice.org.uk/pathways/chronic-obstructive-pulmonary-disease.

REFERENCES

Access Economics 2008. Economic impact of COPD and cost effective solutions. Australian Lung Foundation, Milton, Qld.

Addy KBE 2007. The treatment of depression and anxiety within the context of chronic obstructive pulmonary disease. Clinical Case Studies 6(5), 383–393.

American Thoracic Society 2002. ATS statement: guidelines for the six-minute walk test. American Journal of Respiratory and Critical Care Medicine 166, 111–117.

Antoniu SA, Boiculese LV 2016. Palliative care outcome measures in COPD patients: a conceptual review. Expert Review of Pharmacoeconomics and Outcomes Research 16(2), 267–274.

Australian Institute of Health and Welfare (AIHW) 2020. Chronic obstructive pulmonary disease (COPD) web report. Online. Available: www.aihw.gov.au/reports/chronic-respiratory-conditions/copd/contents/copd

Australian Institute of Health and Welfare (AIHW) 2016. Chronic respiratory conditions including asthma and COPD. COPD-Chronic Obstructive Pulmonary Disease. Online. Available: www.aihw.gov.au/copd.

Australian Institute of Health and Welfare (AIHW) 2015. Leading cause of premature mortality in Australia fact sheet: COPD. Cat. no. PHE 197. AIHW, Canberra.

Australian Physiotherapy Association and Australian Lung Foundation (APA & ALF) 2009. Pulmonary Rehabilitation Toolkit. Online. Available: www.pulmonaryrehab.com.au.

Baker A, Ivers RG, Bowman J et al 2006. Where there's smoke there's fire: high prevalence of smoking among some subpopulations and recommendations for intervention. Drug and Alcohol Review 25, 85–96.

Balcells E, Gea J, Ferrer J, the PAC-COPD Study Group et al 2010. Factors affecting the relationship between psychological status and quality of life in COPD patients. Health and Quality of Life Outcomes 8, 108.

Baraniak A, Sheffield D 2011. The efficacy of psychologically based interventions to improve anxiety, depression and quality of life in COPD: a systematic review and meta-analysis. Patient Education and Counseling 83, 29–36.

Best Practice Advocacy Centre New Zealand (BPACNZ) 2015. The optimal management of patients with COPD – Part 1: The diagnosis. Online. Available: www.bpac.org.nz/BPJ/2015/February/copd-part1.aspx.

Bestall JC, Paul EA, Garrod R et al 1999. Usefulness of the Medical Research Council dyspnoea scale as a measure of disability in patients with chronic obstructive pulmonary disease. Thorax 54, 581–586.

Blanc PD, Toren K 2007. Occupation in chronic obstructive pulmonary disease and chronic bronchitis: an update. The International Journal of Tuberculosis and Lung Disease 11(3), 251–257.

Bratas O, Espnes GA, Rannestad T et al 2010. Pulmonary rehabilitation reduces depression and enhances heath-related quality of life in COPD patients especially in patients with mild or moderate disease. Chronic Respiratory Disease 7(4), 229–237.

Buckingham S, Kendall M, Ferguson S et al 2015. HELPing older people with very severe chronic obstructive pulmonary disease (HELP-COPD): mixed-method feasibility pilot randomised controlled trial of a novel intervention. NPJ Primary Care Respiratory Medicine. 25 Article Number 15020.

Budweiser S, Jorres RA, Riedl T et al 2007. Predictors of survival in COPD patients with chronic hypercapnic respiratory failure receiving non-invasive home ventilation. Chest 131, 1650–1658.

Buist AS, McBurnie MA, Vollmer WM et al 2007. International variation in the prevalence of COPD (the BOLD Study): a population-based prevalence study. Lancet 370, 741–750.

Burgel PR, Escamilla R, Perez T et al 2013. Impact of comorbidities on COPD-specific health-related quality of life. Respiratory Medicine 107(2), 233–241.

Cafarella PA, Effing TW, Usmani Z et al 2012. Treatments for anxiety and depression in patients with chronic obstructive pulmonary disease: a literature review. Respirology (Carlton, Vic.) 17, 627–638.

Carr SJ, Goldstein RS, Brooks D 2007. Acute exacerbations of COPD in subjects completing pulmonary rehabilitation. Chest 132(1), 127–134.

Clarke MP, Coughlin JR 2012. Prevalence of smoking among the lesbian, gay, bisexual, transsexual, transgender and queer (LGBTTQ) subpopulations in Toronto – The Toronto Rainbow Tobacco Survey (TRTS). Canadian Journal of Public Health 103(2), 132–136.

Clini EM, Beghe B 2013. Chronic obstructive pulmonary disease is just one component of the complex multimorbidities inpatients with COPD. American Journal of Respiratory and Critical Care Medicine 187, 668–670.

Corbin JM 1998. The Corbin and Strauss chronic illness trajectory model: an update. Scholarly Inquiry for Nursing Practice 12(1), 33–41.

Disler R, Inglis SC, Currow DC et al 2012. Palliative and supportive care in chronic obstructive pulmonary disease: research priorities to decrease suffering. 1:301. doi:10.4172/scientificreports.301

Doyle C, Dunt D, Ames D et al 2016. Study protocol for a randomised control trial of telephone-delivered cognitive behavioural therapy compared with befriending for treating depression and anxiety in older adults with chronic obstructive pulmonary disease. International Journal of Chronic Obstructive Pulmonary Disease 11, 327–334.

Dunt D, Doyle C 2012. Signs of progress in the Australian post-2000 COPD experience, but some old problems remain. International Journal of Chronic Obstructive Pulmonary Disease 7, 357–366.

Ekici A, Bulcun E, Karakoc T et al 2015. Factors associated with quality of life in subjects with stable COPD. Respiratory Care 60(11), 1585–1591.

Falvo D 2005. Psychosocial aspects of chronic illness and disability, 3rd ed. Jones and Bartlett, Sudbury, MA.

Feller-Kopman D, Schwartzstein R 2012. Use of oxygen in patients with hypercapnia. Online. Available: www.

uptodate.com/contents/use-of-oxygen-in-patients-with-hypercapnia.

Ferreira IM, Brooks D, Lacasse Y et al 2001. Nutritional intervention in COPD: a systematic overview. Chest 119, 353–363.

Fritzsche A, Clamor A, von Leupoldt A 2011. Effects of medical and psychological treatment of depression in patients with COPD – a review. Respiratory Medicine 105, 1422–1433.

Gardiner C, Gott M, Payne S et al 2010. Exploring the care needs of patients with advanced COPD: an overview of the literature. Respiratory Medicine 104(2), 159–165.

Global Initiative for Chronic Obstructive Lung Disease (GOLD) 2020. Global strategy for the diagnosis, management and prevention of COPD. Online. Available: http://goldcopd.org/.

Gore JM, Brophy CJ, Greenstone MA 2000. How well do we care for patients with end stage chronic obstructive pulmonary disease (COPD)? A comparison of palliative care and quality of life in COPD and lung cancer. Thorax 55, 1000–1006.

Guyatt GH, Berman LB, Townsend M et al 1987. A measure of quality of life for clinical trials in chronic lung disease. Thorax 42(10), 773–778.

Hanania NA, Müllerova H, Locantore NW et al 2011. Determinants of depression in the ECLIPSE chronic obstructive pulmonary disease cohort. American Journal of Respiratory and Critical Care Medicine 183, 604–611.

Health Navigator New Zealand 2016. Chronic obstructive pulmonary disease. Online. Available: www.healthnavigator.org.nz/health-a-z/c/chronic-obstructive-pulmonary-disease.

Jennings AL, Davies AN, Higgins JPT et al 2002. A systematic review of the use of opioids in the management of dyspnoea. Thorax 57, 939–944.

Jiang R, Paik DC, Hankinson JL et al 2007. Cured meat consumption, lung function, and chronic obstructive pulmonary disease among United States adults. American Journal of Respiratory and Critical Care Medicine 175, 798–804.

Jones PW, Quirk FH, Baveystock CM et al 1992. A self complete measure of health status for chronic airflow limitation. The St George's Respiratory Questionnaire. American Review of Respiratory Disease 145(6), 1321–1327.

Kara M, Mirici A 2004. Loneliness, depression and social support of Turkish patients with chronic obstructive pulmonary disease and their spouses. Journal of Nursing Scholarship 36(4), 331–336.

Kil SY, Oh WO, Koo BJ et al 2010. Relationship between depression and health-related quality of life in older Korean patients with chronic obstructive pulmonary disease. Journal of Clinical Nursing 19, 1307–1314.

Kilpatrick P, Wilson E, Wimpenny P 2012. Support for older people with COPD in community settings: a systematic review of qualitative research. JBI Library of Systematic Reviews 10(57), 3649–3763. JBL000280 2012.

Lacasse Y, Goldstein R, Lasserson TJ et al 2006. Pulmonary rehabilitation for chronic obstructive pulmonary disease

(review). The Cochrane Database of Systematic Reviews (4), Art. No: CD003793.

Lamprecht B, McBurnie MA, Vollmer WM et al for the BOLD Collaborative Research Group 2011. COPD in never smokers: results from the population-based burden of obstructive lung disease study. Chest 139(4), 752–763.

Livermore N, Sharpe L, McKenzie D 2010. Panic attacks and panic disorder in chronic obstructive pulmonary disease: a cognitive behavioral perspective. Respiratory Medicine 104, 1246–1253.

Lokke A, Lange P, Scharling H et al 2006. Chronic obstructive pulmonary disease. Developing COPD: a 25 year follow up study of the general population. Thorax 61, 935–939.

Lung Foundation Australia 2016a. Fact sheet: A report into the economic impact of chronic obstructive pulmonary disease (COPD) and cost effective solutions report. Online. Available: www.lungfoundation.com.au/health-professionals/clinical-resources/publications/economic-impact-of-copd/

Lung Foundation Australia 2016b. COPD: The statistics. Online. Available: www.lungfoundation.com.au/health-professionals/clinical-resources/copd/.

Lynn J 2001. Serving patients who may die soon and their families. The role of hospice and other services. Journal of the American Medical Association 285(7), 925–932.

Mahler DA, Rosiello RA, Harver A et al 1987. Comparison of clinical dyspnoea ratings and psychophysical measurement of respiratory sensation in obstructive airway disease. American Review of Respiratory Diseases 135, 1229–1233.

Matheson MC, Benke G, Raven J et al 2005. Biological dust exposure in the workplace is a risk factor for chronic obstructive pulmonary disease. Thorax 60, 645–651.

McGinley E 2014. The role of nutrition in the management of COPD patients. Journal of Community Nursing 28(4), 50–58.

Ministry of Health, NZ 2015. Respiratory disease. Chronic obstructive pulmonary disease. Online. Available: www.health.govt.nz.

Ministry of Health NZ 2014. 2013/14 New Zealand Health Survey, Ministry of Health; National Minimum Data Set (NMDS). MoH, Wellington.

Miravitlles M, Rivera A 2017. Understanding the impact of symptoms on the burden of COPD. Respiratory Research 18, 67. https://doi.org/10.1186/s12931-017-0548-3

Murray SA, Kendall M, Boyd K et al 2005. Illness trajectories and palliative care. British Medical Journal 330, 1007–1011.

Mwaiselage J, Bratveit M, Moen BE et al 2005. Respiratory symptoms and chronic obstructive pulmonary disease among cement factory workers. Scandinavian Journal of Work, Environment and Health 31(4), 316–323.

National Institute of Clinical Excellence (NICE) 2020. NICE Pathways. Chronic obstructive pulmonary disease. Online. Available: https://pathways.nice.org.uk/pathways/chronic-obstructive-pulmonary-disease.

Ng TP, Niti M, Tan WC et al 2007. Depressive symptoms and chronic obstructive pulmonary disease. Archives of Internal Medicine 167, 60–67.

Page A, Begg S, Taylor R et al 2007. Global comparative assessments of life expectancy: the impact of migration with reference to Australia. Bulletin of the World Health Organization 85(6), 474–481.

Panagioti M, Scott C, Blakemore A et al 2014. Overview of the prevalence, impact and management of depression and anxiety in chronic obstructive pulmonary disease. International Journal of Chronic Obstructive Pulmonary Disease 9, 1289–1306.

Plant P, Owen JL, Elliott MW 2000. One-year period prevalence study of respiratory acidosis in acute exacerbations of COPD; implications for the provision of non-invasive ventilation and oxygen administration. Thorax 55(7), 550–554.

Poole PJ, Chacko E, Wood-Baker RWB et al 2007. Influenza vaccine for patients with chronic obstructive pulmonary disease. Cochrane Data of Systematic Review 2006(1), Art. No: CD002733.

Pulmar MI, Gray CR, Walsh JR et al 2014. Anxiety and depression – important psychological comorbidities of COPD. Journal of Thoracic Disorders 6(11), 1615–1631.

Qaseem A, Wilt TJ, Weinberger SE et al 2011. Diagnosis and management of stable chronic obstructive pulmonary disease: a clinical practice guideline update from the American College of Physicians, American College of Chest Physicians, American Thoracic Society, and European Respiratory Society. Annals of Internal Medicine 155, 179–191.

Rabe KF, Hurd S, Anzueto A et al 2007. Global strategy for the diagnosis, management, and prevention of chronic obstructive pulmonary disease. American Journal of Respiratory and Critical Care Medicine 176(6), 532–555.

Rau JL 2006. Practical problems with aerosol therapy in COPD. Respiratory Care 51(2), 158–172.

Ries A, Bauldoff GS, Carlin BW et al 2007. Pulmonary rehabilitation: joint ACCP/AACVPR evidence-based clinical practice guidelines. Chest 131, 4–42.

Ries AL, Kaplan RM, Myers R et al 2003. Maintenance after pulmonary rehabilitation in chronic lung disease. American Journal of Respiratory and Critical Care Medicine 167, 880–888.

Rocker G, Cook D 2013. 'INSPIRED' approaches to better care for patients with advanced COPD. Clinical and Investigative Medicine 36(3), E114–E120.

Schols AMWJ, Slangen J, Volovics L et al 1998. Weight loss is a reversible factor in the prognosis of chronic obstructive pulmonary disease. American Journal of Respiratory and Critical Care Medicine 157, 1791–1797.

Seamark DA, Seamark CJ, Halpin DMG 2007. Palliative care in chronic obstructive pulmonary disease. Journal of the Royal Society of Medicine 100, 225–233.

Sherwood Burge P 2006. Preventing exacerbations. How are we doing and can we do better? Proceedings of the American Thoracic Society 3, 257–261.

Singh S, Morgan D, Scott S et al 1992. Development of a shuttle walking test of disability in patients with chronic airways obstruction. Thorax 47, 1019–1024.

Siru R, Hulse GK, Tait RJ 2009. Assessing motivation to quit smoking in people with mental illness: a review. Addiction (Abingdon, England) 104(5), 719–733.

Smith S, Roberts SB, Duggan-Brennan M et al 2009. Emergency oxygen delivery 2: patients with asthma and COPD. Nursing Times 105(11), 22–23.

Toelle BG, Xuan W, Bird TE et al 2013. Respiratory symptoms and illness in older Australians: the Burden of Obstructive Lung Disease (BOLD) Study. Medical Journal of Australia 198(3), 144–148.

Tsiligianni I, Kocks J, Tzanakis N et al 2011. Factors that influence disease-specific quality of life or health status of patients with COPD: a review and meta-analysis of Pearson correlations. Primary Care Respiratory Journal 20, 257–268.

Vanfleteren L, Spruit MA, Groenen M et al 2013. Clusters of comorbidities based on validated objective measurements and systemic inflammation in patients with chronic obstructive pulmonary disease. American Journal of Respiratory and Critical Care Medicine 187, 728–735.

Varraso R, Camargo CA 2015. The influence of processed meat consumption on chronic obstructive pulmonary disease. Expert Review of Respiratory Medicine 9(6), 703–710.

Varraso R, Chiuve SE, Fung TT et al 2015. Alternate Health Eating Index 2010 and risk of chronic obstructive pulmonary disease among US women and men. Prospective Study. British Medical Journal (Clinical Research Ed.) Online. Available: www.bmj.com/content/350/bmj.h286.

Vermylen JH, Szmuilowicz E, Kalhan R 2015. Palliative care in COPD: an unmet area for quality improvement. International Journal of COPD 10(1), 1543–1551.

Watson L, Vonk JM, Lofdahl CG et al 2006. Predictors of lung function and its decline in mild to moderate COPD in association with gender: results from the Euroscop study. Respiratory Medicine 100, 746–753.

Wolkove N, Dajczman E, Colacone A et al 1989. The relationship between pulmonary function and dyspnoea in obstructive lung disease. Chest 96, 1247–1251.

Wood AM, Stockley RA 2006. The genetics of chronic obstructive pulmonary disease. Respiratory Research 7(130). Online. Available: http://respiratory-research.com/content/7/1/130.

World Health Organization (WHO) 2016a. Chronic respiratory disease. Burden of COPD. Online. Available: www.who.int/respiratory/copd/burden/en/.

World Health Organization (WHO) 2016b. Programmes and projects: chronic obstructive pulmonary disease (COPD). Online. Available: www.who.int/respiratory/copd/en/.

World Health Organization (WHO) 2015. WHO Statistical Profile of New Zealand and Australia. Online. Available: www.who.int/countries.

World Health Organization (WHO) 2014. The Ten Top Causes of Death. Fact Sheet 310. Updated May 2014. Online. Available: www.who.int/mediacentre/factsheets/fs310/en/.

World Health Organization (WHO) 1997. WHOQOL; Measuring quality of life. Division of mental health and prevention of substance abuse. WHO, Geneva.

Yang I, Dabscheck E, George J et al on behalf of the Lung Foundation Australia and the Thoracic Society of Australia and New Zealand 2019. COPD-X guidelines: Australian and New Zealand guidelines for management of COPD. Lung Foundation Australia.

Yohannes AM, Willgoss TG, Baldwin RC et al 2010. Depression and anxiety in chronic heart failure and chronic obstructive pulmonary disease: prevalence, relevance, clinical implications and management principles. International Journal of Geriatric Psychiatry 25, 1209–1221.

Yusen R 2001. What outcomes should be measured in patients with COPD? Chest 119, 327–328.

CHAPTER 20

Principles for Nursing Practice: Coronary Heart Disease

JACQUELINE JAUNCEY-COOKE

LEARNING OBJECTIVES

When you have completed this chapter you will be able to:

- recognise conditions associated with obstructive and non-obstructive coronary heart disease
- describe modifiable biomedical and behavioural risk factors for coronary heart disease and secondary prevention strategies to address these risk factors
- discuss the current evidence relating to the relationship of various psychological disorders and coronary heart disease
- recognise factors that increase the risk of developing coronary heart disease and affect outcomes for Aboriginal and Torres Strait Islander people
- describe models of cardiac rehabilitation programs and community supports available to those with coronary heart disease.

KEY WORDS

angina	secondary prevention
coronary heart disease	stress
risk factors	

INTRODUCTION

Coronary heart disease (CHD) is characterised by reduced blood supply to the heart muscle, usually due to a narrowing of the coronary arteries as a result of atherosclerosis. The two major forms of CHD, also known as ischaemic heart disease (IHD), are angina pectoris and myocardial infarction. In Australia and New Zealand, as in most Western nations, CHD is a major public health problem and accounts for a major proportion of health expenditure (Australian Institute of Health and Welfare [AIHW] 2016). Although mortality from CHD has continued to decline over the past two decades (AIHW 2016), we are now facing the challenge of managing chronic heart diseases in the long term.

CHD is usually associated with a condition known as angina pectoris, commonly referred to as 'angina'. Angina is characteristic chest pain associated with myocardial ischaemia that may radiate to the jaw, shoulder, back or arm, and may be associated with dyspnoea, lightheadedness, nausea and diaphoresis. Anginal symptoms may occur due to coronary thrombosis and abrupt occlusion of an epicardial coronary artery resulting in an acute coronary syndrome (acute myocardial infarction or unstable angina). Alternately, if symptoms of angina are present for at least 2 months without changes in severity, character or triggering circumstance, it may be chronic or 'stable' angina. Stable angina occurs due to a reversible myocardial demand/supply mismatch that results in myocardial ischaemia and/or hypoxia (Ohman 2016). It is usually triggered by exertion or emotional stress, and is relieved by nitroglycerin and rest within 10 minutes. For many years it was assumed that the primary cause of stable angina was a fixed blockage in one or more of the larger

- Cardiac Syndrome X (microvascular dysfunction)
- Coronary slow flow phenomenon (CSFP)
- Prinzmetal's angina (coronary artery spasm)
- Aortic stenosis
- Arrhythmia
- Hypertrophic cardiomyopathy
- Takotsubo cardiomyopathy (Broken Heart Syndrome)
- Uncontrolled hypertension
- Non-cardiac causes
- Pulmonary disease
- Anaemia

coronary arteries; however, there is increasing awareness of a number of causes of stable angina that are not related to coronary artery blockages (see Box 20.1).

Angina symptoms in the absence of obstructive coronary artery disease (non-obstructive CHD) have in the past been attributed to psychological problems such as anxiety and depression (Jespersen et al 2013). The relationship between psychological wellbeing and cardiac health remains largely unexplained, although poorly managed angina may contribute substantially to symptoms (De Hert et al 2018). More recently, non-obstructive or vasospastic CHD has been recognised as one of the major causes of stable angina (Agewall et al 2017; Beijk et al 2019). Nearly two-thirds of women and one-third of men undergoing first-time coronary angiography for symptoms of stable angina have been found to have no significant obstructive CHD, but had an increased risk of adverse cardiovascular events and persistent angina symptoms (Beijk et al 2019; Jespersen et al 2013). Angina resulting from obstructive CHD can be managed with revascularisation procedures (coronary artery bypass surgery or percutaneous transluminal coronary angioplasty), medications and lifestyle modifications in most patients (Picard et al 2019). For patients in whom revascularisation is not an option, such as those with non-operable CHD or those with non-obstructive CHD, medication management and lifestyle modifications are the only options for treatment (Picard et al 2019).

Caring for patients with a CHD requires an in-depth knowledge of management options, including strategies for modification of biomedical and behavioural risk factors that contribute to this condition, and the contribution that the multidisciplinary team can make in terms of assisting patients to optimise their quality of life in the presence of this chronic disease.

In the case study, you will be introduced to Brenda Ball. Throughout the chapter, the information presented and learning activities will be related back to Brenda's case where applicable.

CASE STUDY 20.1

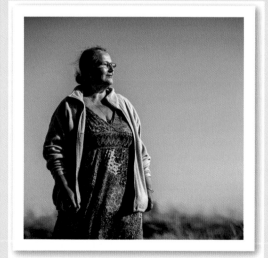

iStockphoto/stevecoleimages.

A COMMON STEMI PRESENTATION

Brenda Ball is a 56-year-old woman who was admitted to the hospital with chest pain. Around an hour before her presentation to the emergency department she had complained of dull chest pain and nausea to her work colleagues. She thought it was indigestion following a 'business lunch' where she had eaten a large meal and consumed two glasses of red wine. Her colleagues noted that she appeared pale and looked unwell, and although Brenda planned to go home, her boss insisted that an ambulance be called. The ambulance personnel obtained an ECG trace from Brenda that showed ST-segment elevation in the anterior leads, indicating an anterior ST-elevation myocardial infarction (STEMI). Brenda was taken directly to the coronary catheter laboratory where she underwent percutaneous coronary angioplasty and placement of a stent to her proximal left anterior descending (LAD) coronary artery. During the procedure it was noted that Brenda had diffuse distal disease in her distal coronary arteries that was not suitable for angioplasty or coronary artery bypass surgery. It was decided that the residual coronary artery disease would be best managed with medical therapy.

Brenda was transferred to the coronary care unit (CCU) where she was referred to the cardiac rehabilitation team and underwent routine screening for cardiovascular disease risk factors. Prior to this presentation, Brenda had rarely consulted with her general practitioner (GP). She admits that 2 years ago she was told she had high cholesterol (total cholesterol 6.5 and HDL of 0.9) and was prescribed some medication, but she developed muscle aches and as she saw on the internet that it was likely a side effect of her cholesterol medication, she stopped taking it. Her blood pressure on admission was 190/100. She was told by her GP that her blood pressure was on the high side and she was advised to lose some weight and was supposed to go back to the GP to have it rechecked in 2 months. She had intended to go back and see the GP, but between working and busy family life, she just did not see it as a priority. Her mother died at 63 years of age following a cardiac arrest at home. The autopsy showed an acute myocardial infarction. Brenda told you that she thought her mother died because medical treatment was not as good in those days as it is now, and she did not seem to realise that her mother dying of CHD at this age increased her own risk. Brenda had never been in contact with her father, who left the family when she was a baby, so she does not know if he is alive or has cardiac disease. She has smoked since she was 16 years of age and has contemplated giving up smoking as her children have been 'nagging' her to quit, but she finds it difficult to stop smoking because of various stressors in her life. She doesn't undertake any regular exercise and she is overweight. As she lives alone, she often buys frozen processed meals or picks up takeaway food on the way home from work. She thinks that

she has never been tested for diabetes. It is noted that her blood sugar level on arrival to hospital was 13 mmol/L.

Brenda recently divorced her husband and now lives on her own, although her five adult children often visit. Her husband left her for someone else and she says that she feels depressed and lonely sometimes, and seems very bitter about the marriage break-up. She discloses that she drinks a bottle of wine every night which helps her to sleep and sometimes drinks during the day on occasions such as business lunches. She says that she is not an alcoholic, but a couple of drinks keeps her from thinking about things that upset her. She has difficulty controlling her stress levels and has a poor self-image and reduced self-confidence since her marriage break-up and has put on more weight. Brenda admits that she has been having chest pains for a few weeks now, but thought it was indigestion or stress.

As Brenda has residual coronary artery disease, it is likely that she may continue to have episodes of angina, particularly at times of higher myocardial oxygen demand, such as during exercise. While stable angina is associated with a low risk of acute coronary events and reduced mortality, the risk is still higher than for those people who do not have stable angina.

Brenda needs to be educated about secondary prevention and participation in a cardiac rehabilitation (CR) program. The goals of management of established disease are to minimise the negative effects of the disease and to reduce the risk of further cardiovascular events. Introducing strategies to address modifiable risk factors that affect health status are core business for nurses involved in the management of patients with CHD. The best time to identify and raise awareness of the impact of the risk of cardiac disease is in the primary care setting. However, in reality, the opportunity to do this often presents following an acute event.

CHD RISK FACTORS AND BEHAVIOURS THAT CONTRIBUTE TO THE DEVELOPMENT OF CHD

A number of clearly defined genetic, behavioural and biomedical risk factors are associated with CHD (see Box 20.2). Risk for CHD rises progressively according to the number of risk factors present in an individual. People with existing CHD are in the highest risk group for future cardiac events, so a more stringent approach to risk factor management through pharmacological and lifestyle interventions will be required.

Some risk factors for cardiovascular disease cannot be modified by lifestyle change or medical treatment. Non-modifiable biomedical risk factors include:

- age – CHD predominantly affects middle-aged and older Australians, but it is not uncommon to have

angina (particularly in relation to non-obstructive cardiac disease) at a younger age
- gender – CHD is more common in men than women due to protective effects of oestrogen; however, after menopause, women have equal risk to men
- family history of CHD, with the risk of CHD increasing if a first-degree relative is diagnosed with heart or blood vessel disease before the age of 55 for males and 65 for females (National Heart Foundation of Australia [NHFA] & Cardiac Society of Australia & New Zealand [CSANZ] 2016).

Although these risk factors cannot be modified, awareness of these risks being present may encourage patients to take positive steps in addressing other risk factors that are modifiable.

BOX 20.2		
Non-Modifiable and Modifiable Risk Factors for Coronary Heart Disease		
Non-Modifiable	**Modifiable Risk Factors: Biomedical**	**Modifiable Risk Factors: Behavioural**
Age	Dyslipidaemia	Tobacco smoking
Gender	Hypertension	Poor nutrition
Family history	Diabetes	Physical inactivity
	Kidney disease	Overweight/obesity
		Psychological disorders
		High alcohol consumption
		Depression and stress

Modifiable risk factors for CHD are those risk factors that can be modified by pharmacotherapy and/or lifestyle change to reduce the risk of a coronary event. Modifiable risk factors may be further divided into biomedical or behavioural risk factors.

Modifiable biomedical risk factors include:

- dyslipidaemia, a metabolic derangement that can be hereditary or acquired, and contributes to many forms of disease, notably CHD
- hypertension, which is responsible for more deaths and disease than any other biomedical risk factor worldwide (NHFA 2016)
- diabetes mellitus, the most prevalent form of which is type 2 diabetes mellitus (type 2 DM) which typically manifests later in life (Vistisen et al 2016)
- kidney disease, which can be either a cause or a consequence of CHD.

Modifiable behavioural cardiovascular risk factors include:

- tobacco smoking, which in all its forms, including low-tar ('mild' or 'light') cigarettes, filter cigarettes, cigars and pipes promotes the development of atherosclerosis and thrombosis (Perk et al 2012)
- smokeless tobacco products, which are associated with deleterious cardiovascular effects (Gupta et al 2019)
- E-cigarettes or vaping, which are linked to an increase in CHD compared with standard combustible cigarettes (Osei et al 2019)
- poor nutrition or excessive food or salt consumption, which can also affect other risk factors including hypertension, overweight and diabetes (Shima et al 2020)
- physical inactivity, which is an independent risk factor for CVD and contributes to around 20% of the CVD disease burden (Nichols et al 2014; Sverre et al 2020)

- being overweight or obese, which is associated with an increased mortality that rises exponentially with the degree of increased body mass index (BMI), and contributes to co-morbid conditions associated with obesity including hypertension, type 2 DM, sleep apnoea (Bastien et al 2014; Cai et al 2018), osteoarthritis (which affects mobility), psychological disorders and social problems (Sverre et al 2020)
- high consumption of alcohol and binge drinking, which may also contribute to hypertension, non-ischaemic dilated cardiomyopathy and atrial fibrillation (Mostofsky et al 2016)
- depression, stress, social isolation, poor social support, which have been associated with the development of CHD (Carney & Freedland 2016).

ABSOLUTE RISK ASSESSMENT

Most cardiac patients tend to have multiple risk factors, thus multiplying the overall extent of the risk. Similarly, the presence of one disease, for example, diabetes, can increase the risk of developing another. Measuring individual cardiovascular risk factors in isolation poorly estimates a person's likelihood of developing new or worsening current cardiovascular disease. Instead, absolute risk, the numerical probability of a cardiovascular event occurring within a 5-year period, is usually used. Visual tools, such as the absolute CVD risk factor assessment tool, may also reinforce to patients the need for change, and provide encouragement to persist with lifestyle modification.

Aboriginal and Torres Strait Islander peoples have significantly higher rates of morbidity and mortality from chronic disease, including CHD, and are more likely to have CHD onset at a younger age and multiple risk factors compared with non-Indigenous Australians (Brown et al 2015). Currently available absolute risk calculators may significantly underestimate cardiovascular risk in Aboriginal, Torres Strait Islander, Māori and Pacific Islander peoples as they do not incorporate many possible factors contributing to CVD among Indigenous Australians, such as cultural and historical factors, environmental and socioeconomic factors, psychosocial stressors and limited access to preventive and clinical healthcare (Chan 2015).

CARDIAC REHABILITATION

The aim of cardiac rehabilitation (CR) is to achieve optimal functioning through improved health behaviour that inhibits the progression of CHD and includes comprehensive long-term services, such as medical evaluation, prescriptive exercise, cardiac risk factor modification, education, counselling and behavioural interventions (Sandesara et al 2015). CR is an important component of CHD management in encouraging patients to develop self-management skills and embrace secondary prevention principles and goals, including adherence to pharmacotherapy regimens. CR traditionally has been associated with recovery following an acute myocardial infarction, but is likely to be useful in a variety of cardiac conditions (Woodruffe et al 2015). Box 20.3 lists the most common conditions for which CR may be useful.

Exercise-based CR has been shown to reduce the risk of cardiovascular mortality and hospital re-admissions, and from a patient perspective, improves quality of life (Anderson et al 2016). Despite the obvious benefits of CR, equity and access to CR in Australia is suboptimal. There are barriers to CR participation that are unique to Australia relating to diverse cultural and linguistic needs and reduced accessibility for those in remote regions of Australia, as most CR programs are based in metropolitan areas (Field et al 2018; Hamilton et al 2018; Woodruffe et al 2015). Technology in the form of CR via a smartphone application has the potential to overcome some geographical challenges. CR participants using a CR application demonstrated improved exercise capacity, compliance with exercise regimes and an overall positive impact on wellbeing (Lunde et al 2020). Access to CR is particularly challenging for Aboriginal and Torres Strait Islander peoples who have higher rates of heart disease but less access to ongoing management after discharge from hospital compared to non-Indigenous people. Participation in CR by Aboriginal and Torres Strait Islander peoples is rare. Some of the reasons put forward for this are extended family responsibilities, sociocultural inappropriateness of the program, poor understanding of CR, and Australian media portrayal of Indigenous fatality and futility leading to an expectation of poor health outcomes that negatively affects motivation to engage with health programs (Hamilton et al 2016).

Developing partnerships between patients and clinicians and assisting patients to understand the long-term impact of risk factors on health may assist and enhance long-term secondary prevention strategies. Consideration of variables that may affect the patient's ability to receive and process information must be taken into account when developing an educational program. Timing of the intervention is often a key factor on how an educational strategy may be received by the patient and family members. Lack of participation is not always the personal choice of the individual: distance from centres that offer CR, culture and language differences, lower socioeconomic status, female gender, and older age are all associated with lower rates of CR attendance. Regular telephone calls, internet resources, nurse-led clinics and community care options are increasingly being used to make CR more cost effective and available for patients. Nurse practitioner-led CR is demonstrating success in relation to attendance and completion rates (O'Toole et al 2020).

Current disparities in outcomes for CHD and access to CR for Aboriginal and Torres Strait Islander people need to be addressed. Culturally appropriate education beginning in hospital, inclusive of family and local Aboriginal liaison officers needs to be available with follow-up in the community and access to CR services and resources that are culturally relevant.

BOX 20.3
Conditions Suitable for Cardiac Rehabilitation

- Cardiac revascularisation procedures
- Medically-managed CHD (stable angina)
- Heart failure and cardiomyopathies
- Valve device, replacement and repair
- Permanent pacemaker and implantable defibrillator insertion
- Heart transplant and ventricular assist device
- Atrial fibrillation
- Those at high risk for coronary artery disease
- Other vascular or heart diseases and interventions
- Familial hypercholesterolaemia

CASE STUDY REFLECTION

Learning Activity

CR programs tend to be under-utilised, particularly by women. Women are less likely to be referred to CR and less likely to complete a CR program, but women completing CR experience a greater reduction in mortality compared with men (Galati et al 2018). Women particularly are less likely to undertake the exercise component of CR (Grace et al 2016). From the case study overview, Brenda may be at risk of not attending CR. From the case study, identify some of the potential barriers to CR attendance in Brenda's case and consider strategies that you might use to encourage Brenda to attend. Remember that you will need to take a person-centred approach and identify goals that are important and achievable for Brenda. The suggested further reading by Resurreccion and colleagues (2018) may assist you in this task.

PATIENT EDUCATION: UNDERSTANDING THE DISEASE

Educational information about the cause of CHD and subsequent management options are usually available to the patient as print or online materials. These materials are supported by counselling and advice by health professionals, including medical and nursing staff, dietitians, pharmacists and social workers. Although it is recognised that patients need information to enable them to actively participate in their rehabilitation and management, in many instances patient education programs fail to influence patients' behaviour in relation to risk factor reduction (Kotseva et al 2016). It is important for the nurse to ascertain which factors the patient considers are the major influences on their illness. Some patients demonstrate an internal locus of control; they feel responsible for becoming ill and believe that their lifestyle behaviour has caused their illness. Others exhibit an external locus of control in that they believe their illness is attributed to external factors over which they had no control. Those with an internal locus of control may be more amenable to behavioural change because they take some responsibility for the state of their health and physical recovery. It is important for nurses to recognise the health beliefs of individual patients with CHD and what they see as important information at each stage of their illness.

Dyslipidaemia

Lipid abnormalities are strongly associated with accelerated development of atherosclerosis. Lipid levels can become abnormal for several reasons, including changes due to ageing, use of certain drugs, being overweight, consuming a diet high in saturated fat, being physically inactive, drinking too much alcohol, smoking or having diabetes. Abnormal lipids may also be due to an inherited disorder, such as familial hypercholesterolaemia. Lipid abnormalities are detected by taking a lipid profile to measure total cholesterol, high density lipoproteins (HDL), low density lipoprotein (LDL) and triglycerides (TG). An elevated level of total cholesterol or LDL and/or a reduced level of HDL are associated with increased risk of CHD. A person's lipid profile is considered in the context of their absolute risk of developing CHD, but statin therapy is recommended for all patients with CHD unless there are exceptional circumstances (NHFA & CSANZ 2016). All patients with abnormal lipids should be given advice on healthy eating.

CASE STUDY REFLECTION

Brenda should receive advice on healthy eating from nursing staff and from a dietitian, but she is also in need of pharmacotherapy, given that she has existing CHD. Statins are the treatment of choice, but Brenda reported that she previously had some muscle aches which she thought were related to statins. Muscle aches and pains are a common side effect in patients taking statins, but rhabdomyolysis is rare. Brenda could try a statin again under close supervision, but if myalgia becomes a problem it may need to be ceased, particularly if serum levels of creatine kinase (CK) rise due to muscle damage. Another type of drug, ezetimibe, is effective in reducing the concentration of LDL cholesterol and may need to be used instead. Fibrates effectively reduce cardiovascular risk in patients who are overweight, have type 2 DM, or high TG and/or low HDL cholesterol, and can be used in combination with statins, but this increases the risk of myalgia and rhabdomyolysis. Although this combination of drugs may be useful given Brenda's risk factor profile, it is unlikely that she would be able to tolerate this combination given her previous myalgia with statin use. As Brenda has elevated TG levels, she should be advised to consume marine omega-3 fortified food and drinks and/or marine omega-F3 capsules (NHFA & CSANZ 2016). Adherence to statins must be an ongoing discussion point with Brenda to ensure that she understands how important it is to her health to reduce her cholesterol levels. Brenda must also understand that medication does not replace the necessity for making lifestyle changes.

Hypertension

Hypertension (HT) has long been known to be an important risk factor for the development of atherosclerosis and CHD, and is associated with myocardial infarction, stroke, heart failure and kidney disease. For most people HT has no symptoms or signs – their blood pressure can be high and yet they feel well, which means that it is common to have HT and not be aware of it. Moreover, when there are no signs or symptoms, people often do not consider HT to be a long-term or current problem (ABS 2019). It is estimated that HT is present in 30–45% of the general population, with a sharp rise in prevalence with increasing age (Mills et al 2016).

The diagnosis of hypertension is not made on a single reading, but rather from multiple readings on separate occasions (National Heart Foundation 2016). As the majority of people with HT have additional risk factors for CHD and these risk factors interact with each other, absolute cardiovascular risk should be assessed in all patients with HT in order to determine the optimal management plan (Gabb et al 2016).

There are a number of pharmacological agents for the management of HT, but the first choice is normally angiotensin-converting enzyme inhibitors (ACEIs), or angiotensin II receptor blockers (ARBs), if ACEIs are not tolerated. Other agents include calcium channel blockers (CCBs) and diuretics. Most patients will require a combination of medications to control HT, and the choice of therapy is often influenced by co-existing medical conditions and patient tolerance. Specialist nurses may be involved in the titration of pharmacotherapy and ongoing monitoring of HT.

CASE STUDY REFLECTION

Brenda's blood pressure was reduced after commencing an ace inhibitor and beta blocker as part of her secondary prevention post-myocardial infarction; however, it will need ongoing monitoring. For patients with CHD, nurses often have an active role in ongoing blood pressure monitoring and should be aware of blood pressure targets. As Brenda has had some difficulty complying in the past, it is important that she understands that hypertension is a major risk in CHD: the higher the blood pressure, the greater the chance of Brenda incurring an adverse event related to CHD.

Brenda has admitted that her diet is not as good as it could be and that she eats a lot of fast foods and prepackaged foods that are high in sodium. As sodium contributes to HT, Brenda needs to be advised how to reduce her sodium intake by avoiding processed foods such as processed meats, commercial sauces, soups, packet seasoning, stock cubes, potato chips, salted nuts and takeaway foods, and increasing her intake of fresh fruit and vegetables (Shima et al 2020). She also needs to be advised how to interpret the 'nutrition information' panel on food purchases and to choose foods labelled with 'no added salt', 'low salt' or 'salt reduced'. Lifestyle modifications are an important component of HT management whether or not pharmacological agents are used. Lifestyle modifications are going to be an integral part of Brenda's HT management, with particular attention to the 'SNAP' (smoking, nutrition, alcohol, physical activity) risk factors (NHFA & CSANZ 2016). Weight reduction is also an important factor. Brenda has had a history of non-adherence to medication and if her blood pressure is difficult to manage, non-adherence with drug therapy should be considered as the potential cause.

Diabetes

Cardiovascular disease is the major cause of morbidity and mortality for individuals with diabetes (Xu et al 2019). Both type 1 and type 2 diabetes mellitus (type 1 DM, type 2 DM) are independent risk factors for CHD, but the most prevalent form is type 2 DM, which typically manifests later in life and is associated with obesity, physical inactivity, hypertension, dyslipidaemia and thrombotic tendencies. Type 2 DM is associated with long-term microvascular and macrovascular complications, and reduced quality of life and life expectancy (National Institute for Health and Care Excellence [NICE] 2019).

CASE STUDY REFLECTION

Brenda has been diagnosed with type 2 DM, which commonly occurs in middle-aged adults and is often linked with obesity. The goal of Brenda's diabetes management is to maintain an optimal blood sugar as indicated by an HbA1c equal to or less than 7% (NHFA & CSANZ 2016). Brenda will need to start oral hypoglycaemics and she will receive education on diet and management of other risk factors that have an impact on her diabetes.

Kidney Disease

With the ageing of the population, the prevalence of chronic kidney disease (CKD) is increasing, and is accelerated by chronic diseases such as diabetes, hypertension and dyslipidaemia (Lu et al 2020; Pinier et al 2020). CKD is closely associated with an increased incidence of CHD, and major cardiac events represent almost 50% of the causes of death in CKD patients (Di Lullo et al 2015). Renal dysfunction is a major predictor of overall and cardiovascular mortality, especially in the elderly. Screening for CKD in those with CHD is important as many cardiac medications will require dose adjustment according to renal function to prevent adverse drug reactions. Appropriate management of HT with nephroprotective drugs, including renin angiotensin system (RAS) blockers, ACEI or ARB, can inhibit the progressive deterioration of renal function (Becquemont et al 2015). Diuretics and RAS blockers are known to reversibly alter renal function particularly in the elderly, and so renal function should be monitored on commencing these drugs and periodically thereafter.

CASE STUDY REFLECTION

Brenda is at risk of having or developing CKD given her CHD risk factor profile. Currently her creatinine, urea and eGFR (estimated glomerular filtration rate) are within acceptable limits, but they will be closely monitored as she has recently had a coronary angiogram and is at risk from contrast nephropathy, and is starting several new medications, some of which may impact upon her renal function.

Smoking

Smoking is associated with long-term harmful effects, including chronic inflammation, dyslipidemia and accelerated atherosclerosis. Smoking also induces acute cardiovascular responses, including endothelial dysfunction, vasoconstriction, platelet activation and increased blood pressure and heart rate, which can lead to destabilisation of coronary artery plaques leading to acute coronary events and sudden death (Prochaska & Benowitz 2015).

Persistent smoking following an acute cardiac event is a major problem, with around 40–50% of smokers continuing to smoke following hospital discharge (Kotseva et al 2015; Sverre et al 2017). Furthermore, continued smoking after a cardiac event predicts lack of attendance in and completion of CR (Gaalema et al 2015). Nicotine, found in cigarette smoke, is highly addictive. The use of pharmacotherapy doubles abstinence rates in patients with a history of cardiovascular disease (Grandi et al 2016). Studies examining the absolute and relative efficacy and cardiovascular safety of tobacco cessation pharmacotherapy, including nicotine replacement therapy (NRT), varenicline, nortriptyline and cytosine, were found to be superior to placebo (Carney et al 2020), with no major adverse cardiovascular events

(Hsia et al 2017). Electronic nicotine delivery systems, on the other hand, are being widely distributed without evidence of safety in their long-term use (Prochaska & Benowitz 2015).

Psychological, as well as physiological, factors contribute to lack of success in quitting smoking. Smoking cessation has a major impact on reducing the risk of a further cardiovascular event or death, and so all cigarette smokers should be offered professional support to stop smoking (Carney et al 2020).

Second-hand smoking also increases cardiovascular risk and complications associated with CHD (Abu-Baker et al 2020). Second-hand smoking exposure at home and having a smoking spouse or peers predicts a lower likelihood of smoking cessation and second-hand smoke may act as a smoking cue by activating acetylcholine receptors in the brain to trigger smoking (Wang et al 2015). Thus the family should be encouraged to stop smoking and the CHD patient should be advised to avoid environments where others actively smoke.

CASE STUDY REFLECTION

The overall goals for addressing Brenda's smoking are complete cessation of smoking and avoidance of second-hand smoke. Brenda needs to understand the impact of smoking on her cardiovascular health and make a positive commitment to quitting. Consideration should be given to referring Brenda to Quitline or a smoking cessation program. These are often offered within CR services and are also available in the community. Tobacco cessation pharmacotherapy may be an option for Brenda, although, given her CHD, the supervision of a medical practitioner, nurse practitioner or pharmacist is advisable. Pharmacotherapy alone will have less chance of success if not accompanied by behavioural and psychosocial support. Brenda's psychosocial problems have to be addressed in planning her quit smoking process to maximise her chance of success.

Nutrition

Being overweight or obese increases a person's risk of developing CHD, HT, type 2 DM, and dyslipidaemia. Being underweight can also be a health risk factor. In the year 2017–18, 67% of Australians aged 18 years and over were overweight or obese (ABS 2019). Healthy diet patterns associated with positive health outcomes include higher intakes of vegetables, fruits, whole grains, low-fat and non-fat dairy, seafood, legumes and nuts. Conversely, consumption of red and processed meats should be lower; and sugar-sweetened foods and drinks and refined grains should be low or avoided (Millen et al 2016). Body mass index (BMI) is a commonly used measure to determine whether a person is underweight, normal weight, overweight or obese. Waist circumference is another commonly used measure of whether a person is of a healthy weight or not and provides a good estimate of body fat. Used in conjunction with BMI, it can indicate a person's potential risk of developing chronic diseases such as heart disease and type 2 DM (ABS 2019). The NHFA and CSANZ (2016) suggest that waist measurements of less than 94 cm for males and 80 cm for females and a BMI between 18.5 and 24.9 should be target goals for healthy weight to reduce cardiovascular risk.

CASE STUDY REFLECTION

Brenda is going to be referred to a dietitian and, in collaboration with nurses and the dietitian, Brenda needs to set intermediate achievable goals. She wants to be able to make assessments of weight change, and so the nurse needs to teach Brenda how to do waist measurement. The waist circumference is measured halfway between the inferior margin of the last rib and the crest of the ilium in the mid-axillary plane at the end of expiration. Brenda's weight and height are measured, and her healthy weight calculated according to BMI. Brenda has already received information on nutrition and exercise, and she is reminded that for weight loss to occur, she must use up more energy (kilojoules) through regular physical activity and consume less energy from food and drinks.

Alcohol

Moderate alcohol intake (1–2 standard drinks per day) appears to have some cardiovascular benefits, whereas heavy drinking (> 3 standard drinks per day) is associated with a higher risk of HT, diabetes mellitus and CHD. However, any level of alcohol use can cause health problems in some people and so even moderate alcohol intake should not be promoted to patients as a good health strategy (Mostofsky et al 2016).

CASE STUDY REFLECTION

It is extremely important to do a thorough alcohol assessment with Brenda to ensure that she is not at risk of alcohol withdrawal during her hospitalisation, and to assist Brenda to recognise how excessive alcohol consumption can contribute to CHD. Patients like Brenda who have hypertension are advised to limit their alcohol intake to no more than two standard drinks per day for men, or one standard drink per day for women (NHFA & CSANZ 2016). For those patients who have a dependence on alcohol, abstinence is recommended following controlled withdrawal. As with smoking, Brenda's psychosocial situation is likely to have an impact upon her alcohol consumption; thus psychological and social management will play a big part in meeting the goal of low-risk alcohol consumption for Brenda.

Physical Activity

Physical inactivity, or sedentary behaviour, is the fourth leading risk factor for global mortality and is responsible for an estimated 3.2 million deaths globally (World Health Organization [WHO] 2016). In Australia only 15% of 18–64-year-olds are regularly meeting the physical activity guideline targets per day (ABS 2019). Increased cardio-respiratory fitness is associated with decreased CHD disease risk, but the effects of exercise on the heart and vascular system are dependent upon the frequency, intensity and duration of the exercise (Wilson et al 2015). The NHFA and CSANZ (2016) advise that patients with CHD set a goal of progressing over time to at least 30 minutes of moderate-intensity physical activity on most, if not all, days of the week. Patients with unstable angina, uncontrolled or severe hypertension, severe aortic stenosis, uncontrolled diabetes, complicated acute myocardial infarction, uncontrolled heart failure, symptomatic hypotension (< 90/60 mmHg), resting tachycardia or arrhythmias, will need to have a clinical assessment of their exercise capabilities and may need to modify or defer physical activity until their condition has stabilised. The positive benefits of physical activity on recovery include improved confidence and morale and it usually enables patients to resume a normal lifestyle, which may include returning to work. Physical activity will also have a significant impact on reducing existing cardiac risk factors, such as HT, dyslipidaemia, obesity and insulin resistance and has demonstrated a proportional improvement in all-cause mortality (Bouisset et al 2020). Physical activity will also have a positive impact on psychological health and wellbeing. A key step in motivating patients to engage in physical activity is to ensure that they are aware of the positive benefits on their heart health.

CASE STUDY REFLECTION

Brenda has had quite a sedentary lifestyle, and so building physical activity into her normal routine may seem quite daunting to her. Brenda will need an assessment prior to undertaking physical activity, and the nurse then needs to discuss her physical activity needs and capabilities with her. Brenda recognises that she has a sedentary lifestyle and feels that her job is a barrier to opportunities for physical activity. The nurse needs to reassure Brenda that physical activity does not have to be completed all at once: short bouts of 10 minutes' duration may be more suited to Brenda's lifestyle. Brenda is wondering how she will know when she is exercising appropriately. Moderate activity should cause a moderate noticeable increase in Brenda's depth and rate of breathing, but she should still be able to talk comfortably. Provision of some written guidelines for Brenda regarding everyday physical activity tasks, such as a light-to-moderate walking program, water aerobics or cycling for pleasure, may encourage her to undertake physical activity regularly. Following discussion, Brenda feels that she is more likely to undertake purposeful walking regularly than activities that need some organisation. During this time, the nurse may take the opportunity to explain to Brenda how to recognise any early warning signs of ischaemia, such as breathlessness or chest discomfort, and together they can discuss strategies that may be used should symptoms reoccur. Brenda should ensure that she carries a supply of sublingual or short-acting nitrate (anginine) during physical activity.

Relatives often become quite anxious when their loved one begins to return to activity as they are concerned that activity may cause another event. It is important that nurses caring for patients with CHD include family members in education consultations wherever possible to allay any fears or misconceptions that may restrict physical activity, including sexual activity, following discharge from hospital.

Early referral to an outpatient cardiac rehabilitation program is recommended for Brenda, so that her progress and response to a physical activity regimen can be monitored.

Medication Adherence

The chronic nature of CHD will require the patient to take numerous medications, attend regular medical appointments and undertake numerous lifelong lifestyle changes. The degree to which the patient is able to commit to this regimen may determine their outcome in terms of ongoing symptoms and quality of life. Medication adherence requires patients to agree to and participate in a treatment program as advised by their treating doctor or health worker and see that the advice or treatment prescribed will add value to their quality

of life. Non-adherence with cardiac medications following discharge from hospital is a huge problem. A lack of awareness or understanding of the importance of taking a number of cardiac drugs is often the case, with many patients stopping their medications when they feel better. Medication regimens are often complicated, and cardiac patients are often required to take several different types of medications for long periods of time. Financially, the cost of purchasing medications, particularly for those on a fixed income, may be seen as prohibitive. Other factors are difficulties with language that affect the patient's ability to read the instructions on medication packaging, cognitive impairment and poor manual dexterity, particularly in the frail, aged patient, which makes them unable to open medication packaging or collect refilled prescriptions. Patients are often labelled as poorly compliant with taking medications and adhering to recommended lifestyle change, without much consideration being given to factors outside the patient's locus of control. These factors can be described as system factors. Poor communication between hospital and community care providers resulting from pressure on institutions to reduce length of stay may see patients being discharged without adequate dialogue between the different sectors of healthcare and the patient. Patients are often discharged with 2 or 3 days of medication and are unable to access general practice due to difficult working hours, or lack of after-hours services.

CASE STUDY REFLECTION

The nurse can encourage Brenda's compliance with medication by involving her in medication administration as soon as she is clinically stable. This will assist her to become familiar with the size, colour and shape of her medication prior to her having to be fully responsible for them. The nurse can then assess how Brenda will be able to manage post-discharge and, if necessary, make recommendations for medications to be prepackaged by a pharmacist. Brenda will be given a medication chart that explains what each of her medications is for, the time of the day that it is to be taken and any other special instructions that may be required. The nurse will discuss with Brenda how she will manage her medications at home. If possible, Brenda's family members will be included in education sessions. Brenda may need to be referred to a community pharmacist for a home medication management review if issues related to poor compliance recur.

Psychosocial Assessment

Psychosocial factors may contribute to the development of CHD and lead to poorer outcomes following a cardiac event. Abnormal psychosocial functioning may be associated with stress-related disorders, such as anxiety, depression, anger and hostility. Internal factors, such as physical health and fitness, genetics and the ability to cope with stress and adapt to change, have an influence on psychosocial health. External factors such as culture, geography and socioeconomic status also have a role.

People often blame stress for causing illness. The impact of psychological stress as a precursor to acute coronary events and determinant of negative cardiac outcomes is now well established. Stress, anger and depressed mood can act as acute triggers of acute cardiac events, and reactions to stress, such as depression, anger, fear, anxiety and sleeping disorders may compound psychological stress. Physical or emotional stress can cause a condition called Takotsubo (stress) cardiomyopathy (see Box 20.4).

Anxiety disorders include conditions such as panic disorder, social anxiety disorder, specific phobias or generalised anxiety disorder. Anxiety disorders have been associated with increased risk of cardiac mortality in individuals with CHD (Jackson et al 2018).

Depression has for some time been known to be a risk factor for adverse outcomes in patients with CHD (Murphy et al 2020). People with anxiety and depression are more likely to have a poor diet with increased dietary cholesterol and total energy intake, an increased prevalence of smoking and a sedentary lifestyle than non-anxious or non-depressed subjects (Hajar 2017).

Outbursts of anger have consistently been found to be associated with a transiently higher risk of an acute cardiovascular event, including acute myocardial infarction (AMI). A study by Smyth and colleagues (2016) found that 13.6% of AMI cases had recently (within 1 hour) engaged in physical activity and 14.4% were angry or emotionally upset. People with severe mental illness have an increased risk of a major adverse cardiac event compared with the general population (Attar et al 2019). Ischemic heart disease is the leading cause of mortality in psychotic disorders (Chang et al 2020). They are also more likely to smoke, be overweight, have high blood pressure, insulin resistance or diabetes, high cholesterol and metabolic syndrome. Reasons for this include symptoms such as low motivation levels; co-occurring mental health issues such as depression, anxiety and substance-use disorders; physical co-morbidities; suboptimal lifestyle factors; low socioeconomic status and unemployment; suboptimal proactive treatment of CVD risk factors by health workers; and the adverse metabolic effects of antipsychotic and mood-stabilising agents used to treat severe mental health disorders (Gladigau et al 2014). Mental illness is also associated with a high rate of medication non-compliance, and so individuals with mental illness and risk factors for CVD are less likely to comply with therapies to reduce risk. See the example of research linking mental and physical co-morbidity and non-adherence to antihypertensive medication in Box 20.5.

CASE STUDY REFLECTION

Brenda has given several clues in her history to suggest that she may be depressed. She needs a professional assessment for depression so that she can receive appropriate psychological and medical management. Nurses caring for patients with CHD should have skills that will assist them to identify patients who may be depressed, and refer them for specialised management as needed. There are a number of validated tools that can aid in this process.

Brenda has already received advice on regular physical activity, which may help to reduce her depression

---

BOX 20.4
Evidence for Practice

Calderón-Larrañaga and colleagues (2016) conducted a study to analyse the association between mental and physical co-morbidity and non-adherence to antihypertensive medication in patients attending primary care. They found that one-fifth of the study population showed poor adherence levels. Patient characteristics and factors associated with poor adherence were female gender, younger age, foreign nationality, living in a rural area, low blood pressure levels, polypharmacy and mental co-morbidities. The researchers concluded that the study emphasised the need for a patient-centred approach rather than focusing on a disease management approach, as well as adequate health worker–patient communication. The significance of this research for nurses is to have an awareness of those patients that are most at risk of poor adherence and the need to ensure that patients have a good understanding of their medications and the need for taking them prior to hospital discharge and in any community interactions with patients. Potential barriers to medication adherence and strategies for overcoming these should be discussed with all patients.

BOX 20.5
Takotsubo Cardiomyopathy: A Challenging Cardiac Condition Associated With Stress

Takotsubo cardiomyopathy (TCM), also known as 'Broken Heart Syndrome' or 'stress cardiomyopathy', is a condition that was first recognised by Japanese researchers over 20 years ago, but it has only attracted interest in Western nations in the past 10 years. TCM transiently affects the ability of the heart to pump efficiently. The symptoms are identical to those of an acute coronary syndrome (myocardial infarction, unstable angina pectoris), but the two conditions do not share the same pathophysiology. ACS is, in most cases, caused by obstructive coronary artery disease (CAD). The pathophysiology of TCM is not yet fully understood, but obstructive CAD is not the cause. In most cases TCM is preceded by an emotional, psychological or physical stressor. Some of the more commonly reported psychological stressors include death of a spouse, family arguments, negative events in the workplace, psychiatric illness, motor vehicle accidents, loss of property, anniversary of a death and traumatic social or environmental events such as war, earthquakes and floods, but TCM can be triggered by seemingly trivial events if they cause stress to an individual. Recently it has been reported that TCM can also occur with positive 'joyful' events (Ghadri et al 2016). Physical triggers of TCM usually include acute medical illness or trauma. TCM is associated with release of stress hormones, such as adrenalin, but it is not clear why some people develop TCM in times of stress while others do not. TCM appears to predominantly affect postmenopausal women with around 90% of reported cases being older women. As the condition becomes more widely recognised, cases are being increasingly reported in other groups, including younger women, men and children.

The diagnosis of TCM is usually made when a person undergoes coronary angiography, a procedure to examine the coronary arteries for blockages. During angiography, it becomes evident that there are no blockages in the arteries to cause the symptoms, and an abnormal contractile pattern of the left ventricle associated with TCM will be seen. TCM may also be diagnosed using echocardiography or cardiac magnetic resonance imaging (MRI).

Although TCM can cause death, it is relatively rare and often associated with a concurrent medical illness. Most people with TCM make a full recovery within a few weeks. It is becoming evident that recurrence of TCM is quite common, and as yet we do not have any therapies to prevent this. TCM is an example of the adverse effects of stress on health. With heightened awareness of the condition, and increasing levels of stress in our society, we are likely to see increasing reports of TCM.

and anxiety, but she may need pharmacological therapy. Selective serotonin uptake inhibitors have been shown to be safe and efficacious in the management of CHD patients with depression. Tricyclic antidepressants should be avoided in CHD patients (NHFA & CSANZ 2016).

Clearly, pharmacological management alone is not going to solve Brenda's problems. The nurse has a role in referring Brenda to a social worker and counselling. It is likely that Brenda will also have input from a psychiatrist or specialist mental health nurse. Cognitive behaviour therapy delivered by a mental health professional specifically trained in this form of therapy is also an effective management strategy (NHFA & CSANZ 2016).

SOCIAL ISOLATION AND LACK OF SOCIAL SUPPORT

A recent meta-analysis to investigate the association between loneliness or social isolation and CHD found that poor social relationships were associated with a 29% increase in the risk of developing CHD (Valtorta et al 2016). The absence of supportive family members and/or friends, participation in work, community or recreational activities and involvement in a social network are also risk factors for adopting an unhealthy lifestyle.

When a crisis such as an acute cardiac event occurs, patients often find themselves surrounded by family members and friends who they would not normally see in their regular day-to-day activities. The actual strength of that social support may not be evident until after discharge, when friends and family members fade into the background, as the crisis is no longer evident. Thus the nurse needs to carefully assess what support is likely to continue after discharge from hospital. If the patient lives alone, the nurse needs to assess how the patient will be able to function, and whether there are people who continuously support that person at home. Asking questions about practical things, such as whether they are able to go to the doctor unaided and who assists with shopping and other activities of daily living, may provide a better insight into their social context.

Aboriginal and Torres Strait Islander people are a particular at-risk group for the negative impact that social isolation and poor social support can have on the recovering cardiac patient. It is a time when they are often in an unfamiliar environment, away from their family members, and experiencing both language and cultural difficulties. Wherever possible, an Aboriginal

Health Worker or Aboriginal Liaison Officer should be included as a member of the healthcare team.

MĀORI AND PACIFIC ISLANDER PEOPLE

In 2010–12 the total cardiovascular disease mortality rate among Māori was more than twice that of non-Māori. A large proportion of Pacific peoples' health disparity is due to their high chronic disease burden, particularly for cardiovascular disease (CVD) and type 2 DM. In 2018 the Ministry of Health published a Consensus statement on cardiovascular disease risk assessment and management for primary care. Screening for Māori, Pacific and South-Asian populations now begins at 30 years of age for men and 40 years for women. Individuals with severe mental illness are screened from 25 years of age. Annual risk assessments are recommended for all high-risk individuals (Ministry of Health NZ 2018).

CONCLUSION

CHD is a chronic disease. Although there are acute phases of CHD (unstable angina and acute myocardial infarction), the precursor of CHD, atherosclerosis, and the reduction of risk factors for the development of atherosclerotic heart disease, must continue to be managed throughout a person's life. There is a good evidence base for primary and secondary prevention strategies and risk reduction for CHD, but health behaviours are very much influenced by social, material and cultural circumstances and can be difficult to change. While changing people's health-related behaviour can have a major impact on cardiovascular mortality and morbidity, attempts to modify health behaviours are often unsuccessful.

Working systematically through the case study presented in this chapter, it can be seen that nurses and other members of the multidisciplinary health team can assist patients and their families to embrace secondary prevention principles and goals, including compliance with pharmacotherapy, and facilitate the development of self-management skills to embrace long-term lifestyle change, particularly with regard to reducing the risk of recurrent cardiac events.

CASE STUDY REFLECTION

Brenda attends the CR sessions and also seems to enjoy the CR exercise program. She joins a gym that specialises in exercise programs for people with CHD. Although she has occasional angina, so far she has managed to control it with anginine and rest. She has adhered to her medication regimen, has lost 10 kg, reduced her LDL and triglycerides, and her diabetes is well controlled. Her blood pressure has continued to be somewhat elevated and she is still undergoing some adjustments to her antihypertensive therapy.

She has cut back on her working hours which has contributed to her being able to eat regular healthy meals (although she confesses that she occasionally has a takeaway meal). Now that she is home more often, she has bought a dog and goes for regular walks in the early morning and evening with it, and her outlook on life seems much improved. She understands that she has a chronic disease and that she is going to have to continue to take medication and maintain a healthy lifestyle for the rest of her life. There will be a lot of challenges in Brenda's future in maintaining this enthusiasm, but continued support from her health carers in managing this chronic disease will enhance Brenda's chances of continuing with a positive outlook.

Reflective Questions

1. Using the information from Brenda's case study, identify her cardiovascular risk factors. Do you think that Brenda's risk factor profile puts her at high risk of a cardiac event?

   a. Once you have identified Brenda's risk factors, go to the Heart Foundation website (www.heartfoundation.org.au). Access the menu 'For Professionals'. Type 'Absolute Risk' into the search bar. The Australian Absolute Risk calculator uses a person's existing risk factor information to calculate the chance of them having a CHD event in the next 5 years. This is expressed as a percentage and is the person's 'risk score'. You may also want to calculate your own risk score.

   b. The Heart Foundation website has a number of resources that can be used to advise patients and also to guide clinical practice. Consider how you might utilise these in caring for patients like Brenda.

2. The case study presented is set in a large tertiary institution with access to all the services required to support recovery and ongoing management. If this case study was set in a rural or remote centre, how do you think the options for management might differ?

3. Lack of compliance with cardiovascular medication regimens is a problem that may lead to re-admissions, recurrent events and poorer outcomes for patients with CHD. Do you think there may be particular groups of patients for whom compliance is a problem, and if so, why?

RECOMMENDED READING

Agewall S, Beltrame JF, Reynolds HR et al 2017. ESC working group position paper on myocardial infarction with non-obstructive coronary arteries. European Heart Journal 38(3), 143–153.

Van den Wijngaart LS, Sieben A, van der Vlugt M et al 2015. A nurse-led multidisciplinary intervention to improve cardiovascular disease profile of patients. Western Journal of Nursing Research 37(6), 705–723.

O'Toole K, Chamberlain D, Giles T 2020. Exploration of a nurse practitioner-led phase two cardiac rehabilitation programme on attendance and compliance. Journal of Clinical Nursing 29, 758–793.

REFERENCES

Abu-Baker N, Al-Jarrah E, Suliman M 2020. Second-hand smoke exposure among coronary heart disease patients. Journal of Multidisciplinary Healthcare 13, 109–116.

Agewall S, Beltrame JF, Reynolds HR et al 2017. ESC working group position paper on myocardial infarction with non-obstructive coronary arteries. European Heart Journal 38(3), 143–153.

Anderson L, Oldridge N, Thompson DR et al 2016. Exercise-based cardiac rehabilitation for coronary heart disease: Cochrane systematic review and meta-analysis. Journal of the American College of Cardiology 67(1), 1–12.

Attar R, Valentin J, Freeman P et al 2019. The effect of schizophrenia on major adverse cardiac events, length of hospital stay, and prevalence of somatic comorbidities following acute coronary syndrome. European Heart Journal 5(2), 121–126.

Australian Bureau of Statistics (ABS) 2019. National Health Survey first results. ABS Cat. No. 4364.0.55.001 ABS, Canberra. Online. Available: www1.health.gov.au/internet/main/publishing.nsf/Content/Overweight-and-Obesity.

Australian Institute of Health and Welfare (AIHW) 2016. Australia's Health 2016. Australia's Health Series no.15. Cat. No. AUS 199. AIHW, Canberra.

Bastien M, Poirier P, Lemieux I et al 2014. Overview of epidemiology and contribution of obesity to cardiovascular disease. Progress in Cardiovascular Diseases 56(4), 369–381.

Becquemont L, Bauduceau B, Benattar-Zibi L et al 2015. Association between cardiovascular drugs and chronic kidney disease in non-institutionalized elderly patients. Basic & Clinical Pharmacology & Toxicology 117(2), 137–143.

Beijk M, Vlastra W, Delewi R et al 2019. Myocardial infarction with non-obstructive coronary arteries: a focus on vasospastic angina. Journal of Netherlands Heart 27, 237–245.

Bouisset F, Ruidavets J-R, Bongard V et al 2020. Long-term prognostic impact of physical activity in patients with stable coronary heart disease. The American Journal of Cardiology 125(2), 176–181.

Brown A, O'Shea RL, Mott K et al 2015. A strategy for translating evidence into policy and practice to close the gap–developing essential service standards for Aboriginal and Torres Strait Islander cardiovascular care. Heart, Lung and Circulation 24(2), 119–125.

Cai A, Zhang J, Wang R et al 2018. Joint effects of obstructive sleep apnea and resistant hypertension on chronic heart failure: a cross-sectional study. International Journal of Cardiology 257, 125–130.

Calderon-Larranaga A, Diaz E, Poblador-Plou B et al 2016. Non-adherence to antihypertensive medication: the role of mental and physical comorbidity. International Journal of Cardiology 207, 310–316.

Carney G, Bassett K, Maclure M et al 2020. Cardiovascular and neuropsychiatric safety of smoking cessation pharmacotherapies in non-depressed adults: a retrospective cohort study. Addiction Feb 19, 1–13.

Carney R, Freedland K 2016. Depression and coronary heart disease. Nature Reviews: Cardiology 181, 1–11.

Chan A 2015. Making the case for a more accurate cardiovascular disease risk assessment tool for Indigenous Australians. Contemporary Nurse 50(1), 92–93.

Chang W, Chan J, Wong C et al 2020. Mortality, revascularization and cardioprotective pharmacotherapy after acute coronary syndrome in patients with psychotic disorders: a population-based cohort study. Schizophrenia Bulletin, Feb 21. doi:10.1093/schbul/sbaa01

De Hert M, Detraux J, Vancampfort D 2018. The intriguing relationship between coronary heart disease and mental disorders. Dialogues Clinical Neuroscience 20, 31–39.

Di Lullo L, House A, Gorini A et al 2015. Chronic kidney disease and cardiovascular complications. Heart Failure Reviews 20(3), 259–272.

Field P, Franklin R, Barker R et al 2018. Cardiac rehabilitation services for people in rural and remote areas: an integrative literature review. Rural and Remote Health 18, 4378.

Gaalema DE, Cutler AY, Higgins ST et al 2015. Smoking and cardiac rehabilitation participation: associations with referral, attendance and adherence. Preventive Medicine 80, 67–74.

Gabb GM, Mangoni AA, Anderson CS et al 2016. Guideline for the diagnosis and management of hypertension in adults – 2016. Medical Journal of Australia 205(2), 85–89.

Galati A, Piccoli M, Tourkmani N et al 2018. Cardiac rehabilitation in women: state of the art and strategies to overcome the current barriers. Italian Federation of Cardiology 19, 689–697.

Ghadri JR, Sarcon A, Diekmann J et al 2016. Happy heart syndrome: role of positive emotional stress in Takotsubo Syndrome. European Heart Journal 37(37), 2823–2829.

Gladigau EL, Fazio TN, Hannam JP et al 2014. Increased cardiovascular risk in patients with severe mental illness. Internal Medicine Journal 44(1), 65–69.

Grace SL, Midence L, Oh P et al 2016. Cardiac rehabilitation program adherence and functional capacity among women: a randomized controlled trial. Mayo Clinic Proceedings 91(2), 140–148.

Grandi SM, Eisenberg MJ, Joseph L et al 2016. Cessation treatment adherence and smoking abstinence in patients after acute myocardial infarction. American Heart Journal 173, 35–40.

Gupta R, Gupta S, Sharma S et al 2019. Risk of coronary heart disease among smokeless tobacco users: results of systematic review and meta-analysis of global data. Nicotine and Tobacco Research 21(1), 25–31.

Hajar R 2017. Risk factors for coronary artery disease. Historical factors. Heart Views 18(3), 109–114.

Hamilton S, Mills B, McRae S et al 2018. Evidence to service gap: cardiac rehabilitation and secondary prevention in rural and remote Western Australia. BMC Health Services Research 18(64), 1–9.

Hamilton S, Mills B, McRae S et al 2016. Cardiac rehabilitation for Aboriginal and Torres Strait Islander people in Western Australia. BMC Cardiovascular Disorders 16(150), 1–11.

Hsia S, Myers M, Chen T 2017. Combination nicotine replacement therapy: strategies for initiation and tapering. Preventative Medicine 97, 45–49.

Jackson JL, Leslie CE, Hondorp SN 2018. Depressive and anxiety symptoms in adult congenital heart disease: prevalence, health impact and treatment. Progress in Cardiovascular Disease 6 1(3–4), 294–299.

Jespersen L, Abildstrøm SZ, Hvelplund A et al 2013. Persistent angina: highly prevalent and associated with long-term anxiety, depression, low physical functioning, and quality of life in stable angina pectoris. Clinical Research in Cardiology 102(8), 571–581.

Kotseva K, Wood D, De Bacquer D et al 2016. EUROASPIRE IV: a European Society of Cardiology survey on the lifestyle, risk factor and therapeutic management of coronary patients from 24 European countries. European Journal of Preventive Cardiology 23(6), 636–648.

Lu T, Forgetta V, Yu O et al 2020. Polygenic risk for coronary heart disease acts through atherosclerosis in type 2 diabetes. Cardiovascular Diabetology 19(1), 1–10.

Lunde P, Bye A, Bergland A et al 2020. Long term follow-up with a smartphone application improves exercise capacity post cardiac rehabilitation: a randomized controlled trial. European Journal of Preventative Cardiology 0(00), 1–11.

Millen BE, Abrams S, Adams-Campbell L et al 2016. The 2015 Dietary Guidelines Advisory Committee Scientific Report: development and major conclusions. Advances in Nutrition 7(3), 438–444.

Mills K, Bundy J, Kelly T et al 2016. Global disparities of hypertension prevalence and control: a systematic analysis of population-based studies from 90 countries. Circulation 134(6), 1–19.

Ministry of Health NZ 2018. Consensus Statement on Cardiovascular Disease Risk Assessment and Management for Primary Care. New Zealand. Online. Available: www.heartfoundation.org.nz/professionals/health-professionals/cvd-consensus-summary

Mostofsky E, Chahal HS, Mukamal KJ et al 2016. Alcohol and immediate risk of cardiovascular events: a systematic review and dose–response meta-analysis. Circulation 133(10), 979–987.

Murphy B, Le Grande M, Alvarenga M et al 2020. Anxiety and depression after a cardiac event: prevalence and predictors. Frontiers in Psychology 10(3010), 1–12.

National Heart Foundation of Australia (National Blood Pressure and Vascular Disease Advisory Committee) 2016. Guidelines for the diagnosis and management of hypertension in adults. Online. Available: www.heartfoundation.org.au/images/uploads/publications/PRO-167_Hypertension-guideline-2016_WEB.pdf

National Heart Foundation of Australia and the Cardiac Society of Australia and New Zealand 2016. Australian Clinical Guidelines for the Management of Acute Coronary Syndromes. Heart, Lung and Circulation 25, 895–951.

National Institute for Health and Care Excellence (NICE) 2019. Type 2 diabetes in adults: management. NICE Guidelines (NG28). Online. Available: www.nice.org.uk/guidance/ng28.

Nichols M, Brendason K, Alston L et al 2014. Australian heart disease statistics 2014. National Heart Foundation of Australia, Melbourne. Online. Available: https://heartfoundation.org.au/images/uploads/publications/HeartStats_2014_web.pdf.

Ohman EM 2016. Chronic stable angina. New England Journal of Medicine 374(12), 1167–1176.

Osei A, Mirbolouk M, Orimoloye O et al 2019. Association between E-cigarette use and cardiovascular disease among never and current combustible-cigarette smokers. The American Journal of Medicine 132(8), 949–954.

O'Toole K, Chamberlain D, Giles T 2020. Exploration of a nurse practitioner-led phase two cardiac rehabilitation programme on attendance and compliance. Journal of Clinical Nursing 29, 785–793.

Perk J, De Backer G, Gohlke H et al 2012. European Guidelines on cardiovascular disease prevention in clinical practice (version 2012). European Heart Journal 33(13), 1635–1701.

Picard F, Sayah N, Spagnoli V et al 2019. Vasospastic angina: a literature review of current evidence. Archives of Cardiovascular Disease 112(1), 44–55.

Pinier C, Gatault P, Fauchier L et al 2020. Specific impact of past and new major cardiovascular events on acute kidney injury and end-stage renal disease risks in diabetes: a dynamic view. Clinical Kidney Journal 13(1)17–23.

Prochaska JJ, Benowitz NL 2015. Smoking cessation and the cardiovascular patient. Current Opinion in Cardiology 30(5), 506–511.

Resurreccion D, Motrico E, Rubio-Valera M et al 2018. Reasons for dropout from cardiac rehabilitation programs in women: a qualitative study. PLoS ONE 13(7) 1–14.

Sandesara PB, Lambert CT, Gordon NF et al 2015. Cardiac rehabilitation and risk reduction: time to 'rebrand and reinvigorate'. Journal of the American College of Cardiology 65(4), 389–395.

Shima A, Miyamatsu N, Miura K et al 2020. Relationship of household salt intake level with long-term all cause and cardiovascular disease mortality in Japan: NIPPON DATA80. Hypertension Research 43, 132–139.

Smyth A, O'Donnell M, Lamelas P et al and INTERHEART investigators 2016. Physical activity and anger or emotional upset as triggers of acute myocardial infarction: the INTERHEART study. Circulation 11(134), 1059–1067.

Sverre E, Otterstad J, Gjertsen E et al 2017. Medical and sociodemographic factors predict persistent smoking after coronary events. BMC Cardiovascular Disorders 17(1), 1–9.

Sverre E, Peersen K, Weedon-Fedkaer H et al 2020. Preventable clinical and psychosocial factors predicted two out of three recurrent cardiovascular events in a coronary population. BMC Cardiovascular Disorders 20(61), 1–9.

Valtorta NK, Kanaan M, Gilbody S et al 2016. Loneliness and social isolation as risk factors for coronary heart disease and stroke: systematic review and meta-analysis of longitudinal observational studies. Heart 102(13), 1009–1016.

Vistisen D, Andersen GS, Hansen CS et al 2016. Prediction of first cardiovascular disease event in type 1 diabetes mellitus: the steno type 1 risk engine. Circulation 133(11), 1058–1066.

Wang MP, Chen J, Lam TH et al 2015. Impact of secondhand smoke exposure on smoking cessation in cardiac patients. Journal of the American College of Cardiology 66(5), 592–593.

Wilson MG, Ellison GM, Cable NT 2015. Basic science behind the cardiovascular benefits of exercise. Heart (British Cardiac Society) 101(10), 758–765.

Woodruffe S, Neubeck L, Clark RA et al 2015. Australian Cardiovascular Health and Rehabilitation Association (ACRA) core components of cardiovascular disease secondary prevention and cardiac rehabilitation 2014. Heart, Lung and Circulation 24(5), 430–441.

World Health Organization (WHO) 2016. Physical activity. Online. Available: www.who.int/topics/physical_activity/en/.

Xu G, You D, Wong L et al 2019. Risk of all-cause and CHD mortality in women versus men with type 2 diabetes: a systematic review and meta-analysis. European Journal of Endocrinology (180), 243–255.

CHAPTER 21

Principles for Nursing Practice: Chronic Heart Failure

PHILLIP J. NEWTON • SUNITA R. JHA • SERRA E. IVYNIAN • PATRICIA M. DAVIDSON

LEARNING OBJECTIVES

When you have completed this chapter you will be able to:

- describe the epidemiology and pathophysiology of chronic heart failure
- appreciate the burden of heart failure on the individual, their family and society
- discuss evidence-based strategies for the diagnosis and management of chronic heart failure
- reflect on the role of the nurse in the multidisciplinary care team
- identify the need for communication across the care continuum to improve outcomes for people with chronic heart failure.

KEY WORDS

chronic heart failure	self-care
nurse coordinated care models	symptom management
nursing	

INTRODUCTION

Chronic heart failure (CHF) is a growing public health problem, both in Australia and globally, and is associated with significant morbidity, mortality and economic burden. This is particularly the case among those aged 65 years and older (Carlsen et al 2012; Cook et al 2014). Epidemiological data estimates the lifetime risk of developing CHF as one in five (Bui et al 2011). The prevalence of CHF is predicted to increase in parallel with the ageing of the population and the continuing decrease in fatal coronary heart disease (CHD) (Jugdutt 2010; National Heart Foundation of Australia 2005; National Heart Foundation of Australia and the Cardiac Society of Australia and New Zealand 2011). Rising rates of inactivity, smoking, hypertension, diabetes, atrial fibrillation and obesity threaten to change the contemporary epidemiology of CHF and have significant implications for nursing management.

It is important to recognise that nurses and other health professionals play a critical role in preventing CHF, as well as treating and managing the condition. Several key principles underpin the structure of this chapter. Firstly, it is important to appreciate the pathophysiological and epidemiological basis of CHF to undertake informed clinical practice; secondly, the role of the nurse in evidence-based practice strategies to prevent and manage CHF is emphasised; and thirdly, the process of reflection in developing clinical knowledge from prevention to palliation of CHF is emphasised.

There are no definitive data on the incidence and prevalence of CHF in Australia and available information is largely modelled from clinical trial and international data sets. In 2000 it was estimated that 325,000 Australians had symptomatic heart failure and another 214,000 Australians had asymptomatic left ventricular dysfunction (2.8% of the population) (Clark et al 2004). A survey of randomly selected residents in Canberra, aged between 60 and 86 years, was conducted between February 2002 and June 2003 (Abhayaratna et al 2006). Participants enrolled in the study had a comprehensive clinical history, were examined by a cardiologist and received an echocardiogram. Consistent with other data sets, the incidence of CHF in the Canberra Heart Study increased with age (4.4-fold increase from the 60–64 years group to the 80–86 years group, p < 0.0001) (Abhayaratna et al 2006). More recent data using linked, administrative data sets from Western Australia suggest that while the incidence (new onset) of CHF has decreased over the preceding two decades, the number of hospitalisations per year has increased during this same period (Teng et al 2010), and these findings are consistent with other contemporary studies.

The most recent data on hospitalisation of heart failure in Australia comes from the NSW Heart Failure Snapshot study (Newton et al 2016). This study enrolled consecutive patients admitted to 24 hospitals around New South Wales over a 1-month period with an admission diagnosis of acute failure (either decompensation of CHF or new onset heart failure). A total of 811 patients were enrolled into the snapshot, with hospitals enrolling between 4 and 81 patients during the month. This study highlighted the complexity of patients and the treatment received and outcomes of people admitted to Australian facilities with acute heart failure across a broad range of facilities.

Although CHF is seen across the lifespan from paediatrics to gerontology, the majority of people that will be seen will be older and suffering from multiple concurrent conditions, such as diabetes, depression, arthritis and chronic obstructive pulmonary disease (COPD). Preventing illness, as well as assisting individuals to cope and adjust to living with a chronic illness is an important part of the nurse's role.

The prevalence and likely burden of CHF is important to consider given the ageing of the Australian population, which is consistent with other Western societies. In the coming decades we will see a three- to fourfold increase in the number of Australians living over the age of 65 years (Australian Bureau of Statistics [ABS] 2013). This predicted increase will also be seen in those over the age of 85 years, which will considerably require the further incorporation of a cardiogeriatric approach to care. A cardiogeriatric approach involves the combination of best practice cardiovascular and gerontological management that tailors and targets appropriate interventions to meet the needs of individuals and their families. The ageing demographic of CHF patients has resulted in the high prevalence of previously denoted geriatric syndromes, such as frailty. While frailty is common among elderly populations, concomitance with CHF is especially precarious and is associated with an increased risk of morbidity and mortality above that of non-frail CHF patients (Jha et al 2015). However, as frailty is a dynamic syndrome, management strategies (such as exercise and nutritional intervention, mechanical circulatory support implantation and cardiac transplantation) can mitigate the associated risk of being frail.

It is therefore important to consider the range of physical, social, cultural, psychological and spiritual factors that impact on living with a chronic condition and not merely focus on the biomedical dimensions of CHF management. Considering issues such as cognitive impairment, depression and physical frailty is just as important in developing nursing care plans for patients with CHF as a cardiovascular physical assessment. Over the past decade there has been an increasing focus on managing CHF because of the high costs to the individual and the healthcare system, primarily stemming from frequent hospitalisations, many of which are avoidable through targeted disease management interventions (Maru et al 2015).

DEFINITION OF CHRONIC HEART FAILURE

In spite of the burden and prevalence of CHF, there is no international consensus on the definition of CHF. The National Heart Foundation/Cardiac Society of Australia and New Zealand defines CHF as a:

> … *complex clinical syndrome with typical symptoms (e.g. dyspnoea, fatigue) that can occur at rest or on effort, and is characterised by objective evidence of an underlying structural abnormality or cardiac dysfunction that impairs the ability of the ventricle to fill with or eject blood (particularly during physical activity). A diagnosis of CHF may be further strengthened by improvement in symptoms in response to treatment (Krum et al 2011).*

CAUSES OF CHRONIC HEART FAILURE

CHF is a complex clinical syndrome characterised by evidence of an underlying structural abnormality or cardiac dysfunction that impairs the ability of the ventricle to either fill or eject blood. The most common cause of CHF is CHD, which is present in over 50% of newly diagnosed patients (Krum et al 2011). Hypertension is present in approximately two-thirds of people with CHF. Less common is idiopathic dilated cardiomyopathy, representing 5–10% of the cases of CHF. Left ventricular hypertrophy contributes to the development of CHF, due to changes in the heart muscle caused by the stress of pressure and volume overload. Remodelling is characterised by a change in the dimensions of the left ventricle and the ventricular wall causing myocardial fibrosis, myocyte hypertrophy and hypertrophy of the coronary artery smooth muscle cells. The causes of CHF are broadly attributed to ventricular function and the capacity of the ventricles to contract and relax.

Systolic Heart Failure: Impaired Ventricular Contraction

CHD, resulting in decreased perfusion of the myocardium, is the most common cause of systolic heart failure. Essential hypertension may also contribute to CHF through increasing afterload and accelerating the progression of CHD. People with non-ischaemic idiopathic dilated cardiomyopathy are often younger and there is often a familial association. Less common causes of systolic heart failure (where the heart does not pump effectively) include valvular heart disease, alcoholic dilated cardiomyopathy, peripartum cardiomyopathy, myocarditis and thyroid dysfunction.

Heart Failure With Preserved Ejection Fraction: Impaired Ventricular Relaxation

Impaired ventricular relaxation results in the lack of ability of the ventricles to fill with blood, rather than a problem of pumping: this is why it is described as heart failure with preserved ejection fraction. The most common cause of heart failure with preserved ejection fraction is hypertension and is most common in elderly women. Diabetes is an important contributing factor for CHF and can also be associated with myocardial ischaemia (Lind et al 2012). Heart failure with preserved ejection fraction can occur in conditions such as aortic stenosis (a condition where the opening of the aortic valve is narrowed), hypertrophic (enlargement of constituent heart cells) and restrictive cardiomyopathy (where the heart chambers are unable to fill).

Modifiable and non-modifiable risk factors

Given the high patient and societal burden of CHF, it is important to identify modifiable risk factors to develop strategies for the prevention of incident CHF, as well as slowing disease progression. Advancing age, male sex, CHD, hypertension, diabetes, obesity and tobacco use are several important risk factors in CHF (Del Gobbo et al 2015).

Modifiable

- *Hypertension*: Hypertension is prevalent in 60% of all CHF cases, especially in elderly HFpEF women. Hypertension increases the risk of developing CHF 2- to 3-fold. While it may be easy to detect, successful management can be difficult and may require more than one antihypertensive agent, as well as lifestyle changes and other strategies.
- *Tobacco use*: Smoking is strongly associated with incident CHF in both men and women, with female tobacco users particularly at risk. Tobacco use is also associated with the development of CHD, a major cause of CHF. Smoking cessation therapy is an essential element to CHF management.
- *Physical inactivity*: Physical activity reduces the risk of CHD, obesity, hypertension and diabetes, as well as CHF. Lifestyle changes to improve physical activity are integral in CHF management and prevention. Physical inactivity is also a large determinant of physical frailty, sarcopenia and cachexia in CHF, and is thus a target of many interventions.
- *Obesity*: Overweight (BMI 25–29.9) and obese (BMI ≥ 30 or greater) patients are at a greater risk of incident CHF. Malnourishment and poor diet (high salt and fat intake) are also risk factors. Anaemia is common in heart failure patients.
- *Frailty*: Frail patients are seven times more likely to develop CHF, and vice versa. This cyclical relationship between frailty and CHF is likely due to overlapping inflammatory, metabolic and autonomic abnormalities across both syndromes. With the ageing CHF population, frailty is key in identifying 'biological age' as opposed to 'chronological age', and is increasingly being used as a screening tool for patient vulnerability (Jha et al 2016).

Non-modifiable

- *Age*: 10% of people aged ≥ 65 years have CHF, with an exponential increase in prevalence and incidence thereafter.
- *Gender*: The incidence and prevalence of CHF is higher in men than women across all ages. However, as the incidence increases greatly with age, and there are more elderly women, the overall prevalence of CHF is similar in both sexes (Mehta & Cowie 2006).

DELETERIOUS COMPENSATORY MECHANISMS IN CHRONIC HEART FAILURE

Systolic heart failure is associated with a decrease in cardiac output due to left ventricular dysfunction. The body, in response to the reduced cardiac output, activates several neurohormonal compensatory mechanisms. While the activation of these systems is effective in the short term, in the longer term they become ineffective and even deleterious, leading to further progression of CHF. The activation of these systems stresses the failing ventricle, resulting in further reduction in cardiac output and stroke volume. These systems also cause further changes in the structure of myocardium, which is known as remodelling. Two of these mechanisms will now be considered.

Renin-Angiotensin-Aldosterone System

When the cardiac output falls, the kidneys respond by stimulating the renin-angiotensin-aldosterone system. This system leads to the retention of sodium and water. The mechanism of sodium and water is designed to compensate for a low-volume state. In individuals with CHF, alterations in tissue and organ perfusion are the consequence of lower circulation volume as a result of either reduced cardiac output caused by left ventricular dysfunction (systolic CHF) or abnormal filling (heart failure with preserved ejection fraction). Fluid retention is a common sign of CHF. If left untreated, retained fluid may manifest as oedema. The long-term activation of the renin-angiotensin-aldosterone system may also contribute to the cardiac remodelling seen in CHF (Jackson et al 2000).

Sympathetic Nervous System Response

An early compensatory mechanism in CHF is the stimulation of the sympathetic nervous system. Cardiac output is initially maintained through vasoconstriction and increased heat rate. Again, while effective in the short term, the resulting increase in preload and afterload further reduces cardiac output, which results in further ventricular dysfunction. The resulting tachycardia may increase the vulnerability of the CHF myocardium to arrhythmias.

The activation of the compensatory mechanisms in CHF, while effective in the short term, results in detrimental effects on heart function when prolonged.

To prevent this detrimental cyclical stimulation, these compensatory mechanisms have become the target of pharmacological management of CHF, particularly with the introduction of angiotensin converting enzyme (ACE) inhibitors, beta blockers and aldosterone antagonists, three of the common classes of drugs prescribed in CHF, particularly systolic CHF (Lindenfeld et al 2010; National Heart Foundation of Australia and the Cardiac Society of Australia and New Zealand 2011).

SIGNS AND SYMPTOMS OF CHRONIC HEART FAILURE

CHF is a condition that is associated with numerous signs and symptoms. Dyspnoea (shortness of breath) is the most common symptom associated with CHF. Initially dyspnoea occurs on exertion, but as CHF worsens it may occur with minimal activity or at rest. Breathlessness that occurs at night, waking the individual, is known as orthopnoea. When pulmonary congestion is present, patients may need to sleep on a number of pillows to decrease the sensation of dyspnoea. This may indicate fluid congestion in the lungs. Other signs and symptoms associated with CHF include fatigue and cachexia. Oedema can be present and reflected in a raised jugular venous pressure, ankle and sacral oedema, ascites and hepatomegaly indicating fluid retention. Other signs, including tachycardia, displaced apex beat and a third heart sound, are indicative of CHF. Heart murmurs can also be present, indicating structural heart disease, such as mitral regurgitation. The New York Heart Association (NYHA) Scale, as described in Table 21.1, is a common way to classify the severity of CHF through the impact of symptoms on physical activity.

Living With Symptom Burden

Living with signs and symptoms of CHF can be a daily struggle, particularly for patients classified as NYHA III or IV, who experience considerable physical limitation due to symptoms (Table 21.1). Dyspnoea and fatigue overshadow daily activities, which makes it difficult for patients to carry out routine tasks such as household chores, dressing, bathing, and even walking. Patients will often adapt their daily routine by limiting or pacing activities in order to accommodate symptoms. It is important to note that the consequences of these limiting symptoms extend beyond the physical. Increased dependence on others as a result of reduced mobility can make patients feel useless and negatively impact on a person's self-concept. Maintaining a social life is also challenging for patients, as lack of energy and mobility impedes the ability to see family and friends. Consequently, social isolation, loss of independence and self-worth ensue due to the restrictive nature of CHF symptoms. It is therefore not surprising that CHF patients are particularly vulnerable to depression. Over 20% of all patients with CHF suffer from depression, with this rate only increasing as severity of CHF increases; that is, higher rates of depression as NYHA classification increases (Rutledge et al 2006). Patients with CHF are also commonly forced to give up hobbies, travel and employment roles due to physical limitations. This further affects how patients view

TABLE 21.1
New York Heart Association Functional Class

CLASS I	No limitation: ordinary physical exercise does not cause undue fatigue, dyspnoea or palpitations.
CLASS II	Slight impairment of physical activity: comfortable at rest, but ordinary activity results in fatigue, palpitations.
CLASS III	Marked limitation of physical activity: comfortable at rest, but less than ordinary activity results in symptoms.
CLASS IV	Unable to carry out any physical activity without discomfort: symptoms of CHF are present even at rest with increased discomfort with any physical activity.

Reprinted with permission. Adapted from Dolgin M, Association NYH, Fox AC, Gorlin R, Levin RI, New York Heart Association. Criteria Committee. Nomenclature and criteria for diagnosis of diseases of the heart and great vessels. 9th ed. Boston, MA: Lippincott Williams and Wilkins; March 1, 1994. Original source: Criteria Committee, New York Heart Association, Inc. Diseases of the Heart and Blood Vessels. Nomenclature and Criteria for diagnosis, 6th ed. Boston, Little, Brown and Co. 1964, p 114.

themselves, as they must unwillingly give up activities that once brought great pleasure, meaning and purpose. Giving up activities that were once a large part of a person's identity can also lead to reduced self-concept and quality of life. The impact of symptom burden on patient wellbeing and quality of life must be highlighted, as studies have shown that depression and poor quality of life are both independent predictors of worse outcomes (death and re-hospitalisation) in patients with CHF (Hoekstra et al 2013; Jiang et al 2001).

DIAGNOSIS OF CHRONIC HEART FAILURE

The diagnosis of CHF is based on clinical features, chest X-ray and assessment of ventricular function using methods such as echocardiography. The signs and symptoms of CHF, such as fatigue and dyspnoea, can reasonably be associated with a range of other conditions, including physical deconditioning. As a consequence, it is important that astute physical examination and appropriate diagnostic tests be instituted in order to:
- confirm the clinical diagnosis
- determine the structural or biochemical anomalies responsible for CHF
- identify exacerbating and precipitating factors and treat accordingly
- instigate appropriate therapeutic interventions
- determine the probable clinical course and prognosis.

Physical Examination

The physical examination is important not only in diagnosing CHF, but also in monitoring the condition. Key steps in the physical examination include:
- measuring blood pressure and heart rate, both lying and standing

- assessment of heart rate and rhythm
- checking peripheral pulses and tissue perfusion
- examining the veins in the neck for elevated venous pressure
- listening to breath sounds and auscultation of the chest cavity
- listening to the heart for murmurs or extra heart sounds
- checking the abdomen for swelling caused by fluid build-up and for enlargement or tenderness over the liver
- assessing the legs and ankles for swelling caused by oedema
- measuring and recording body weight.

Whenever CHF is suspected, the individual should undergo an electrocardiogram (ECG), chest X-ray and echocardiogram, even if the physical examination is normal. Biochemical and haematological tests, such as full blood count, plasma urea, creatinine and electrolytes, should be measured during the investigation period and subsequently if there are any changes in clinical status.

B-type natriuretic peptide (BNP) is secreted by the ventricles of the heart in response to excessive stretching of cardiac myocytes in the ventricles. Two forms of BNP (BNP and NT pro BNP) are currently able to be measured. The plasma concentrations of both forms of BNP are increased in patients with asymptomatic and symptomatic left ventricular dysfunction. Initially, BNP has been used in the emergency department to differentiate shortness of breath as being caused by CHF or by some other cause (Singer et al 2009). Further research has demonstrated the feasibility and effectiveness of BNP levels as a biomarker, as well as an independent predictor of CHF (Biswas et al 2012; Yamamoto et al 2012). Higher BNP levels at admission have been associated with increased risk of acute myocardial infarction (AMI) and mortality (Kociol et al 2012). Moreover, animal studies have suggested that elevated levels of BNP contribute to the progression of CHF after AMI (Thireau et al 2012). As further research is undertaken, further uses of BNP are being proposed including screening for CHF, treating CHF patients according to the BNP level and monitoring the effectiveness of the treatments. Box 21.1 summarises some of the key diagnostic approaches in CHF.

Electrocardiogram

The electrocardiogram depicts the electrical activity of the heart. It is unusual in CHF for the patient to have a normal ECG, although identification of abnormalities is not diagnostic. Common anomalies identified on the ECG include ST and T wave changes, atrial fibrillation and bundle branch blocks.

Chest X-Ray

In CHF, the chest X-ray (CXR) can show an enlarged heart (cardiomegaly) and pulmonary venous congestion with upper lobe blood diversion. In severe cases, interstitial oedema may be present and prominent vascular markings present in the perihilar region. The presence of pleural effusions in the basal areas may obscure the costophrenic angle. Kerley B lines (thin

linear pulmonary opacities caused by fluid or cellular infiltration into the interstitium of the lungs) may be indicative of lymphatic oedema due to raised left atrial pressure. It is important to consider that a normal CXR does not exclude a diagnosis of CHF.

Echocardiogram

All patients with suspected CHF should have an echocardiogram. A standard echocardiogram is also known as a transthoracic echocardiogram (TTE) or a cardiac ultrasound. The echocardiogram gives information about the size, volume and thickness of the atria and ventricles, as well as the presence or absence of regional wall motion abnormalities. An echocardiogram involves placing a transducer on the chest wall to capture images of the heart. The echocardiogram allows imaging of valves and the degree of heart muscle contraction, which can allow the determination of the indicator of the ejection fraction. The left ventricular ejection fraction is the amount of blood ejected in each heart beat and is an important predictor of outcome with a diagnosis of CHF. The echocardiogram can also allow detection of potentially correctable causes of CHF, such as valvular disease.

MANAGEMENT OF CHRONIC HEART FAILURE

Management of CHF involves prevention, early detection, slowing of disease progression, relief of symptoms, minimisation of exacerbations and prolongation of survival. Key therapeutic approaches or considerations include the implementation of both non-pharmacological and pharmacological strategies.

Pharmacological therapy

The pharmacological management of CHF aims to relieve symptoms and improve prognosis of CHF, primarily through modification of activation of the renin-angiotensin system that occurs in response to a decrease in cardiac output. The following pharmacological treatments are used:

- angiotensin-converting enzyme inhibitors (ACEIs) or angiotensin II receptor antagonists (ARBs) that prevent disease progression and prolong survival
- beta blockers that prolong survival in symptomatic patients
- diuretics that provide symptom relief and restoration or maintenance of euvolaemia; often aided by daily self-recording of body weight and adjustments of diuretic dosage
- aldosterone receptor antagonists (aldosterone antagonists) in patients who remain symptomatic

---

BOX 21.1
Diagnosis of Heart Failure

- An echocardiogram should be undertaken to confirm a clinical diagnosis, identify structural abnormalities and potentially reversible pathology such as valvular dysfunction or ischaemia.
- Coronary angiography should be considered in people with suspected myocardial ischaemia following the weighting of risks and benefits.
- Plasma B-type natriuretic peptide has been shown to improve diagnostic accuracy with a high negative predictive value.
- Endomyocardial biopsy may be indicated in patients where an inflammatory or infiltrative process is suspected.
- Diagnostic test to identify viable myocardium and reversible ischaemia such as radionuclide ventriculography, stress echocardiography or positive electron tomography.
- Assessment of thyroid function and assessment for concomitant conditions such as diabetes and hypertension.

- direct sinus node inhibitor (ivabradine) in patients who have a resting heart rate above 70 and are on a maximum dose of beta blocker, or cannot tolerate beta blockers.

Device Therapy

Technological advances have assisted in improving the quality of life of people with CHF. The cost and complexity associated with implantation limit the access of these therapies to large numbers of people with CHF.

- Biventricular pacing has been shown in patients with NYHA Class II or IV and wide QRS complexes to improve activity tolerance and quality of life, as well as reducing mortality (Cleland et al 2013).
- Implantable cardioverter defibrillators, which have been shown to reduce the risk of sudden cardiac death in patients with CHF, and low left ventricular ejection fractions (Pokorney et al 2015).
- Ventricular assist devices (VADs) are designed to assist either the right (RVAD) or left (LVAD) ventricle, or both at once (BiVAD). These are mechanical pumps that are implanted to help the heart's weakened ventricle pump blood throughout the body. In Australia, VADs are used as a bridge to transplantation, while in countries such as the United States they are also used as destination therapy.

Surgical Therapy

Surgical approaches in CHF include myocardial revascularisation and cardiac transplantation. Although cardiac transplantation is an effective option, access to this therapy is limited through donor shortage and issues in patient selection (Mehra et al 2016).

TEAM MANAGEMENT APPROACH TO CHRONIC HEART FAILURE MANAGEMENT

An important focus on CHF care is supporting individuals in the community. As a consequence, CHF is often managed away from acute hospitals by community-based teams and general practitioners. Current CHF guidelines recommend the use of a team management approach to CHF. While the composition of this team will vary between institutions due to a number of reasons, including resources and models of care, a typical CHF team will generally include CHF specialist nurses, cardiologists and the GP. Other allied health workers who may be involved include pharmacists, social workers, occupational therapists, physiotherapists and dietitians.

Based on evidence from systematic reviews and meta-analyses, it is possible to identify broad elements that are common to the most effective programs. These include:

- involvement of health professionals and other providers from a range of disciplines using a team approach across healthcare sectors
- implementation of evidence-based management guidelines, including systems for optimisation of pharmacological and non-pharmacological therapy
- monitoring of signs and symptoms to enable early identification of decompensation and/or deterioration, and effective protocols for symptom management
- inclusion of patients and their families in negotiating the aims and goals of care
- development and implementation of individualised management plans
- promotion of and support for self-care (e.g. taking medicines, following lifestyle management advice about smoking cessation, physical activity and exercise programs, nutrition and limiting alcohol use and monitoring and interpreting symptoms), the use of behavioural strategies to support patients in modifying risk factors and adhering to their management plans
- continuity of care across healthcare services, including acute care, primary care and community care
- monitoring of program outcomes and systems to ensure continuous quality improvement.

A range of challenges are faced by health professionals in educating CHF patients, including cognitive impairment and co-morbidities. These challenges highlight the need to move away from traditional education strategies to a model with multiple sessions and reinforcing of information. In fact, a failure to adhere to the recommended treatment regimen is a major cause for decompensation and hospitalisation. There is massive potential for health professionals to intervene during clinical encounters to promote treatment adherence and empower patients to carry out recommended self-management behaviours through effective health communication. A range of supplementary tools, including written, audio and visual strategies, are available to provide and reinforce information. When undertaking this process it is important to consider factors such as impaired vision and hearing or health literacy issues, which may impact upon the ability of the patient to interact with this information. A recent review has revealed that approximately 39% of CHF patients have low levels of health literacy (Cajita et al 2016). This means that a large proportion of CHF patients have difficulty understanding and acting upon health information presented to them. It is therefore essential that information about CHF be delivered at a level that is suitable for CHF patients. Ineffective patient/provider communication involving complex medical terminology and inconsistent information further compounds confusion, which can lead to huge gaps in patient knowledge (Ivynian et al 2015). This is problematic as patients must be able to understand attributes of their condition in order to make decisions about how to effectively self-manage and develop action plans involving professional intervention when necessary. The nurse should engage with the patient to be sure that they are able to:

- identify key health providers, particularly their general practitioner, and have current methods of contacting these people
- engage family members as much as possible in their care plan
- demonstrate knowledge of the name, dose and purpose of each medication, or at least have a comprehensive list of medications and a reliable system of dosing and monitoring adherence, such as a dosette box
- understand the rationale of daily weights and have a system of recording these
- have a mechanism for monitoring signs and symptoms of worsening CHF
- have an action plan to contact providers or undertake self-management strategies in response to specific symptoms, such as dyspnoea and orthopnoea, or weight changes.

MANAGING ACUTE DECOMPENSATED HEART FAILURE

The aim of supportive and disease management strategies in CHF is to prevent decompensation, particularly to the extent requiring hospitalisation. Effective symptom management and recognition are key factors in decreasing the risk of decompensation. There is great potential to minimise the rate of 'preventable' hospitalisations and re-admissions by enabling patients to recognise CHF symptoms early, act appropriately, and in a timely manner (Ivynian et al 2015). The management of acute decompensated heart failure is complex and involves recognition of precipitants, such as pneumonia. Symptomatic management involves the use of oxygen, diuretics, vasodilators such as morphine and nitrates, and, where indicated, inotrope therapy. Adjunctive therapies include non-invasive mechanical therapies, such as continuous positive airway pressure (CPAP) via mask, or bilevel non-invasive positive-pressure (BiPAP) ventilation to decrease pulmonary congestion. When the exacerbation is associated with haemodynamic decompensation, patients may require

inotropic support, intubation and ventilation, intra-aortic balloon counter pulsation. In severe cases of decompensated heart failure, VADs may be indicated as a bridge to transplantation or as destination therapy.

STRATEGIES TO MANAGE CHRONIC HEART FAILURE ON A DAILY BASIS ACROSS THE DISEASE CONTINUUM

Optimally, the approach to CHF management should reflect a team management approach. This should occur from the primary care setting, where the practice nurse collaborates with the general practitioner through to the specialist setting where nurses coordinate a range of health professionals in providing evidence-based management. A range of nurse-coordinated programs, including home-based and clinic-based strategies, as well as telephone support and internet-based strategies have been shown to improve the outcomes of people with heart failure (Dendale et al 2012; Inglis et al 2010; Stewart et al 2012).

Box 21.2 summarises key considerations in CHF management. The important role of nurses in coordinating

---

BOX 21.2
Key Characteristics of Coordinated Chronic Heart Failure Programs

- Comprehensive assessment of the needs of patients and their family focusing on physical, social, cultural, psychological and existential issues.
- Negotiation of goals of treatment and the developing of a treatment plan.
- Promotion of adherence to evidence-based therapies and strategies to promote access.
- Coordination and communication between patients, their families and care providers.
- Provision of information and counselling strategies, tailored to individual needs.
- Promotion of self-care, including titration of diuretic therapy in appropriate patients (or with family member/caregiver assistance).
- Adoption of behavioural strategies to increase adherence, such as diaries and medication management strategies.
- Monitoring and follow-up after hospital discharge or after periods of instability.
- Instigation of action plans and processes for monitoring signs and symptoms, particularly fluid overload as monitored by daily weights.
- Implementation of social support and consideration of financial considerations.

and managing care of the person with CHF cannot be overemphasised. As can be seen in Box 21.2, the successful management of these complex patients requires the skills and knowledge of a range of professionals, including physicians, surgeons, specialist heart failure nurses, practice and community nurses and allied health professionals. Part of the success of heart failure disease management programs has been the coordination of care provided by the heart failure specialist nurses and the development of action plans in consultation with the patient, family, cardiologist, primary healthcare team and allied health professionals.

EVIDENCE-BASED TREATMENT GAP

Despite the evidence for the improvement of morbidity and mortality for both pharmacological and non-pharmacological management strategies for CHF, utilisation of these therapies is often sub-optimal (Newton et al 2016). Possible explanations for this are the complexity of CHF management and the increasing evidence that there needs to be an established infrastructure to support the implementation of evidence-based practice into usual clinical care (Caldwell & Dracup 2001; Clark et al 2007; Hancock et al 2014).

Many contemporary healthcare systems are configured for acute, reactive care rather than planned, proactive, systematic management of chronic conditions (Hancock et al 2014). Further, the perceived disparity between clinical trial and community populations potentially precludes doctors from prescribing therapies, particularly within elderly populations (Clark et al 2007; Hancock et al 2014; Lloyd-Williams et al 2003; McMurray 2000).

PALLIATIVE AND SUPPORTIVE STRATEGIES IN CHRONIC HEART FAILURE

People with severe CHF and those of advanced age are treatable and are fortunate to have access to a range of therapies. The poor prognosis associated with heart failure mandates that clinicians engage with patients and their families in advance care planning and providing adequate symptom management (Davidson et al 2010). Living with a life-limiting illness means that people may experience a range of physical, psychological and existential symptoms impacting on functional status and diminished quality of life (Denfeld et al 2015). In addition, families and significant others also experience a significant treatment burden. Therefore, people should only be considered palliative when all therapeutic options have been explored within the context of the clinical condition and the patient's needs and value systems (Pantilat & Steimle 2004). The treatment gap in CHF means that many people fail to receive evidence-based treatments and, as a consequence, many people suffer and die unnecessarily. Therefore, whenever assessing patients with CHF for a palliative approach it is important that clinicians consider whether the patient has been assessed for reversible conditions, particularly ischaemia and anaemia, if they have had a trial of evidence-based therapies appropriate to their condition and, importantly, undergone specialist CHF assessment from both the medical and the nursing perspectives. Increasingly, it is evident that communication strategies, such as advance care planning, are integral in ensuring that patients and their families are aware of their condition and prognosis, yet are supported to manage their condition within a context of hope. Supporting patients and their families to negotiate transitions in the CHF illness trajectory are critical roles of nurses and should be prominent goals of therapy. A summary of the main points appears in Box 21.3. Case Studies 21.1, 21.2 and 21.3 describe scenarios for three different patients with CHF.

BOX 21.3
Summary Points

- CHF is a common condition primarily affecting older people and is associated with poor prognosis, significant symptom burden and high healthcare costs.
- The most common cause of CHF is CHD, which can largely be prevented through addressing modifiable risk factors, such as smoking, inactivity and obesity.
- Diagnosis of CHF should be undertaken using objective measures such as echocardiography.
- Promoting self-management is an important part of CHF care planning.
- Symptom monitoring and treatment is important in avoiding decompensation.
- Heart failure has a substantial evidence base to guide management and nurses play a critical role in care.
- People with CHF often have a poor prognosis so that palliative care is an important component of management.

CASE STUDY 21.1

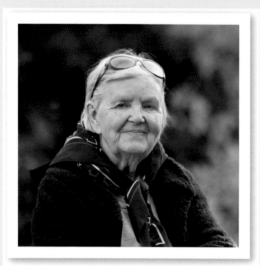

iStockphoto/itsmejust.

Mavis Brown, a 74-year-old female patient, was admitted from home with progressive increase in breathlessness, orthopnoea and ankle oedema over the previous 3 weeks. She has a history of diabetes, osteoarthritis and glaucoma. Her ECG confirmed sinus tachycardia and evidence of a previous acute myocardial infarction. Her chest X-ray confirmed cardiomegaly and interstitial oedema. Chest auscultation revealed bibasal crepitations and her jugular venous pressure was elevated. Her current medications included aspirin, a lipid lowering agent and ACE-inhibitor therapy.

CASE STUDY QUESTIONS

1. What do you consider is the most likely cause of Mavis's breathlessness?
2. Do you think it is probable that Mavis has CHF? If so, how will this be definitively diagnosed?
3. What would be the treatment strategies to relieve her symptoms?
4. What are the key self-management strategies that prevent fluid overload in people with CHF?

CASE STUDY 21.2

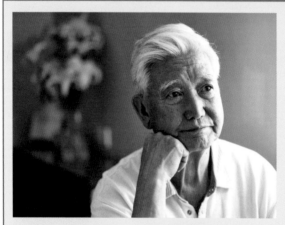

Shutterstock/imtmphoto.

Bruce Fletcher is an 81-year-old retired plumber who presents to his GP complaining of chronic fatigue, and with a

4-week history of breathlessness when walking his dog. He has recently started using three pillows in his bed due to night-time wheeze and coughing. On examination his blood pressure (BP) is 135/85 mmHg, his heart rate is 80 beats per minute at rest and regular and a third heart sound can be heard. His weight is 80 kg, increased by 4 kg since it was last measured 6 months ago. Echocardiography documents global systolic dysfunction and his left ventricular ejection fraction is 28%. He is referred to the nurse-led heart failure clinic for education and support.

CASE STUDY QUESTIONS

1. What are the important self-management strategies to discuss with Bruce?
2. What is the likely structural abnormality in the heart contributing to Bruce's symptoms?
3. What would be the medication regimen you would anticipate that Bruce would be prescribed?
4. What are considerations for medication adherence in CHF?

CASE STUDY 21.3

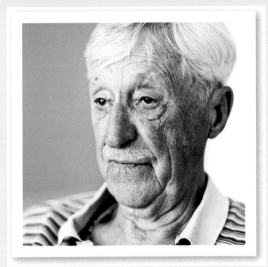

iStockphoto/RapidEye.

Bill Evans is a 78-year-old gentleman who has been admitted for the third time in the last 6 months with an acute exacerbation of his heart failure. He was first diagnosed with ischaemic cardiomyopathy 3 years ago, and had responded well to therapy (ACE inhibitor, beta blocker, loop diuretic) and, with the assistance of his wife, was managing well. Eight months ago Mr Evan's wife passed away and he has been living on his own since. He has two adult children who visit regularly on the weekends. Since his wife's passing, he has not been interested in going to the bowling club anymore and now spends most days at home reading the newspapers, watching television and listening to music. He is referred to the community heart failure nurse who visits Bill at home. Bill tells the nurse that he has been managing his condition well and cannot understand why he has had the exacerbations. The nurse asks him about his diet and he says that he finds it difficult to cook for just one so has been eating a big bowl of canned soup for lunch and dinner. He is aware of his fluid restriction (1.5 L) and always makes sure to drink this much water with the occasional beer (2–3 nights a week). His children help him with the shopping and general cleaning. The nurse finds numerous medication boxes and Bill says there have been so many changes to his medications in the last 6 months that he has found it difficult to remember what he is supposed to take and when, so he just takes the pills that he was on before his wife passed away. Bill is adamant that he wants to stay living in his home.

CASE STUDY QUESTIONS

1. In addition to the water, what else has been contributing to Bill's total daily fluid intake? What is wrong with this?

2. In addition to the standard physical examination, what other screening assessments would be worth considering?

3. What community services are available to assist Bill maintain his independence?

4. What strategies would you consider implementing to help Bill take his medications as prescribed? What other health professional(s) would you consult to help manage this?

CONCLUSION

CHF is a common and burdensome condition, particularly in the elderly. The high risk of mortality and the co-morbidity burden underscore the importance of providing accurate information about prognosis and advance care planning to avoid unnecessary and futile treatments. As health professionals negotiate the plan of care with patients and their families, it is important to consider the aetiological and pathophysiological factors that impact on disease progression as well as psychological and social factors that impact on the capacity to adhere to recommended treatment strategies. We are fortunate to have evidence-based practice guidelines to guide the management of CHF, yet a treatment gap challenges optimal outcomes for people with CHF. As hospitalisation for decompensated CHF is a frequent event, discharge planning and follow-up in the outpatient and community setting using an interdisciplinary approach are critical. Integrating optimal medical therapy with strategies to promote self-care and communication across the care continuum is necessary to optimise patient outcomes. Monitoring and enhancing adherence with the treatment plan and promoting symptom monitoring and action plans are important strategies in improving patient outcomes, including improving quality of life, increasing functional status, reducing hospitalisation and health service utilisation and cost, as well as prolonging survival.

Reflective Questions

1. What are the factors contributing to the burden of CHF in contemporary society?
2. What role do nurses play in the effective prevention and management of CHF?
3. What is the role of advance care planning and shared decision-making in CHF?

RECOMMENDED READING

Allen LA, Stevenson LW, Grady KL et al 2012. Decision making in advanced heart failure: a scientific statement from the American Heart Association. Circulation 125(15), 1928–1952.

Lainscak M, Blue L, Clark AL et al 2011. Self-care management of heart failure: practical recommendations from the Patient Care Committee of the Heart Failure Association of the European Society of Cardiology. European Journal of Heart Failure 13(2), 115–126.

Page K, Marwick TH, Lee R et al 2014. A systematic approach to chronic heart failure care: a consensus statement. The Medical Journal of Australia 201(3), 146–150.

REFERENCES

Abhayaratna WP, Smith WT, Becker NG et al 2006. Prevalence of heart failure and systolic ventricular dysfunction in older Australians: the Canberra Heart Study. The Medical Journal of Australia 184(4), 151–154.

Australian Bureau of Statistics (ABS) 2013. Population projections, Australia 2012 to 2101. Canberra. Online. Available: www.abs.gov.au/Ausstats/abs@.nsf/mf/3222.0.

Biswas SK, Sarai M, Toyama H et al 2012. Role of 123I-BMIPP and serum B-type natriuretic peptide for the evaluation of patients with heart failure. Singapore Medical Journal 53(6), 398–402.

Bui AL, Horwich TB, Fonarow GC 2011. Epidemiology and risk profile of heart failure. Nature Reviews. Cardiology 8(1), 30–41.

Cajita MI, Cajita TR, Han HR 2016. Health literacy and heart failure. The Journal of Cardiovascular Nursing 31(2), 121–130.

Caldwell MA, Dracup K 2001. Team management of heart failure: the emerging role of exercise, and implications for cardiac rehabilitation centers. Journal of Cardiopulmonary Rehabilitation 21(5), 273–279.

Carlsen CM, Bay M, Kirk V et al 2012. Prevalence and prognosis of heart failure with preserved ejection fraction and elevated N-terminal pro brain natriuretic peptide: a 10-year analysis from the Copenhagen Hospital Heart Failure Study. European Journal of Heart Failure 14(3), 240–247.

Clark RA, Driscoll A, Nottage J et al 2007. Inequitable provision of optimal services for patients with chronic heart failure: a national geo-mapping study. The Medical Journal of Australia 186(4), 169.

Clark RA, McLennan S, Dawson A et al 2004. Uncovering a hidden epidemic: a study of the current burden of heart failure in Australia. Heart, Lung and Circulation 13, 266–273.

Cleland JG, Abraham WT, Linde C et al 2013. An individual patient meta-analysis of five randomized trials assessing the effects of cardiac resynchronization therapy on morbidity and mortality in patients with symptomatic heart failure. European Heart Journal 34(46), 3547–3556.

Cook C, Cole G, Asaria P et al 2014. The annual global economic burden of heart failure. International Journal of Cardiology 171(3), 368–376.

Davidson PM, Macdonald PS, Newton PJ et al 2010. End stage heart failure patients – palliative care in general practice. Australian Family Physician 39(12), 916.

Del Gobbo LC, Kalantarian S, Imamura F et al 2015. Contribution of major lifestyle risk factors for incident heart failure in older adults: the Cardiovascular Health Study. JACC. Heart Failure 3(7), 520–528.

Dendale P, De Keulenaer G, Troisfontaines P et al 2012. Effect of a telemonitoring-facilitated collaboration between general practitioner and heart failure clinic on mortality and rehospitalization rates in severe heart failure: the TEMA-HF 1 (TElemonitoring in the MAnagement of Heart Failure) study. European Journal of Heart Failure 14(3), 333–340.

Denfeld QE, Mudd JO, Hiatt SO et al 2015. Physical symptoms and depression interact in predicting quality-of-life in heart failure. Circulation 132(Suppl. 3), A12322.

Hancock HC, Close H, Fuat A et al 2014. Barriers to accurate diagnosis and effective management of heart failure have not changed in the past 10 years: a qualitative study and national survey. British Medical Journal Open 4(3), e003866.

Hoekstra T, Jaarsma T, Veldhuisen DJ et al 2013. Quality of life and survival in patients with heart failure. European Journal of Heart Failure 15(1), 94–102.

Inglis S, Clark R, McAlister F et al 2010. Structured telephone support or telemonitoring programmes for patients with chronic heart failure. The Cochrane Database of Systematic Reviews (8), Art. No.: CD007228.

Ivynian SE, DiGiacomo M, Newton PJ 2015. Care-seeking decisions for worsening symptoms in heart failure: a qualitative metasynthesis. Heart Failure Reviews 20(6), 655–671.

Jackson G, Gibbs C, Davies M et al 2000. ABC of heart failure. Pathophysiology. British Medical Journal 320(7228), 167–170.

Jha SR, Ha HS, Hickman LD et al 2015. Frailty in advanced heart failure: a systematic review. Heart Failure Reviews 20(5), 553–560.

Jha SR, Hannu MK, Chang S et al 2016. The prevalence and prognostic significance of frailty in patients with advanced heart failure referred for heart transplantation. Transplantation 100(2), 429–436.

Jiang W, Alexander J, Christopher E et al 2001. Relationship of depression to increased risk of mortality and rehospitalization in patients with congestive heart failure. Archives of Internal Medicine 161(15), 1849–1856.

Jugdutt BI 2010. Aging and heart failure: changing demographics and implications for therapy in the elderly. Heart Failure Reviews 15(5), 401–405.

Kociol RD, Greiner MA, Hammill BG et al 2012. B-type natriuretic peptide level and postdischarge thrombotic events in older patients hospitalized with heart failure: insights from the Acute Decompensated Heart Failure National Registry. American Heart Journal 163(6), 994–1001.

Kossman CE (ed.) 1964. Diseases of the heart and blood vessels; nomenclature and criteria for diagnosis, 6th ed. Little Brown, Boston, p. 112. (36) © Wolters Kluwer.

Krum H, Jelinek MV, Stewart S et al 2011. Update to National Heart Foundation of Australia and Cardiac Society of Australia and New Zealand Guidelines for the prevention, detection and management of chronic heart failure in Australia, 2006. The Medical Journal of Australia 194(8), 405.

Lind M, Olsson M, Rosengren A et al 2012. The relationship between glycaemic control and heart failure in 83,021 patients with type 2 diabetes. Diabetologia 55(11), 2946–2953.

Lindenfeld J, Albert N, Boehmer J et al 2010. HFSA 2010 comprehensive heart failure practice guideline. Journal of Cardiac Failure 16(6), e1–e194.

Lloyd-Williams F, Mair F, Shiels C et al 2003. Why are patients in clinical trials for heart failure not like those we see in everyday practice? Journal of Clinical Epidemiology 56(12), 1157–1162.

Maru S, Byrnes J, Carrington MJ et al 2015. Cost-effectiveness of home versus clinic-based management of chronic heart failure: extended follow-up of a pragmatic, multicentre randomized trial cohort – the WHICH? study (Which Heart Failure Intervention Is Most Cost-Effective & Consumer Friendly in Reducing Hospital Care). Internal Journal of Cardiology 201, 368–375.

McMurray J 2000. Heart failure: we need more trials in typical patients. European Heart Journal 21, 699–700.

Mehra MR, Canter CE, Hannan MM et al 2016. The 2016 International Society for Heart Lung Transplantation listing criteria for heart transplantation: a 10-year update. The Journal of Heart and Lung Transplantation 35(1), 1–23.

Mehta PA, Cowie MR 2006. Gender and heart failure: a population perspective. Heart (British Cardiac Society) 92(s3), iii14–iii18.

National Heart Foundation of Australia 2005. The shifting burden of cardiovascular disease in Australia. National Heart Foundation of Australia, Melbourne.

National Heart Foundation of Australia and the Cardiac Society of Australia and New Zealand 2011. Guidelines for the Prevention, Detection and Management of Chronic Heart Failure in Australia (Chronic Heart Failure Guidelines Expert Writing Panel). National Heart Foundation of Australia, Melbourne.

Newton PJ, Davidson PM, Reid CM et al 2016. Acute heart failure admissions in New South Wales and the Australian Capital Territory: the NSW HF Snapshot Study. The Medical Journal of Australia 204(3), 113.

Pantilat SZ, Steimle AE 2004. Palliative care for patients with heart failure. JAMA: The Journal of the American Medical Association 291(20), 2476–2482.

Pokorney SD, Miller AL, Chen AY et al 2015. Implantable cardioverter-defibrillator use among medicare patients with low ejection fraction after acute myocardial infarction. JAMA: The Journal of the American Medical Association 313(24), 2433–2440.

Rutledge T, Reis VA, Linke SE et al 2006. Depression in heart failure: a meta-analytic review of prevalence, intervention effects, and associations with clinical outcomes. Journal of the American College of Cardiology 48(8), 1527–1537.

Singer AJ, Birkhahn RH, Guss D et al 2009. Rapid Emergency Department Heart Failure Outpatients Trial (REDHOT II): a randomized controlled trial of the effect of Serial B-type natriuretic peptide testing on patient management. Circulation. Heart Failure 2(4), 287–293.

Stewart S, Carrington MJ, Marwick T et al 2012. Impact of home versus clinic based management of chronic heart failure: the Which Heart failure Intervention is most Cost-effective & consumer friendly in reducing Hospital care (WHICH?) multicentre, randomized trial. Journal of the American College of Cardiology 60(14), 1239–1248.

Teng T-HK, Finn J, Hobbs M et al 2010. Heart failure: incidence, case-fatality and hospitalization rates in Western Australia between 1990 and 2005. Circulation. Heart Failure 3, 236–243.

Thireau J, Karam S, Fauconnier J et al 2012. Functional evidence for an active role of B-type natriuretic peptide in cardiac remodelling and pro-arrhythmogenicity. Cardiovascular Research 95(1), 59–68.

Yamamoto E, Sato Y, Sawa T et al 2012. Correlation between serum concentrations of B-type natriuretic peptide and albumin in patients with chronic congestive heart failure. International Heart Journal 53(4), 234–237.

CHAPTER 22

Principles for Nursing Practice: Chronic Kidney Disease

ANN BONNER • LEANNE BROWN

LEARNING OBJECTIVES

When you have completed this chapter you will be able to:
- understand the stages and trajectory of chronic kidney disease
- understand the physical, psychological and social impact of chronic kidney disease
- consider the effects of chronic kidney disease on quality of life
- understand the importance of patient self-management in achieving optimal health
- understand the role of nurses in providing patient education.

KEY WORDS

chronic kidney disease (CKD)	quality of life
kidney replacement therapy (KRT)	self-management
patient education	

INTRODUCTION

Globally, chronic kidney disease (CKD) affects about 10–16% of adults (Hill et al 2016), and in Australia one in three adults are at risk of developing CKD. It is a serious worldwide health problem, and in its later stages requires people to invest considerable time to manage their health, including modifying their diet, managing numerous medications, undergoing kidney replacement therapy (KRT) (if required) and attending medical and hospital appointments. CKD, its treatment and concomitant complications has a significant impact on a person's lifestyle, family responsibilities, ability to work and financial status (Webster et al 2017). CKD endures for the rest of a person's life, often for many decades, so the burden on an individual and their family is immense and frequently under-recognised by health professionals (Crews et al 2019). CKD requires an integrated multidisciplinary care pathway commencing with good primary healthcare.

This chapter includes a review of CKD and its effects on symptom burden and quality of life. CKD is also associated with numerous co-morbid chronic conditions, particularly cardiovascular disease and diabetes. The importance of adherence; patient education, including treatment options; and the impact on families and carers will be discussed. Nurses have a crucial role in providing healthcare and may lead the multidisciplinary CKD team. The goal of the multidisciplinary team is to support people to engage in effective self-management of CKD, its associated, complex treatment regimens, and for advance care planning. As CKD is a major concern for Indigenous people in Australia and New Zealand, Case Study 22.1 examines the development, impact and consequences of living with reduced kidney function for an Aboriginal and Torres Strait Islander (ATSI) man.

UNDERSTANDING CKD

The kidneys have remarkable functional reserve (Hryciw & Bonner 2018). Up to 80% of the glomerular filtration rate (reflected in creatinine clearance measurements)

CASE STUDY 22.1

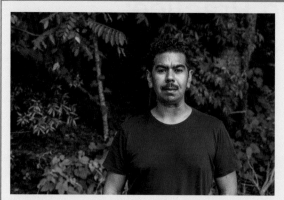

iStockphoto/davidf.

PART 1

David is a 35-year-old Aboriginal and Torres Strait Islander (ATSI) man. He recently attended the primary healthcare centre to address flu-like symptoms. The general practitioner opportunistically undertook an adult health check as David has type 2 diabetes. At that visit several issues were identified. David had been previously identified as having stage 3a CKD with macroalbuminuria secondary to diabetes nephropathy. He had a history of poorly controlled diabetes and difficulty engaging with the primary healthcare centre as he works shift work as a fly-in fly-out (FIFO) plant operator. He was identified as being at high risk of progressive kidney failure due to macroalbuminuria, poorly controlled diabetes and hypertension. His kidney function had deteriorated rapidly as he had normal kidney function 2 years ago. David lives with his partner in a rental property with their two children and three grandchildren and two adopted children. His partner is trying to find employment and is currently on New Start payments. David has a couple of his extended family members on dialysis and his brother is currently undertaking peritoneal dialysis.

	At Last Visit	Notes/Comments
Weight	85 kg	Weight gain of 5 kg over past year
Height	164 cm	
Body mass index (BMI)	31.6 kg/m²	Obese*
Blood pressure	185/110	Target BP < 130/80
Urinalysis	Protein positive, otherwise no abnormalities	
Urine albumin/creatinine ratio (ACR) (RR < 1.0)	680 mg/mmol	This is defined as macroalbuminuria
Smoking status	1 pack /day	
Haemoglobin (RR 115–160)	105 g/L	
Serum creatinine (RR 60–110)	204 micromol/L	
eGFR (RR > 60)	23 mL/min/1.73 m²	
HbA1c IFCC (NGSP)	78 mmol/mol (9.3%)	Target ≤ 53 mmol/mol < 7.0%
Estimated average glucose	12.2 mmol/L	
Alcohol	Between 1 – 2 cases of rum and cola every fortnight	Drinks these on his days off – Binge drinking
Drugs	Marijuana	$100 per fortnight on days off

*The current World Health Organization (WHO 2006) definition maintains the cut-off points for BMI classification should be maintained across different population groups.

David is prescribed metformin, irbesartan and amlodipine, hydrochlorothiazide, atorvastatin, and vitamin D. He does not know the names of his tablets and is vague about why each were prescribed. He wonders if he really needs to keep taking them and he is not sure if they are doing him any good. He also struggles to remember to take them when he is working night shift and regularly misses his medication about 30% of the time.

David was referred to the nurse practitioner-led, multidisciplinary CKD clinic at the local hospital. The referral was made due to his deteriorating kidney function over the last year. The irbesartan is used to not only assist with controlling his blood pressure but it also assists with reducing albuminuria. Albuminuria is a recognised marker of risk for kidney disease progression. The referral to specialist healthcare, in this case led by a CKD nurse practitioner, is consistent with the best practice guidelines for the management of CKD in primary healthcare (Kidney Health Australia [KHA] 2020).

may be lost with few obvious changes in the functioning of the body. A person is born with about 2 million nephrons and can survive without dialysis until almost 90% of the nephrons are lost. In the majority of cases the individual passes through the early stages of CKD without recognising the disease state, because the remaining nephrons hypertrophy to compensate. CKD is defined as either kidney damage or a glomerular filtration rate (GFR) $\leq$ 60 mL/min/1.73 m^2 for more than 3 months. There may be the presence of pathological abnormalities or markers of damage, including abnormalities in blood or urine tests or imaging studies (KHA 2020).

CKD is characterised by a progressive loss of kidney function over time, and the development and progression of cardiovascular disease (Webster et al 2017). It results from a number of conditions that cause permanent loss of nephron function and a decrease in GFR. A five-stage classification system for describing the severity of CKD has been developed. This uses GFR to describe the phases of CKD and guides clinical interventions. Stage 3 is subdivided into 3a (GFR 46–60 mL/min/1.73 m^2) and 3b (GFR 30–60 mL/min/1.73 m^2). End-stage kidney disease (ESKD) or stage 5 (GFR $\leq$ 15 mL/min/1.73 m^2) is also divided into 5 or 5D, which indicates dialysis (see Table 22.1). Globally, most people are in CKD stages 3–4 (Crews et al 2019), although the most visible group are those receiving dialysis, who actually account for the smallest number of people with CKD.

In the early stages of CKD, polyuria results from the decreased ability of the kidneys to concentrate urine. This is most noticeable at night, and the patient must rise several times to urinate (nocturia). During stage 3, when about 50% of nephron function has been destroyed, signs and symptoms such as hypertension, elevated urea and creatinine levels and anaemia develop (KHA 2020). Deterioration of kidney function affects all body systems (see Fig. 22.1).

The progression of CKD is highly variable and depends on the age, underlying aetiology, co-morbid conditions, ethnicity, and adequacy of healthcare follow-up. Some individuals live normal, active lives with stable CKD, whereas others may progress to ESKD. Haemodialysis, peritoneal dialysis or kidney transplantation, collectively known as kidney replacement therapy (KRT), are required when the clinical manifestations become life-threatening; this is during the later parts of stage 5 when the GFR is <10 mL/min/1.73 m^2.

In Australia and New Zealand, the exact number of people with CKD regardless of stage is not known, but Kidney Health Australia estimates that one in nine people over the age of 25 years have at least one clinical sign of CKD (KHA 2020). A registry for those with CKD was established in Queensland for those not receiving kidney replacement therapy (Venuthurupalli et al

TABLE 22.1
Staging of CKD. Combines Kidney Function Stage (Stages 1–5) with Description of Kidney Damage (albuminuria) and Clinical Diagnosis to Specify CKD Fully (e.g. Stage 2 CKD with Microalbuminuria, Secondary to Diabetic Kidney Disease). Colour Coding Refers to Clinical Action Plan Applicable

Kidney function stage	GFR (mL/min/1.73 m^2)	ALBUMINURIA STAGE		
		Normal (urine ACR mg/mmol) Male: < 2.5 Female: < 3.5	Microalbuminuria (urine ACR mg/mmol) Male: 2.5–25 Female: 3.5–35	Macroalbuminuria (urine ACR mg/mmol) Male: > 25 Female: > 35
1	$\geq$ 90	Not CKD unless haematuria, structural or pathological abnormalities present		
2	60–89			
3a	45–59			
3b	30–44			
4	15–29			
5	< 15 or on dialysis			

Kidney Health Australia 2020.

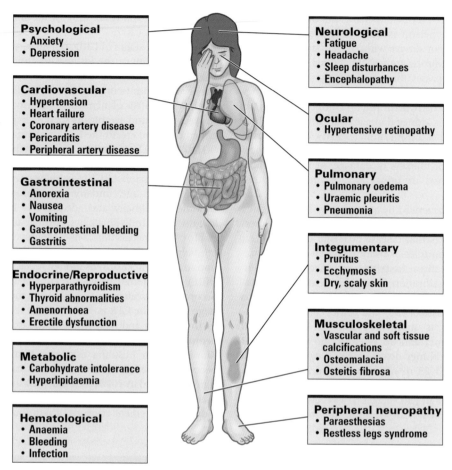

Psychological
• Anxiety
• Depression

Cardiovascular
• Hypertension
• Heart failure
• Coronary artery disease
• Pericarditis
• Peripheral artery disease

Gastrointestinal
• Anorexia
• Nausea
• Vomiting
• Gastrointestinal bleeding
• Gastritis

Endocrine/Reproductive
• Hyperparathyroidism
• Thyroid abnormalities
• Amenorrhoea
• Erectile dysfunction

Metabolic
• Carbohydrate intolerance
• Hyperlipidaemia

Hematological
• Anaemia
• Bleeding
• Infection

Neurological
• Fatigue
• Headache
• Sleep disturbances
• Encephalopathy

Ocular
• Hypertensive retinopathy

Pulmonary
• Pulmonary oedema
• Uraemic pleuritis
• Pneumonia

Integumentary
• Pruritus
• Ecchymosis
• Dry, scaly skin

Musculoskeletal
• Vascular and soft tissue calcifications
• Osteomalacia
• Osteitis fibrosa

Peripheral neuropathy
• Paraesthesias
• Restless legs syndrome

FIG. 22.1 **Clinical manifestations of uraemia.** Brown & Edwards 2019.

2019). However, the major causes of ESKD are well known, as all people starting dialysis or receiving a kidney transplant are entered into a registry, and these are diabetes mellitus (38% Australia, 47% NZ), glomerulonephritis (16% Australia, 18% NZ) and hypertension (13% Australia, 7% NZ) (Australian and New Zealand Dialysis and Transplant Registry [ANZDATA] 2019). Other significant causes include polycystic kidney disease, reflux nephropathy and analgesic nephropathy.

Aboriginal and Torres Strait Islander (ATSI) peoples in Australia and New Zealand Māori are three to eight times more likely to be affected by CKD (AIHW 2019; Walker et al 2019). While the high prevalence of diabetes in ATSI peoples is a factor in the high rate of CKD, low birth weight, cigarette smoking, as well as social and economic disadvantage, are significant contributors to adverse health outcomes (AIHW 2019). CKD also affects children and adolescents, with 353 young people between

0 and 19 receiving KRT at the end of 2014. The cause of CKD in young people varies with age, but glomerulonephritis is the most common (20%) (ANZDATA 2018).

CKD AND ACCELERATED CARDIOVASCULAR DISEASE

While people are understandably concerned about the risk of progression of CKD to ESKD, even in the early stages of CKD the risk of cardiovascular disease is even more significant. In fact, for people with CKD, the risk of dying from a cardiovascular event is much greater than requiring dialysis or a transplant (Webster et al 2017). The key goals of management of CKD are to:
• identify the cause of CKD to exclude any treatable kidney disease
• reduce progression of kidney disease by treating high blood pressure and albuminuria

- reduce cardiovascular risk
- avoid acute kidney injury as this accelerates progression of CKD and increases the risk of mortality and ESKD (i.e. nephrotoxic medications or volume depletion).

SCREENING FOR CKD

An annual kidney health check is recommended for those at risk of CKD (see Table 22.2). A kidney health check has three components:

1. urine albumin creatinine ratio (ACR)
2. serum creatinine measurement, leading to an estimated GFR (eGFR)
3. blood pressure (BP) measurement.

CKD can only be diagnosed if the urine ACR or eGFR tests are abnormal on at least two out of three separate occasions. Since 2005, all pathology services in Australia and New Zealand automatically report eGFR for adults having serum creatinine measurements. This calculates

TABLE 22.2
Early Detection of CKD Using Kidney Health Check

Indication For Testing*	Recommended Tests	Frequency Of Testing
Smoker		
Diabetes		
Hypertension		
Obesity	Urine ACR§	
Established cardio-vascular disease†	eGFR blood pressure	Every 1–2 years**
Family history of CKD		
Aboriginal or Torres Strait Islander origin aged ≥ 30 years‡		

*While being aged 60 years of age or over is considered to be a risk factor for CKD, in the absence of other risk factors it is not necessary to routinely test these individuals for kidney disease.
**1 year for individuals with hypertension or diabetes.
†Established cardiovascular disease is defined as a previous diagnosis of coronary heart disease, cerebrovascular disease or peripheral vascular disease.
‡See source text for more detail re: indications for testing in ATSI peoples.
§If urine ACR positive, arrange two further tests over 3 months (preferably first morning void). If eGFR < 60 mL/min/1.73 m² repeat within 14 days.
Kidney Health Australia 2020.

an eGFR using the patient's age and sex, as well as the creatinine (Johnson et al 2013). Like all clinical measurements, there are many variables that influence eGFR.

DELAYING PROGRESSION

The single-most important intervention to delay progression of CKD is to achieve good blood pressure control. The target BP for people with diabetes and/or albuminuria is consistently < 130/80. Otherwise, BP should be consistently < 140/90 (KHA 2020). Glycaemic and lipid control, along with routine monitoring of kidney function, is also required (KHA 2020).

Lifestyle change is an important element of delaying progression and preventing complications of CKD (Evangelidis et al 2019). Lifestyle changes include cessation of smoking, increased physical activity, weight loss and reduced dietary sodium intake. The nurse should encourage the patient to set realistic goals, plan strategies and give positive reinforcement for achievements (Nguyen, Douglas et al 2019). Smoking cessation is an important goal for anyone with CKD.

Patients with CKD and albuminuria (see Case Study 22.1) may be prescribed an angiotensin-converting enzyme inhibitor (ACEI) or an angiotensin receptor blocker (ARB), even if their BP is normal. These classes of drugs have been shown to protect the kidneys by reducing albumin loss as well as through the blood pressure-lowering effect (Ku et al 2019).

There is limited evidence that intensive treatment of other co-morbidities such as diabetes actually slows progression of CKD once it has developed. However, achieving good glycaemic control is an important goal for patients with CKD, because it helps to prevent other complications of diabetes, such as retinopathy. Recently, the use of SGLT2 inhibitors to lower glucose has also demonstrated reduced cardiovascular disease risk as well as the progression of kidney disease associated with type 2 diabetes (Bakris 2019).

Not all people with CKD require a referral to a renal unit. Indications for referral to specialist nephrology care are:

- eGFR < 30 mL/min/1.73 m²
- persistent significant albuminuria (urine ACR ≥ 30 mg/mmol)
- a consistent decline in eGFR from a baseline of < 60 mL/min/m² (a decline of > 5 mL/min/m² over a 6-month period which is confirmed on at least three separate readings)
- glomerular haematuria with macro-albuminuria
- CKD and hypertension that is hard to get to target, despite at least three antihypertensive agents.

These indications for referral should also take into consideration the individual patient's circumstances and preferences.

The book *Chronic Kidney Disease Management in Primary Care* provides contemporary evidence-based explanations useful for nurses working in either primary healthcare or acute hospitals across Australia and New Zealand regarding care for people with CKD (KHA 2020). Kidney Health Australia also provides a range of other resources for healthcare professionals (e.g. CKD GO app) and patients (fact sheets, chat rooms, etc). Anyone presenting with signs of acute nephritis (oliguria, haematuria, hypertension and oedema) should be treated as a medical emergency and referred without delay to a nephrologist.

PREVENTING COMPLICATIONS

Those with CKD, particularly older people, are susceptible to deterioration in remaining kidney function due to dehydration and nephrotoxic substances. It is important for nurses to be aware that the kidneys are less able to regulate urinary concentration and are more sensitive to dehydration. Intravenous fluids may be needed for diagnostic and/or therapeutic interventions that require fasting. In addition, radio-opaque contrast used in coronary angiography (and similar procedures) is nephrotoxic, and decisions to use contrast will be weighed up in view of the risks and benefits to the individual patient. Many medications (e.g. gentamicin, vancomycin) will require dose adjustment and monitoring to ensure patient safety. Others, such as metformin, must be used with caution in the earlier stages of CKD and discontinued in patients with a creatinine clearance of less than 30 mL/min (KHA 2020).

TREATING COMPLICATIONS

As CKD progresses, the symptoms and complications of CKD manifest, usually around late stage 3 and into stage 4. These complications are a result of anaemia and abnormal bone and mineral metabolism (Webster et al 2017). Management involves medication (iron supplements and erythropoietin-stimulating agents for anaemia; calcitriol and phosphate binders for bone and mineral metabolism) (Bonner 2019). Some patients will need sodium bicarbonate to correct acidosis or Resonium A for hyperkalaemia.

The patient may require dietary advice to maintain a healthy nutrition status. The broad guidelines for patients with CKD are in line with the recommendations for the general population. They need to be particularly conscious of limiting sodium (salt) and avoiding saturated fats. Referral to a dietitian is required if the patient needs specific advice about managing protein or potassium intake or if there are several conditions that have an impact on nutrition. Those in stages 4 and 5 CKD should be referred to a dietitian to prevent malnutrition and to manage alterations in electrolytes (particularly potassium and phosphate) and water homeostasis (Bonner 2019). It is important to note that protein restriction (< 0.8 g/kg/day) is not a recommended practice in Australia.

THE PERSON WITH END-STAGE KIDNEY DISEASE

When renal function deteriorates to the point of ESKD (stage 5), people decide about the type of treatment they would like. There are essentially two options: supportive (also called conservative or palliative) care or KRT. Supportive care is likely to be chosen by people aged over 70 years who have several co-morbid chronic health conditions and who are likely to have shorter life expectancies (Purtell et al 2018). Supportive care involves providing symptom support, often in collaboration with a palliative team. From a patient and family perspective, symptom management and quality of life are deemed important when considering this option (Metraiah & Brown 2019).

KRT includes haemodialysis, peritoneal dialysis (PD) and kidney transplantation. The choice of dialysis modality is influenced by several factors, including the preference of a fully informed patient, absence of medical and surgical contraindications and resource availability. If the patient is willing and suitable it is suggested that PD is preferable to haemodialysis to better preserve residual kidney function and allow graded introduction of dialysis (Nguyen et al 2019). PD is performed by introducing 2–3 litres of a sterile dextrose-containing solution (dialysate) into the peritoneal cavity. There are several different techniques for PD; the most common is automated peritoneal dialysis (APD) where the patient connects to a small machine every night.

Haemodialysis (HD) involves access to the vascular system (usually an arteriovenous fistula is formed and cannulated), an extracorporeal circuit, dialyser and technological equipment. Typically, a patient will receive a minimum of 4 hours of treatment on three occasions each week. HD can be undertaken in three different clinical settings: 'in-centre', in satellite HD units or at home (Chan et al 2019). 'In-centre' refers to therapy provided to people who are medically unstable and require significant care with on-site nephrology support; the centre is located in a hospital within a recognised renal unit. Satellite HD encompasses lower acuity care located in hospitals with no formal nephrology unit or community-based units where self-care is encouraged. If a person is suitable to undertake HD at home, then the number of hours is flexible and they are encouraged to dialyse for five or six times a week, often overnight (Choo et al 2018).

The last type of KRT is kidney transplantation, and is an option for most patients with ESKD, either before or after the initiation of dialysis. The donor kidney is placed in the iliac fossa and native kidneys are not removed. Immunosuppression (e.g. prednisone, mycophenolate and cyclosporin) is required to prevent rejection.

SYMPTOM BURDEN OF CKD

No matter what the stage of CKD, people experience a range of burdensome symptoms (often worse than those experienced by terminal cancer sufferers) that affect all body systems. Those in CKD stages 4 and 5 are likely to experience up to 20 different symptoms, most of which are very severe and distressing (Almutary et al 2016a). The burden arising from symptoms is responsible for the poor quality of life of people, particularly during the more advanced stages of CKD. The most prevalent symptom is fatigue (feeling weak or tired), experienced by approximately 70–97% of people with CKD. Other common symptoms are pain, pruritus, sleep disturbance and poor appetite (Rhee et al 2020). Recent research seems to suggest that fatigue is interconnected with most other symptoms (Almutary et al 2016b). Factors associated with the fatigue experienced in CKD include prescribed medications and their side effects; nutritional deficiencies; physiological alterations, such as obstructive sleep apnoea, needing dialysis; abnormal urea and haemoglobin levels; and psychological factors such as depression, sleep dysfunction and those associated with HD treatment (Rhee et al 2020). Not surprisingly, fatigue impacts on everyday life, and there is reduced capacity to perform routine living chores, going to work (if not retired), enjoying a normal social life, and the ability to undertake physical activity.

However, the most prevalent symptoms are not always the most severe or distressing. This is why symptoms are now considered to be multidimensional, and indeed may cluster together (Almutary et al 2017). For example, depression could cause fatigue and may result in worse sleep quality in people with CKD. All members of the multidisciplinary healthcare team ought to routinely assess for physical and psychological symptoms using valid and reliable assessment tools so that support and treatment can be commenced in a timely way. Multidimensional assessment tools such as the chronic kidney disease symptom burden index (CKD-SBI; Bonner, Chambers et al 2018) and the IPOS-Renal (Morton et al 2019) are used.

Those who are in CKD stages 4 and 5 are likely to develop anaemia due to the kidneys' reduced ability to produce erythropoietin (Hryciw & Bonner 2018). Anaemia causes decreased energy, tiredness, shortness of breath and weakness. In addition, anaemia in CKD contributes to significant co-morbid complications, such as left ventricular hypertrophy, congestive heart failure and ischaemic heart disease. Management involves assessment of iron levels and prescribing an erythropoietin stimulating agent (KHA 2020).

PSYCHOSOCIAL BURDEN OF CKD

The experience of living with CKD (a chronic, life-altering illness) involves many challenges for patients and their families in achieving a satisfactory health-related quality of life. Having CKD and deteriorating kidney function requires people to invest considerable time in managing their health, including modifying their diet, managing numerous medications, undergoing KRT (if required) and attending medical and hospital appointments. CKD, its treatment and concomitant complications, also impact significantly on a person's lifestyle, family responsibilities, their ability to work and financial status. The impact of CKD and its treatment on physical, emotional, social and overall health-related quality of life, therefore, is profound.

Poor health-related quality of life is due to CKD symptoms and its treatment, which affects the physical, cognitive, psychological and social aspects of lives (Van der Willik et al 2020). Regardless of the stage of CKD, it is crucial for healthcare professionals to strive to keep the person's health-related quality of life at the highest possible level.

It is difficult to adequately assess health-related quality of life, as it is a subjective and individual experience. For example, a person who is blind with bilateral leg amputations, diabetes, ESKD and requiring HD may well rate their health-related quality of life as being quite good. Nevertheless, health-related quality of life is important to assess in routine practice using validated patient-reported outcome measures (Van der Willik et al 2020). Overall, it is well documented that people with CKD have much lower quality of life scores compared with people of normal health, due to physical, psychological and social changes to daily life.

The many symptoms and complications of CKD can adversely affect health-related quality of life (Yapa et al 2019). These include fatigue, restless legs, sleep disturbance, anaemia, challenges of fluid and dietary restrictions (see Fig. 22.1), other health problems (e.g. diabetes, heart failure, infection, etc.) and chronic pain. All contribute to the stress associated with living and coping with CKD and its treatment.

BODY IMAGE

CKD can result in both physical and psychological changes in body image. There is limited research, however, exploring the patient's perception of body image in CKD. Physical changes are common and are not restricted to those directly affecting the renal system, as other body systems are also involved (see Fig. 22.1). Alterations in body image are often due to external changes in skin, body weight, mobility, side effects of medications and the presence of KRT devices. In children, growth retardation occurs because of the effects of uraemia on growth hormone production (Drube et al 2019). Internal or psychological alterations, such as fatigue, depression and altered feelings of wellbeing, also occur. Both external and internal alterations in body image may contribute to a decreased health-related quality of life and adherence with treatment.

When CKD progresses to stage 5 and KRT is commenced, other physical alterations to a person's body image occur due to the presence of dialysis access devices and several surgical procedures. These access devices could be one or more of (or in some situations both) a PD catheter, an arteriovenous fistula (AVF) or an external vascular catheter. A PD catheter and extension set protrudes from the body by approximately 15–30 cm and often requires adjustments to the type of clothing worn to accommodate its presence (e.g. underpants, location of belts or waist bands). An AVF is an internal surgical anastomosis of an artery and a vein (commonly radial artery and cephalic vein), and results in arterial blood flowing straight into the vein. The AVF causes the vein to dilate, and when repeatedly cannulated for HD, can result in tortuous and/or aneurysmal dilations which can be noticeable particularly if the AVF is in the arm. Vascular catheters can be temporary or permanent and are often visible. Lastly, scars as a result of previous, and often numerous, occasions of surgery for access devices and/or kidney transplantation can also affect an individual's body image.

Nurses need to understand, assess and recognise the impact of CKD on an individual's actual or perceived alterations in body image. Assisting individuals to verbalise their feelings and to provide supportive strategies are important facets of providing renal nursing care.

Alterations in body image, together with the physical and psychosocial complications of CKD, have an impact on an individual's sexuality. Diabetes (a leading cause of CKD), as well as a number of medications (e.g. antihypertensive agents), interfere with sexual function. Other factors, such as endocrine, vascular and hormonal changes, are also involved in sexual dysfunction. Patients describe decreased interest in and frequency of intercourse and difficulties with erection. Difficulties with sexual arousal are among the most bothersome of symptoms reported by people with CKD, particularly for those on dialysis (Yapa et al 2019). Using a non-judgemental approach will assist nurses in early identification of sexual dysfunction and timely referral for support.

The impact of CKD on the psychological wellbeing of people is significant. For example, those with CKD report high levels of stress and anxiety, feeling scared or fearful and experience feelings of guilt, frustration, worry and powerlessness (Pascoe et al 2017). Depression is the most common psychological symptom, affecting one in five people with CKD (KHA 2020), and there is strong evidence linking depression and CKD with a reduced quality of life (Shirazian 2019). There are many causes of depression in CKD patients, such as stresses associated with the disease, medications used to treat CKD, the increased need to see health professionals and hospitalisation, or simply as a result of feeling unwell. Depression can be a response to loss, and CKD patients have sustained multiple losses, including their role within the family and workplace, renal function and mobility, physical skills, cognitive abilities and sexual function. At present, there is a reliance on pharmacotherapy to treat depression in CKD, although there is growing evidence to support the effectiveness of psychosocial interventions in the treatment of depression in patients with CKD (Pascoe et al 2017). Selective serotonin reuptake inhibitors (SSRIs) are commonly prescribed as these drugs are extensively metabolised in the liver, making them safe for patients with CKD.

The social impact of CKD is immense (Hoang et al 2019). People with CKD may experience social isolation, relationship difficulty, decreased autonomy and financial difficulties. People with CKD may have difficulties re-establishing normal relationships. It interferes with an individual's ability to work, engage in social activities, participate in family and enjoyment of hobbies. Many people suffer loss of income due to unemployment, which affects themselves and their families. Unemployment and reliance on government social welfare benefits are high (Krishnasamy & Gray 2018). Loss of income leads to changes in spending patterns as household finances are directed towards care and welfare costs. There are high out-of-pocket costs associated with the care and management of CKD, despite availability of a comprehensive government funded healthcare system, and that financial hardship is experienced by Australians with CKD (Gorham et al 2019; Walker et al 2017). For children and adolescents, these complications affect their ability to attend and actively participate at school (Agerskov et al 2019). Temporary or permanent relocation to larger regional or urban healthcare facilities is also experienced by people living in rural and remote locations and this also affects quality of life. This is especially evident for ATSI people where dislocation from Country and family is associated with loss and disempowerment and this can lead to adverse health outcomes and affect their social and emotional wellbeing (Conway et al 2018). Being able to take vacations when and where an individual desires is also affected by CKD and its treatment. Being unable to take a holiday is particularly problematic for those needing HD across Australia, and to address the social impact on patients and their families, the Big Red Kidney Bus, an initiative of KHA, is available. At the family level, there is an impact on the quality of life of caregivers, as well as financial impact on the family (Hoang et al 2019). Having adequate social support networks (home, work and renal unit) has been consistently linked to improved health outcomes (Sajadi et al 2017).

At a societal level, the most obvious effect is the enormous financial cost and loss of productivity associated with CKD. CKD poses a significant financial burden to healthcare systems around the world. In Australia CKD is responsible for 13% of all hospitalisations and 10% of all deaths (AIHW 2019) and by 2030 the cost of dialysis is predicted to outstrip the health budget. Box 22.1 summarises the common psychological and sociological problems experienced by people with CKD and ESKD.

The effect of adding KRT into the demands of daily life with ESKD is considerable for most people and is one of the most stressful of all illnesses and treatment

---

BOX 22.1
Common Psychological and Sociological Problems

Psychological	Sociological
Depression	Role change in family
Anger	Employment status
Denial	Ability to continue education
Helplessness	Financial status
Anxiety	Reduced social network and activities
Loss of control	Change in residential location
Burden	Holiday and recreation
Fear of death	
Feelings of guilt	

---

regimens (Crews et al 2019). While HD treatment itself typically lasts for 4 hours, three times per week, every week of the year, there are also other demands, such as travelling to and from the dialysis unit, waiting for staff/machine availability, completing pre-dialysis assessment, cannulation of fistula, and so on. This often means 8–10 hours need to be allowed for each treatment session, and this allocation of time needs to fit around the usual activities of daily life, such as work, family and school commitments. PD makes similar demands on time (approximately 4 hours per day), but PD treatment is typically undertaken on a daily basis (i.e. 365 days of the year). Consequently, the demands of KRT are considerable and result in a highly abnormal everyday life.

Rehabilitation is about the return of lost function and is an aspect of nursing care provided to people with CKD/ESKD (Yamagata et al 2019). Given the repeated and frequent contact nephrology nurses have with people over long periods of time, they are in an ideal position to provide rehabilitation. Common rehabilitative interventions include the teaching, coaching and supporting strategies that assist people to increase their movement along a continuum towards self-management. The self-management continuum typically begins with teaching people about CKD and its management through to complete independence by undertaking dialysis self-care at home. The point on this continuum is individualised for each person depending on their health, personal and home situations.

CASE STUDY 22.1

PART 2

The nurse practitioner (NP) determined several short- and long-term treatment priorities. Because of the presence of macroalbuminuria, David's BP target was established as < 130/80 mmHg. On discussion with the NP, David said he was not taking his tablets every day because he didn't know if they were really necessary and because he was feeling weak and tired. The NP explained the importance of achieving good blood pressure control and the need for indefinite treatment with tablets. They also discussed the ways to ensure a routine, so he would remember to take them each day with strategies such as providing the medications in a Webster pack and prescribing all the medications to be taken in the morning (as this was identified by David as a time he would most likely remember to take his medications. The NP arranged a joint appointment with a pharmacist to review medications. At that appoint the pharmacist also spent time explaining the purpose of all medications and side effects. Additional medications that were commenced was an additional antihypertensive (alpha blocker [Prazosin]) and a DPP-4 inhibitor (linagliptin) to assist with lowering blood pressure to target range and assisting with BGL management due to the removal of metformin from his medication regimen. The use of metformin is not recommended when the eGFR is < 30 mL/min/1.73 m^2 (KHA 2020). An initial discussion was also had regarding the use of a GLP1 receptor agonist (once weekly injection) to reduce cardiovascular risk, improve glucose management and assist with weight loss (Bakris 2019). David was reluctant to have any form of injection so this medication was not commenced but would be revisited at his next appointment with the NP.

David had gained 5 kg in weight and the NP also referred him to the dietitian. Weight reduction was more challenging for David as he finds fruit and vegetables expensive and when working, eats the meals that are provided for him. The dietitian also discussed portion control, low salt options, healthy meal choices and incorporation of bush tucker.

David said that the company he works for provides exercise classes on a daily basis. He needed a medical certificate to allow him to access this service which the NP provided. It was agreed he would join these classes three times a week and on days off walk regularly with his partner. The NP also discussed smoking and marijuana cessation strategies and reducing alcohol intake. Importantly, the NP and David collaborated on important lifestyle modifications and improving adherence with CKD self-management which will all assist in slowing the progression of his CKD.

Promoting quality of life is a key aspect of nursing care for people with CKD. Adequate and timely assessment and working collaboratively with patients is necessary to optimise quality of life. No single strategy or plan will work for everyone, but support, encouragement, education, rehabilitation and promoting self-care, are fundamental elements of renal nursing care. Of importance for nurses is to assist patients to acquire and maintain a sense of control as they adjust to living with CKD. Learning to manage the illness, finding a balance between illness and normalcy and reaching an acceptance of the illness are crucial to achieving an optimal quality of life. It is crucial that nurses ask people for their own assessments of how they are doing, what their relationships are like in their families and what life is like for them. The challenge for all health professionals involved in caring for people with CKD is to devise interventions that meaningfully increase quality of life.

SUPPORTING EFFECTIVE SELF-MANAGEMENT IN CKD

National and international clinical practice guidelines recommend that supporting patients and their families to effectively self-manage and to adhere to treatment regimens requires a multidisciplinary CKD healthcare team (KHA 2020). The team comprises general and specialist medical practitioners, nurses (and increasingly nurse practitioners), a dietitian, pharmacist, social worker and psychologist. One of the most important functions is to provide patient education, as many people with CKD have poor knowledge of their condition. They do not know what their kidneys do, why kidney function deteriorates, what treatment is needed to prevent dialysis, the options available if their kidneys fail, or how to follow their treatment plans.

People frequently report being shocked by their diagnosis and are largely unaware of where to find information or how to judge its veracity.

CKD, regardless of stage, requires people to adhere to complex treatment regimens. Initially they are asked to modify their lifestyle (stop smoking, reduce weight, limit alcohol intake and increase exercise), take numerous medications (e.g. antihypertensive agents, statins, glycaemic agents, etc.) and possibly perform self-monitoring activities at home (e.g. blood pressure, weight, blood glucose levels, etc.). As their CKD progresses, they will be asked to make further adjustments, have regular pathology investigations performed and attend clinic appointments more frequently (see Table 22.3). To successfully self-manage CKD, individuals need to know how to monitor their disease, manage symptoms, interpret

TABLE 22.3
Outline of Expected Self-Management Behaviours for CKD/ESKD

	CKD	Home Dialysis (Haemodialysis and Peritoneal Dialysis)	Hospital Haemodialysis	Transplant
Therapeutic Lifestyle Change	Stop smoking* Healthy diet, no added salt Safe alcohol More exercise +/− fluid restriction	Stop smoking Healthy diet plus adjustments as indicated by blood results Safe alcohol More exercise +/− fluid restriction, depending on urine output	Stop smoking Healthy diet plus adjustments as indicated by blood results – likely to need potassium restriction Safe alcohol More exercise Most likely to need fluid restriction	Continue to be a non-smoker Healthy diet, no added salt Safe alcohol More exercise Unlikely to need fluid restriction – have to avoid dehydration Sun protection
Home Observations	BP Weight (if fluid management an issue)	Temperature, pulse, BP Weight		Temperature, pulse, BP Weight Urinalysis
Medications	Antihypertensives, diuretics Lipid-lowering agents Phosphate binders Vitamin D analogue Sodium bicarbonate Iron Folic acid Erythropoietin-stimulating agent Other medications as required by the individual	Antihypertensives, diuretics – can often be decreased Lipid-lowering agents Phosphate binders Vitamin D analogue Iron Folic acid Erythropoietin-stimulating agent Other medications as required by the individual	Antihypertensives, diuretics – can often be decreased Lipid-lowering agents Phosphate binders Vitamin D analogue Iron Folic acid Erythropoietin-stimulating agent Other medications as required by the individual	Immunosuppressive drugs (usually a combination of three) plus a number of other drugs to minimise the side effects. These are weaned as the transplant is established, but some medication continues for the duration of the transplant Other medications as required by the individual
Dialysis Access	Once dialysis is imminent	Care of AVF/Tenckhoff catheter. Self-cannulation for home haemodialysis	Care of AVF. Some patients self-cannulate	Once transplant is working, Tenckhoff catheter will be removed. AVF remains in situ
Dialysis Procedure		Have to do procedure, maintain equipment, problem-solving to the ability of the individual	In many centres patients are encouraged to participate in self-care as able	

*In most transplant centres, current smokers will not be accepted for the active transplant waiting list.

results of home-monitoring therapies, and to carry out daily treatment plans, and for some, perform dialysis at home. Rarely are patients consulted about what they need help with, and the renal multidisciplinary team needs to shift towards developing and implanting self-management support programs that are person-centred (Havas et al 2018).

Active patient involvement in making decisions is important. Patients need to be informed of the options available and supported to make this decision (Brown et al 2019). The choices are whether to have dialysis or not, where to do it, and whether to be considered for a kidney transplant. Organisations such as Kidney Health Australia (KHA) provide information to support both patients and staff with decision-making. Once they start KRT, their schedule is dominated by the activities required to stay alive.

With the increasing number of patients experiencing reduced kidney function has come the need to develop new roles for nurses to help manage this group of patients. Nurses are actively involved in patient care at all stages of CKD: as practice nurses in primary healthcare settings, and nurses working in renal outpatient clinics and dialysis units. Increasingly, CKD clinics are being led by nurse practitioners, including across Australia and New Zealand (Coleman et al 2017). In Australia, the CKD nursing role has coincided with the development of the advanced and extended role of nurse practitioner. These advanced practice roles demonstrate safety and efficacy in achieving clinical targets, improved self-management behaviours and high levels of patient satisfaction (Bonner, Havas et al 2019).

The principles and strategies developed in other chronic disease areas, such as asthma, diabetes and heart failure, are similar to those required to develop and support effective CKD self-management (Havas et al 2018). For the nurse working with patients with CKD, this means that assessment must include consideration of the social environment and supports available. Often multiple therapeutic lifestyle changes are indicated, but it is unrealistic to expect that all can or will be adopted. The nurse will assess the patient's readiness to self-manage and work collaboratively with them to set goals. Compromise is often necessary to make sure goals are achievable. Information giving must be at a level and pace appropriate for the individual (Havas et al 2018). (See 'Education for the person and family' below.)

On return visits, the patient should be given positive reinforcement for their achievements, and encouragement to persevere. It is important to build confidence and self-efficacy, as each gain is an opportunity to set new goals (Havas et al 2018). Active and sustained follow-up by the nurse helps maintain momentum and provide support. This may be through telephone calls, reminder notices and invitations to patient education seminars. For those now in ESKD, home dialysis patients are followed up with home visits and may be able to get access to telephone assistance out of hours. However, more research on interventions designed to increase the level of self-efficacy to change self-management behaviours that adhere with treatment is required (Peng et al 2019).

Not everyone can self-manage effectively. The approach described makes assumptions about and demands on health literacy, cognitive and social skills, motivation and self-efficacy. For patients who are unable or unwilling to engage in self-management, the multidisciplinary healthcare team must develop strategies that will provide the best possible outcome for the individual.

Blaming and labelling patients who do not follow their healthcare providers' advice should be avoided. In CKD and ESKD patient care, the label of 'non-compliance' (a paternalistic term that should not be used) can have far-reaching repercussions. For example, it may be viewed unfavourably when a person is being assessed for transplantation as it is assumed that a person who is non-adherent with CKD and dialysis treatments will not follow post-kidney transplant instructions.

FAMILY AND CARERS

People with CKD often require the support of family and friends to manage their illness and treatment (particularly KRT) at home and be the principal caregiver. Existing family and marital relationships are altered by the complex and burdensome treatments associated with CKD and its treatment (Moore et al 2020). The moment CKD and its treatment regimen enter the lives of family members and friends, significant adjustments must be made to the roles they have in the relationship. There is the uncertainty about whether the person's health will become worse, how long treatment will be needed for, whether dialysis will effectively manage the condition or cause more problems, whether the person will die from CKD and when or if the person will get a kidney transplant. In addition, family members may experience guilt if the CKD is as a result of an inherited condition (such as polycystic kidney disease, Alport's syndrome).

Although home dialysis, whether peritoneal or HD, can be performed independently, evidence suggests that adult caregivers often assume some, and in some situations total, responsibility for the dialysis regimen (Moore et al 2020). Caregivers not only provide physical and technical support, but they also provide emotional support. For these caregivers, particularly spouses, KRT contributes to additional stress, fatigue, home responsibilities and, for some, a negative reaction to their partner's situation (Hoang et al 2018). Family members are constantly watching the person under care, juggling activities to meet all responsibilities, advocating or intervening on behalf of their loved one, modifying home routines to fit in with the KRT and encouraging their loved one to perform self-care and to adhere to the treatment regimen (Hoang et al 2019).

With the shortage of deceased donors, living related and living unrelated kidney organ donation rates have increased in both Australia and New Zealand (ANZ-DATA 2019). Living relatives (i.e. parents, child, sibling, etc.) are still the most common source of living donors, but living unrelated donors (e.g. spouse, significant other, close friend, etc.) have also increased the pool of available kidneys. While the donor's autonomy must be respected by healthcare professionals, the explicit or implicit pressure on family members, spouses or close friends to donate is an additional burden associated with the experience of living with someone with CKD that is not well understood or acknowledged.

It is not surprising that the burden of CKD on caregivers has been the focus of research, but there are rewards for being a caregiver; for many families, interpersonal relationships can be sustained and developed further. Nurses require an understanding of the impact of CKD on family members and others. Ongoing assessment, assisting family members and exploring the degree to which an individual family caregiver is involved in the care of their loved one are important components of providing holistic care. The type and amount of care provided by family members may alter over time due to the changing burden of CKD (i.e. different stages of CKD). Strategies such as providing professional support and early intervention to reduce the burden, strain and fatigue, increased social support services in the home and referral to other health professionals are important components of renal nursing care.

Education for the Person and Family

The patient with CKD has a continuum of education needs. From the diagnosis of CKD to dialysis and transplantation there is much to learn in relation to their disease and how to manage it. Pre-dialysis education is particularly important (Brown et al 2019). Older patients remember less and patients misconstrued 48% of what they thought they remembered. Importantly, the more information that was given, the less that was correctly recalled (Fortnum et al 2015). Bonner and Lloyd (2012) found that those with ESKD are likely to be either information receivers or engagers. 'Receivers' are those who do not interact with information but merely acquire it passively; being passive is their way of coping with kidney disease. In contrast, 'engagers' actively sought out and interacted with information and used it to better understand and cope with kidney disease and its treatment. Frequent and multifaceted educational sessions for patients and their family members are likely to improve knowledge about CKD and its treatment,

develop confident self-management behaviours, and improve patient outcomes such as quality of life (Nguyen, Douglas et al 2019).

Teach-back is a technique whereby the health educator verifies whether learning has occurred by asking the learner to teach it back to them (Yen & Leasure 2019). The technique assists with helping patients to be actively engaged in education and is likely to improve self-efficacy. It is also likely to reduce the risk of people misunderstanding critical information. In a systematic review, Dinh and colleagues (2016) found that when teach-back is used for people with chronic disease there are improvements in the patient's knowledge, adherence and self-management skills, and a reduction in hospital re-admissions.

There are many potential sources of information for patients and their carers (see, for example, Kidney Health Australia website). Even if the patient doesn't access websites, it is almost certain that friends and/or family do. Some of the information on websites is excellent, but much is confusing, misleading or even dangerous (Bonner, Gillespie et al 2018). It is useful to ask patients what they know and create opportunities to clarify incorrect or misunderstood information. Social media sites such as Facebook are also an increasing source of information.

When teaching patients about CKD or KRT, information is provided at a level and pace appropriate for the individual. This is easier to do when in a one-on-one situation. If conducting group education, attention must be given to meeting a variety of individual needs. Education seminars involving the renal multidisciplinary team are also provided. There is growing recognition that involving patients and their family in choosing the most suitable KRT for them improves health outcomes (Chan et al 2019).

One of the challenges of nursing patients with ESKD is to provide effective patient education to people who are uraemic, often elderly and almost always very anxious. If a patient begins dialysis in a hospital HD unit, the dialysis nurses will explain what is happening to them. The patient will learn about how their self-care practices will have to adapt and change as they make the transition to their new treatment modality. They will be shown the dialysis area and where the patients are weighed and introduced to the pre-dialysis assessment (weight, temperature, pulse, blood pressure).

The patient will be told not to take any antihypertensive medications before the first dialysis, but to bring all medications so the nursing staff can obtain a complete list. Some 'antihypertensives' may be taken for heart failure and the patient will need to have a personalised medication plan. There will be further teaching as medications are adjusted (e.g. sodium bicarbonate may be stopped, water-soluble medications should be taken after dialysis) and new ones are started.

Initial concerns are likely to relate to the AVF which is being cannulated for the first time and may be soft and inclined to 'blow'. Patients should be shown how to apply pressure to the needle sites and given extra sterile gauze to take home in case of bleeding.

Once their dialysis routine is established, their diet and fluid intake will be reviewed by a dietitian. Depending on residual kidney function, the patient will be given diet advice that will maintain safe blood levels of potassium between treatments without compromising their nutritional status and that takes into account individual and cultural preferences.

PD home training is usually done as an outpatient (Maley et al 2019). The patient has the Tenckhoff catheter inserted about a month before the anticipated need to start dialysis. The PD nurses are involved in teaching about preoperative preparation and postoperative care of the catheter site. It is especially important to prevent and treat constipation as this interferes with the functioning of the catheter.

Learning to perform the PD exchange, connect to the APD machine and associated procedures is done at the patient's own pace. Most patients are ready to self-manage at home within 2 weeks. However, if there are barriers to learning (e.g. language, anxiety, etc.), it may take longer. The degree to which problem-solving is taught is determined by the nurses' assessment of the patient's ability to take this on. For some patients the main focus is to make sure they recognise when problems occur, such as an infected catheter exit site or peritonitis, and what action to take; for example, contact the GP or ring the PD unit.

Patients starting PD will also have changes to their medications and diet and fluids. Because APD provides dialysis constantly, the diet tends to be more relaxed in relation to potassium, but they must be careful to have adequate protein intake to replace the protein lost in the dialysate. Also, because of the dextrose in the dialysate there is a tendency to gain body weight.

Home HD training is a more complex series of learning activities and commonly takes about 3 months to complete. In addition to everything that the hospital HD patient learns about their self-management, the home HD patient must master a range of technical activities as well. This includes water treatment and machine maintenance as well as the dialysis procedure itself. The patient and their support person will be competent in emergency procedures, such as what to do in case of adverse reactions (such as hypotension), power or water failure.

Following transplantation, the kidney transplant recipient stays in hospital until they have recovered from the surgery. The patient will have a period of daily outpatient appointments, which then taper off to alternate daily, to weekly and so on until the kidney function is well established and stable. Before discharge, the patient will be educated about their new immunosuppressive medications, including what each one is for, how to recognise them, when they should be taken and which side effects to be aware of. In addition, a patient will learn to monitor the wellbeing of the kidney by doing a daily weight, urinalysis and BP.

CONCLUSION

This chapter has explained the key aspects of CKD, ESKD and KRT and their effect on aspects of daily life. This was followed by a discussion of symptom burden, quality of life, and the impact of CKD and KRT on family and carers. Nurses should develop strategies that better support people to self-manage this chronic and complex health condition, and strategies for effective patient education as this is of prime importance when providing nursing care to people with CKD.

Reflective Questions

1. What are the different stages of CKD and what are the priorities of healthcare for each stage?
2. How does CKD impact on the individual, family and wider community?
3. How can models of care such as nurse practitioners and multidisciplinary team members improve health outcomes for the person with CKD?

RECOMMENDED READING

Havas K, Douglas C, Bonner A 2017. Closing the loop in person-centred care: patient experiences of a chronic kidney disease self-management intervention. Patient Preference and Adherence 11, 1963–1973.

Lim WH, Johnson DW, McDonald SP et al 2019. Impending challenges of the burden of end-stage kidney disease in Australia. Medical Journal of Australia 211(8), 374–380.

Peng S, He J, Huang J et al 2019. Self-management interventions for chronic kidney disease: a systematic review and meta-analysis. BMC Nephrology 20, Article number: 142.

REFERENCES

Agerskov H, Thiesson HC, Pedersen BD 2019. Everyday life experiences in families with a child with kidney disease. Journal of Renal Care 45(4) 205–211.

Almutary H, Douglas C, Bonner A 2016a. Symptom burden in advanced stages of chronic kidney disease. Journal of Renal Care 42(2), 73–82.

Almutary H, Douglas C, Bonner A 2016b. Multidimensional symptom clusters: an exploratory factor analysis in advanced chronic kidney disease. Journal of Advanced Nursing 72(10), 2389–2400.

Almutary H, Douglas C, Bonner A 2017. Towards a symptom cluster model in chronic kidney disease: a structural equation approach. Journal of Advanced Nursing 73, 2450–2461.

ANZDATA 42nd Annual Report 2019. Incidence of renal replacement therapy for end stage kidney disease. Australia and New Zealand Dialysis and Transplant Registry, Adelaide, Australia.

ANZDATA Registry 2018. 41st Report, Chapter 11: Paediatric patients with end stage kidney disease requiring renal replacement therapy. Australia and New Zealand Dialysis and Transplant Registry, Adelaide, Australia.

Australian Institute of Health and Welfare (AIHW) 2019. Chronic kidney disease web report. Online. Available: https://www.aihw.gov.au/reports/chronic-kidney-disease/chronic-kidney-disease/contents/how-many-australians-have-chronic-kidney-disease.

Bakris GL 2019. Major advancements in slowing diabetic kidney disease progression: focus on SGLT2 inhibitors. American Journal of Kidney Diseases 74(5), 573–575.

Bonner A 2019. Adaptation of nursing management: acute kidney injury and chronic kidney disease. In: D Brown, H Edwards, L Seaton et al (eds), Lewis's medical–surgical nursing, 5th edn. Elsevier, Sydney.

Bonner A, Chambers S, Healy H et al 2018. Tracking patients with advanced kidney disease in last 12 months of life. Journal of Renal Care 44(2), 115–122.

Bonner A, Gillespie K, Campbell K et al 2018. Evaluating the prevalence and opportunity for technology use in chronic kidney disease patients: a cross-sectional study. BMC Nephrology 19, Article number 28.

Bonner A, Havas K, Tam V et al 2019. Evaluation of an integrated chronic disease nurse practitioner clinic: rationale, service model and baseline characteristics. Collegian, 26(2), 227–234.

Bonner A, Lloyd AM 2012. Exploring the information practices of people with end stage kidney disease. Journal of Renal Care 38(3), 124–130.

Brown D, Edwards H, Seaton L et al 2019. Lewis's medical surgical nursing, 5th edn. Elsevier, Sydney.

Brown L, Gardner G, Bonner A 2019. A randomized controlled trial testing a decision support intervention for older patients with advanced kidney disease. Journal of Advanced Nursing 75, 3032–3044.

Chan CT, Blankestijn PJ, Dember LM et al 2019. Dialysis initiation, modality choice, access, and prescription: conclusions from a Kidney Disease: Improving Global Outcomes (KDIGO) controversies conference. Kidney International 96(1), 37–47.

Choo SZ, See EJ, Simmonds RE et al 2018. Nocturnal home haemodialysis: the 17 years experience of a single Australian dialysis service. Nephrology 24(10), 1050–1055.

Coleman S, Havas K, Ersham S et al 2017. Patient satisfaction with nurse-led chronic kidney disease clinics: a multicentre evaluation. Journal of Renal Care 43(1), 11–20.

Conway J, Lawn S, Crail S et al 2018. Indigenous patient experiences of returning to country: a qualitative evaluation on the Country Health SA Dialysis bus. BMC Health Services Research 18(1), 1010.

Crews DC, Bello AK, Saadi G et al 2019. Burden, access, and disparities in kidney disease. Kidney International 95, 242–248.

Dinh TTH, Bonner A, Clark R et al 2016. The effectiveness of health education using the teach-back method on adherence and self-management in chronic disease. JBI Database of Systematic Reviews & Implementation Reports 14(1), 210–247.

Drube J, Wan M, Bonthuis M et al 2019. Clinical practice recommendations for growth hormone treatment in children with chronic kidney disease. Nature Reviews Nephrology 15, 577–589.

Evangelidis N, Craig J, Bauman A et al 2019. Lifestyle behaviour change for preventing the progression of chronic kidney disease: a systematic review. BMJ Open 9, e031625.

Fortnum D, Grennan K, Smolonogov T 2015. End-stage kidney disease patient evaluation of the Australian 'My Kidneys, My Choice' decision aid. Clinical Kidney Journal 8(4), 469–475.

Gorham G, Howard K, Zhao Y et al 2019. Cost of dialysis therapies in rural and remote Australia – a micro-costing analysis. BMC Nephrology 20, 231.

Havas K, Douglas C, Bonner A 2018. Meeting patients where they are: improving outcomes in early chronic kidney disease with tailored self-management support (the CKD-SMS study). BMC Nephrology 19, 279.

Hill NR, Fatoba ST, Oke JL et al 2016. Global prevalence of chronic kidney disease – a systematic review and meta-analysis. PloS One 11(7), e0158765.

Hoang LV, Green T, Bonner A 2018. Informal caregivers' experiences of caring for people receiving dialysis: a mixed-methods systematic review. Journal of Renal Care 44(2), 82–95.

Hoang VL, Green T, Bonner A 2019. Informal caregivers of people undergoing haemodialysis: associations between activities and burden. Journal of Renal Care 45(3), 151–158.

Hryciw D, Bonner A 2018. Alterations of renal and urinary tract function across the lifespan. In J Craft, C Gordon, SE Huether et al (eds), Understanding pathophysiology, 3rd edn. Elsevier, Sydney.

Johnson DW, Atai E, Chan M et al 2013. KHA–CARI Guideline: early chronic kidney disease: detection, prevention and management. Nephrology 18, 340–350.

Kidney Health Australia 2020. Chronic Kidney Disease (CKD) management in primary care, 4th edn. Kidney Health Australia, Melbourne.

Krishnasamy R, Gray NA 2018. Low socio-economic status adversely affects dialysis survival in Australia. Nephrology 23(5), 453–460.

Ku E, Lee BJ, Wei J et al 2019. Hypertension in CKD: core curriculum 2019. American Journal of Kidney Disease 74(1), 120–131.

Maley MAL, Patel RS, Lafferty NT et al 2019. A theory-driven, evidence-based approach to implementing the ISPD syllabus – patients as learners. Peritoneal Dialysis International: Journal of the International Society for Peritoneal Dialysis 39(5), 409–413.

Metraiah EH, Brown E 2019. Comprehensive conservative care for patients with advanced chronic kidney disease. Medicine 47(9), 614–617.

Moore C, Skevington S, Wearden A et al 2020. Impact of dialysis on the dyadic relationship between male patients and their female partners. Qualitative Health Research 30(3), 380–390.

Morton RL, Lioufas N, Dansie K et al 2019. Use of patient-reported outcome measures and patient-reported experience measures in renal units in Australia and New Zealand: a cross-sectional survey study. Nephrology 25(1), 14–21.

Nguyen ANL, Kafle MP, Sud K et al 2019. Predictors and outcomes of patients switching from maintenance haemodialysis to peritoneal dialysis in Australia and New Zealand: strengthening the argument for 'peritoneal dialysis first' policy. Nephrology 24(9), 958–966.

Nguyen NT, Douglas C, Bonner A 2019. Effectiveness of self-management program in people with chronic kidney disease: a pragmatic randomized controlled trial. Journal of Advanced Nursing 75(3), 652–664.

Pascoe MC, Thompson DR, Castle DJ et al 2017. Psychosocial interventions for depressive and anxiety symptoms in individuals with chronic kidney disease: systematic review and meta-analysis. Frontiers in Psychology 8, 992.

Peng S, He J, Huang J et al 2019. Self-management interventions for chronic kidney disease: a systematic review and meta-analysis. BMC Nephrology 20, Article number: 142.

Purtell L, Sowa M, Berquier I et al 2018. The kidney supportive care program: baseline results from a new model of care for advanced chronic kidney disease. BMJ Supportive & Palliative Care, Epub ahead of print, doi: 10.1136/bmjspcare-2018-001630.

Rhee EP, Guallar E, Hwang S et al 2020. Prevalence and persistence of uremic symptoms in incident dialysis patients. Kidney360 1(2), 89–92

Sajadi SA, Ebadi A, Moradian ST 2017. Quality of life among family caregivers of patients on hemodialysis and its relevant factors: a systematic review. International Journal of Community Based Nursing and Midwifery 5(3) 206–218.

Shirazian S 2019. Depression in patients undergoing haemodialysis: time to treat. Kidney International 94, 1264–1266.

Van der Willik EM, Hemmelder MH, Bart HAJ et al 2020. Routinely measuring symptom burden and health-related quality of life in dialysis patients: first results from the Dutch registry of patient-reported outcome measures. Clinical Kidney Journal, 1–10.

Venuthurupalli SK, Healy H, Fassett R et al 2019. Chronic kidney disease, Queensland: profile of patient with chronic kidney disease from regional Queensland, Australia: a registry report. Nephrology 24(12), 1257–1264.

Walker RC, Howard K, Morton RL 2017. Home hemodialysis: a comprehensive review of patient-centered and economic considerations. Clinico Economics and Outcomes Research 9, 149–161.

Walker RJ, Tafunai M, Krishnan A 2019. Chronic kidney disease in New Zealand Maori and Pacific people. Seminars in Nephrology 39(3), 297–299.

Webster AC, Nagler EV, Morton RL et al 2017. Chronic kidney disease. The Lancet 389(10075), 1238–1252.

World Health Organization (WHO) 2006. BMI classification. Online. Available: http://www.euro.who.int/en/health-topics/disease-prevention/nutrition/a-healthy-lifestyle/body-mass-index-bmi.

Yamagata K, Hoshino J, Sugiyama H et al 2019. Clinical practice guidelines for renal rehabilitation: systematic reviews and recommendations of exercise therapies in patients with kidney disease. Renal Replacement Therapy 5, 28.

Yapa H, Chambers S, Purtell L et al 2019. The relationship between chronic kidney disease, symptoms and health-related quality of life: a systematic review. Journal of Renal Care 46(2), 74–84.

Yen PH, Leasure AR 2019. Use and effectiveness of the teach-back method in patient education and health outcomes. Federal Practitioner 36(6), 284–289.

CHAPTER 23

Principles for Nursing Practice: Chronic Diseases of the Bowel

MICHELLE WOODS

LEARNING OBJECTIVES

When you have completed this chapter you will be able to:

- explain the pathophysiology of irritable bowel syndrome and inflammatory bowel disease, including Crohn's disease and ulcerative colitis
- outline the nursing role when caring for a patient diagnosed with irritable bowel syndrome or inflammatory bowel disease
- describe the clinical manifestations of inflammatory bowel disease
- describe the effects that altered body image may have on a patient diagnosed with inflammatory bowel disease
- highlight the patient-centred interventions that may be considered when working with patients diagnosed with irritable bowel syndrome.

KEY WORDS

biopsychosocial condition	supportive care
Crohn's disease	ulcerative colitis
inflammatory bowel disease	

INTRODUCTION

This chapter discusses chronic diseases of the bowel, including Crohn's disease (CD) or regional enteritis, ulcerative colitis (UC) and irritable bowel syndrome (IBS). More specifically, the principles and practices of supportive care for patients who have been diagnosed with inflammatory bowel disease (IBD) or with irritable bowel syndrome will be presented.

IBD is a collective group of disorders that are chronic and incurable and characterised by inflammation in the intestinal tract. CD and UC are two prominent and distinctive inflammatory bowel disorders. The disorders share the challenging characteristics of being largely unpredictable in the cycle of relapses (acute exacerbations), remission and in the severity in symptoms. Both are associated with high morbidity and decreased quality of life (QOL) (Jäghult et al 2011).

Epidemiological studies across developed countries highlight a rise in prevalence of these two disorders (Cosnes et al 2011). IBD is said to affect one in 400 people in the United Kingdom (Reid et al 2010), and smaller population studies in New Zealand and Australia (Wilson et al 2010) indicate a rising annual incidence rate of IBD. Interestingly, the increased prevalence in Asia (Molodecky et al 2012), which previously had a low incidence rate, supports the hypothesis of environmental factors associated with the aetiology of IBD.

IBS is a chronic functional bowel disorder and is identified as having a similar rise in prevalence to IBD. It is estimated that IBS prevalence is 10–15% in the UK and 20–25% in the United States (Canavan et al 2014). In Australia, a population-based study found that approximately 9% of participants meet the Rome III criteria for IBS (Boyce et al 2006; see Box 23.1). The prevalence of IBS has been described as markedly

> **BOX 23.1**
> **Rome III Diagnostic Criteria for Irritable Bowel Syndrome**
>
> At least 3 months, with onset at least 6 months previously, of recurrent abdominal pain or discomfort* associated with two or more of the following:
> - improvement with defecation; and/or
> - onset associated with a change in frequency of stool; and/or
> - onset associated with a change in form (appearance) of stool.

*Discomfort means an uncomfortable sensation not described as pain.
Boyce et al 2006.

increased in recent decades, with the age of onset in early adulthood and a corresponding increase in severity of complications and relapses (Gibson 2009).

INCIDENCE/PREVALENCE: NURSING IMPACT

In addition to the patient toll of living with IBD and/or IBS, the rising prevalence for both IBD and IBS has a substantial impact on the global economic burden (Access Economics 2007).

The nature of chronic bowel diseases and the age of onset tend to hinder the normal evolution of independent adulthood. This impingement affects psychological wellbeing and creates challenges for health professionals, patients and families in the provision of best practice of care for sustaining an optimal QOL. The issues arising from psychological, nutritional and other life issues that are associated with chronic illness and IBD have been noted as the most challenging for clinicians (Gibson 2009). Nurses play an integral role in facilitating patients' treatment goals (Reid et al 2010). These goals involve non-pharmacological and pharmacological interventions and aim for intervals that are long in remission and short in acute exacerbations.

The role of the nurse in caring for people at risk and living with IBD and IBS is directly involved with primary, supportive and restorative care. For example, a patient may confide in a primary care nurse, completing a chronic conditions care plan, that she is having multiple bowel motions per day, is periodically bloated and these symptoms are interfering with her capacity to work effectively in her current employment. Through further subjective assessment questions, the nurse identifies that the patient meets the Rome III criteria

(see Box 23.1) for IBS and discusses these concerns with the patient and a medical practitioner for further review.

An acute care nurse may look after a patient experiencing an acute exacerbation of UC that results in a total colectomy with an ileal pouch–anal anastomosis, who requires intravenous medications and supportive parenteral feeding. A specialist IBD nurse and/or nurse practitioner may monitor and provide support for a CD patient post-ileostomy. Additional interventions over time may include supporting the patient and their family in a collaborative plan that foresees strategies to decrease their risk for future exacerbation of CD.

Specific interventions vary depending on the nurse's practice arena, level of specialisation and advancement in practice. Intervention range may include, but is not limited to, initial assessment of IBD and IBS; preparations and ordering of diagnostic investigations; prescribing and titration of medications; education and identification of factors contributing to the patient's capacity to adhere to medication; and providing and referring patients to support services. Central to all nurses is their role in facilitating the patient and their family/carer's understanding and efficacy that is necessary for living with a functionally challenging disease. Specialisation as an IBD nurse in a tertiary setting in Australia is relatively new and has arisen from the need for short-term management of the disease and inequitable access to support and education (Australian Crohn's & Colitis Australia 2013). From a health service delivery viewpoint, Australian research outlined the economic value and impact of an IBD nurse. Outcomes included avoidance of hospital, emergency admissions and outpatient reviews (Leach et al 2014).

As with all chronic conditions, patients may become complex in their care needs and need a multidisciplinary care team to provide optimal care. An IBD patient may interact with the following healthcare providers: general practitioner (GP); medical specialist; gastroenterologist; rheumatologist; practice nurse; nurse practitioner; stoma and/or IBD specialist nurse; dietitian; and psychologist. Further discussion and guidance regarding multidisciplinary teams can be found in Chapter 2.

INFLAMMATORY BOWEL DISEASE: TWO DISTINCTIVE DISORDERS

A nurse's capacity to provide quality nursing care for patients living with IBD is enhanced by a sound understanding of the aetiology, pathophysiology, disease trajectory and treatment options. CD and UC come under the heading of IBD as two distinct diseases with similar characteristics and symptoms. The main difference between Crohn's disease and ulcerative colitis is the location and nature of the inflammatory changes (Nurgali et al 2015). CD is a chronic inflammatory condition non-specific to a single area of the gastrointestinal (GI) system, affecting the whole bowel wall and resulting in transmural lesions (Cullen 2014). The most common sites affected are the terminal ileum, jejunum and colon (Schmelzer 2011). The inflammation process is frequently discontinuous with normal bowel separating portions of diseased bowel.

In the earliest stages of the disease, inflammation promotes lesion formation in the intestinal sub-mucosa, which over time traverses the intestinal wall to eventually involve the mucosa and serosa (Nurgali et al 2015). These lesion formations lead to thickening of the intestinal wall and on inspection can be likened to a cobblestone (Nurgali et al 2015). This leads to intestinal wall lumen narrowing and associated stricture development. The affected areas are in many cases regional, as they may affect one particular area of the bowel, skip a section and then re-present as another affected area. These discontinuous areas are classified as 'skip lesion' (Schmelzer 2011).

The diagnosis of CD is confirmed by symptom history and clinical evaluation. Patient symptoms will vary due to the severity of inflammation and the area of bowel affected (Hompson & Read 2015). Symptoms include increased frequency of bowel motions, abdominal pain, rectal bleeding (although rare), weight loss, reduced appetite and faecal incontinence (Nurgali et al 2015).

The urgency of diarrhoea (bloody in colonic Crohn's) is often associated with mucus. Stricturing or narrowing of the intestine in CD can lead to obstructive symptoms associated with abdominal pain, constipation and vomiting. In more severe exacerbations, anorexia, weight loss and anaemia lead to fatigue.

To exclude anaemia and infections, both acute and chronic, pathology investigations include full blood count and inflammatory markers such as C-reactive protein and erythrocyte sedimentation rate (ESR). Stool cultures provide evidence to exclude infections such as *Clostridium difficile* toxin (Mowat et al 2011). Confirmation of a diagnosis is through the utilisation of ileocolonoscopy and biopsy of the colonic and terminal ileal disease (Morrison et al 2009).

UC is a chronic disease of the bowel that affects the mucosa and sub-mucosa of the colon and rectum. In most cases, the inflammatory process is confined to the rectum and sigmoid colon. However, it may progress to involving the entire colon, stopping at the ileocaecal junction (Schmelzer 2011). The inflamed mucosa becomes oedematous, abscesses form and eventually the bowel mucosa becomes ulcerated. The ulcerations destroy the bowel mucosa and subsequently the patient may experience the primary symptom of bloody diarrhoea with the passage of mucus. Associated symptoms are lower abdominal cramping associated with urgency, called tenesmus (Reid et al 2010). Similar to CD, other manifestations include fatigue, weakness, nausea and anorexia. Typically the symptoms may last for days or weeks, followed by a period of remission. UC can be mild, moderate or severe. Classification is based on the number of bowel motions per day, associated abdominal pain, bleeding from the rectum, elevated temperature, elevated ESR and a drop in haemoglobin (Gastroenterological Society of Australia [GESA] 2013). See Table 23.1, which summarises the distinguishing features of CD and UC.

Manifestations

The underlying autoimmune process of IBD does not confine itself to the bowel and extra intestinal manifestations occur in other body systems and organs. These may involve the dermatological system, ocular system, joints or the hepatobiliary system. Complications of IBD can be the result of severity in inflammation, such as small bowel obstruction, toxic megacolon, fistulas and fissures, perforation and GI blood loss (Orchard et al 2011).

Both UC and CD are associated with an equivalent increased risk of colonic carcinoma (Schmelzer 2011). Patients with UC have 7–30 times more prevalence of carcinoma of the colon than the general population. Factors attributing to increased risk of carcinoma of the colon are the duration of the colitis and the extent of colitis involvement (Orchard et al 2011).

Demographics and Aetiology

The exact cause of IBD is not known, but rather the model in understanding the aetiology is multifactorial, where an autoimmune response is strongly correlated with a genetic predisposition and triggered by modifiable and environmental risk factors. Recently, a greater understanding has been articulated in the literature regarding the interplay of the intestinal microbiota (microbial community) composition and an overactive immune response that leads to chronic inflammation in genetically susceptible individuals. Intestinal inflammation induces dysbiosis, providing a selective growth advantage for disease-producing pathobionts (e.g. facultative anaerobes). A limited immune response allows

TABLE 23.1
Distinguishing Features of Crohn's Disease and Ulcerative Colitis

Key Features	Crohn's Disease	Ulcerative Colitis
Symptoms	Diarrhoea, fever, sores around the anus, abdominal pains and cramps, pain and swelling in the joints, anaemia, fatigue, loss of appetite, weight loss	Bloody diarrhoea, mild fever, inflamed rectum, abdominal pains and cramps, fatigue, loss of appetite, weight loss, pain and swelling in joints
Affected area	Mouth to anus	Colon only
Rectum involvement	Rectum sparing	Always
Inflammation of GI layers	Transmural	Mucosal layers only
Lesions	Granulomas	Granulomas are rare
Frank and occult bleeding per rectum	Up to 1/3 no evidence of bleeding	Most often frank blood
Cure	Incurable	Through colectomy only
	Maintenance therapy is used to reduce the chance of relapse	Maintenance therapy is used to reduce the chance of relapse

Gastroenterological Society of Australia (GESA) 2013.

for outgrowth and invasion of colitogenic microbes, leading to the initiation and perpetuation of chronic gut inflammation (Kostic et al 2014).

Non-Modifiable Risk Factors

The non-modifiable risk factors (Orchard et al 2011) are detailed below.
- Gender: females tend to have a predominance of CD, whereas males tend to have a higher incidence of UC.
- Age: both CD and UC are most commonly diagnosed in late adolescence and early adulthood; however, the diagnosis may occur at any age.
- Race/ethnicity: studies comparing the prevalence of IBD among different ethnic groups suggests genetic predispositions. There is also strong evidence to suggest that CD does have some genetic predisposition, with between 12 and 18% of patients having some family history of the disease (Cullen 2014).
- IBD has been recorded to be 2–4 times greater in Jewish populations as compared to other ethnic groups. Caucasians have a higher incidence of IBD. Ethnic and racial differences may be more related to lifestyle and environmental influences than genetic differences.

Modifiable Risk Factors

Modifiable risk factors (behaviours that contribute to disease probability) are detailed below.
- Cigarette smoking: implications for increased risk for CD (Orchard et al 2011).

- Dietary: considerable speculation but inconsistent findings regarding the role that food antigens may have as a trigger for the inflammatory reaction in IBD. A number of studies have implicated cow's milk, refined sugar, decreased vegetable intake and high fat intake as dietary risk factors for the development of IBD (Punyanganie de Silva et al 2011).
- Non-steroidal anti-inflammatories: studies linked to a risk for the development of IBD and may exacerbate underlying IBD (Ananthakrishnan et al 2012).
- Psychosocial factors: stress as an independent factor does not appear to directly contribute to a diagnosis of IBD. However, stress may play a role in the exacerbation of symptoms possibly via activation of the enteric nervous system and the elaboration of pro-inflammatory cytokines (GESA 2013).

Treatment
Non-pharmacological

Nutritional therapy becomes a central focus in treatments of IBD (Mowat et al 2011). It is essential for patients to have a referral and access to a specialised dietitian with appropriate supplementation instituted as indicated (Lomer et al 2014). Patients are at risk for malnutrition secondary to the disease by avoiding foods perceived by the patient as triggering symptoms and pain and disease sequelae of malabsorption. In addition, long-term administration of steroids adversely results in poor bone mineralisation, resulting in osteoporosis and predisposing children and adolescents to retarded growth (Mowat et al 2011). Osteoporosis is due to the relationship between inflammatory responses and an increase in bone breakdown; the use of corticosteroids as a treatment option; and diminished vitamin D and calcium levels due to malabsorption (Lomer et al 2014).

Patients are particularly at risk for malnutrition in times of acute exacerbations – pain, nausea and diarrhoea. Malnutrition is the result of anorexia, malabsorption, fluid and electrolyte disturbance and side effects from medications (Lomer et al 2014). Patients with CD are susceptible to large amounts of fluid loss due to malabsorption and consequently a reduction of essential electrolytes, especially potassium and magnesium (Ruthruff 2007). Fluid and electrolyte balances are of paramount concern and, if possible, patients should be encouraged to drink between 1 and 2 litres of fluid per day to counteract these large losses (Ruthruff 2007). Due to the involvement of all layers of the GI wall and subsequent damage to intestinal mucosa, diets high in fat or milk and milk products are poorly absorbed (Schmelzer 2011) and are therefore often avoided.

Subsequently, malnutrition leads to fatigue and an inability to carry out some activities of daily living. Assessment for risk for malnutrition can be validated through such tools as the Malnutrition Universal Screening Tool (MUST) available online (www.bapen.org.uk/pdfs/must/must_full.pdf). Of particular importance is the distal bowel's involvement and receptor sites in the absorption of solely bile salts, vitamin B_{12} and magnesium. With both CD and UC, impaired absorption results in nutritional deficiencies.

The most common nutritional deficiencies are:
- calories, protein and fat
- calcium
- vitamin D
- iron
- folic acid
- vitamin B_{12}
- electrolytes and fluid.

Dietary guidelines for IBD are general and highlight recommendations for a balanced and nutritionally dense diet as tolerated and based on preferences. Specific macronutrient and food types are dependent on a person's staging and/or remission and/or relapse of condition. A comprehensive global review of dietary guidelines identifies specific categories for recommendations based on avoiding nutritional deficits, decreasing the risk of flare-ups by omitting foods and chemicals that are known to exacerbate symptoms, such as alcohol and caffeine, eliminating food intolerances such as lactose, maintenance of nutritional needs by amounts and frequency of meals and/or dependent on presence of bowel stricture/luminal narrowing and ostomies (Brown et al 2011).

Over the past 10 years the implications of the gut microbiome role in IBD has been investigated.

The human microbiome (MB) is a diverse and complex microbial community that resides in our GI tracts and has been coined a forgotten target metabolic 'organ' (Blaser 2014).

The capacity to investigate the MB function and its role in disease and health has come to attention through the development of culture independent approaches and has been made possible through advances in gene sequencing technology (Evans et al 2013). The impact of the MB is implicated in a number of human metabolic and physiological functions. These include energy harvesting through nutrient extraction and fermentation of indigestible food substances, synthesis of key substances such as vitamins (B_{12} and K), neurotransmitters such as serotonin, maintenance of gut barrier (mucosa), immune functions, such as protection against infection, systemic immunity–inflammatory and autoimmune disease protection (Blaser 2014).

All of these functions have implications for IBD, onset, prevention or promotion of a flare-up, supportive therapy and the rate of disease progression (Knight-Sepulveda et al 2015).

MB research is in its infancy and a large metagenome project (National Institute of Health Human Microbiome Project [HMP] https://commonfund.nih.gov/hmp/index) is identifying the 'who and what' of the MB (Blaser 2014). What is appreciated is that the MB is a complex and dynamic internal ecosystem. Various ecological principles provide a new appreciation of a dynamic interplay between health and diseases (Rook 2013). For example, in a biome of over 100 trillion microbes, representing 500 different species, symbiosis allows for a relationship between two or more organisms that live closely together as commensal, mutualistic or independent.

Alternatively, dysbiosis is an imbalance (compositional and/or diversity) in the intestinal bacteria that precipitates changes in the normal activities of the GI tract.

Associated with chronic intestinal symptoms of gas, bloating, diarrhoea and constipation that may predispose a person to chronic diseases and contribute to 'leaky gut' syndrome (hypermerable tight junctions), the question is not whether the MB has a role in IBD, but rather for current research to provide insight into how the MB contributes to, promotes or aids in resolving IBD. For people living with IBD, non-pharmacological approaches have focused on how to create a healthy biome. This includes knowledge on what factors contribute to dysbiosis such as environmental toxins, diets that are high in fat/sugar, low in fibre, and a reduction in the overuse of antibiotics and what factors aid in creating and sustaining a health biome (Calafiore et al 2012).

Beyond energy harvesting, the MB has a primary function of maintaining the integrity of the intestinal membrane. The intestinal membrane comprises protein and a cytoskeletal structure with intracellular tight junctions and is in a constant state of remodelling. The intestinal membrane is essential for necessary absorptive functions without compromising barrier exclusion while regulating intestinal permeability (Blaser 2014).

MB contributes to the integrity of the intestinal membrane through the metabolism of dietary plant-derived polysaccharides to short chain fatty acids such as acetate and butyrate. These short chain fatty acids are recognised as 'probiotic' in the provision of nutrients for colonic epithelial cells, antimicrobial secretion, and regulation of apoptosis and proliferation of the mucosa (Sanders 2008). In a state of dysbiosis there is both hypermerable tight junctions of the intestinal membrane and an increase in Gram-negative bacteria that release endotoxin fragments from the cell wall called lipopolysaccharides. Passive diffusion across the hyperpermeable tight junctions leads to a two- to threefold increase of lipopolysaccharides in blood circulation, identified as metabolic toxaemia. Lipopolysaccharides are incorporated into chylomicrons fractions and pro-inflammatory cytokines. The increases in lipopolysaccharides have been positively associated with obesity and type 2 diabetes (Neves et al 2013).

From a nutritional perspective, there has been much speculation about the benefits of probiotic foods and supplements as a means of improving the health of biome. Prebiotics are defined as a non-living non-digestible special form of fibre or carbohydrates and probiotics are referred to as live active microorganisms which, when administered in adequate amounts, will have beneficial effects on its host (Sanders 2008). Although the current research on probiotics as a therapy is promising, there is no regulation of probiotic supplements. Recommendations were not endorsed by professional bodies such as the World Gastroenterology Organization in their Practice Guidelines for the Diagnosis and Management of IBD in 2016 for patients

living with IBD (Bernstein et al 2015). This is partly due to conflicting data and a lack of sufficiently rigorous studies on CD to yield evidence to support or reject probiotic use for this condition (Calafiore et al 2012). Additional placebo-controlled double-blind studies in CD and UC, active and inactive, taking into account other medical therapy, are required before recommendations can be offered on routine use of probiotics in IBD (Knight-Sepulveda et al 2015).

At this time it is well recognised in the gastroenterology literature that patients commonly consume probiotic products with the intent of restoring intestinal microbiota for their health benefits. There are a number of clinical trials that have assessed the therapeutic effects of probiotics for several disorders, including antibiotic or *C. difficile*-associated diarrhoea, IBS and the inflammatory bowel diseases.

To aid in navigation and application of probiotic use, Ciorba (2012) provides an extensive review of the literature to help clinicians decipher condition-specific rationale for using probiotics as therapy and utilising literature-based recommendations. In doing so, a central theme of probiotic use is that in disease states (e.g. IBD) probiotic use may be beneficial as an adjunct to pharmacological treatment. The capacity of probiotics to modify disease symptoms is modest, and for treatment effects to be substantiated, specific strains should be investigated. In addition, not all probiotics are right for all disease states (Ciorba 2012).

Providing patients with specific guidance on what to eat in relation to a diet that influences the onset or course of IBD can be challenging based on the nature of the IBD, but more specially that no IBD diet is supported by robust data. Trials have been limited by noncomparative placebo groups and in controlling for specific dietary macronutrients in taking and ruling out and/or investigating the potential complex interactions between foods and withdrawal and additions of medication (Knight-Sepulveda et al 2015).

Referrals to a dietitian can ensure that specific patient nutritional needs are being met and that patients gain efficacy and confidence in choosing and cooking meals that support their preferences and reduces the risk of flare-ups. Other important sources of dietary information are available through Crohn's and Colitis Australia and the Crohn's and Colitis Foundation of America.

In specific circumstances, protein and caloric support are indicated, such as in perioperative care of patients with significant weight loss. In severe cases of CD, intestinal failure is an indication for parenteral nutrition due to the extremely poor absorption rates of fluids and electrolytes (Schmelzer 2011). Element liquid feeding is an alternative to steroids and may be a consideration for children and adolescents to ensure optimal growth before fusion of epiphyses prohibits growth. This treatment option appears to have an anti-inflammatory effect and does require considerable motivation and dietetic support (Alastair et al 2011).

The chronic nature of CD and UC results in many patients exploring and engaging in alternative treatment options and remedies to relieve their symptoms. While acupuncture, reflexology and aromatherapy are considered appropriate stress reduction techniques, some therapies may interact with prescribed medications, and therefore the patient should be instructed to discuss these therapies with their medical provider, nurse or pharmacist in the first instance (Schmelzer 2011). Notably, patients are at risk of overnight remedies promising 'quick relief' from IBD. Many products marked as 'bowel cleansing' can put patients at further risk for electrolyte imbalances and disruption to bowel flora.

Pharmacological

The goals of IBD treatment are to induce and maintain remission of both clinical symptoms and mucosal inflammation and to re-establish the intestinal barrier. In addition, long-term medical management includes regular monitoring of therapy to minimise medication side effects and long-term adverse effects; eliminate symptoms (abdominal pain, diarrhoea and rectal bleeding); and correct nutritional deficiencies (GESA 2013). A patient's medication regimen is a tailor-made approach where adverse drug reactions and efficacy of treatment are individualised in order to sustain corticosteroid-free remission, decrease complications and to improve quality of life (QOL) (Gastrointestinal Expert Group 2011).

The treatment goal for long remission and symptom-free intervals is often enhanced by the anti-inflammatory and immunosuppressant agents. Treatment is initiated and monitored through a stepwise approach and a top-down approach (Morrison et al 2009). The newer therapeutic classes of medications (i.e. immuno-modulators and biological therapies) enhance treatment goals to change the natural history of the disease and its long-term outcomes, rather than simply to achieve symptomatic control (Gastrointestinal Expert Group 2011). The medical management of IBD (indication of medication class, formulations) is determined by the location of inflammation within the GI tract, the degree of involvement, severity of symptoms, extra-intestinal complications, and response or lack of response to previous treatment (GESA 2013).

5-Amino salicylic acid (5-ASA) drugs, such as sulfasalazine and mesalazine, are anti-inflammatory drugs (oral, enema, suppository formulations). They are prescribed for treating flare-ups and maintaining remission, and are indicated for mild-to-moderate symptoms of UC. The maintenance of remission of intestinal inflammation in CD is controversial and tends to be limited to reduction of post-surgical recurrence limited to the small bowel if used in high doses (Gearry et al 2007).

The use of antibiotic therapy is important in treating secondary complications in IBD, such as abscess and bacterial overgrowth. However, due to the anatomical location of UC, antibiotic treatment has limited efficacy, and an increased risk for antibiotic-associated pseudomembranous colitis. For CD, metronidazole and ciprofloxacin are the most commonly used antibiotics for complications such as perianal disease, fistulas, inflammatory mass and bacterial overgrowth in the setting of strictures (Bernstein et al 2015). Long-term administration (more than 3 months) of antibiotics has been used in CD patients with fistulas or recurrent abscesses near their anus. Patients presenting on antibiotics are at risk for *C. difficile*-associated disease (CDAD), and if presenting with a flare-up of diarrhoeal disease should be checked for *C. difficile* and other fecal pathogens.

Corticosteroids are generally administered for severe exacerbations or 'flare-up' periods of the disease, and are usually continued for up to 3 weeks before being slowly tapered prior to discontinuation (Irving et al 2007; Ruthruff 2007). The route and dose of corticosteroids are determined by the severity of the symptoms and therapeutic response to other drug therapies (Schmelzer 2011). The anti-inflammatory properties of corticosteroids suppress the symptoms of the disease and allow for affected areas to repair; however, patients require close monitoring due to the serious side effects of these drugs (Mayberry et al 2013).

Notable steroid adverse reactions include changes to body appearance, such as acne, weight gain and distribution of fat deposits to the face, neck and abdomen. Daily disturbance in function include poor quality of sleep and metabolic changes, which can lead to impaired glucose tolerance and steroid-induced diabetes.

Immune-system-modifying medications is a category of medications with specific indications for the suppression of the immune system; such as ciclosporin, which is usually used for UC, and anti-metabolite medications such as methotrexate (MTX), used for CD. Thiopurines, such as azathioprine and mercaptopurine, are the long-term maintenance medication therapy for patients with more than mild CD and for chronically active or frequently relapsing UC where 5-ASA drugs sustain maintenance (Mowat et al 2011). The goal of using this class of medication is to control active inflammation, allow for the withdrawal of steroids and ultimately to maintain long-term remission of CD and UC. Because immunomodulators weaken or modulate the activity of the immune system, decreasing the inflammatory response, patients are at risk for serious and opportunistic infections (Moshkovska et al 2011).

Tumor necrosis factor α (TNF-α) is a potent proinflammatory cytokine that plays a pivotal role in the development of Crohn's inflammation. Biological agents, such as anti-tumor necrosis factor (anti-TNF) agents, infliximab and adalimumab, can be first-line therapy in patients who present with aggressive disease and in those with perianal CD. Infliximab and adalimumab can be used concurrently with either thiopurines or methotrexate to enhance the effectiveness and reduce the likelihood of antibody formation (Dassopoulos et al 2013).

Surgery

Surgical intervention for IBD provides an important treatment role when medical treatment is inadequate at providing symptom relief or complications to disease arise. For example, approximately 30–40% of patients with UC will require surgical treatment for complications, such as GI haemorrhage, toxic megacolon, or if there is a disease progression to colorectal carcinoma. Some patients with UC, who have refractory disease, may require a total colectomy with an ileal pouch–anal anastomosis (Schmelzer 2011). For patients living with CD for up to 20 years, 80% will have at least one bowel surgery (Orchard et al 2011). Over the course of the past 20 years, decreases in morbidity and mortality from IBD have been associated with the combination of medical–surgical therapies and the advancement of surgical approaches. The indications leading to surgery have not changed significantly; however, improved knowledge of the course of both CD and UC has led to an evolving surgical approach. For example, complex fistulas require aggressive immunomodulating therapy in combination with surgery. Surgical therapy for complex fistulas involves less invasive techniques for closure of high fistulas to prevent incontinence associated with damage to the anal sphincters (Nandivad et al 2012).

Irritable Bowel Syndrome

It's terrible. The symptoms are sometimes constant. There's diarrhoea and abdominal pain or constipation and bloating. I can't commit to anything too far in advance or anything that is regularly occurring. Wherever I go I need to find out where the toilets are; I often feel embarrassed (Patient quote).

Irritable bowel syndrome (IBS) is a functional bowel disorder in which abdominal pain or discomfort is associated with defecation and/or a change in bowel habit. Sensations of discomfort (bloating), distension and disordered defecation are commonly associated features (National Institute for Health and Clinical Excellence [NICE] 2015). In developed countries the majority of patients diagnosed with IBS are women, and typically first present with clinical symptoms between 30 and 50 years of age (Boyce et al 2006). IBS is one of the most common GI diseases and accounts for approximately 50% of referrals to gastroenterology outpatient clinics (Ness 2011). The aetiology of IBS is understood as a biopsychosocial disorder and multifactorial in nature (El-Salhy 2012). It is also not uncommon for patients with IBS to have other functional GI disorders, such as functional dyspepsia and extraintestinal symptoms, including irritable bladder, fibromyalgia and chronic pelvic pain (Gibson 2012). Multiple factors predisposing a person to IBS have been identified and categorised as genetics; dietary factors, such as lactose intolerance; inflammation, such as yeast infection; and neurotransmitter, such as serotonin imbalances (El-Salhy 2012). Recent research has been influential in the understanding of IBS as partly a function of low-grade systemic inflammation. Underlying IBS pathophysiology related to inflammations has been identified as an interplay between the GI immune system, microbial antigens and food (Mansueto et al 2015).

The perception of stress initiates and/or exacerbates the intensity of GI motility that leads to a heightened perception of sensation. The altered bowel function, motility and sensation in the small bowel and colon are modulated from the central nervous system, referred to as the brain–gut axis (Ness 2011). Unaddressed chronic and severe psychosocial factors result in poor resolution of IBS symptoms (Drossman et al 2011), which exemplifies the biopsychosocial relationship of chronic conditions (van Tilburg et al 2013). It is unlikely that psychological factors cause IBS, but the evidence suggests that depression and anxiety exert a strong influence on patients living with

IBS compared to non-IBS sufferers. Associations have been made between psychiatric disturbances and IBS pathogenesis. Seeking consultation for IBS symptoms is clearly dependent on the number of symptoms reported (especially abdominal pain), and has also been shown to correlate with high depression and anxiety scores (El-Salhy 2012). Sexual and physical abuse may play a role in IBS as well. Reports from specialty clinics to which patients with severe cases of IBS are referred indicate that a significant percentage of women with IBS have a history of abuse (Leserman & Drossman 2007). Difficulty arises in interpreting the implications of co-morbidity between IBS and psychiatric disorders as primary or secondary (reactionary) (Ness 2011).

Treatment
Non-pharmacological
Foods can be related to symptoms where GI stimulants or irritants, such as spicy and fatty foods, caffeine and unrefined carbohydrates, cause contraction of the intestine and cramping (Böhn et al 2013). The GI deficiency of lactulose reduces intolerance to dairy foods and patients with lactose intolerance find that symptoms decrease when they have a limited amount of dairy products (GESA 2006).

Gibson and Shepherd (2010) provide evidence of clinical trials restricting rapidly fermenting short-chain carbohydrates (FODMAP) in the control of functional gut symptoms. It is now widely accepted that this approach in restriction for a patient with nil persistent symptoms has a durable effect in controlling symptoms (Halmos et al 2014; Gibson et al 2013). Referral to a dietitian is warranted if patients need advice on the application of an elimination diet to assess trigger foods.

Similarly with IBD: non-pharmacological strategies such as relaxation therapy, hypnotherapy, short-term psychodynamic psychotherapy and cognitive behaviour therapy have been shown to decrease symptom distress (Taylor & Taylor 2011).

Pharmacological
Medications provide partial relief of symptoms, depending on the patient's symptom presentation. Therapy focuses on symptomatic relief of pain, diarrhoea and constipation (Gastrointestinal Expert Group 2011; GESA 2006). However, many IBS patients have no long-lasting relief of symptoms after drug treatment. Over-the-counter medications, such as paracetamol and ibuprofen, can provide some relief for pain, but ibuprofen can cause gastritis.

CHRONIC DISEASES OF THE BOWEL: NURSING IMPLICATIONS
Nursing is a discipline that focuses on the understanding of human responses to the human conditions of illness, disease and injury. As a prime caregiver and advocate for patient self-management, the nurse needs to be able to demonstrate patient-centred care that is responsive to complex and challenging disorders. The nurse works in partnership with patients towards the patient outcome of self-management, which is:

engaging in activities that protect and promote health, monitoring and managing of symptoms and signs of illness, managing the impacts of illness on functioning, emotions and interpersonal relationships and adhering to treatment regimens (Grunman & Von Korff 1996, p. 1).

The effects of IBD and IBS on QOL include overall health; vitality; sexual function; sleep; social functioning; and bodily pain. Nursing assessment identifies how these factors are related to behaviours that contribute to the development of the condition, alter mobility and body image and behaviours that sustain remission.

Behaviours that Contribute to the Development of the Condition or Sustain Remission
Assessment of a patient's knowledge and understanding of their disease, its process, triggers, support systems and a patient's attributes of resilience and capacity to sustain treatment protocols in remission are key to establishing a collaborative care plan. Furthermore, the role in chronic condition management may be one of identifying lifestyle behaviours that put the patient at risk for optimal health, such as cigarette smoking. A chronic condition management plan is only as good as the level of patient engagement in problem-solving and negotiating achievable actions that are patient-centred. The role of the nurse, therefore, is in facilitation, whereby through a process of negotiation and information sharing, treatment options and choices are discussed (Whayman 2011).

Document the plan in the patient's notes and give the patient a copy. This may be in the form of a formal care plan into which other healthcare providers have input, a diagnosis-specific diary or monitor, or a centre-specific record (Royal Australian College of General Practitioners 2008).

Small achievable steps are as follows (but not limited to):
- ensuring sufficient rest and sleep and avoiding exhaustion

- chewing food very slowly, and avoiding overeating
- ingesting food only when emotionally calm and real hunger is present
- avoiding foods that are known triggers, such as coffee, tea, soft drinks, alcohol and so forth
- maintaining relationships with friends and family
- engaging in work and activities that are rewarding.

The chronic nature of IBD and at times increased disease activity are indicators of stress, depression and poor psychological health for patients (Goodhand et al 2012). Anxiety may not only relate to the diagnosis and symptom control, but also be associated with issues such as loss of income and an increase in family expenditure due to the cost of medical appointments, hospitalisation and medications (Park & Jeen 2016). Nurses are in a prime position to assess patients and provide an environment where the patient and caregiver can freely discuss concerns, worries and fears. During times when the patient is not managing with sustaining a plan or is exhibiting signs and symptoms of depression and anxiety, a referral to a psychologist may aid the patient and their family in developing coping skills.

For patients living with IBS, the nature of the problems can be identified by the patient writing a diary of their food intake and symptoms, including the number and type of stools (Bristol Stool tool, available at www.continence.org.au/pages/bristol-stool-chart.html) and the presence, severity and duration of pain. Patient awareness of these factors and symptom pattern recognition will greatly enhance self-assessment and provide the impetus to change behaviours and treatment options that can ultimately affect their condition. For example, in menstruating women, symptoms typically increase in severity immediately before or at onset of menses (Lim et al 2013). Over the course of managing IBS, patients also need to learn the signs and symptoms that would indicate further investigation. These have been identified as rectal bleeding, significant weight loss, fat substances in stool, diarrhoea at night and fever. Faecal occult blood testing is not an appropriate test for people with IBS symptoms (GESA 2006).

Altered Mobility, Body Image and Fatigue

The stigma attached to bowel disease, as for any disease that is not visible, often means that the patient may decline to discuss symptoms, fears and concerns (Chelvanayagam 2014). Altered body image (which may lead to low self-esteem) due to either the disease itself (pallor, skin lesions) or the side effects of treatment (weight gain from drug therapy) has a huge impact on wellbeing.

During an acute exacerbation, patients may feel lethargic or dirty, and changes in their physical appearance, secondary to weight gain due to corticosteroid treatment or weight loss due to chronic diarrhoea and malnutrition, may affect their willingness to engage in social activities. Diarrhoea and the subsequent odour are often a concern. Deodorisers and wipes should be kept close by to ensure that the dignity of the patient is maintained. Another factor to consider is perianal skin care, because often this area becomes excoriated and uncomfortable due to frequent diarrhoea (Schmelzer 2011). Skin integrity should also be a strong focus for the nurse. Redness and tenderness near the anus and surrounding perineum are aggravated by diarrhoea (Ruthruff 2007).

Faecal incontinence and urgency for bowel movements can inhibit patients' confidence in employment, travel and social interactions. Consumer support web-based organisations such as Crohn's and Colitis Australia offer patients support with problem-solving ideas. For example, the Can't Wait Card aids people living with Crohn's or colitis (IBD) to gain access to a toilet in times of urgency (available at www.cantwait.net.au/). The National Institute of Clinical Excellence (2015) recommends that the patient continuing to have faecal incontinence should be referred to a specialist. Practical advice for patients with faecal incontinence includes, but is not limited to:

- eat small, frequent meals
- reduce intake of fibre, spicy and fried foods
- avoid caffeine and other stimulants (artificial sweeteners)
- use simple pelvic floor exercises
- try neutralising sprays
- take an emergency kit when you go out
- wear clothes that conceal accidents
- when travelling, know your journey and plan your route.

Fatigue is multifactorial and can be attributable to a number of reasons, requiring a comprehensive assessment and investigative pathology. Fatigue can be attributable to poor sleep throughout the night due to nocturnal diarrhoea and abdominal pain. Other factors include malnutrition and iron deficit anaemia. In times of an acute exacerbation, restricted activity and bed rest are to be encouraged (Schmelzer 2011) during symptomatic episodes. Surgical interventions, such as a resection of the affected area or formation of a stoma, can lead to impaired body image and is a challenging impairment to bodily function (Cullen 2016). Nurses can aid in stoma management and/or refer the patient to specialist nurses.

The impact of IBD and IBS on sexuality and sexual function is significant (Access Economics 2007). Principles in assessing and addressing QOL and altered body image pertaining to sexuality and sexual function are addressed in Chapter 7. See Box 23.2 regarding how to measure the QOL.

Interventions to Attain Adherence

A key component of the treatment regimen for IBD is medication management, because medication therapy may induce remission (Hompson & Read 2015) and reduce the incidence of relapse. In addition, the adherence of oral vitamins such as vitamin D and calcium is recommended to promote bone health (Punyanganie de Silva et al 2011). Clear review of the patient's and family's knowledge and verification of medications is necessary to enhance their understanding of the indication and rationale. Equally important is assessing the patient's beliefs in medication administration and side effects experienced. In addition, assessment of complementary alternative therapies is necessary to identify the drug interactions (Schmelzer 2011).

Notably the efficacy of medications in sustaining patients in remission is enhanced through the consistency of administration. Improving patient understanding of the disease may assist in identifying the precursory signs and symptoms, which may in turn reduce relapse rates (Greenley et al 2013). For example,

studies have shown 5-ASA drug regimens have a relatively low compliance rate (Moshkovska et al 2011). Problem-solving with a UC patient who does not adhere to daily administration may involve changing the delivery from twice-daily administration to once a day and/or highlighting the association of decreased risk of colorectal cancer with the consistent administration of 5-ASA drugs (Mowat et al 2011).

Core interventions that may promote compliance include access to support groups; rapid access and triage to health services; and patient and family educational strategies (Ruthruff 2007). Support groups provide an avenue for patients to share their experiences and have the ability to develop coping skills and strategies (Cullen 2016). Support groups can attempt to overcome the isolation and fear associated with IBD and offer additional support to that provided by family and friends (Greenley et al 2013).

Education and Family and Carer Support

While medical treatment aims at controlling inflammation, education centres on patient self-management, where the patient ultimately becomes the expert in managing their condition with the assistance of support networks. As with any chronic disease, patients with IBD must manage their treatment regimens as well as any symptoms that may arise. This requires focus and commitment while they still try to maintain a 'normal' life (IBD Standards Group 2013).

Anticipatory guidance related to outcomes and disease process, as well as disease trajectory and management may also be provided. However, it is important to discuss this information once the patient has demonstrated a readiness to learn more (Panés et al 2014). Ongoing support and education pertaining to medication management, diet nutrition and lifestyle changes are the prime focus of the nurse. Keeping patients informed about recommended dietary intakes, pain management, fluid intake and associated stress management techniques, including low-impact exercises and relaxation strategies, will provide significant emotional support (Ruthruff 2007).

The role of the nurse specialist in the field of IBD is now recognised in many countries (Reid et al 2010), with nurses working alongside patients and their families to provide support, assistance and education. However, if access to a clinical nurse specialist is not available it is important for the patient and their family to have regular contact with their GP, and to visit a dietitian. The patient and family may also choose to join a community support group related to IBD.

BOX 23.2
Measuring Quality of Life
Validated Questionnaires Useful to Assess Quality of Life and Gut Health

IBS-Quality of life (IBS-QOL)	Validated for assessment of QOL specific to IBS: 34 questions
Inflammatory Bowel Disease Questionnaire (IBDQ)	Validated for assessment of health-related quality of life (HRQOL) in adult patients with IBD
Bowel Disease Questionnaire (BDQ)	Validated to distinguish patients with functional and organic GI disease
Health Status Questionnaire (HSQ-12)	Validated for assessment of HRQoL in the general population
Short Form Health Survey SF-12 (SF-12)	Validated for assessment of HRQoL in the general population

Bischoff 2011.

Family support and education in conjunction with patient education are essential areas of focus. For example, families of patients with Crohn's disease must not only deal with the debilitating effects of this condition, but also the possible long-term effects, which include ongoing hospital admissions and, at times, surgical interventions and stoma formation (Reid et al 2010).

Quality of Life

Panés and colleagues (2014) suggest that 88.5% of individuals with Crohn's disease experience a significantly diminished QOL due to the chronic nature of the condition. It is therefore a disease that is difficult for the patient to deal with because, as mentioned previously, most patients are diagnosed during the prime of their life. QOL may become affected due to the isolating nature of the disease, as some individuals claim they have lost control over their body.

Although IBS is not a life-threatening condition, it can have a disabling impact upon the patient's health and lifestyle (Gethins et al 2011). Patients with IBS commonly report that symptoms interfere with work, social activities and personal relationships (Ness 2011). The patients who experience constipation-dominant IBS describe the straining of stool as leaving them with the feeling of incomplete evacuation. Patients in the diarrhoea-predominant group experience an increase in gut motility and secretions, often leading to urgency and often faecal incontinence (Hompson & Read

2015). Non-gut symptoms reported include lethargy, heartburn, backache, nausea, urinary problems, weakness, palpitations and loss of appetite (GESA 2006). It is the summation and chronicity of these symptoms and presence of pain that reduces patients' QOL on multiple levels, including diminished physical, social and emotional wellbeing (Hompson & Read 2015).

Finally, the evaluation of QOL in living with a chronic condition can be further validated, measured through the utilisation of QOL surveys and assessment tools (see Box 23.2) that include disease-specific questions. These can be utilised to support a program targeted at the patient living with IBD and IBS or as individual markers in living with a chronic and challenging condition.

CONCLUSION

Living with a chronic bowel disease can be a debilitating and frustrating experience, as the patient and their family members come to terms with symptom control and management. While there is no one single treatment modality, supportive care of patients and their family members focuses on careful explanation, reassurance and education relating to diet, lifestyle factors and pharmacological interventions. Continuity of care is of utmost importance for these patients, and nurses are in a prime position where they can provide this care, based on individualised managed care plans.

CASE STUDY 23.1

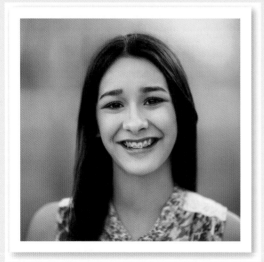

iStockphoto/aldomurillo.

You are a school nurse at a high school and Amy, a 15-year-old female student, comes into your clinic because she cannot complete her exams. She states that she has terrible diarrhoea – foul smelling and bloody. She is fearful of faecal incontinence, as this would be humiliating and embarrassing. She states that this happened a year ago and she was diagnosed with UC. Amy states, 'I went on medications and then it went away and I thought I would not have to worry about it again'. She states that she has hidden the symptoms of abdominal pain and weight loss for the past month, but she cannot continue to hide them. She did recall that her parents and boyfriend had pestered her to take the medications, but she did not see the point.

Amy says she is feeling isolated and none of her friends know that she has this 'disease'. She asks for your help. She currently does have a GP, but has not kept up with appointments.

In assessment, you confirm that Amy has a fair understanding of UC, but does not understand the chronic nature of UC. She has not taken her sulfasalazine for 6 months.

(Crohn's & Colitis Australia [CCA] 2013)

CASE STUDY 23.1 – cont'd

CASE STUDY QUESTIONS

1. What are the knowledge deficits and behaviours contributing to Amy's reason for seeking care?
2. Discuss how you would establish a collaborative management plan with Amy.
3. Discuss the specifics of the following nursing interventions you would utilise when working with Amy: clinical; educational; advocacy; referral; case management.

CASE STUDY 23.2

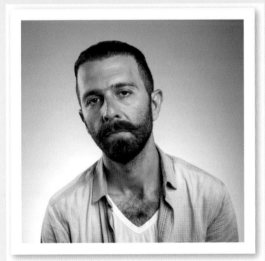

iStockphoto/Barcin.

You are a community nurse taking care of Allan, who is 4 days postoperative for a bowel resection. He had resection of the terminal ileum and a hemicolectomy, removing the caecum and appendix surgery, and did not necessitate an ostomy.

Allan is a 33-year-old male with a 10-year history of Crohn's disease. He has his own business and has managed his Crohn's via conservative therapy with medications and diet. Intermittent flare-ups have increased substantially over the past 2 years and he attributes this to increased stress with his business. He has controlled episodes of relapses with steroids. Over the past year he has lost 15 kg and is malnourished.

Post-surgery Allan is now taking immunosuppressants, immunomodulators (mercaptopurine and azathioprine) and antibody therapy (infliximab) for prevention of recurrence after surgery.

As you change his dressing Allan states that he is overwhelmed and does not know how he is going to manage. Allan confides in you: 'It has just hit me – I am worried that my children will get this ...'. In addition, he was told by the gastroenterologist that his bone density test is showing signs of osteoporosis.
(Schmelzer 2011)

CASE STUDY QUESTIONS

1. Describe what you would assess to aid Allan in his adjustment postoperatively and his setback with Crohn's disease.
2. Explain the rationale for his new medication regimen.
3. What focus and resources would you utilise to problem-solve with Allan and his family?
4. Allan shares that he is fearful of losing his relationship with his wife secondary to sexual dysfunction. How would you explore this further with Allan?

Reflective Questions

1. Describe the differences between Crohn's disease (CD) and ulcerative colitis (UC).
2. Outline the disease management goals for IBD.
3. List and expand on nursing strategies/interventions you would demonstrate to decrease a patient's susceptibility to relapse or remission. What resources would you utilise?

RECOMMENDED READING

Brown AC, Rampertab SD, Mullin GE 2011. Existing dietary guideline for Crohn's disease and ulcerative colitis. Expert Review of Gastroenterology & Hepatology 5(3), 411–425.

Czuber-Dochan W, Norton C, Bredin F et al 2014. Assessing fatigue in patients with inflammatory bowel disease. Gastrointestinal Nursing 12(8).

Ramdeen M, Poullis A, Gupta S et al 2014. Motivational interviewing to improve inflammatory bowel disease outcomes. Gastrointestinal Nursing 12(4).

RECOMMENDED WEBSITES

American Gastroenterological Association: www.gastro.org/.

Crohn's & Colitis Australia: www.crohnsandcolitis.com.au/.

Gastroenterological Society of Australia (GESA): www.gesa.org.au/about.asp?id=5.

International Foundation for Functional Gastrointestinal Disorders: www.iffgd.org.

Irritable Bowel Syndrome Association: www.aboutibs.org; www.ibsassociation.org/.

Self-help and support groups

IBD Support Australia: www.ibdsupport.org.au/about-ibd.

Irritable Bowel Syndrome Self-help and Support Group: www.IBSgroup.org.

REFERENCES

Access Economics Pty Limited for the Australian Crohn's and Colitis Association 2007. The economic costs of Crohn's disease and ulcerative colitis. Improving Inflammatory Bowel Disease Care Across Australia. March 2013. Online. Available: www.crohnsandcolitis.com.au/research/studies-reports/.

Alastair F, Emma G, Emma P 2011. Nutrition in inflammatory bowel disease. JPEN. Journal of Parenteral and Enteral Nutrition 35(5), 571–580.

Ananthakrishnan A, Higuchi L, Huang E et al 2012. Aspirin, nonsteroidal anti-inflammatory drug use, and risk for Crohn disease and ulcerative colitis: a cohort study. Annals of Internal Medicine 156, 350.

Australian Crohn's and Colitis Association 2013. Improving inflammatory bowel disease care across Australia. PriceWaterhouseCoopers. Online. Available: www.crohnsandcolitis.com.au/research/studies-reports/.

Bernstein C, Fried M, Krabshuis J et al 2015. World Gastroenterology Organization practice guidelines for the diagnosis and management of IBD. Inflammatory Bowel Diseases 16(1), 112–124.

Bischoff S 2011. Gut health – a new objective medicine? BioMed Central 9, 24. Retrieved May 2016. Online. Available: www.biomedicentral.com/1741-7015/9/2/4 © Bischoff; licensee BioMed Central Ltd.

Blaser MJ 2014. The microbiome revolution. The Journal of Clinical Investigation 124(10), 4162–4165.

Böhn L, Störsrud S, Törnblom H et al 2013. Self-reported food-related gastrointestinal symptoms in IBS are common and associated with more severe symptoms and reduced quality of life. American Journal of Gastroenterology 108(5), 634–641.

Boyce P, Talley N, Burke C et al 2006. Epidemiology of the functional gastrointestinal disorders according to Rome II criteria: an Australian population-based study. International Medicine Journal 36, 28–36.

Brown A, Rampertab S, Mullin G 2011. Existing dietary guidelines for Crohn's disease and ulcerative colitis. Expert Review of Gastroenterology & Hepatology 5(3), 411–425.

Calafiore A, Gionchetti P, Calabrese C et al 2012. Probiotics, prebiotics and antibiotics in the treatment of inflammatory bowel disease. Journal of Gastroenterology and Hepatology Research 1(6).

Canavan C, West J, Card T 2014. The epidemiology of irritable bowel syndrome. Clinical Epidemiology 6, 71–80.

Chelvanayagam S 2014. Stigma, taboos, and altered bowel function. Gastrointestinal Nursing 12(1), 16–22.

Cosnes J, Gower-Rousseau C, Seksik P et al 2011. Epidemiology and natural history of inflammatory bowel diseases. Gastroenterology 140(6), 1785–1794.

Crohn's and Colitis Australia (CCA) 2013. Students with IBD: a guide for primary, secondary, and tertiary educators. Online. Available: www.crohnsandcolitis.com.au/site/wp-content/uploads/CCA-IBD-Education-Information-Booklet-Final.pdf.

Cullen M 2016. Crohn's disease. Nursing Standard 28(48), 19.

Dassopoulos T, Sultan S, Falck-Ytter T et al 2013. American Gastroenterological Association Institute technical review on the use of thiopurines, methotrexate, and anti-TNF-α biologic drugs for the induction and maintenance of remission in inflammatory Crohn's disease. Gastroenterology 145, 1464–78.e1-5.

Drossman D, Chang L, Bellamy N et al 2011. Severity in irritable bowel syndrome: a Rome Foundation Working Team report. American Journal of Gastroenterology 106, 1749–1759.

El-Salhy M 2012. Irritable bowel syndrome: diagnosis and pathogenesis. World Journal of Gastroenterology 18(37), 5151–5163.

Evans JM, Morris LS, Marchesi JR 2013. The gut microbiome: the role of a virtual organ in the endocrinology of the host. The Journal of Endocrinology 218(3), R37–R47.

Gastroenterological Society of Australia (GESA) 2013. Australian guidelines for general practitioners and physicians inflammatory bowel disease, 3rd ed. Online. Available: http://membes.gesa.org.au/membes/files/Clinical%20Guidelines%20and%20Updates/Inflammatory_Bowel_Disease_2013.pdf.

Gastroenterological Society of Australia (GESA) 2006. Irritable bowel syndrome, 2nd ed. Online. Available: www.gesa.org.au/index.cfm//resources/clinical-guidelines-and-updates/irritable-bowel-syndrome/.

Gastrointestinal Expert Group 2011. Functional lower gastrointestinal disorders. In: Therapeutic Guidelines: Gastrointestinal. Version 5. Therapeutic Guidelines Ltd, Melbourne. Inflammatory Bowel Disease (rev. 2014 Oct).

Gearry R, Ajlouni Y, Nandurkar S et al 2007. 5-Aminosalicylic acid (mesalazine) use in Crohn's disease: a survey of the opinions and practice of Australian gastroenterologists. Inflammatory Bowel Diseases 13(8), 1009–1015.

Gethins S, Duckett T, Shatford C et al 2011. Self-management programme for patients with long-term inflammatory bowel disease. Gastrointestinal Nursing 9(3).

Gibson P 2012. How to treat irritable bowel syndrome. Australian Doctor. Online. Available: www.australiandoctor.com.au.

Gibson P 2009. Overview of inflammatory bowel disease in Australia in the last 50 years. Journal of Gastroenterology and Hepatology 24(Suppl. 3), S63–S68.

Gibson P, Barrett J, Muir J 2013. Functional bowel symptoms and diet. Internal Medicine Journal 43(10), 1067–1074.

Gibson P, Shepherd S 2010. Evidence-based dietary management of functional gastrointestinal symptoms: The FODMAP approach. Journal of Gastroenterology and Hepatology 25, 252–258.

Goodhand J, Wahed M, Mawdsley JE et al 2012. Mood disorders in inflammatory bowel disease: relation to diagnosis, disease activity, perceived stress, and other factors. Inflammatory Bowel Diseases 18(12), 2301–2309.

Greenley RN, Kunz JH, Walter J et al 2013. Practical strategies for enhancing adherence to treatment regimen in inflammatory bowel disease. Inflammatory Bowel Diseases 19(7), 1534–1545.

Grunman J, Von Korff M 1996. Indexed bibliography on self management for people with chronic disease. Centre for Advancement in Health, Washington DC.

Halmos E, Power V, Shepherd S et al 2014. A diet low in FODMAPs reduces symptoms of irritable bowel syndrome. Gastroenterology 146(1), 67–75.

Hompson J, Read N 2015. Managing the symptoms of irritable bowel syndrome. Nurse Prescribing 13(5), 230–234 5p.

Inflammatory Bowel Disease (IBD) Standards Group 2013. Standards for the healthcare of people who have inflammatory bowel disease (IBD Standards) 2013 update. Online. Available: www.ibdstandards.org.uk.

Irving P, Gearry B, Sparrow P et al 2007. Review article: appropriate use of corticosteroids in Crohn's disease. Alimentary Pharmacology & Therapies 26, 313–329.

Jäghult S, Saboonchi F, Johansson U et al 2011. Identifying predictors of low health related quality of life among patients with inflammatory bowel disease: comparison between Crohn's disease and ulcerative colitis with disease duration. Journal of Clinical Nursing 20, 1578–1587.

Knight-Sepulveda K, Kais S, Santalolalla R 2015. Diet and inflammatory bowel disease. Gastroenterology and Hepatology 11(8), 511–520.

Kostic A, Xavier R, Gevers D 2014. The microbiome in inflammatory bowel diseases: current status and the future ahead. Gastroenterology 146(6), 1489–1499.

Leach P, De Silva M, Mountifield R et al 2014. The effect of an inflammatory bowel disease nurse position on service delivery. Journal of Crohn's & Colitis 8(5), 370–374.

Leserman J, Drossman D 2007. Relationship of abuse history to functional gastrointestinal disorders and symptoms: some possible mediating mechanisms. Trauma, Violence and Abuse 8, 331–343.

Lim S, Nam C, Kim Y et al 2013. The effect of the menstrual cycle on inflammatory bowel disease: a prospective study. Gut and Liver 7(1), 51–57.

Lomer M, Gourgey R, Whelan K 2014. Current practice in relation to nutritional assessment and dietary management of enteral nutrition in adults with Crohn's disease. Journal of Human Nutrition and Dietetics 27(Suppl. 2), 28–35.

Malnutrition Universal Screening Tool (MUST). Online. Available: www.bapen.org.uk/pdfs/must/must_full.pdf.

Mansueto P, D'Alcamo A, Seidita A et al 2015. Food allergy in irritable bowel syndrome: the case of non-celiac wheat sensitivity. World Journal of Gastroenterology 21(23), 7089–7109.

Mayberry J, Lobo A, Ford A et al 2013. NICE clinical guideline (CG152): the management of Crohn's disease in adults, children and young people. Alimentary Pharmacology and Therapies 37, 195–203.

Molodecky N, Soon S, Rabi D et al 2012. Increasing incidence and prevalence of the inflammatory bowel diseases with time, based on systematic review. Gastroenterology 142(1), 46–54.

Morrison G, Headon B, Gibson P 2009. Update on inflammatory bowel disease. Australian Family Physician 38(12), 956.

Moshkovska T, Stone M, Smith R et al 2011. Impact of a tailored patient preference intervention in adherence to 5-Aminosalicylic acid medication in ulcerative colitis: results from an exploratory randomized controlled trial. Inflammatory Bowel Diseases 17, 1874–1881.

Mowat C, Cole A, Windsor A et al 2011. Guidelines for the management of inflammatory bowel disease in adults. Gut 60(5), 571–607.

Nandivada P, Poylin V, Nagle D 2012. Advances in the surgical management of inflammatory bowel disease. Current Opinion in Gastroenterology 28(1), 47–51.

National Institute for Health and Clinical Excellence (NICE) 2015. Clinical practice guideline: irritable bowel syndrome in adults: diagnosis and management of irritable bowel syndrome in primary care. Online. Available: www.nice.org.uk/guidance/cg61/resources/irritable-bowel-syndrome-in-adults-diagnosis-and-management-975562917829.

Ness W 2011. Individual treatment for irritable bowel syndrome. Nursing Times 108(30-31) 20.

Neves AL, Coelho J, Couto L et al 2013. Metabolic endotoxemia: a molecular link between obesity and cardiovascular risk. Journal of Molecular Endocrinology 51(2), R51–R64.

Nurgali K, Wildbore C, Craft J et al (eds) 2015. Understanding pathophysiology, 2nd ed. Mosby, Elsevier Australia, Chatswood.

Orchard TR, Goldin RD, Tekkis PP et al 2011. An atlas of investigation and management. UK Atlas Medical Publishing, Oxford.

Panés J, O'Connor M, Peyrin-Biroulet L et al 2014. Improving quality of care in inflammatory bowel disease: what changes can be made today? Journal of Crohn's & Colitis 8(9), 919–926.

Park SC, Jeen YT 2016. The mental health state of quiescent inflammatory bowel disease patients. Gut and Liver 10(3), 330–331.

Punyanganie de Silva S, Lund E, Chan S et al 2011. Is diet involved in the etiology of ulcerative colitis and Crohn's disease? A review of the experimental and epidemiological literature. Inflammatory Bowel Disease Monitor 12(1), 14–22.

Reid L, Chivers S, Plummer V et al 2010. Inflammatory bowel disease management: a review of nurses' roles in Australia and the United Kingdom. The Australian Journal of Advanced Nursing 27(2), 19–26.

Rook GA 2013. Regulation of the immune system by biodiversity from the natural environment: an ecosystem service essential to health. Proceedings of the National Academy of Sciences of the United States of America 110(46), 18360–18367.

Royal Australian College of General Practitioners 2008. Chronic condition self-management guidelines – summary for nurses and allied health professionals. RACGP, South Melbourne, Vic.

Ruthruff B 2007. Clinical review of Crohn's disease. Journal of the American Academy of Nurse Practitioners 19, 392–397.

Sanders ME 2008. Probiotics: definition, sources, selection, and uses. Clinical Infectious Diseases: an Official Publication of the Infectious Diseases Society of America 46 (Suppl. 2), S58–S61.

Schmelzer M 2011. Nursing management: lower gastrointestinal problems. In: D Brown, H Edwards et al, Lewis's medical–surgical nursing: Assessment and management of clinical problems, 5th edn. Elsevier, Chatswood.

Taylor NS, Taylor KM 2011. Complementary and alternative medicine in inflammatory bowel disease. Gastrointestinal Nursing 9(6), 32–39.

van Tilburg M, Palsson O, Whitehead W 2013. Which psychological factors exacerbate irritable bowel syndrome? Development of a comprehensive model. Journal of Psychosomatic Research 74(6), 486–492.

Whayman K 2011. Supporting and educating patients. In: K Whayman, J Duncan, M O'Connor (eds), Inflammatory bowel disease nursing. MA Healthcare Ltd, London.

Wilson J, Hair C, Knight R et al 2010. High incidence of inflammatory bowel disease in Australia: a prospective population-based Australian incidence study. Inflammatory Bowel Diseases 16(9), 1550–1556.

CHAPTER 24

Principles for Nursing Practice: Keratinocyte Cancers and Melanoma

ISABELLE SKINNER • KERYLN CARVILLE

LEARNING OBJECTIVES

When you have completed this chapter you will be able to:

- describe the risk factors for skin cancer
- outline the diagnostic procedures for skin cancer
- discuss the principles of management for keratinocyte cancer and melanoma
- outline health education strategies for the prevention of skin cancer.

KEY WORDS

cutaneous squamous cell carcinoma	Marjolin's ulcer
basal cell carcinoma	skin cancer
melanoma	keratinocyte cancer

INTRODUCTION

Skin cancer is the most common form of cancer, especially in Australia and New Zealand. In 2019 it was estimated that 145,000 new cancer cases would be diagnosed, excluding basal cell and cutaneous squamous cell carcinoma (AIHW 2019). Skin cancer can be broadly classified as either melanoma or keratinocyte cancer. The Australian Institute of Health and Welfare (AIHW) estimated that in 2016 there would be 13,280 new cases of melanoma, which makes it one of the three most common forms of registrable cancer (AIHW 2016). Comparisons can be made with other malignant conditions: for men the most common cancer estimate in 2019 was prostate cancer, with 19,508 new cases expected; colorectal cancer was next with 9069 new cases; followed by melanoma of the skin with 8899 new cases. Women most commonly were estimated to be diagnosed with breast cancer, 19,371 new cases; followed by colorectal cancer, 7329 new cases; and, again, third was melanoma of the skin with 6330 new cases (AIHW 2019). Incidence data on keratinocyte cancer is not routinely collected

by the Australian state and territory cancer registries. However, in 2013–14 there were 114,722 hospitalisations for keratinocyte cancer, up 39% from 2002–03. The age standard hospitalisation rate was 44 hospitalisations per 10,000 (AIHW 2016). This makes the incidence of skin cancer in Australia more than 10 times that of the other three major forms of cancer combined. In Australia about 80% of all new cases of cancer are skin cancers (AIHW 2016).

BEHAVIOURS THAT CONTRIBUTE TO THE DEVELOPMENT OF SKIN CANCER

Skin cancer is generally thought to be preventable. Exposure to ultraviolet radiation (UVR) is now accepted as the highest environmental risk factor for all types of skin cancer. The International Agency for Research on Cancer classified UVR as carcinogenic in 2012 and specifically classified UVR from arc welding as carcinogenic in 2017 (Falcone & Zeidler-Erdely 2019). The causative relationship between UVR exposure and skin cancer is still not fully understood. Kanavy and Gerstenblith (2011) have identified that there are multiple detrimental effects from sunlight or tanning beds on human skin, including DNA damage, gene mutations, oxidative stress, inflammation and immunosuppression. A person's susceptibility to sunburn is related to the amount of sun exposure and their skin tone. Fair-skinned and auburn-haired people experience sunburn more readily than people with darker complexions given the same exposure (Carter et al 1999). Keratinocyte cancer development is known to be strongly associated with the cumulative effect of UVR skin exposure. Head and neck melanomas are also associated with cumulative UVR exposure, while truncal melanoma is more associated with intermittent patterns of sun exposure (Nikolaou & Stratigos 2014). Climate change and ozone depletion have both increased the risk of skin cancer. Kaffenberger and colleagues (2017) estimate that a 2°C increase in temperature may increase the number of skin cancers annually by 10%. Arc welding, as an occupation, has also been shown to increase the risk of skin cancer (Falcone & Zeidler-Erdely 2019).

Although information about the risk of sun exposure is believed to be readily available, research has shown that 70% of children and adults are not adequately protected from exposure to sunlight in the high-risk areas of northwest Australia, where the UV index reaches 11 on most days during the dry season between May and October (Woloczyn et al 2010). A recent survey of schools in Queensland also identified that despite more than a decade of SunSmart Schools Accreditation, most schools only had policies addressing two of the 12 SunSmart criteria (Harrison et al 2016). The Cancer Council of Australia (2020d) recommends that UVR exposure requires a balance between the amount needed to reduce the risk of skin cancer and enough to reduce the risk of vitamin D deficiency. They recommend protective measures should be employed throughout life, noting that sunscreen use does not impede vitamin D production. They also recommend banning solariums in all Australian states (Cancer Council 2020d).

KERATINOCYTE CANCER

Keratinocyte cancer encompasses basal cell carcinoma (BCC) and cutaneous squamous cell carcinoma (cSCC) (Cancer Council Australia 2020b). BCC is the most common form of skin cancer and accounts for two-thirds of all keratinocyte skin cancers. It is most commonly found in males and those aged over 40, and is usually found on the face (AIHW 2016). A BCC usually presents as a persistent non-healing lesion, scaly spot or pinkish-red growth. It usually begins as a small waxy nodule with rolled translucent pearly borders and telangiectatic vessels may be visible. The BCC arises from the single layer of basal cells that line the basement membrane which separates the dermis from the epidermis. It is categorised as a nodular, pigmented, superficial, morpheaform or sclerotic lesion and fortunately it rarely metastasises; instead it invades and erodes adjoining tissues (Vargo 2006). Left unchecked, a BCC can cause destruction to the tissues and result in significant loss of tissue and disfigurement.

Cutaneous squamous cell carcinoma (cSCC) is also a common form of skin cancer. It tends to be of greater concern than BCC as it is an invasive cancer and may metastasise via the lymphatic system and bloodstreams. Virtually all reported cases are among people over 40 years of age, with a higher incidence among persons 70 years and above (AIHW 2016). An cSCC usually presents as a rough, thickened, scaly lesion. The lesion may be asymptomatic or may tend to bleed. Although a cSCC usually appears on sun-damaged skin, it may arise from a pre-existing skin lesion, such as scarred or ulcerated lesions or actinic keratoses (lesions of sun-exposed skin) or leukoplakia (premalignant lesions of the mucous membranes). Alternatively, it may first appear on areas of skin with no evident sun damage. An cSCC is a tumour of the keratinising cells of the epidermis. It can appear anywhere on the skin or mucous membranes and it is characterised as non-invasive (superficial) or invasive (Vargo 2006).

PRESENTATION AND DIAGNOSIS OF KERATINOCYTE CANCERS

General medical practitioners (GPs) are the gatekeepers to the health system in Australia and elsewhere; most people will access diagnostic services for skin lesions through their GP (Youl et al 2011). Nurse practitioners (NPs) also provide diagnostic services, in particular NPs with a generalist scope of practice and those working in rural and remote areas. The patient may present to their primary care health practitioner with a sinister-looking lesion or a non-healing ulcer. According to Winterbottom and Harcourt (2004), there are a number of factors that lead people to seek medical advice, but none of the participants with skin cancer interviewed for their study sought medical help until others persuaded them to do so, despite significant symptoms. These authors revealed that most of the participants in their study self-diagnosed their lesions and considered them to be relatively minor problems.

Two participants' comments illustrate this point well (Winterbottom & Harcourt 2004, p. 229):

It started like a pimple ... and I thought I had been bitten. I was putting antiseptic on it, trying to get rid of it (participant with BCC).

Certain members of my family used to have various bits and pieces like that, so I wondered if it was hereditary (participant with cSCC).

A diagnosis of BCC and cSCC requires a biopsy of the lesion and histopathological examination of the tissue. Regional lymph nodes should be examined for suspected cSCC metastases.

Medical Treatment

The definitive goal of medical interventions for keratinocyte cancers is to remove the tumour completely. The guidelines for BCC treatment recommend wide margin surgical excision or Moh's micrographic surgery, in which the tumour is removed layer by layer until the tissue margins are tumour-free for all patients with high-risk recurrent facial BCCs (Cancer Council 2020b).

Surgery for most keratinocyte cancer is conducted as a minor outpatient procedure or admission to a day surgery unit. However, the visible nature of the disease and the types of treatment available mean that patients are often left with visible scars or disfigurement. Although not as life-threatening as a diagnosis of melanoma, keratinocyte cancers, and in particular cSCC, have the potential to be fatal if they go untreated. Adjuvant radiotherapy may be employed in the treatment of advanced cSCC. Radiotherapy can also be used alone in the treatment of keratinocyte cancer when surgery is not possible, or the patient does not want to undergo surgery (Cancer Council 2020b). It has been identified that patients who received their surgery soon after diagnosis experience reduced stress when compared to those who have to wait for treatment (Winterbottom & Harcourt 2004).

MELANOMA

Melanoma is a serious form of skin cancer. Apart from breast cancer and prostate cancer, melanoma is the most common cancer and affects males more commonly than females (AIHW 2019). Melanoma is classified into subtypes based on histologic and morphologic characteristics. The most common subtype is superficial spreading melanoma, which accounts for 55–60% of cases (Cancer Council 2020a). It typically presents on the trunk of people who are prone to naevi or moles. It is strongly associated with intermittent sun exposure. The ABCDE classification (asymmetry, border irregularity, colour variation, diameter greater than 6 mm and elevation of the lesion) is a useful prompt for identification of skin changes related to superficial spreading melanomas and aids clinical diagnosis (Cancer Council 2020a). Melanoma prognosis is highly dependent on the subtype, the clinical stage or extent of the tumour burden at diagnosis (Markovic et al 2007). Other subtypes of melanoma include nodular, lentigo maligna, desmoplastic, acral lentiginous and subungal. These vary in location, depth, colour variation and association with sun exposure. The most important feature is the changing nature of the lesion, regardless of their other clinical features (Cancer Council 2020a).

Presentation and Diagnosis of Melanoma

As with keratinocyte cancer, patients usually access melanoma diagnosis through their primary care practitioner. Patients self-refer or can be referred by a skin clinic. Delay in seeking treatment is considered to be one of the factors that influences prognostic outcomes. Research by Tsao and colleagues (2003), which used a population-based approach to calculate the risk of moles turning into melanomas, estimated that there was a very low likelihood of moles becoming melanomas in the Caucasian or white population for people under the age of 20; however, with increasing age, the risk rose sharply. Men over the age of 60 years were most likely to develop melanoma. They calculated the risk per mole as approximately 1:33,000 in this age group. Moles are common and even in high-risk groups, there is a low likelihood that any one mole will become a melanoma. However, any suspicious, changing raised lesion should be excised rather than being monitored, as there is a narrow window to detect rapidly growing lesions while they are still thin (Cancer Council 2020a).

There is little research on the factors that lead people to access their primary care practitioner for a skin cancer diagnosis. In a study by Walter and colleagues (2014), it was found, as was the case for BCC and cSCC, that many people needed to be urged by others to seek help. Many of their study participants failed to recognise the significance of their presenting lesions. Eleven of the 63 participants in their study who had a melanoma diagnosis reported previous reassurance about the skin changes from a healthcare professional. The guidelines recommend that clinicians who are conducting skin examinations for detecting skin cancer should be trained in and use dermoscopy (Menzies et al 2018).

A diagnosis of melanoma is confirmed by biopsy and histopathological examination of the lesion. The optimal biopsy approach for a suspicious lesion is a complete excision with a 2 mm margin (Kelly et al 2018). Detailed inspection of the skin is also performed to identify satellite or in-transit metastases. Satellites are discontinuous foci of the tumour located within 5 cm of the primary tumour and in-transit metastases are discontinuous foci found more than 5 cm from the primary tumour. Follow-up for early detection of recurrences after definitive treatment is important as there is 2–8% incidence of new primaries and a high lifetime risk of a second primary invasive melanoma (Barbour et al 2018).

Medical Treatment

The principal medical intervention for melanoma depends on the stage of the disease at diagnosis. The surgical intervention for a small lesion of less than 1 mm thickness with no ulceration, involves complete excision of the tumour. Research has shown that a margin of 2 mm is sufficient for patients with a small lesion.

Up to 10% of people with melanoma will develop in-transit metastases with a median time of 12–18 months. Because of the variability of the regional and distal spread, management is difficult. In a large Australian study of 505 people with in-transit metastates, 42% developed regional recurrence (Henderson et al 2018). The guidelines recommend radiotherapy for palliation for larger symptomatic lesions and systemic therapies, targeted and immune therapies for recurrent or progressive disease.

Lymph node involvement detected by sentinel node biopsy or clinical examination indicates a poorer prognosis. Five-year survival rates for people with no lymph involvement (N1c) was 81%; with one lymph node involved (N2c) was 69%; and more than one lymph node involved (N3c) was 52% (Henderson et al 2018).

The interdisciplinary team will assess patients for Stage IV tumours and, if identified, a decision will be made on the likelihood of surgical excision rendering the patient disease-free. In this case, a complete surgical resection will be considered. If surgery is unlikely to be successful, the patient will be considered for palliative care.

MARJOLIN'S ULCER

A Marjolin's ulcer is the relatively rare but aggressive transformation of a chronic wound into a degenerative malignant skin lesion (Cohen et al 1992). The resultant epidermoid cancer is more frequently a cSCC, although BCCs and melanomas have also been reported (Dupree et al 1998). Jean Nicolas Marjolin gave his name to this malignant transformation in 1828 when he noted the malignant degeneration of a burn scar (Trent & Kirsner 2003). Since then the term has been used to describe malignant alterations in all types of chronic wounds and includes burns, osteomyelitis, leg ulcers, pressure ulcers and fistulae. It has been estimated that 1.7% of chronic wounds will transform into a Marjolin's ulcer (Trent & Kirsner 2003), and 30–40% of these will metastasise (Habif 2004). The aetiology of Marjolin's ulcers is considered to be the prolonged cellular mitotic activity that occurs during attempts to re-epithelialise the chronic wound (Menendez & Warriner 2006). The diagnosis and treatment of a Marjolin's ulcer is aligned with that of cSCC, BCC and melanoma.

CASE STUDY 24.1

Living with melanoma has been frustrating and frightening. My name is Mandy Lewis, and I live in a town in Northern Australia with my husband Stewart and my three gorgeous daughters. My journey with melanoma started with a mole on the outside of my right calf, which was fairly ugly looking.

Before I was diagnosed with melanoma, each year we had been to the local skin clinic for a check. My husband and I are very conscious of our skin. My dad has had a lot of treatment for skin cancers, which he has had burnt off. He has worked outside all his life. Each visit they looked at my mole and said it was fine. This time my husband didn't think it was fine; he insisted on me going to the GP. I have been going to the same GP for the last 10 years and I trusted her. She had seen the mole before and was reassured that the skin clinic thought it was fine. My husband wasn't convinced and pushed her to remove it, which she reluctantly agreed to do. She was concerned that the scar would be very visible. I agreed to go on holidays and think about it. On my return, I made another appointment by myself and had the procedure done. A week later I got a call from the GP who said I needed to come in that day to see her. The results had come back as melanoma, but not to worry as there were only slight changes. I was given a referral to a general surgeon.

CASE STUDY 24.1 – cont'd

I rang the surgeon and he managed to fit in an appointment for 2 days' time. He had planned to take a larger margin in his rooms; however, I was admitted to hospital for day surgery as I had private health insurance. I have two very strong memories about that experience. First, the nurse gave me a dressing that was just a bit bigger than a standard bandaid and said that I should re-dress the wound in 3 days. After 3 days I took down the dressing and it looked like I had been attacked by a shark. I had a 15 cm cut on my leg. Second I was sitting next to a lovely young man in recovery whose fiancée had insisted he have a mole checked and he had been diagnosed with melanoma too. We agreed to become FaceBook friends to support each other through the treatment. Unfortunately he died very quickly after diagnosis. That brought home how serious this all could be.

My GP referred me to another surgeon who specialised in cancer treatment. He wasn't a melanoma specialist and I was invited to sit in on a consultation between himself and the melanoma referral clinic in the tertiary referral centre. I would be required to have a check-up every 3 months to check the site for any return and to check the lymph nodes for any swelling. All went well for 3 years.

Then in January I had a painful lump come up on the front of my leg. It just kept getting bigger. The GP thought it was an infection and prescribed antibiotics. After 3 weeks it was still getting bigger, so I was referred back to the surgeon who confirmed that the melanoma had returned. I was booked for surgery to have it removed and then sent to the tertiary referral centre for a PET scan. The radiologist stopped halfway through as he had identified more cells. I asked him for more details but he couldn't tell me anything as he said he wasn't my doctor. This was a terribly anxious time. I returned home and cried for about a month until I could get back in to see the surgeon. He confirmed the melanoma had spread to my bowel and I was booked in for laparoscopic surgery to remove the lesions. Again it was a short stay. Nobody asked me about the pain, which was awful. I was discharged without a prescription for pain medication.

The worst part is the pain. The ongoing pain from the leg is excruciating. There has been lots of nerve damage. If it's not painful there is a horrible crawling feeling under the skin. The leg pain extends up into my hip and back. These are the things you are left with. At no time has anyone talked about the pain or offered a prescription for pain relief. This has always made me think they can't consider it to be too serious. It wasn't until the PET scan that it really hit me. This is serious. I couldn't even walk or think. My husband was in shock. I had to pay and I couldn't even remember the PIN for my card. Luckily my husband held it together till we got home. My three girls were waiting for me. It was the worst afternoon. My husband refuses to talk about it now. He's in denial. He won't come to appointments. I feel helpless. We haven't been offered any family counselling.

My only options are surgical, as we live a long way from the tertiary referral centre. Now I am being monitored for a lesion on my liver and I am having investigations for a lesion on my lip.

My advice to health professionals is patients are human; we are going through a difficult time. A smile and some empathy goes a long way.

CASE STUDY 24.2

Max Smart is a 70-year-old man who has had poorly controlled diabetes type II for more than 15 years. Max retired about 5 years ago and lives on his own in a small cottage. Max has two cats and a dog who he is very fond of and a lovely garden that occupies most of his time.

Max has a history of peripheral vascular disease and peripheral neuropathy and is prone to lower limb ulcers, which can be difficult to heal. In the last 6 months Max has had an ulcer on his left lower leg that has been particularly difficult to heal despite visits to the GP twice a week for dressings. The wound margins of the ulcer are poorly demarcated and there appears to be a nodular lump next to the distal edge. The nurse in the clinic has been measuring the wound area using a clear acetate sheet and the wound appears to be getting larger. The clinic nurse has been taking a digital image of the wound once a fortnight.

The GP thinks it is time to admit Max to hospital to try to get his diabetes under control and to facilitate education by the diabetes educator and review by the podiatrist and the nutritionist. Prior to admission a wound swab and a wound biopsy are taken.

Max's wound biopsy results come back positive for squamous cell carcinoma. He will require cryosurgery to treat the lesion.

Nursing Management

The nursing management of patients who are to undergo treatment for potentially life-threatening skin cancer should be directed towards enhancing patients' coping skills. Strategies that can be used include hopeful and goal-oriented thinking. The provision of comprehensible information about the disease has also been shown to alleviate anxiety (Dolan et al 1997; Winterbottom & Harcourt 2004). In Janine's case, information on the stage of the tumour and the existence of satellite metastases will be needed. Janine may be shocked to discover that her mole is actually a potentially life-threatening skin cancer. The nurse would manage information-giving in the following ways:

- Develop a trusting therapeutic relationship with Janine and her husband to alleviate anxiety and increase information uptake.
- Provide answers to the questions relating to the medical diagnosis and the treatment options that have been outlined to Janine.
- Maintain and communicate a positive outlook to assist Janine and her family to remain hopeful.

Max also has a potentially life-threatening skin cancer. Although his prognosis is better than Janine's, he will also require the nurse to manage information-giving sensitively. Janine has family responsibilities and Max has three pets that he cares for. It is important for the nurse to recognise they may be more concerned about the impact of their conditions on their loved ones than on themselves in the early stages of their care journey.

Optimal wound management is also a prime requisite.

WOUND MANAGEMENT

The presence of a malignant wound is visible evidence of the existence and progression of the malignancy. Anxiety and depression are frequently associated with the presence of these wounds and can impact significantly on the individual's coping mechanisms and quality of life. The care of a person with a malignant wound can present considerable challenges to the patient, their carers and health professionals as the disease exacerbates. Malignant wounds can present as either fungating or ulcerating lesions and at times protruding nodular growths and cavity formation may co-exist. Comprehensive and ongoing assessment of the person, their wound and their healing environment is a fundamental requirement for planning and implementing optimal wound management. In Max's case,

the healing environment is compromised by his poorly controlled diabetes. The nurse would promote wound healing in the following ways:

- Encourage Max to maintain his blood sugar within normal limits.
- Encourage Max to consume a diet high in essential vitamins and minerals.
- Apply the appropriate pressure bandages to reduce lower limb oedema.
- Assist with ambulation to maintain the calf pump.

A holistic and multidisciplinary approach to symptom control of presenting problems is a principal activity. Potential problems associated with malignant wounds include:

- alterations in body image
- discomfort or wound pain
- bleeding
- infection
- increased exudate
- malodour.

ALTERATIONS IN BODY IMAGE

Preservation of body image and self-esteem are overriding principles in the care of persons with malignant wounds. Quality of life can be severely reduced by ineffectual wound management protocols. Bulky dressings or those that require frequent changes because they fail to contain exudate or malodour, significantly impair a person's psychological and physical wellbeing, while the use of conformable, skin-toned dressings may help to camouflage visible lesions on exposed sites. Head and neck tumours are particularly confronting, and wound management protocols should be directed towards optimising osmesis. Skilled orthotists employed within many specialised maxillo-facial units may assist in producing custom-made cosmetic orthotics, which can assist with the camouflage of significant facial defects. In cases of facial lesions, significant removal of tissue and extensive reconstructive surgery may be required. Surgical reduction or 'debulking' of extensive fungating tumours may be a possibility and can improve bodily function and appearance, although this may prove to be a temporary solution.

In Janine's case, the nurse would instigate care to manage the situation in the following ways:

- Recognise that Janine may be distressed by the large scar on her leg.
- Encourage family members to continue to visit.
- Schedule dressing changes prior to visiting times to maximise Janine's comfort and reduce her distress.

- Assist with fitting and maintenance of any orthotic devices that have been fashioned.

Discomfort or Wound Pain

Comprehensive assessment will indicate whether discomfort or pain is related to the disease process or wound management protocols, and both aetiologies require appropriate and adequate pain relief. Pain related to wound management regimens or dressing changes must be eradicated or minimised. Analgesia should be offered prior to dressing changes. Irradiated skin can also be very sensitive or itchy, and should be assessed for signs of inflammation, desquamation and ulceration (Carville 2012). Patients with irradiated skin require gentle skin care protocols and the frequent application of moisturisers in the form of lotions or emollients to exposed skin. If they are undergoing active radiation therapy, they should avoid all metallic agents, including silver- and zinc-impregnated dressings. All patients with irradiated skin damage should be advised to avoid skin trauma, sun exposure and irritant chemicals. An increasing range of non-adherent and silicon-backed dressings and tapes can lessen deafferentation pain associated with removal of adhesive agents. The use of roller or tubular bandages and secure garments for dressing retention may be a more acceptable option.

In the cases of both Janine and Max, the nurse would assess any discomfort or pain relating to their surgical procedure and prior to any dressing changes.

Bleeding

Disseminated disease can result in erosion of capillaries or major blood vessels, with resulting haemorrhage. Potential or actual bleeding in malignant wounds can be extremely distressing for patients, carers and staff. Protection of fragile tissues and avoidance of local trauma or unnecessary debridement of tissues in close approximation to major blood vessels is warranted. Dry eschar can protect underlying vascular structures, while debridement can increase the risk of haemorrhage. However, increased bacterial proliferation and autolysis of moist necrotic tissue may increase malodour and the risk of infection. Therefore, conservative debridement of moist necrotic tissue may be required. Autolytic debridement offers a more conservative approach and the use of topical antimicrobial agents, such as cadexomer iodine or honey dressings, affords additional antimicrobial protection. However, hydrogels and wound honey do add to the fluid burden of some wounds and this may be undesirable. Hypertonic

saline agents should be avoided when there is potential bleeding. Topical agents that promote haemostasis in malignant wounds include the firmer calcium alginate dressings, cautery with silver nitrate sticks or solution and ostomy hydrocolloid powders that contain gelatine or pectin (Stomahesive and Hollihesive powders). Surgical haemostatic agents such as Surgicel are also useful but expensive and not readily available in many care settings. Topical adrenaline 1:1000 solution is occasionally prescribed. However, its vasoconstriction properties can lead to tissue necrosis if not used with due care. The prescribed use of oral or topical fibrinolytic inhibitors have also proved to be useful in controlling bleeding. Application of dressings such as foams and absorbent pads, as well as the wearing of loose-fitting garments, may offer the wound some added protection against friction forces.

Infection

The presence of necrotic tissue and hypoxia in a malignant wound increases the risk of wound infection. Anaerobic and aerobic bacteria can proliferate in moist necrotic tissues and can exacerbate malodour and lead to an increase in exudate. The classic local signs of pain, erythema, oedema, heat, increased exudate or purulence indicate infection. However, other local signs may indicate a level of increased colonisation, commonly referred to as 'critical colonisation'. These changes include changes in the nature (friable and hypergranulated) and colour (bright red or grey) of granulation tissue; increased pain, pain or exudate; static healing; rolled edges of the wound; and possible bridging of the tissues (Gardner et al 2001; Sibbald et al 2003). Systemic antibiotics may be required, but the efficacy is reduced when infection presents in poorly vascularised tumours. The use of topical antimicrobials in the form of 'tissue-friendly' solutions and dressings is prudent in suspected wound infection. Cadexomer iodine (Iodosorb), silver impregnated dressings, 'wound' honey, hypertonic saline impregnated dressings and povidone-iodine or chlorhexidine-impregnated tulle gras are some of the antimicrobial dressings available.

Increased Exudate

Uncontrolled exudate and the need for frequent dressing changes reduce the person's quality of life, increase fatigue and increase the resources needed to care appropriately. There is also an increased risk of infection, maceration of tissues and malodour. Extra-absorbent dry dressings such as Zetuvit, Mesorb or Exu-Dry are useful, as are a large range of incontinent or sanitary pads. Wound or ostomy appliances for containment of fistulae output or large amounts of exudate that may be associated with fungating tumours provide a cost-effective and less fatiguing alternative to frequent dressing changes.

Malodour

Malodour is a particularly distressing complication of malignant wounds for all involved in the care or support of patients. Malodour can result from infection, faecal fistulae drainage, autolysis of necrotic tissue or poor wound hygiene. Malodour impacts significantly upon body image and quality of life, and wound management should be directed towards eliminating or controlling malodour (Young 2005). Identification and management of the causative problem is crucial. Malodour is managed environmentally, systemically (when the aetiology is infection) and topically. Environmental control of malodour is best achieved by providing good ventilation, disposal of waste products and prudent use of air deodorisers. Topical management options include: the use of topical antiseptic dressings (as previously discussed) and activated charcoal dressings such as Actisorb Plus, Lyofoam C and CarboFlex. Topical antimicrobial dressings reduce the bacterial load in the wound and the activated charcoal dressings adsorb or attract volatile odours, gases and microorganisms (Lee et al 2006). A wide variety of ostomy or wound appliances is useful for containment of offensive exudate. Dry black tea bags used as a secondary or tertiary dressing have been reported to provide an additional benefit in the control of malodour when more orthodox dressings prove ineffectual or are not available (Ng & Lee 2002).

EDUCATION FOR THE PERSON, FAMILY AND COMMUNITY

There is a large body of evidence that reducing sun exposure reduces the risk of skin cancer of all types. Carter and colleagues (1999) proposed that a 20% reduction in lifetime UVR exposure would have more than a 30% reduction in non-melanocytic skin cancers and a 30% reduction in melanoma skin cancers, with a decreased number of deaths in Australia. This is supported by the Australian Radiation Protection and Nuclear Safety Agency in their submission to the House of Representatives Inquiry into Skin Cancer in Australia (2015). Most of the mass media campaigns promote the use of sunscreen and the wearing of protective clothing and hats as personal protective measures. The Cancer Council's 'slip slop slap' campaign ('slip on a shirt, slop on sunscreen and slap on a hat') is an example of this. These campaigns have been effective at raising awareness of the key messages (Smith et al 2005): a telephone survey of a random sample of 800 parents of children under 12 in New South Wales reported a 95% awareness of the key messages. However, the most effective measure to reduce sun exposure is sun avoidance, particularly between the hours of 10 am and 3 pm. Studies have shown that intermittent sun exposure rather than chronic exposure increases the risk of melanoma. Childhood sun exposure has been shown to be a significant risk factor in the development of keratinocyte cancer and melanoma (Balk 2011). Like all health promotion campaigns targeting behaviour modification, the key is to translate awareness of the benefits into personal action. Nurses have a role in this in a number of ways:

- providing accurate information to parents and prospective parents in the antenatal and early childhood settings
- providing targeted brief interventions to reinforce messages in primary care settings and during clinical contact
- conducting local health promotion campaigns to reinforce mass media messages in community settings.

Cancer Council Australia does not distinguish between keratinocyte cancer and melanoma in its sun protection messages:

- If the solar UV rating is 3 or above, people should wear a wide-brimmed hat and clothing to cover exposed skin.
- Apply sunscreen with a sun protection factor (SPF) of 30 or higher to all exposed skin surfaces daily and for children before any outdoor play.
- Adequate sunscreen is 2 mg of sunscreen for each square centimetre of exposed skin: approximately 1 teaspoon per limb.
- Wear close-fitting glasses to protect eyes against sun damage.

CONCLUSION

Skin cancer is a major cause of morbidity and mortality. Reducing the incidence of skin cancer requires individuals to take lifelong personal protective action for themselves and their children. Early detection is the key to a good outcome for keratinocyte cancer and melanoma. This can be achieved by regular skin inspection and needs to be accompanied by personal action, supported by encouragement to seek treatment when suspect lesions are found.

Reflective Questions

1 A woman with varicose veins has a non-healing leg ulcer. You have taken a swab and it comes back with normal commensals. What other investigations are warranted?

2 What strategies could be used to encourage teenagers to adopt 'SunSmart' behaviours?

3 What features of a melanoma may lead you to suspect that the patient may have a poor prognosis?

RECOMMENDED READING

Cancer Council Australia 2020. Keratinocyte Cancers Guideline Working Party. Clinical practice guidelines for keratinocyte cancer. Cancer Council Australia, Sydney. https://wiki.cancer.org.au/australia/Guidelines:Keratinocyte_carcinoma.

Carville K 2012. Wound care manual. Silver Chain Foundation, Perth.

Young C 2005. The effects of malodorous fungating malignant wounds on body image and quality of life. Journal of Wound Care 14(8), 359–361.

REFERENCES

Australian Institute of Health and Welfare (AIHW) 2019. Cancer in Australia 2019. Cancer series no. 119. Cat no. CAN 123. AIHW, Canberra.

Australian Institute of Health and Welfare (AIHW) 2016. Skin cancer in Australia. Cat no. CAN 96. AIHW, Canberra.

Balk S 2011. Ultraviolet radiation: a hazard to children and adolescents. Pediatrics 127(3), 791–817.

Barbour A, Guminski A, Liu W et al 2018. Cancer Council Australia Melanoma Guidelines Working Party. Follow-up after initial definitive treatment from each stage of melanoma. Online. Available: https://wiki.cancer.org.au/australia/Clinical_question:How_should_patients_at_each_stage_of_melanoma_be_followed_after_initial_definitive_treatment%3F

Cancer Council 2020a. Clinical practice guidelines for the diagnosis and treatment of melanoma. Online. Available: https://wiki.cancer.org.au/australia/Guidelines:Melanoma

Cancer Council Australia 2020b. Keratinocyte Cancers Guideline Working Party. Clinical practice guidelines for keratinocyte cancer. Cancer Council Australia, Sydney. Online. Available: https://wiki.cancer.org.au/australia/Guidelines:Keratinocyte_carcinoma.

Cancer Council Australia 2020c. Position statement – private ownership and use of solariums in Australia. Online. Available: https://wiki.cancer.org.au/policy/Position_statement_-_Private_solariums

Cancer Council Australia 2020d. Position statement – risks and benefits of sun exposure. Online. Available: http://wiki.cancer.org.au/policy/Position_statement_-_Risks_and_benefits_of_sun_exposure#_ga=1.159489790.2135240054.1470190719

Carter R, Marks R, Hill D 1999. Could a national skin cancer primary prevention campaign in Australia be worthwhile? An economic perspective. Health Promotion International 14(1), 73–82.

Carville K 2012. Wound care manual. Silver Chain Foundation, Perth.

Cohen K, Dieglemann R, Lindblad W 1992. Wound healing: biochemical and clinical aspects. Saunders, Philadelphia.

Dolan N, Ng J, Martin G et al 1997. Effectiveness of skin cancer control educational intervention for internal medicine housestaff and attending physicians. Journal of Internal Medicine 12, 531–536.

Dupree M, Boyer J, Cobb M 1998. Marjolin's ulcer arising from a burns scar. Cutis 62(1), 49–51.

Falcone LM, Zeidler-Erdely PC 2019. Skin cancer and welding. Clin Exp Dermatol 44(2), 130–134.

Gardner S, Frantz R, Doebbeling B 2001. The validity of the clinical signs and symptoms used to identify localised chronic wound infection. Wound Repair and Regeneration 9, 178–186.

Habif T 2004. Clinical dermatology: a colour guide to diagnosis and therapy, 4th edn. Elsevier, St Louis.

Harrison S, Garzón-Chavez D, Nikles C 2016. Sun protection policies of Australian primary schools in a region of high sun exposure. Health Education Research 31(3), 416–428.

Henderson M, Cancer Council Australia Melanoma Guidelines Working Party 2018. What are the most effective treatments of satellite and in-transit metastases? Online. Available: https://wiki.cancer.org.au/australia/Clinical_question:What_are_the_most_effective_treatments_for_satellite_and_in-transit_metastatic_melanoma%3F

House of Representatives Standing Committee on Health. Skin Cancer in Australia: Our National Cancer 2015. Parliament of the Commonwealth of Australia.

Kaffenberger B, Shetlar D, Norton S et al 2017. The effect of climate change on skin disease in North America. Journal of the American Academy of Dermatology 76(10), 140–147.

Kanavy H, Gerstenblith M 2011. Ultraviolet radiation and melanoma. Seminars in Cutaneous Medicine and Surgery 30(4), 222–228.

Kelly J, Beer T, Damian D et al Cancer Council Australia Melanoma Working Party 2018. What type of biopsy should be performed for a pigmented lesion suspicious for melanoma? Online. Available: https://wiki.cancer.org.au/australia/Clinical_question:What_type_of_biopsy_should_be_performed_for_a_suspicious_pigmented_skin_lesion%3F

Lee G, Anand S, Rajendran S et al 2006. Overview of current practices and future trends in the evaluation of dressings for malodorous wounds. Journal of Wound Care 15(8), 344–346.

Markovic S, Erickson L, Rao R et al 2007. Malignant melanoma in the 21st century, part 2: staging, prognosis and treatment. Mayo Clinic Proceedings 82(4), 490–513.

Menendez M, Warriner R 2006. Marjolin's ulcer: report of two cases. Wounds 18(3), 65–70.

Menzies S, Chamberlain A, Soyer P et al, Cancer Council Australia Melanoma Guidelines Working Party 2018. What is the role of dermascopy in melanoma diagnosis? Online. Available: https://wiki.cancer.org.au/australia/Clinical_question: What_is_the_role_of_dermoscopy_in_melanoma_diagnosis%3F

Ng PL, Lee GY 2002. A case report of an innovative strategy using tea leaves in the management of malodorous wounds. Singapore Nurses Journal 29(3), 16–18.

Nikolaou V, Stratigos AJ 2014. Emerging trends in the epidemiology of melanoma. British Journal of Dermatology 170(1), 11–19.

Sibbald RG, Orsted H, Schultz G et al 2003. Preparing the wound bed: focus on infection and inflammation. Ostomy/Wound Management 49(11), 24–51.

Smith L, Pope C, Botha J 2005. Patients' help-seeking experiences and delay in cancer presentation: a qualitative synthesis. The Lancet 366(9488), 825–831.

Trent J, Kirsner R 2003. Wounds and malignancy. Advances in Skin and Wound Care 16(1), 31–34.

Tsao H, Bevona C, Goggins W et al 2003. The transformation rate of moles (melanocytic nevi) into cutaneous melanoma: a population based estimate. Archives of Dermatology 139(3), 282–288.

Vargo N 2006. Cutaneous malignancies: BCC, SCC, and MM. Dermatology Nursing 18(2), 183–200.

Walter F, Birt L, Cavers D et al 2014. 'This isn't what mine looked like': a qualitative study of symptom appraisal and help seeking in people recently diagnosed with melanoma. BMJ Open 2014; 4:e005566.

Winterbottom A, Harcourt D 2004. Patients' experience of the diagnosis and treatment of skin cancer. Journal of Advanced Nursing 48(3), 226–233.

Woloczyn M, Trzesinski A, Takahashi M et al 2010. Sun protective behaviours of beach goers in the North West. Health Promotion Journal of Australia 21(2), 146–148.

Youl PH, Janda M, Aitken JF et al 2011. Body-site distribution of skin cancer, pre-malignant and common benign pigmented lesions excised in general practice. British Journal of Dermatology 165(1), 35–43.

Young C 2005. The effects of malodorous fungating malignant wounds on body image and quality of life. Journal of Wound Care 14(8), 359–361.

CHAPTER 25

Principles for Nursing Practice: Osteoarthritis and Osteoporosis

TIFFANY NORTHALL • STEVEN A. FROST

LEARNING OBJECTIVES

When you have completed this chapter you will be able to:

- outline the major risk factors for the development of osteoarthritis and osteoporosis in the ageing population
- describe the impact that osteoarthritis and osteoporosis have on the function and wellbeing of ageing persons within the community
- outline current approaches to reducing the impact of these conditions on members of the older population
- suggest nursing practices that will promote health and mobility in older persons experiencing the effects of osteoarthritis and osteoporosis
- develop strategies to support the families of clients experiencing the effects of osteoarthritis and osteoporosis.

KEY WORDS

activities of daily living (ADLs)	nursing practice
ageing	wellbeing
education	

INTRODUCTION

The majority of the population in Australia and New Zealand anticipate a lifetime of independence and good health that allows them to maintain a self-directed lifestyle. However, living a healthy and productive life does not necessarily protect the individual from varying levels of disability later in life due to the natural changes of ageing, life's physical stressors and individual genetic make-up. Osteoarthritis, rheumatoid arthritis and other musculoskeletal conditions, such as osteoporosis and back pain, affect more than 6.9 million Australians, mostly among people aged 65 years and over (Australian Institute of Health and Welfare [AIHW] 2018). As populations age, more people are likely to experience disability as a result of these conditions. Even if the disability does not interfere with daily function and mobility, in combination with other changes of ageing and age-related diseases, the effects of these conditions and their management can

prove to be challenging for the person, their family and health providers, and result in increased levels of disability.

In this chapter there will be a discussion of osteoarthritis, rheumatoid arthritis and osteoporosis. There will be a focus on the effects of osteoarthritis and osteoporosis on two older people and their families through the use of case studies. The case studies will assist you to understand how nursing practices can promote health and wellbeing for persons experiencing disability and challenge as a result of the effects of these conditions.

OSTEOARTHRITIS

Osteoarthritis is a disease that becomes more common in people over the age of 45. Worldwide, osteoarthritis affects 9.6% of men and 18% of women and is one of the 10 most disabling diseases in developing countries

(WHO 2016). It affects 2.2 million Australians and is more common in women (10%) than men (6.1%) (AIHW 2019). Indigenous Australians are more likely to have osteoarthritis than other Australians (AIHW 2011). In New Zealand, 17% of the population is affected by arthritis, with osteoarthritis being the most common form (Arthritis New Zealand 2018). Māori adults are 1.3 times more likely to have arthritis compared to non-Māori adults (Ministry of Health NZ 2016). Osteoarthritis is characterised by the deterioration of the articular cartilage that covers and protects the ends of the bones in joints. A person who does not have osteoarthritis has a balance between cartilage breakdown and production, while a person with osteoarthritis loses this balance and degeneration exceeds regeneration. This results in painful bone-on-bone contact in the joints, synovial inflammation and joint deformity (Kapoor et al 2015). Pain in osteoarthritis can also include stiff joints, swelling and lack of strength (Anand 2017).

Behaviours that Contribute to the Development of Osteoarthritis

Lifestyle behaviours that are known to contribute to the development of osteoarthritis are obesity, misalignment of bones and joints, joint trauma and injury, repetitive occupational joint use and physical inactivity (Glyn-Jones et al 2015). Age, however, is a strong predictor of osteoarthritis, which may be due to

increased risk factors and the inability of joints to regenerate (Glyn-Jones et al 2015). Lifestyle choices can help prevent osteoarthritis. Eating a healthy diet, not smoking and doing moderate exercise can reduce the risk even in the presence of uncontrollable risk factors (Roos & Arden 2016). Case Study 25.1 highlights some of the factors that contribute to the development of osteoarthritis. Adelina's situation illustrates a number of controllable and uncontrollable factors that have placed her at greater risk of developing osteoarthritis. The uncontrollable factors include her age, gender and genetic disposition or family history. Controllable factors include her weight, smoking status and activity levels.

Comprehensive holistic nursing assessment is needed when looking after people with chronic conditions. For people with osteoarthritis, it is important for nurses to consider its effect on the person: mobility; mood; body image; relationships; and quality of life (see Case Study 25.1).

Altered Mobility and Fatigue

Each person with osteoarthritis experiences their own challenges in maintaining mobility and managing the activities of daily living (ADLs). The most problematic issue in the development of osteoarthritis is pain, and it is the pain that limits mobility and function and contributes to fatigue, affecting activity levels (Medina

---

CASE STUDY 25.1

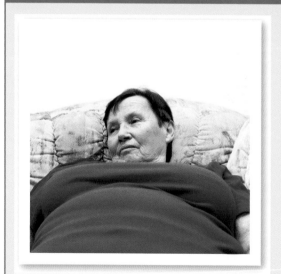

iStockphoto/JanMika.

Adelina is a 68-year-old retired teacher. She began teaching when she was 20 and continued to work until her retirement 2 years ago. Adelina is married to Harry and has two children. She and her husband have worked hard, they own their own home and have income from their superannuation. Adelina enjoys looking after their five grandchildren and loves gardening.

Adelina has always exercised regularly. She does not like strenuous exercise, but prefers to walk to help keep her fit. Despite this exercise, Adelina has been overweight for the last 20 years. Her current body mass index (BMI) is 34. Over the last few years she has had increasing pain in her spine and knees and has recently been diagnosed with osteoarthritis. Sometimes she finds it difficult to walk as far as she used to without pain. Recently, she has found that the pain is limiting her ability to play and look after her grandchildren. Adelina smokes 10 cigarettes per day and has done so for 20 years; she does not drink alcohol. She has a family history of osteoarthritis and heart disease.

2016). Nursing assessment of people with osteoarthritis should include frequency and duration of joint pain, as well as the durations, type and severity of pain (Roberts 2017).

In Australia 48% of people with osteoarthritis report that they feel the disease impacts on their ability to work and they more commonly experience anxiety and depression (AIHW 2019). At this time Adelina is not experiencing severe limitations on bathing, grooming or dressing, although she has made some changes to her clothing to compensate for reduced spinal mobility and she is no longer able to get in or out of a bathtub. Showering is not a problem for Adelina as there is no need to step into a raised shower and the alcove is large enough to move around freely.

The impact of osteoarthritis means that it has become the leading cause of disability worldwide (Cross et al 2014). With the projected global increase in ageing and obesity, it is expected that there will be significant increases in people who are affected by osteoarthritis and therefore experience some form of disability (Cross et al 2014). Adelina is experiencing some mobility deficits as a result of her pain and joint restrictions. Living with Harry offers the potential for support with ADLs, yet Adelina finds it difficult as she likes to look after and play with her grandchildren. This increases the physical demands on her that have the potential to increase her fatigue on particularly 'bad' days, when her pain becomes disabling. Adelina's outward responses to her pain include periods of solitude and silence, and a feeling of irritation that she is unable to perform some of the activities she planned around the house. Due to pain, a decreased ability to exercise and medications, people with osteoarthritis have an increased risk of developing depression and anxiety (Stubbs et al 2016). Fatigue is also a significant problem for people with osteoarthritis. This can be as a result of pain, and impacts on a person's mood (Hegarty et al 2016).

One of society's benchmarks of outward independence is the ability to drive, but driving necessitates getting in and out of a car and sitting for extended periods. In addition, driving requires manipulation and coordination of the joints, especially the knees (Latz et al 2019). It also requires the driver to sit in a restricted space. Limiting physical activity for older people with osteoarthritis can increase joint stiffness and pain (Fertelli et al 2019). Some evidence shows that aquatic exercise can reduce pain and improve physical function for older people with osteoarthritis (Fertelli et al 2019). Adhering to an exercise regime can be challenging, although positive reinforcement and reminders may encourage adherence.

The pain of osteoarthritis is not limited to the hours a person is awake and mobile. The ageing adult will experience changes in sleep patterns, including shorter, less deep sleep and overall a poorer quality of sleep than younger people (Cooke & Ancoli-Israel 2011). The resulting fatigue can impact on the older person's quality of life and mood (Tang et al 2017). Adelina finds that she must get out of bed more frequently due to pain and age-related nocturia and this reduces the duration of her restorative sleep. The pain and stiffness she experiences in her spine from sleeping in a single position for a prolonged time further interferes with the duration and quality of her sleep. Fewer hours of sleep, more frequent awakenings and physical discomfort have a cumulative effect on her vitality the following day. She experiences greater levels of fatigue with daytime pain and thus has less energy to mobilise, which is necessary to reduce joint stiffness and pain, and prevent further disability. Comprehensive nursing assessment is needed to support Adeline to be able to do the things she wants to do.

Key points

- Worldwide, osteoarthritis affects 9.6% of men and 18% of women and is one of the 10 most disabling diseases in developing countries (WHO 2016).
- Pain and joint stiffness affect mobility, independence, sleep and lifestyle.
- Holistic nursing assessment should be practised.

Body Image

People can experience an alteration in their body image as a result of the ageing process and functional decline (Jankowski et al 2016). Adelina has struggled to maintain her optimum weight for many years; she enjoys walking and the exercise not only has helped with her overall fitness, but it has helped to alleviate pain, promote confidence and improve her quality of life. However, she is concerned about her weight and her future wellbeing and mobility. She has seen her contemporaries develop deformities of the knee joint (genu valgum and genu varum), necessitating the use of canes or walking aids, and a number have needed joint replacements of the knees or hips.

The outward changes are apparent to her family, including her hesitancy and deliberate movements with position change, her need to ensure that there is a suitable chair to support her back at family outings, but mostly they notice her slow walking pace after she rises from a chair because of the discomfort, which improves within a short distance. This change in pace frequently causes her family to be concerned when they see the physical changes in their once active and energetic mother, whom they saw as invincible during their growing years. Adelina worries that her mobility problems and pain are making her look and act old. She worries that she may need to use a walking frame or walking sticks to move around. This affects the way she sees herself and her body image. As part of a comprehensive health assessment, nurses should include assessment of a person's view of their body image, which can impact on their overall mental health.

Quality of Life

Quality of life (QOL) has been studied among many populations and is an individual or personal measure. Little is known of the effect of osteoarthritis on the quality of life of older persons. However, the associated pain and loss of mobility significantly reduces a person's ability to attend to the ADLs (Hunter & Riordan 2014). In a survey of adults 75 years and older with osteoarthritis ($n = 168$) and those without osteoarthritis ($n = 246$), Jakobsson and Hallberg (2006) found that pain and reduced ability to perform ADLs significantly reduced the older person's QOL. However, there was no difference in reports of mood depression between those who did and did not have osteoarthritis. It is suggested that as a person ages they develop alternative views on life that assist in accommodating health and physical change. The reasons for this, as suggested by Dziechcia and colleagues (2013), is that older adults are more likely to feel pain than younger people.

Some evidence suggests that older persons with osteoarthritis who have control over their disease experience improved QOL (Sunden et al 2013). Although this may be challenging with arthritis, as symptoms are often unpredictable (Willis 2014). Strategies to support self-management of osteoarthritis include education about pain management, weight reduction, exercise and physical therapies (Fertelli et al 2019; Nicolson et al 2017; Roos & Arden 2016).

Harry and Adelina have a close relationship with their two adult children, but there is no extended family support other than their children and grandchildren. As they both worked throughout their adult lives, there was little time or opportunity to develop social relationships outside of work and family. Retirement has meant selling their property and moving away from lifetime neighbours and occupational contacts. Both Harry and Adelina face increasing social isolation that can have a negative impact on their QOL, especially as they are not actively involved in social activities outside their immediate family and small circle of lifetime friends.

Where pain and reduced ability to perform ADLs interfere with independence, there will be a negative impact on the QOL. Participating in leisure activities can provide a diversion from the symptoms of arthritis; however, it may be necessary to modify some activities. Janke and colleagues (2011) found that people with arthritis were willing to find new standards of participating in leisure activities if pain or symptoms became a limiting factor. As prolonged periods of immobility can increase pain, people with arthritis reported a need to take more regular stops when travelling and driving so that they could exercise (Janke et al 2011).

Key points

- Stiffness, fatigue and pain from osteoarthritis can affect the ability to carry out ADLs.
- Symptoms of osteoarthritis can cause anxiety, depression and feelings of helplessness which affect QOL.

Interventions to Attain Self-Management

Increasing interest in health self-management in our community is also associated with increasing availability of health information, especially through the internet. More seniors are looking for non-invasive approaches to manage their chronic health conditions, especially osteoarthritis. There are a number of non-pharmacological and pharmacological interventions that people such as Adelina can use to manage the pain and retain optimum mobility. Non-pharmacological interventions include exercise, physical therapy, joint protection, heat and cold therapy, hydrotherapy, acupuncture, nutrition and weight reduction (Swift 2012).

Exercise has been found to have both psychological and physiological benefits for older adults. In the presence of osteoarthritis, exercise strengthens the supporting skeletal muscles that stabilise the joints, which can help reduce pain and improve mobility and QOL (Swift 2012). Exercise also increases muscle strength, flexibility and may also reduce weight, all of which can help to manage the pain and disability associated with osteoarthritis (Harris & Crawford 2015). Exercise may be low impact, such as stretching to maintain the flexibility of the joints and swimming, but for more able older adults it can include power walking or aerobic exercise. There are a number of programs and opportunities for older community members to participate in, such as aqua-aerobics and aquatic exercise (also known as hydrotherapy). Aquatic exercise has been found to reduce pain, stiffness, and improve self confidence and muscle strength in older people with osteoarthritis (Fertelli et al 2019).

Rest is needed to reduce pain and to allow recovery after exercise (Walker 2011). It is also suggested that joints can be protected through attention to body mechanics and posture, and avoiding prolonged use of individual joints such as digging in the garden for long periods. More intensive or heavier activities should be broken down into shorter periods, alternating with rest and lighter activities (Walker 2011). The use of assistive devices, such as garden trolleys and washing trolleys, will protect joints from heavier workloads. Footwear that has a wide heel and uppers that cover the foot provide more structural protection to the foot bones and ankle joints and can reduce the pain of walking and exercise. Thermal therapy, such as the application of heat packs, can reduce muscle spasm and improve circulation, but care must be taken with their use for older clients due to the risks of thermal burns associated with reduced peripheral sensation.

Adelina has made some home modifications to accommodate her reduced mobility. Rather than bathing she showers, and rather than wearing high-heeled shoes she finds that flat slip-on shoes are easier to put on. At this stage she does not need home aids such as rails in the shower and toilet.

Over-the-counter (OTC) medications are frequently used to self-treat the milder symptoms associated with osteoarthritis. While some non-steroidal anti-inflammatory medications (NSAIDs) require a prescription, many people self-medicate with readily available analgesics and herbal supplements. Paracetamol is a commonly used pharmacological treatment for osteoarthritis pain (Swift 2012). However, there is some evidence that non-prescription NSAIDs (such as ibuprofen) are more effective on moderate pain but carry a greater risk of gastric ulcers or bleeding with their use (Shmerling 2016). Medications to manage osteoarthritis pain also include COX 2 selective inhibitors which can minimise the gastric issues associated with NSAIDs, but have been linked to an increased risk of stroke or heart attack (Shmerling 2016). Opioids are rarely used in the treatment of pain associated with osteoarthritis. If oral medications are not providing adequate pain relief, corticosteroid injections may be considered (Harris & Crawford 2015). People experiencing chronic pain should see their doctor or a medical professional before taking any analgesics to ensure that they are taking the medication that is best suited to their pain and any other medical conditions.

Adelina has been influenced by media advertising to try glucosamine with chondroitin as a self-treatment for the pain of osteoarthritis. While this OTC preparation as a combination supplement is more expensive than glucosamine alone, she is willing to try it. She has found that this medication reduces her knee pain significantly. However, a meta-analysis of all available randomised control trials on the effectiveness of glucosamine for people with osteoarthritis found that there was no significant benefits on pain or function (Runhaar et al 2017).

There is increasing access to alternative therapies for people with osteoarthritis, but individuals should be advised to seek the services of qualified practitioners of these therapies to ensure that there will be no interactions with other prescribed medications or adverse effects on other physical disorders. While Adeline is able to access many non-pharmacological treatments and adopt those that are suited to her resources and lifestyle, these should also be discussed collaboratively with her general practitioner (GP).

Key points

- Promote self-management by providing information.
- Comprehensive treatment regimens should be developed in consultation with the person's GP.
- Non-pharmacological interventions include exercise, physical therapy, alternative therapies, joint protection, heat and cold therapy, hydrotherapy, nutrition and weight reduction.
- Pharmacological interventions include OTC and prescription medications.

Family and Carers

Adelina remains an independent retiree with mobility and physical limitations. Her disability has little direct impact on her family, except for her inability to look after her grandchildren on days when her mobility is affected by pain. While she remains physically capable she is able to control her lifestyle to a high degree. However, her increasing frailty and vulnerability place her at risk of becoming physically less able to manage and also of having a fall.

While her children have families of their own, they also work to support themselves and maintain their own homes. Their ability to provide supportive or full-time care for their parents in the near future appears limited at this time. Harry and Adelina would do well to plan for such a contingency or look for alternative living arrangements (a smaller residence or access to home care/support), should one of them become disabled.

As Adelina sees her GP for regular health assessments and has her annual influenza immunisations with the practice nurse, she has had an ideal opportunity to discuss non-pharmacological options and evaluate her self-management strategies with her multidisciplinary team. She has found the input from her doctors, dietitian, nurse, occupational therapist and physiotherapist helpful to help keep her as active and well as possible.

Education for the Person and Family

Adelina, like many of her contemporaries, has access to information about osteoarthritis through the internet. However, the large amount of information can prove to be confusing and conflicting at times. Individuals like Adelina and her family would be best advised to use the resources of established support groups such as Arthritis Australia, My Joint Pain and Arthritis New Zealand, which provide up-to-date information sheets on varying self-management strategies, as well as the latest medical and scientific evidence presented in accessible language. Education should include an understanding of the processes of osteoarthritis, pain and mobility management, strategies to maintain mobility (such as activity and exercise), and short- and long-term therapies (pharmacological and surgical). Community health centres and practice nurses, as part of a multidisciplinary team, can provide information about free community education on self-management of osteoarthritis within the individual's own community for those who feel unable to use internet resources.

RHEUMATOID ARTHRITIS

Rheumatoid arthritis is a chronic condition that affects 1.9% of the Australian population (AIHW 2019), while rheumatoid arthritis makes up 14% of the prevalence of arthritis in New Zealand (Arthritis New Zealand 2018). Women and those over 65 are more likely to develop rheumatoid arthritis (AIHW 2013). Rheumatoid arthritis is characterised by chronic inflammation of the joints, usually the hand, but can affect the whole body, including the circulatory and pulmonary systems. Rheumatoid arthritis is a chronic inflammatory immune disease that causes joint damage and increased mortality (Smolen et al 2016). Joints become inflamed as a result of the immune system attacking the synovial membrane in the joint, and as a result the joint becomes inflamed and often permanently damaged (Vollenhoven 2016). People with rheumatoid arthritis may experience a decline in mobility and function, which impacts on their QOL and increases their risk of developing co-morbidities (Kitas & Gabriel 2011). A family history of rheumatoid arthritis increases the likelihood of developing the disease.

Treatment for rheumatoid arthritis includes medications to manage pain and control the inflammatory response (Smolen et al 2016). The effects of rheumatoid arthritis lead to increasing disability and isolation, and a holistic nursing assessment that includes the family is needed. While there is currently no cure for rheumatoid arthritis, over the last 20 years treatment options have improved (Storheim & Zwart 2014). Early diagnosis and intervention is important as the disease left untreated can lead to bone and joint damage, reduced QOL and high morbidity and mortality (Drosos et al 2019).

OSTEOPOROSIS

The term osteoporosis is derived from French, *osteoporose*, literally meaning porous bone. The earliest use of the term has been attributed to the French pathologist Jean George Chretien Martin Lobstein in the early nineteenth century (Schapira & Schapira 1992). It was later in the nineteenth century that more rigorous descriptions of osteoporosis included: (1) the absolute decrease in bone tissue, and (2) the abnormal draining of minerals from the bone. The modern application of the term includes the clinical manifestation of osteoporosis of skeletal fragility and increased risk of fracture. Currently, osteoporosis is defined as a disease characterised by low bone mass, micro-architectural deterioration of bone tissue leading to bone fragility, and increased fracture risk (Anonymous 1991). Bone mass and the micro-architecture of the bone are two important determinants of bone strength. Bone strength is the primary predictor of fragility fracture. Bone strength can be indirectly measured by several techniques, including dual-energy X-ray absorptiometry (DXA) in the form of bone mass or bone mineral density (BMD) (Cummings et al 2002).

Significance

Osteoporosis has been estimated to affect over 200 million women worldwide, with one-third of these women aged 60 to 70 years of age and the remaining aged over 70 (Cooper 1999). Approximately one-third of postmenopausal women have osteoporosis in North America and Europe (Hernlund et al 2013; Wade et al 2014). Although osteoporosis was often thought to be a disease mainly affecting elderly women, epidemiological studies have found that the disease also affects elderly men (Orwoll & Klein 1995).

The lifetime risk of osteoporotic fracture (from the age of 60) for a man and woman is 25% and 44% respectively (Nguyen et al 2007). It has been estimated that among elderly women and men around the world, an osteoporotic fracture occurs every 3 seconds (Johnell

& Kanis 2006). In women, the lifetime risk of hip fracture is equivalent to or even higher than that of breast cancer (Feuer et al 1993; Nguyen et al 2007). Importantly, sustaining an osteoporotic fracture increases the risk of subsequent fracture (Kanis et al 2004). Hip fracture is the most serious consequence of osteoporosis, because it is associated with an increased risk of mortality (Cauley et al 2000; Center et al 1999; Ensrud et al 2007). In Australia, osteoporosis currently affects 2.2 million elderly women and men (Ebeling et al 2013). The total direct cost of osteoporosis in Australia is estimated to be over $1.9 billion per year, with an additional $5.6 billion in indirect costs, based on an Access Economics report commissioned by Osteoporosis Australia (Ebeling et al 2013).

Bone Mass and the Diagnosis of Osteoporosis

'Bone mass' is a generic term, which is commonly used to describe the amount of tissue and mineral (calcium) in bone. An individual's current bone mass represents the cumulative effect of many factors, both present and past, some genetic and some due to lifestyle. Bone mass in the elderly is determined by peak attainment between the ages of 20–30 years and the rate of bone loss, with women having a significant loss in bone mass following menopause. The most common estimate of bone mass status is via a BMD from a DXA scan. For diagnostic purposes BMD is transformed into a T-score, which reflects the number of standard deviations (SD) above or below the mean in healthy young adults. The thresholds for each bone mass category are shown in Table 25.1 (Kanis 1994).

Fracture

The incidence of fracture in the community shows a bimodal relationship with age. Peaks are evident in youth and the elderly (Marcus et al 1996). In the young, more so in males, fractures incorporate long bones, and are due to significant trauma. While after the age of 50, fracture incidence climbs steeply in women (Donaldson et al 1990). The three main sites associated with osteoporotic fractures in elderly women and men are of the hip, spine and distal forearm (Jones et al 1994).

Risk Factors

During the past three decades numerous epidemiological studies have been undertaken to identify risk factors for fracture. Initial studies focused on hip fracture, but subsequent studies also considered non-hip fractures. Factors to date that have consistently been shown to be associated with increased risk of osteoporotic fracture are older age and being a female; a family history of fracture; low bone mass; low body weight; hormonal factors such as low oestrogen or testosterone levels; lifestyle factors such as smoking, excessive alcohol consumption and reduced physical activity; nutritional factors such as a low calcium diet; decreased vitamin D levels; a history of corticosteroid use; and falls. The strongest predictor of osteoporotic fracture is low bone mass, with measurements at the specific skeletal site having the highest risk. Therefore, low bone mass at the proximal femur is the strongest indicator of hip fracture risk. Outside of age and sex, one of the strongest risk factors is having a history of low-trauma fracture. This initial fracture related to low trauma, indicates bone fragility.

Timely diagnosis and the initiation of optimal treatment, when indicated, has been shown to reduce the risk of re-fracture (Ganda et al 2013; Huntjens et al 2014; Inderjeeth et al 2018; Lih et al 2011; Nakayama et al 2016). Unfortunately the majority of elderly women and men with an initial low-trauma fracture do not receive appropriate assessment for the presence of osteoporosis, or optimal treatment to prevent re-fracture (Andrade et al 2003; Leslie et al 2012). For this reason, the identification of osteoporotic fractures among adults, the screening for osteoporosis, and initiation of treatment where indicated has become a worldwide priority (Eisman et al 2012). This is why it is important to ensure that all adults who experience a low-trauma fracture are screened for the presence of osteoporosis and receive treatment when indicated to reduce the risk of a subsequent fracture.

TABLE 25.1
WHO Criteria for Clinical Diagnosis of Osteoporosis

BMD T-score	Diagnosis
T-score ≥ −1	Normal
−1 > T-score > −2.5	Low bone mass
T-score ≥ −2.5	Osteoporosis
T-score ≤ −2.5 with existing fracture	Severe osteoporosis

Kanis 1994.

Therapeutic Decisions

The basis of any therapeutic decision is the fracture probability assessed from evaluation of clinical risk factors jointly, if possible, with BMD measured by DXA. It is necessary to exclude other causes of low bone mass that may need treatment, for example, osteomalacia or primary hyperparathyroidism. The potential causes of secondary osteoporosis should be evaluated and treated if possible, such as thyrotoxicosis or multiple myeloma. Assessment of modifiable lifestyle factors should not be neglected, including smoking, excessive alcohol intake and nutritional habits. The patient should be informed that these factors also influence bone fragility. The choice of specific medications to decrease the risk of fracture will depend on the drugs available, their reimbursement status, personal preferences of the patient and contraindications.

Key points

- Risk factors linked to the development of osteoporosis include ageing, being a post-menopausal woman, family history of the disease, decreased vitamin D levels, low bone mass and a history of low trauma fracture.
- Lifestyle factors that can increase the potential for developing osteoporosis include low calcium intake, reduced physical activity, tobacco consumption and excessive consumption of alcohol.

- Therapeutic decisions should be made by incorporating the overall risk of osteoporotic fracture, using a validated risk assessment tool: www.garvan.org.au/promotions/bone-fracture-risk/calculator/

When considering Leila's health and social history, as described in Case Study 25.2, it can be seen that she has a history of nutritional deficits from her childhood which may have affected the attainment of peak bone mass. Maintaining a diet that is high in calcium and ensuring adequate vitamin D levels is of particular importance for women over the age of 45 to help maintain bone health (Nazarko 2011). A full nursing history of her intake with a focus on her intake of calcium-rich foods (milk, cheese, yoghurt, nuts and bread) will highlight any current deficiency. Vitamin D is found in oily fish and dairy foods; however, most of the vitamin D we need is produced by exposing the skin to sunlight (Nazarko 2011). Leila's history of working outdoors had stood her in good stead, but the nursing assessment should focus on current outdoor activity to maintain her vitamin D levels. Most significantly, Leila underwent a hysterectomy and bilateral oophorectomy almost 20 years ago. This is also the expected age for menopause, which results in decreased production of

---

CASE STUDY 25.2

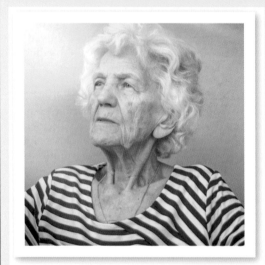

iStockphoto/ivanastar.

Leila is a 73-year-old widow who lives with her extended family in an urban area. Following the death of her husband Thomas 10 years ago, Leila moved in with her daughter and son-in-law, assisting with the care of Leila's three

grandchildren, who have now completed their education and left home. Throughout her early childhood and young adulthood Leila experienced periodic economic and nutritional deprivations because of the transient work habits of her family. She felt fortunate to have met and married Thomas, who had a trade and provided for her and her young family. Leila cared for her family and worked locally in a market garden. She developed strong relationships with the other women who worked in the garden.

Leila has been generally well during her life, plagued only by seasonal influenza complicated by her ongoing cigarette smoking. She was smoking up to two packets per week from the age of 14 until her first hospitalisation. At age 55 she underwent a hysterectomy and bilateral oophorectomy because of fibroid growth with associated uterine bleeding.

Leila has had several falls at home, two that resulted in fractures and the need for hospitalisation. Three years ago Leila sustained a Colles' fracture of the right wrist that required closed reduction. At the time she was assessed for osteoporosis, which was confirmed. Six months ago Leila fell while getting out of the car and sustained a fractured head of femur that was repaired with a hemiarthroplasty. Her recovery from surgery was problematic and she has returned to her daughter's home frail and highly anxious when mobilising.

oestrogen, a hormone that is central to maintaining bone mass (Simon et al 2007). Her decision to stop smoking almost 20 years ago and her minimal intake of alcohol at periodic family celebrations have eliminated these as risks to the development of osteoporosis. Perhaps the most telling factors in Leila's history are the two fractures she sustained as a result of minimal trauma and the subsequent diagnosis of osteoporosis. Unfortunately these initial low-trauma fractures were not followed by an assessment of BMD via a DXA scan and referral to a dedicated fracture liaison service.

Altered Mobility and Fatigue

Leila and her family face a number of challenges in relation to her mobility. Immobility increases the impact and severity of osteoporosis; an appropriate exercise program for Leila has the potential to maintain or improve bone strength, and as a consequence reduce the risk of falls through stronger muscles and improved balance. The appropriate exercise program would be developed in consultation with Leila's treating doctor and employing the skills of a physiotherapist who has experience in treating older women with a history of osteoporotic fracture (www.iofbonehealth.org/exercise-recommendations). The previous hip and Colles' fractures that Leila has experienced are indicators of osteoporosis, as they are often caused by a fall from standing height or less.

Leila has returned from hospital where she received assistance and instruction on using a walking frame from the physiotherapist and nurses. However, her right wrist has residual weakness from the previous Colles' fracture, and this adds to her insecurity with walking. Leila requires someone to walk beside her because she fears her right hand will not grip the walker securely; her loss of independent mobility has become a source of personal stress, as she is acutely aware of the demands she is making on her family. This acts as a disincentive to walking distances because of her slow pace and she has declined suggestions that she go outdoors and sit in the garden because she is afraid that her daughter will not hear her if she falls. The self-imposed limitations on her walking have reduced Leila's exercise tolerance and increased her levels of fatigue during activities such as bathing and walking to the kitchen for meals.

Leila's hip fracture is not the only source of her daily activity problems. The loss of strength from the fracture of her wrist has reduced her ability to turn on taps in the shower and bathroom, to be able to button or tie clothing and to grip the hairbrush to brush her own hair into the style she prefers. Where Leila once enjoyed preparing and cooking meals, she is no longer able to manipulate kitchen utensils or carry heavy pots or containers of food.

Body Image

Leila accepts most of the changes of ageing that she is experiencing, but her family take pains to ensure that her clothing is suitable for her ability. Her family pretend not to notice her occasional dishevelled appearance, as they know she has difficulty dressing herself and she cannot brush her hair well with her left hand. However, they take pains not to restrict her attempts to complete her own care.

Quality of Life

Leila's increasing frailty and reliance upon others for her safety and care have reduced her perception of her quality of life. She had imagined that she would share her later years in the company of her husband sharing memories and their achievements raising their family. Her loss of her husband, Thomas, and her loss of independence related to her osteoporosis have contributed to an alteration in her perceived quality of life. These responses are similar to those reported by Adachi and colleagues (2010), where pain, fatigue and mobility impairments were linked to lower reported quality of life among women with osteoporosis.

Interventions to Attain Self-Management

Because of her increasing age and decreased mobility, Leila and her family have accepted that she will need support to maintain and strengthen her current level of self-management. An assessment by the Aged Care Assessment Team (ACAT) of the home and family resources (structural, physical and emotional) has identified that there are no structural changes to be made as Leila's son-in-law has made some changes to facilitate her movement around the house. There are gentle ramps where there were previously access steps; the shower and toilet have handrails; and tiled flooring throughout the home is non-slip, although it is a hard surface to fall on. These all facilitate Leila's mobility and participation in family and outdoor activities.

Leila also needs a referral to the hospital's fracture liaison service (FLS), which will also refer on to the falls clinic, or community-based falls prevention programs, when indicated.

While Leila had been managing her medications independently, since her last fall her daughter has been monitoring the medications by dispensing daily doses in labelled containers kept on the kitchen table within her easy reach.

Education for the Person and Family

Following the ACAT assessment, Leila and her family participated in a conference with her doctor, nurse, occupational therapist and physiotherapist, at which they learned about a number of strategies they could implement to support Leila's recovery and reduce further disability. The family were helped to understand how the osteoporosis has developed, and its link to pain, disability and fractures. One of their primary goals as a family became the prevention of further falls and fractures; the dedicated FLS will coordinate DXA follow-up and medications management in an ongoing capacity. Leila's risk of falling was assessed against factors identified by Flores (2012). The factors include previous history of falling, diseases and disorders that affect balance and strength, sensory deficits, environmental factors and medication use (Flores 2012). Leila has a previous history of falls and while she does not have orthostatic hypotension or arthritis, she has some gait impairment and muscle weakness as a result of her previous fractures. Leila does not take any medication that may increase her risk of falls, and her home environment has been adjusted to reduce environmental falls. While this was of some comfort to Leila, it was only one factor. To improve posture, muscle strength and coordination, and so prevent future falls, Leila and her daughter began day rehabilitation at a local health centre where the physiotherapist taught Leila how to use and exercise her muscles effectively. The occupational therapist taught Leila how to exercise and use her right hand more effectively to dress and groom herself. Leila's daughter learned effective ways of getting her mother in and out of the shower and chairs at home and the types of utensils that would allow her mother to participate in food preparation again.

Leila and her family also learned that to prevent fractures and further bone loss, Leila needed to maintain an exercise program that actually challenged her bones. As she had already sustained two fractures, she was not a suitable candidate to undertake high-impact or resistance exercises, but they learned that weight-bearing exercises were most effective (www.iofbone-health.org/exercise-recommendations). Although Leila found the exercise regimen tiring at first, over time her endurance increased and she gained greater confidence in walking and self-care.

A review of the prescribed medications by the nurse identified the need for some further education on their effective use. Medications specifically related to the osteoporosis included a bisphosphonate preparation and paracetamol. The bisphosphonate preparation is used to reduce bone loss, but it can cause pain when swallowing (McBane 2011). Bisphosphonate has been associated with gastrointestinal complications and administration recommendations include taking it with a full glass of water and remaining upright for 30 minutes after administration (Lewiecki 2011). The nurse encouraged Leila to talk to her doctor about developing a comprehensive medication regimen, including an individual pain management plan to help her self-manage her disease, and follow-up by the FLS.

Information and contact details for Osteoporosis Australia (OA) (www.osteoporosis.org.au) in their state, and the International Osteoporosis Foundation (www.iofbonehealth.org/) were provided so that Leila and her family could access further information and advice on the disease. Leila's daughter was also provided with information, as having family history of maternal osteoporosis is a risk factor for developing the disease (Swann 2012).

CONCLUSION

In this chapter you have seen how two older people have experienced disability as a result of lifestyle diseases that affect and will continue to affect millions of Australians directly or indirectly in the future. Many residents in aged care facilities have one or both of these diseases, which limits their mobility and participation in wider society. Too often these limitations are considered a 'natural' part of ageing and thus not amenable to change and improvement. As this chapter has illustrated, there are a number of strategies that individuals and families can implement to prevent the onset of these diseases or reduce the severity of them. Nurses have a critical role in promoting independence and mobility through education and considered physical support.

Reflective Questions

1. What are the nursing considerations when looking after a client who has osteoarthritis in both hips and knees?
2. Consider strategies that a person with osteoarthritis may adopt at home to promote independence.
3. What are the risk factors for developing osteoporosis?

Acknowledgement

The author would like to thank Leonie Williams and Belinda Harpin for their contribution to this chapter.

RECOMMENDED READING

Australian Institute of Health and Welfare (AIHW) 2019. Osteoarthritis. AIHW, Canberra.

Australian Institute of Health and Welfare (AIHW) 2013. A snapshot of rheumatoid arthritis 2013. AIHW, Canberra.

Chiodo B 2007. Preventing osteoporosis – healthy bones for life. Journal of Community Nursing 21(5), 22–26.

Swift A 2012. Osteoarthritis 2: pain management and treatment strategies. Nursing Times 108(8), 25–27.

REFERENCES

Adachi JD, Adami S, Gehlbach S et al 2010. Impact on prevalent fractures on quality of life: baseline results from the global longitudinal study of osteoporosis in women. Mayo Clinic Proceedings 85(9), 806–813.

Anand A 2017. Management of osteoarthritis – a holistic view. Frontiers in Arthritis, Vol. 1. Bentham Publishers, Sharjah.

Andrade SE, Majumdar SR, Chan KA et al 2003. Low frequency of treatment of osteoporosis among postmenopausal women following a fracture. Archives of Internal Medicine 163(17) 2052–2057.

Anonymous 1991. Consensus development conference: prophylaxis and treatment of osteoporosis. The American Journal of Medicine 90(1), 107–110.

Arthritis New Zealand 2018. The economic cost of arthritis in New Zealand in 2018. Deloitte Access Economics.

Australian Institute of Health and Welfare (AIHW) 2019. Osteoarthritis. AIHW, Canberra.

Australian Institute of Health and Welfare (AIHW) 2018. Australia's Health. AIHW, Canberra.

Australian Institute of Health and Welfare (AIHW) 2013. A snapshot of rheumatoid arthritis 2013. AIHW, Canberra.

Australian Institute of Health and Welfare (AIHW) 2011. Population differences in health-care use for arthritis and osteoporosis in Australia. AIHW, Canberra.

Cauley JA, Thompson DE, Ensrud KC et al 2000. Risk of mortality following clinical fractures. Osteoporosis International 11(7), 556–561.

Center JR, Nguyen TV, Schneider D et al 1999. Mortality after all major types of osteoporotic fracture in men and women: an observational study. Lancet 353(9156), 878–882.

Cooke J, Ancoli-Israel S 2011. Normal and abnormal sleep in the elderly. Handbook of Clinical Neurology 98(C), 653–665.

Cooper C 1999. Epidemiology of osteoporosis. Osteoporosis International 9(Suppl. 2), S2–S8.

Cross M, Smith E, Hoy D et al 2014. The global burden of hip and knee osteoarthritis: estimates from the Global Burden of Disease 2010 Study. Annals of Rheumatic Diseases 77, 1323–1330.

Cummings SR, Bates D, Black DM 2002. Clinical use of bone densitometry: scientific review. JAMA: The Journal of the American Medical Association 288(15), 1889–1897.

Donaldson LJ, Cook A, Thomson RG 1990. Incidence of fractures in a geographically defined population. Journal of Epidemiology and Community Health 44(3), 241–245.

Drosos A, Pelechas E, Voulgari P 2019. Rheumatoid arthritis treatment. A back to the drawing board project or high expectations for low unmet needs? Journal of Clinical Medicine 8(8), 1237.

Dziechciaż M, Balicka-Adamik L, Filip R 2013. The problem of pain in old age. Annals of Agricultural and Environmental Medicine: AAEM, Spec no. 1, 35–8.

Ebeling PR, Daly RM, Kerr DA et al 2013. Building healthy bones throughout life: an evidence-informed strategy to prevent osteoporosis in Australia. MJA 2(Suppl. 1), 1–47.

Eisman JA, Bogoch ER, Dell R et al and ASBMR Task Force on Secondary Fracture Prevention 2012. Making the first fracture the last fracture: ASBMR task force report on secondary fracture prevention. Journal of Bone and Mineral Research 27(10) 2039–2046.

Ensrud KE, Ewing SK, Taylor BC et al 2007. Frailty and risk of falls, fracture, and mortality in older women: the study of osteoporotic fractures. Journal of Gerontology: Biological Sciences. Medical Science 62(7), 744–751.

Fertelli TK, Mollaoglu M, Sahin O 2019. Aquatic exercise program for individuals with osteoarthritis: pain, stiffness, physical function, self-efficacy. Rehabilitation Nursing 44(5), 290–299.

Feuer EJ, Wun LM, Boring CC et al 1993. The lifetime risk of developing breast cancer. Journal of the National Cancer Institute 85(11), 892–897.

Flores EK 2012. Falls risk assessment and modification. Home Health Care Management & Practice 24(4), 198–204.

Ganda K, Puech M, Chen JS et al 2013. Models of care for the secondary prevention of osteoporotic fractures: a systematic review and meta-analysis. Osteoporosis International 24(2), 393–406.

Glyn-Jones S, Palmer AJR, Price AJ et al 2015. Osteoarthritis. The Lancet 386, 376–387.

Harris H, Crawford A 2015. Recognizing and managing osteoarthritis. Nursing 45(1), 36–42.

Hegarty R, Treharne G, Stebbings S et al 2016. Fatigue and mood among people with arthritis: carry-over across the day. Health Psychology: Official Journal of the Division of Health Psychology, American Psychological Association 35(5), 492–499.

Hernlund E, Svedbom A, Ivergård M et al 2013. Osteoporosis in the European Union: medical management, epidemiology and economic burden. Archives of Osteoporosis 8(1), 1–115.

Hunter D, Riordan E 2014. The impact of arthritis on pain and quality of life: an Australian survey. International Journal of Rheumatic Diseases 17(2), 149–155.

Huntjens KM, van Geel TA, van den Bergh JP et al 2014. Fracture liaison service: impact on subsequent nonvertebral fracture incidence and mortality. The Journal of Bone and Joint Surgery (America), 96(4), e29.

Inderjeeth CA, Raymond WD, Briggs AM et al 2018. Implementation of the Western Australian Osteoporosis Model of Care: a fracture liaison service utilising emergency department information systems to identify patients with fragility fracture to improve current practice and reduce re-fracture rates: a 12-month analysis. Osteoporosis International 29(8), 1759–1770.

Jakobsson U, Hallberg IR 2006. Quality of life among older adults with osteoarthritis. Journal of Gerontological Nursing (August), 51–60.

Janke MC, Jones JJ, Payne LL et al 2011. Living with arthritis: using self management of valued activities to promote health. Qualitative Health Research 22(3), 360–372.

Jankowski G, Diedrichs P, Williamson H et al 2016. Looking age-appropriate while growing old gracefully: a qualitative study of ageing and body image among older adults. Journal of Health Psychology 21(4), 550–561.

Johnell O, Kanis JA 2006. An estimate of the worldwide prevalence and disability associated with osteoporotic fractures. Osteoporosis International 17(12), 1726–1733.

Jones G, Nguyen T, Sambrook PN et al 1994. Symptomatic fracture incidence in elderly men and women: the Dubbo Osteoporosis Epidemiology Study (DOES). Osteoporosis International 4(5), 277–282.

Kanis JA 1994. Assessment of fracture risk and its application to screening for postmenopausal osteoporosis: synopsis of a WHO report. WHO Study Group. Osteoporosis International 4(6), 368–381 with permission of Springer.

Kanis JA, Johnell O, De Laet C et al 2004. A meta-analysis of previous fracture and subsequent fracture risk. Bone 35(2), 375–382.

Kapoor M, Mahomed Nizar N 2015. Osteoarthritis: pathogenesis, diagnosis, available treatments, drug safety, regenerative and precision medicine. Springer International, Switzerland.

Kitas GD, Gabriel SE 2011. Cardiovascular disease in rheumatoid arthritis: state of the art and future perspectives. Annals of Rheumatic Diseases 70(8), 8–14.

Latz D, Schiffner E, Schneppendahl J et al 2019. Doctor, when can I drive? Range of motion of the knee while driving a car. The Knee 26(1), 33–39.

Leslie WD, Giangregorio LM, Yogendran M et al 2012. A population-based analysis of the post-fracture care gap 1996–2008: the situation is not improving. Osteoporosis International 23(5), 1623–1629.

Lewiecki M 2011. Safety of the long term bisphosphonate therapy for the management of osteoporosis. Drugs 71(6), 791–814.

Lih A, Nandapalan H, Kim M et al 2011. Targeted intervention reduces refracture rates in patients with incident non-vertebral osteoporotic fractures: a 4-year prospective controlled study. Osteoporosis International 22(3), 849–858.

Marcus R, Feldman D, Kelsey JL 1996. Osteoporosis. Academic Press, San Diego.

McBane S 2011. Osteoporosis: a review of current recommendations and emerging treatment options. Formulary (Cleveland, Ohio) 46, 432–439.

Medina S 2016. Knee osteoarthritis (orthopedic research and therapy). Nova Biomedical, New York.

Ministry of Health NZ 2016. Annual update of key results 2015–16: New Zealand Health Survey. Ministry of Health, Wellington.

Nakayama A, Major G, Holliday E et al 2016. Evidence of effectiveness of a fracture liaison service to reduce the re-fracture rate. Osteoporosis International 27(3), 873–879.

Nazarko L 2011. Silent epidemic: helping people live with osteoporosis. British Journal of Healthcare Assistants 5(3), 111–116.

Nguyen ND, Eisman JA, Center JR et al 2007. Risk factors for fracture in nonosteoporotic men and women. Journal of Clinical Endocrinology and Metabolism 92(3), 955–962.

Nicolson P, Bennell K, Dobson F et al 2017. Interventions to increase adherence to therapeutic exercise in older adults with low back pain and/or hip/knee osteoarthritis: a systematic review and meta-analysis. British Journal of Sports Medicine 51(10), 791–799.

Orwoll ES, Klein RF 1995. Osteoporosis in men. Endocrine Reviews 16(1), 87–116.

Roberts D 2017. Arthritis and connective tissue disease. In: Medical–surgical nursing: assessment and management of clinical problems, 10th edn. Elsevier, St Louis, Missouri.

Roos E, Arden N 2016. Strategies for the prevention of knee osteoarthritis. Nature Reviews. Rheumatology 12(2), 92–101.

Runhaar J, Rozendaal R, Van Middelkoop M et al 2017. Subgroup analyses of the effectiveness of oral glucosamine for knee and hip osteoarthritis: a systematic review and individual patient data meta-analysis from the OA trial bank. Annals of the Rheumatic Diseases 76(11), 1862–1869.

Schapira D, Schapira C 1992. Osteoporosis: the evolution of a scientific term. Osteoporosis International 2(4), 164–167.

Shmerling R 2016. Living well with osteoarthritis: a guide to keeping your joints healthy. Harvard Health Publications, Boston.

Simon JA, Murphy D, Ravnikar VA et al 2007. Hysterectomy and surgical menopause. A management plan based on expert opinion. Contemporary OB/GYN 52(9), 1–8.

Smolen JS, Aletaha D, McInnes IB 2016. Rheumatoid arthritis. The Lancet 16, 30173–30178.

Storheim K, Zwart JA 2014. Musculoskeletal disorders and the global burden of disease study. Annals of the Rheumatic Diseases 73(6), 949–950.

Stubbs B, Aluko Y, Myint PK et al 2016. Prevalence of depressive symptoms and anxiety in osteoarthritis: a systematic review and meta-analysis. Age and Ageing 46, 228–235.

Sunden A, Ekdahl C, Magnusson SP et al 2013. Physical function and self-efficacy – important aspects of health related quality of life in individuals with hip arthroplasty. European Journal of Physiotherapy 15, 151–159.

Swann JI 2012. Osteoporosis: the fragile bone disease. British Journal of Healthcare Assistants 6(2), 59–62.

Swift A 2012. Osteoarthritis 2: pain management and treatment strategies. Nursing Times 108(8), 25–27.

Tang H-Y, McCurry SM, Pike KC et al 2017. Differential predictors of nighttime and daytime sleep complaints in older adults with comorbid insomnia and osteoarthritis pain. Journal of Psychosomatic Research 100, 22–28.

Vollenhoven R, ProQuest 2016. Biologics for the treatment of rheumatoid arthritis. Springer Science, London.

Wade SW, Strader C, Fitzpatrick LA et al 2014. Estimating prevalence of osteoporosis: examples from industrialized countries. Archives of Osteoporosis 9, 182.

Walker J 2011. Management of osteoarthritis. Nursing Older People 23(9), 14–19.

Willis E 2014. The making of expert patients: the role of online health communities in arthritis self-management. Journal of Health Psychology 19(12), 1613–1625.

World Health Organization (WHO) 2016. Chronic diseases and health promotion. Chronic rheumatic conditions. Online. Available: www.who.int.en.

CHAPTER 26

Principles for Nursing Practice: Diabetes

TRISHA DUNNING

LEARNING OBJECTIVES

When you complete this chapter you will be able to:

- differentiate between type 1, type 2 and gestational diabetes mellitus
- state the principles of management for each type of diabetes
- state the acute and chronic complications of diabetes mellitus
- state the key principles of dietary management
- state precautions to be adopted prior to, during and following exercise
- understand the main action profiles and side effects of glucose-lowering medicines
- list the key issues that need to be discussed when educating people with diabetes mellitus.

KEY WORDS

diabetes complications

diabetes education

diabetes mellitus

dietary management and exercise management

GLOSSARY

AGEs: Advanced glycosylation end-products

BGL: Blood glucose level

CSII: Continuous subcutaneous insulin infusion

DKA: Diabetic ketoacidosis

DM: Diabetes mellitus

GDM: Gestational diabetes mellitus

GLM: Glucose lowering medicines

HbA1c: Glycosylated haemoglobin

HBGM: Home blood glucose monitoring

IGT: Impaired glucose tolerance

OGTT: Oral glucose tolerance test

SBGM: Self-blood glucose monitoring

INTRODUCTION

Diabetes mellitus (DM) is an epidemic of the twenty-first century. It is a metabolic disorder of increasing prevalence that affects an estimated 9.3%, 463 million people worldwide, and is projected to increase to 578 million (10.2%) by 2030 and 700 million (10.9%) by 2045 (International Diabetes Federation [IDF] 2019). In addition, an estimated >193 million people are at risk of diabetes but are undiagnosed (IDF 2019).

One person with diabetes dies every 6 seconds (IDF 2015). There are cultural and age-related differences in the prevalence and impact of diabetes among and within countries.

In Australia, 1.2 million people have diabetes as the initial diagnosis or an associated co-morbidity; 6% of the population, and 100,447 people are diagnosed each year. One million have type 2 diabetes, 117,000 have type 1 and 35,000 have gestational diabetes mellitus (GDM). Diabetes costs over $14.6 billion per year (Diabetes Victoria 2016). Men had a higher prevalence than women, at 6% and 4% respectively (Australian Institute of Health and Welfare [AIHW] 2019). GDM occurs in over 58% of births and women aged 45–49 are at greatest risk (AIHW 2018). Prevalence increased from 5% in 2000 to 15% in 2016–17 (AIHW 2019).

Australian Aboriginal and Torres Strait Islander (ATSI) people are at high risk of pre-diabetes and diabetes, with an overall prevalence rate of 13% in 2017–18 (one in eight people); rates are higher in ATSI women than men (Australian Bureau of Statistics [ABS] 2019; AIHW 2019). The prevalence is four times higher than in the general population.

Diabetes was present in one million hospital admissions in 2017–18, most of which concerned type 2 diabetes. Deaths were due to cardiovascular disease, cancer, stroke and renal disease (AIHW 2014). Diabetes is the second leading cause of death among ATSI people (Lalor et al 2014) and is particularly prevalent in rural areas (ABS 2014).

In New Zealand, based on the New Zealand Adult Nutrition Survey in 2018–19, the overall prevalence of diabetes was 7% and was more common among men than women: 8.3% and 5.8% respectively. A further 18.6% had pre-diabetes and the prevalence was higher in Māori and South Asian people (Ministry of Health NZ 2019). Like other countries, the prevalence of diabetes in New Zealand increases with age and is specifically linked to obesity.

Māori also have a higher prevalence of diabetes complications, especially renal failure and foot pathology and lower limb amputations, similar to ATSI peoples and First Nations people in the United States.

Significantly, diabetes prevalence increases in people over age 65 and a corresponding number in this age group are at risk of diabetes but are undiagnosed. In Australia, 43% of people over age 65 and 14% of those over age 80 have diabetes (AIHW 2011). The global prevalence in older people >65 is 112 million: 19.9% of diagnosed cases and a further 75% of older people have pre-diabetes (IDF 2019).

Approximately 20–25% of residents in aged care facilities have diabetes (Care Quality Commission 2014/2015; Sinclair et al 2001). These people are a vulnerable group and are likely to have functional deficits and between three and five co-morbidities and polypharmacy. Prevalence data varies depending on how data are collected. Many countries use self-report data. The IDF analyses the data collected from countries and literature searches. Thus, data can vary to some extent,

but it is useful to look at the trends in order to plan prevention and management strategies. Significantly, family members and carers who also live with diabetes provide significant support and assistance with self-care.

Diabetes encompasses many disorders characterised by hyperglycaemia, but there are two primary forms: type 1 and type 2 (World Health Organization [WHO] 2019). About 10–15% of people have type 1 and 85–90% have type 2 DM (WHO 2019). Type 2 DM is typically regarded as a disease that occurs in adults; however, there is increasing prevalence among children and adolescents (Alberti et al 2004; Saeedi et al 2019). Unless the blood glucose is kept close to normal, young people with diabetes will develop complications in early to late adulthood.

A third form that is increasing in prevalence, gestational diabetes mellitus (GDM), refers to diabetes that is first diagnosed during pregnancy. GDM is increasingly common in developed countries. GDM is also considered to be a precursor to type 2 DM, and up to half the women diagnosed with GDM go on to develop type 2 DM over the 20 years following pregnancy (Australian Diabetes In Pregnancy Study Groups [ADIPS] 2013; Lee et al 2007).

A rare form of diabetes, Maturity Onset Diabetes of the Young (MODY), refers to several specific genetic variants. Consequently, the underlying nature of MODY is heterogeneous (Fajans & Bell 2011; WHO 2019). While MODY is similar to type 2 DM in many respects, there are inherent differences among the genetic variants in presentation and treatment. MODY is not discussed in detail in this chapter.

The World Health Organization (WHO) proposed a new classification of diabetes in 2019 that encompassed the existing types 1 and 2, hybrid form, other specific types, unclassified diabetes, hyperglycaemia first diagnosed in pregnancy, and provided some guidance for diagnosing the various types in clinical settings (WHO 2019). Understanding the genetic and molecular basis of diabetes has implications for treatment.

Regardless of the type, diabetes is characterised by changes in normal glucose homeostasis that lead to chronic hyperglycaemia and altered carbohydrate, fat and protein metabolism. The changes arise from defects in insulin secretion or insulin action or a combination of both. The gastrointestinal tract plays a major role in regulating blood glucose after meals (postprandial glucose) through hormones called incretins, which are released when digested nutrients enter the small intestine. Incretins regulate gastric emptying and insulin release, which controls postprandial blood glucose and reduces the output of glucose from the liver (Holst

& Gribble 2016). The YouTube video, 'How insulin and glucagon control blood glucose levels' (4 minutes) (www.youtube.com/watch?v=e-3N7w2sWps20) outlines glucose homeostasis. Note the clip uses the term 'blood sugar', which is incorrect. The correct term is 'blood glucose'.

This chapter focuses on the management of type 1 and type 2 DM. Guidelines for the management of GDM can be found in midwifery textbooks and journal articles and on the Australian Diabetes In Pregnancy Study Group (ADIPS) website.

TYPE 1, TYPE 2 AND GESTATIONAL DIABETES

Type 1 and type 2 DM are traditionally regarded as different disease processes. However, the accelerator hypothesis suggests that type 1 and type are caused by the same three factors (Fourlanos et al 2008). The three factors are:

- lower beta cell replacement rate, the faster the cells are damaged
- modern environments that put high demands on beta cells, such as high fat, calorie-dense diets, reduced activity and environmental toxins
- autoimmune systems that aggressively attack stressed beta cells. The rate of immune system destruction of beta cells results in the different onset and presentation of the two types of diabetes. Generally, if the immune system reaction is aggressive, type 1 diabetes occurs. Type 2 diabetes occurs when the immune reaction is smaller or does not occur.

According to the accelerator hypothesis, all three factors affect everybody with diabetes, but different people have different 'mixes' of the three accelerator factors. In addition, genetic predisposition may play a role, especially in type 2 diabetes.

An individual can have type 1 or type 2 diabetes, but not both. People with type 1 diabetes require exogenous insulin to sustain life because their pancreatic beta cells do not produce any insulin; that is, they depend on insulin. Type 2 diabetes occurs when the pancreatic beta cells do not produce sufficient insulin and/or the body cannot use insulin effectively (insulin resistance). People with type 2 and GDM do not require exogenous insulin to sustain life in the early stages of the disease, but women with GDM are commenced on insulin if their blood glucose levels are close to the normal range, and over time more than 75% of people with type 2 require insulin to control their blood glucose due to beta cell exhaustion and other physiological changes. That is, type 2 diabetes is

associated with slow progressive loss of beta cell function and, consequently, insulin production. This does not mean they become type 1 diabetics. They remain type 2 and are referred to as having insulin-requiring diabetes because they usually still produce some insulin, which prevents them from developing ketoacidosis (DKA), unless they are very ill.

Type 2 DM is not distributed equally across the community: some ethnic groups have a higher prevalence. As mentioned previously, Australians from ATSI communities are particularly at risk. One in 12 ATSI peoples has diabetes (data based on ever being told they have diabetes by a doctor) (ABS 2014). Diabetes is prevalent in ATSI peoples from age 25 and prevalence increases with age to 39% after age 55. The prevalence of GDM is also increasing in ATSI women, where rates as high as 20% are reported (ABS 2019; AIHW 2018). Women from high-risk populations, such as the Indian sub-continent, Asia and Pacific islands, are at increased risk of GDM (AIHW 2019).

COMMON SYMPTOMS AND MANAGEMENT GOALS

DM presents as a combination of symptoms and signs which include thirst, polyuria, polydipsia, vision changes, and, in type 1 diabetes, weight loss. If the symptoms are not recognised and diabetes diagnosed, individuals with type 1 diabetes can develop and present with DKA. Hyperglycaemic hyperosmolar states (HHS) can occur in type 2 DM. Individuals who develop HHS have very high blood glucose levels, dehydration and often cognitive changes.

DKA is an emergency and requires fluid and insulin treatment to prevent death. HHS often has a slower onset and is more common in people over age 60 who often do not have a diagnosis of diabetes. Fluid and insulin are required treatments. HHS can also lead to death if it is not treated. HHS often occurs in older people in residential aged care facilities, and may be the first presentation of diabetes.

All diabetes treatments must be individualised and designed with the individual and sometimes their families, for example, children and older people with dementia. The goal of treatment is to assist the person with DM to achieve and maintain a blood glucose level (BGL) as close to normal physiological levels as possible (3.5–6.5 mmol/L) (Australian Diabetes Society [ADS] 2017), depending on their age, functional status and life expectancy (Dunning et al 2013; IDF 2013). Blood glucose needs to be controlled to delay the onset and reduce the severity of diabetes-related complications and reduce the associated morbidity and mortality. A combination of diet, medication and exercise/activity, supported by education designed to meet the needs of each person, are the most effective ways to achieve these goals.

It is important to realise that the person needs to undertake a great deal of self-care to meet their management goals. Self-care is challenging and burdensome for many people with diabetes and families caring for people with diabetes, particularly children and older people.

Two large landmark studies demonstrated an association between poor long-term blood glucose control and the onset and progression of complications for type 1 DM (The Diabetes Control and Complications Trial [DCCT] Research Group 1993) and type 2 DM (Stratton et al 2000) and identified the optimal BGLs for both types of DM. These studies remain the benchmark, because the cost and scale of these studies will probably preclude them from being replicated. However, the intervention and control groups are still being followed up.

The 10-year post-study follow-up shows the intensive blood glucose control group had lower rates of microvascular complications and mortality than the usual control group. This is referred to as the 'legacy effect' (Brett & Holman 2008). Interestingly, the beneficial effects of tight blood pressure control did not continue at the 2-year follow-up (Brett & Holman 2008).

Research and technological advances led to recognition of other factors that need to be considered when planning care and deciding on treatment target. For example, tight BGL control is unsafe and associated with significant adverse events, such as hypoglycaemia, and falls in older people (Dunning et al 2013; McCulloch & Munshi 2016). Research also indicates that glucose variability, swings between high and low blood glucose, is associated with inflammatory processes that lead to oxidative stress and complications, even when the glycosylated haemoglobin (HbA1c) is within the target range (Monnier et al 2008).

Type 1 Diabetes

Type 1 DM is the result of destruction of beta cells in the pancreas following some triggering event. The trigger event generally occurs some time before enough beta cells are destroyed to cause clinical symptoms. Symptoms seem to appear rapidly once the remaining beta cells are unable to meet the body's demand for insulin (American Diabetes Association [ADA] 2019; Craig et al 2011; De Fronzo et al 2004). Type 1 is the most common form of DM among children and young

adults, although the onset can occur at any age (ADA 2019; Craig et al 2011). The incidence of type 1 varies around the world. The highest incidence occurs in Scandinavian countries and the lowest among Asian people and populations living in the tropics, and it is extremely rare among First Nations people (Karvonen et al 2000; WHO 2019).

Type 1 DM has been associated with genetic determinants, environmental factors and acquired factors, including autoimmune reactions, which appear to play a significant role, because up to 70% of newly diagnosed people have islet cell antibodies that lead to beta cell destruction (De Fronzo et al 2004). Common antibodies include GAD65 and IA-2 (Pihoker et al 2005).

Some researchers have identified a peak in diagnosis in the winter months, although the finding is not consistent across all countries. Nevertheless, the seasonal incidence of the onset to type 1 suggests viral infections could be one triggering factor (De Fronzo et al 2004). The term idiopathic diabetes describes forms of type 1 diabetes with no known aetiology (ADA 2007). Idiopathic diabetes still occurs clinically but is not listed in the 2019 WHO classification. Discovering a cure for type 1 DM has been a priority for people with type 1 diabetes, their families and researchers for over 50 years. Although significant progress towards understanding the underlying causes has occurred, currently no cure or preventative measures are available.

Studies focusing on curing type 1 diabetes include gluten-free diets, vitamin D in combination with various other substances such as Diamicron, a sulphonylurea, and Etanercept, 'diabecell' encapsulated cell technology, Metformin, and stem cell research (Current Research into Cures for Type-1 diabetes 2016). The Accelerator Hypothesis, mentioned earlier, suggests trying to prevent the immune attack on the beta cells to prevent or cure type 1 diabetes might not cure it, but might change the rate and progression of beta cell destruction.

It is important for nurses to be aware that, unlike type 2 DM, obesity and lack of exercise do not contribute to the development of type 1 DM. However, people with type 1 are becoming heavier, in line with general population trends towards overweight and obesity (KidsHealth 2016; WHO 2019).

Type 2 Diabetes

Type 2 is the most common form of DM and in some groups, such as the First Nations people and South Pacific Islander peoples, it is the only form of diabetes (De Fronzo et al 2004; IDF 2019). People with type 2 DM do not usually require insulin to survive, although many (over 75%) do require insulin over time to compensate for declining beta cell function and declining insulin production (ADA 2019; Pihoker et al 2005; WHO 2019).

Although the aetiology of type 2 DM is not clear, there is a strong familial tendency to develop type 2 DM, particularly when combined with lifestyle factors, such as inactivity and inadequate diets that lead to obesity. Women who previously developed GDM are at increased risk of developing type 2 DM (IDF 2019), as are their offspring (ADIPS 2013; IDF 2019). Unlike type 1 DM, the beta cells are not destroyed by autoimmune processes and DKA rarely occurs in type 2 DM, but can develop in the presence of stress or other illnesses such as infection (ADA 2019; IDF 2019).

Overweight individuals, those who do not exercise and eat a diet high in fat, those from particular ethnic groups, those with a family history of diabetes, those using diabetogenic medicines and previous GDM are particularly at risk of developing type 2 DM (The Australian Type 2 Diabetes Risk Assessment Tool – AUSDRISK). People with excess abdominal body fat may not be obese according to traditional measures, but they are at risk because abdominal obesity is strongly associated with insulin resistance. Abdominal fat increases the risk of cardiovascular disease (Aguilar-Salinas et al 2006; Riddle & Karl 2012). Increasing age is also a diabetes risk factor; therefore some lean older people will develop type 1 DM or latent autoimmune diabetes in adults (LADA).

Metabolic Syndrome

The metabolic syndrome, which is strongly associated with insulin resistance, describes a cluster of symptoms and signs associated with type 2 DM and cardiovascular disease, namely abdominal obesity, dyslipidaemia, insulin resistance, hyperglycaemia, impaired fibrinolysis and hypertension (Katzmarzyk et al 2005; Riddle & Karl 2012, p. 2101; Rewers et al 2004). The risk of developing diabetes or a cardiovascular event increases as the levels for these indicators increase above the normal range (Aguilar-Salinas et al 2006; Bonadonna et al 2006). DM is associated with increased morbidity and mortality, and people with DM and insulin resistance are at higher risk of dying from cardiovascular disease (Bonadonna et al 2006; Riddle & Karl 2012).

There are two myths about type 2 DM, which unfortunately continue to be perpetuated by some health professionals, despite the evidence that DM is a common cause of death in Australia where it was linked to 11% of deaths as the principal or associated cause in 2017 (AIHW 2019). The blood glucose may not be very high, but hyperglycaemia of any level results in an inflammatory response that causes damage to body tissues. You may hear individuals say that they have '... a touch of sugar, but nothing to worry about'. In fact, any blood glucose above the normal range places the person at risk of developing all of the chronic complications discussed later in this chapter.

The Member States, including Australia, participated in a United Nations General Assembly convened to develop goals for managing chronic disease up to 2030, known as the Sustainable Development Goals. Seventeen goals and 169 targets were developed with the aim of reducing complications and premature mortality from non-communicable disease, including diabetes, by 33%, as well as achieving universal health coverage and access to essential medicines (United Nations 2015).

The second myth is that type 2 DM can be cured, although pre-diabetes can be reversed with effective management, including weight loss, regular aerobic and anaerobic exercise, and an appropriate diet. Sometimes glucose-lowering and other medicines are required. Increasingly, bariatric surgery is considered for very overweight individuals. However, the pathological processes associated with type 2 diabetes can manifest at any time if the individual does not continue to follow a healthy lifestyle.

DIAGNOSTIC CRITERIA

DM must be considered as the cause when the fasting BGL is above 7.0 mmol/L or random BGL is 11.1 mmol/L or higher on two occasions (ADS 2019). Generally, oral glucose tolerance tests (OGTT) are no longer routinely performed. However, a 75 gram OGTT at 24–28 weeks is still being performed to confirm GDM in at-risk groups (Diabetes Australia 2020). HbA1c is increasingly being used as a screening or diagnostic test in place of or as well as fasting BGL: HbA1c > 6.5% or 48 mmol/mol is diagnostic (ADS 2019).

Type 1 Diabetes

The signs and symptoms of type 1 DM develop rapidly (over days to weeks) and include hyperglycaemia; excessive thirst; frequent urination; excessive hunger; nausea and vomiting; weight loss; and blurred vision (ADS 2019; Craig et al 2011; WHO 2019). However, the initial triggering event that has led to beta cell destruction usually occurs years before symptoms develop. People with type 1 DM may be acutely ill when diagnosed, frequently presenting as a medical emergency with hyperglycaemia over 15 mmol/L, ketone bodies in the blood or urine, signs of acidosis and severe dehydration. The diagnosis is made on clinical signs and laboratory BGL and ketones and sometimes tests for GAD antibodies are used. OGTT tests are not usually performed in type 1 diabetes.

A detailed description of the signs, symptoms and management of severe hyperglycaemia will not be provided; therefore you are advised to consult one of your texts if you need to revise that information.

Type 2 Diabetes

The onset of type 2 DM is usually insidious and may occur over years. The symptoms are similar to type 1 (hyperglycaemia; excessive thirst; frequent urination; excessive hunger; nausea and vomiting and blurred vision), although weight loss is rarely a feature: in fact, the majority of people with type 2 DM are overweight or obese. However, many people do not experience these symptoms and may present with tiredness/lethargy or a complication of diabetes, such as a cardiac event.

As previously stated, DKA is rare in people with type 2 DM, but they may present with HHS. Opportunistic screening using the AUSDRISK tool is often used to detect people at risk of diabetes before they develop diabetes, because early detection may prevent or delay the onset of type 2 diabetes and its related complications. Nurses are encouraged to assess their personal and/or family diabetes risk using the AUSDRISK tool, which is available on www.diabetesaustralia.com.au/risk-calculator. The diagnosis is confirmed by a fasting BGL, a non-fasting BGL or HbA1c.

The prevalence of type 2 DM in children and adolescents is increasing globally (IDF 2019). A rare form of type 2 DM in young people called Maturity Onset Diabetes of the Young (MODY) occurs in particular genetic forms and in families.

MANAGING DIABETES

Diabetes management involves medications (insulin and/or oral glucose-lowering medicines [GLM] or other injectable GLMs), dietary modification, exercise and self-management education. While the principles of dietary modification and exercise are common to all types of DM, the medication regimen depends on the type of diabetes the person has and the risks and benefits of the medicine for the individual, the BGL pattern and life expectancy. People with type 1 DM are not treated with oral GLMs (ADA 2019; Craig et al 2011), although, as indicated earlier, trials using Metformin to prevent type 1 DM are underway. People must have an individualised insulin regimen designed to maintain their BGL as close as possible to physiological levels and that also reflects their lifestyle. People with type 2 DM may be prescribed oral or injectable GLMs and/or insulin, depending on their BGL pattern (Colagiuri et al 2009; NHMRC 2014).

Medication Management

This section provides an overview of management. DM is a complex disorder that is associated with other disease processes, for example, cardiac disease and stroke, and leads to complications in almost all body systems. Therefore, you are advised to consult specialised and relevant resources to assist you to develop personalised care plans for people with DM and their families that suit their goals and care preferences, metabolic disturbance, age, and life expectancy: one care plan does not suit everybody and is not safe for everybody.

Type 1 diabetes

In the person without DM, insulin release is stimulated by the ingestion of food containing carbohydrates and the incretin hormones in the gut. The objective of treatment is to have small amounts of insulin circulating at all times (basal insulin), supplemented by larger doses after meals (prandial insulin). A regimen of insulin injections is prescribed to mimic the physiological insulin secretion pattern of people who do not have DM.

The most common regimens for people with type 1 DM are either:

1. a combination of meal-time (rapid-acting) and background (long-acting) insulin
2. continuous subcutaneous infusion of insulin (CSII) of rapid-acting insulin.

Insulin requirements can increase during illness. Extra insulin may be given with meals in both regimens.

Insulin is administered by subcutaneous injection using a needle and syringe, an insulin pen device or more CSII through an infusion pump which is programmed to deliver basal insulin and bolus doses when needed, for example, with meals. CSII is more commonly used for younger individuals, but some older people also use CSII. Insulin is destroyed in the gut, therefore insulin needs to be injected.

New forms of oral (The Diabetes Prevention Trial – Type 1 Study Group 2005) and inhaled (McElduff & Yue 2007; Rosenstock, Cappelleri et al 2004; Rosenstock, Lorber et al 2010; Skyler et al 2004) insulin are being tested, but are not widely used.

Insulin was originally extracted from the pancreas of cattle or pigs. Current forms of insulin are produced in a laboratory, which overcomes some of the side effects

TABLE 26.1
Types of Insulin

	Onset	Peak	Duration
Premixed Insulin Preparations (Biphasic)			
Insulin Neutral 30% + Isophane 70% Brand name: Mixtard 30/70	30 mins	2–12 hrs	24 hrs
Insulin Neutral 30% + Isophane NPH 70% Brand name: Humulin 30/70	More rapid than NPH alone	2–12 hrs	16–18 hrs
Insulin Neutral 50% + Isophane 50% Brand name: Mixtard 50/50	30 mins	4–8 hrs	24 hrs
Analogue Insulin Preparations			
Rapid-Acting Insulin (Prandial)			
Insulin Aspart 100 units/mL Brand name: NovoRapid	0–20 mins	1–2 hrs	4–5 hrs
Insulin Lispro 100 units/mL Brand name: Humalog	0–20 mins	1–2 hrs	4–5 hrs
Insulin Glulisine 100 units/mL Brand name: Apidra	0–20 mins	1–2 hrs	4–5 hrs
Long-Acting Insulin (Basal)			
Insulin Detemir 100 units/mL Brand name: Levemir	0.5–1 hr	3–8 hrs	Up to 24 hrs
Insulin Glargine 100 units/mL Brand name: Lantus	1–2 hrs	None	24 hrs
Ultra Long-Acting			
Toujeo	1–2 hrs	8–10 hrs	Up to 24 hours
Human Insulin Preparations			
Short-Acting Insulin			
Insulin Neutral HM 100 units/mL inject subcutaneous Brand name: Humulin R	30 mins	2–4 hrs	6–8 hr
Insulin Neutral HM 100 units/mL inject subcutaneous Brand name: Actrapid	30 mins	2.5–5 hrs	8 hrs
Intermediate-acting insulin			
Insulin Isophane 100 units/mL inject subcutaneous Brand name: Protaphane	1.5 hrs	4–12 hrs	24 hrs
Insulin Isophane NPH 100 units/mL inject subcutaneous Brand name: Humulin NPH	1 hr	4–10 hrs	16–18 hrs

Insulin is given subcutaneously. In acute illness short-acting insulin can be given via intravenous infusion.

associated with insulin from animal sources. The name and time of onset, peak and duration of action of insulin available in Australia is presented in Table 26.1 (Australian Medicines Handbook 2015).

Insulin doses are individualised depending on the person's blood glucose pattern and HbA1c. It is important to note that insulin requirements are dynamic and therefore require frequent BGL monitoring and insulin dose adjustment to achieve the best possible, safe glycaemic control. Early in the diagnosis of type 1 DM there is often a phase when there is some residual insulin secretion and insulin doses may be very small or not required for a brief period of time. This phenomenon is commonly referred to as the 'honeymoon' period (Harmel & Mathur 2004), and is a result of the reduced stress on the beta cells in the pancreas, which enables them to produce some insulin prior to their complete destruction. The honeymoon phase may not occur in toddlers. This phenomenon can prove challenging for patients and their families as they sometimes regard the remission as a cure. For this reason, insulin is usually not stopped once it is commenced. Support and education are the keys to successfully negotiating this period in the disease process.

Basal or long-acting insulin

Long-acting insulin is used specifically to control the release of stored glucose from the liver, and therefore control the fasting BGL. Long-acting insulin analogues include Insulin Glargine (Lantus®), Insulin Detemir (Levemir®) and Insulin Toujeo. They are usually in the form of daily or twice-daily injections as basal insulin therapy (Australian Medicines Handbook 2015). These insulin analogues have largely replaced premixed insulins: Isophane (Protaphane®, Humulin NPH®) (intermediate-acting insulin) and Lente (Ultralente®, Humulin L®) and Ultratard® (long-acting insulin). Glargine (Ratner et al 2000) and Detemir (Hermansen et al 2001) are associated with fewer hypoglycaemic events.

Glargine, Detemir and Toujeo provide a prolonged and reasonably consistent level of insulin, which more accurately mimics insulin secretion in people without DM (Garber et al 2012). Glargine, Detemir and Toujeo cannot be mixed in the same syringe as other insulins because the action profile will be affected.

The onset of action of intermediate-acting insulin is around 90 minutes after injection, with the peak action at 4–12 hours and duration of 24 hours. The onset of action for long-acting insulin is around 4 hours, followed by a broad peak of action that lasts for 8–16 hours with a duration ranging from 20 to 36 hours.

Rapid-acting (prandial) insulin

The preferred option for mealtime insulin in adults is one of the rapid-acting analogues: Insulin Aspart (NovoRapid®) or Insulin Lispro (Humalog®) or Insulin Glulisine (Apidra®). All have rapid onset of action (10–20 minutes) and short duration (3–5 hours), thus mimicking natural secretion of insulin following meals. Rapid-acting insulin is administered before meals and large snacks of more than 15 grams carbohydrate (equivalent to one slice of sandwich-thickness bread). It is ideal for adults with type 1 DM to have flexible insulin doses depending on their carbohydrate intake. Therefore, it is important that management regimens for people with type 1 DM allow for a flexible

lifestyle and that they have the opportunity to attend specific education programs to provide them with the skills and knowledge required to assume a self-care role.

Education programs such as DAFNE (Dose Adjustment For Normal Eating) (McIntyre 2006) have been designed specifically for people with type 1 DM, while a similar program called DESMOND was designed for people with type 2 diabetes (Diabetes UK). A detailed description of the characteristics of various types of insulin can be found in pharmacology texts such as the Australian Medicines Handbook.

Continuous subcutaneous infusion of insulin (CSII)

The advent of portable and reliable subcutaneous infusion pumps revolutionised the management of type 1 DM. Insulin pumps reduce the need for multiple daily injections and achieve better glucose control because the insulin doses can be adjusted frequently. One drawback of using CSII is that equipment failure, including blockage or disconnection of the tube, can result in a rapid elevation of BGL. The pumps and the necessary consumables are expensive and not always covered by private health insurance, although consumables are available through the government-subsidised National Diabetes Services Scheme. Cost does prevent some people from using pump therapy. Successful use of a pump depends on frequent, accurate BGL testing and the person's ability to accurately count carbohydrate intake (National Institute for Health and Clinical Excellence [NICE] 2011).

Either rapid- or short-acting insulin is used in insulin pumps (CSII). There are two specific modes of administration:

- basal rate, meaning the continuous rate of insulin infused as a background dose
- bolus rate, meaning the mealtime dose of insulin given as a bolus to cover the carbohydrate intake.

Specific education programs are required to enable people to use CSII effectively and safely and assistance should be available when required (NICE 2011).

Type 2 Diabetes

Unlike people with type 1 DM, people with type 2 DM do not usually require exogenous insulin to sustain life early in the course of the disease. Dietary modification and increased exercise are the first approaches for managing type 2 DM, particularly those who are overweight and whose BGL is just above the normal range.

Over the past decade the medication management of type 2 has changed significantly. Insulin is now commonly used when hyperglycaemia persists and the person is taking maximum doses of oral GLMs, and new categories of GLMs have been introduced (ADA 2019; Colagiuri et al 2009; Kamp 2007; NICE 2011). Most GLMs reduce the HbA1c by 0.5 to 2% depending on the medicine class.

Insulin-sensitising medicines

These medications lower BGLs by sensitising the muscle and liver cells to insulin, which may improve the insulin resistance present in type 2 DM and increase the uptake of glucose by cells (Kamp 2007). Insulin-sensitising medicines have the advantage of lowering BGL without placing the person at risk of hypoglycaemia and are effective for people who are overweight or obese. Commonly used medications are Biguanide (Metformin®), the medicine of choice, or a thiazolidinedione (TZD). However, TZDs are not commonly used because of the associated risk of oedema, and are contraindicated in the presence of cardiac disease.

Metformin can significantly reduce the incidence of both microvascular and macrovascular complications, although it can also cause gastrointestinal upset, such as nausea, abdominal pain and diarrhoea. These medications are not suitable for all people and they should be introduced at a low dose, which is slowly increased until the recommended dose is achieved (Australian Medicines Handbook 2016) (see Table 26.2).

Insulin-stimulating medicines

Sulfonylurea derivatives are a class of GLMs that are used to manage type 2 DM. These are short-acting forms of these medicines (see Table 26.2), which act by stimulating insulin release from the beta cells in the pancreas. A side effect of these GLMs is their potential to cause hypoglycaemia, therefore the doses of these medicines may be increased gradually to assess the dose response. They also cause weight gain. Therapeutic dose adjustment is usually guided by SBGM patterns results. Sulfonylureas are often used in combination with the insulin-sensitising medicines to address the major features of type 2 DM: reduced insulin production and insulin resistance in the cells. The common forms of oral GLMs are shown in Table 26.2 (Australian Medicines Handbook 2016).

Incretin medicines

The oral dipeptidyl peptidase 4 (DPP4) inhibitors enhance circulating concentrations of glucagon-like peptide-1 (GLP1) and glucose-dependent insulinotropic polypeptide (GIP) (Richter et al 2008). This causes an increase in glucose-dependent insulin secretion and reduces glucagon secretion. There is little risk of hypoglycaemia when using incretin medications alone or in combination with Metformin. A specific benefit of incretins is that they are weight neutral (AMH 2016; Inzucchi et al 2012; NHMRC 2014).

Injectable GLP1-receptor agonists mimic endogenous GLP1, therefore they stimulate the pancreatic beta cells to produce insulin in a glucose-dependent manner. In addition, they reduce appetite and slow gastric emptying. The major advantage of the incretins is modest weight reduction in most cases; however, the side effects of nausea and vomiting may limit their tolerability for some people. It is important to consider the prescribing precautions and potential side effects when administering GLMs (see Table 26.2).

Insulin therapy

Insulin therapy is usually commenced when oral GLMs do not keep the BGLs within the individual's target range or when there are contraindications to their use; for example, declining renal function.

It is important to note that commencing insulin for a person with type 2 DM does not change the diagnosis. People with type 2 DM who inject insulin are referred to as 'insulin requiring' and people with type 1 DM are 'insulin dependent'. Insulin therapy can be combined with oral GLMs or as a replacement therapy depending on the individual's circumstances. Often less intense insulin regimens are used. Premixed insulin preparations are still used to manage type 2 DM. Insulin therapy is used in combination with Metformin, a sulfonylurea or both. Goals for glucose control are individualised and may be higher than normal for frail older people with diabetes (Dunning et al 2013; IDF 2013).

There is no consensus about when to prescribe insulin for people with type 2 DM, although HbA1c levels of more than 7% on more than one occasion are regarded by clinicians as an appropriate time to commence insulin.

Frequently a small dose of insulin is required to start. As insulin production declines over time the insulin dose may need to be increased with longer duration of diabetes. Insulin reduces an individual's

TABLE 26.2
Glucose-Lowering Medicines, Doses, Side Effects and Duration of Action

Medicine	Usual Daily Dose	Frequency	Possible Side Effects	Duration of Action (DA)
Sulphonylureas Reduce HbA1c by 1–2% used alone			Some reduce myocardial ischaemic preconditioning	
Euglucon 5 mg Glimel 5 mg		>10 mg in divided doses Taken with, or before, food	Nausea, anorexia, skin rashes Severe hypoglycaemia especially in older people and people with renal dysfunction	
Glipizide				
Minidiab 5 mg	2.6–40 mg	Up to 15 mg as a single dose Taken before meals	GIT disturbances Skin reactions Hypoglycaemia (rare)	Up to 24 hours Peak: 1–3 h
Gliclazide				
Diamicron MR (a sustained release form)	30–120 mg Dose increments should be 1–2 weeks apart Should not be crushed	Daily	Hypoglycaemia	Released over 24 hours
Glimepiride (Amaryl)	1–4 mg	2–3 per day	Hypoglycaemia	5–8 h
Biguanides Reduce HbA1c by 1–2% used alone				
Metformin				
Diaformin 500 mg Diabex 500 mg Glucophage 500 mg	0.5–1.5 g May be increased to 3–0 g	1–3 times/day Taken with or just after food	GIT disturbances Lactic acidosis Reduce B12 absorption	5–6 h
Combination medicines				
Metformin and gyburide: Glucovance Metformin and rosiglitazone: Avandamet Metformin and sitagliptin: Janumet XS Saxagliptin and metformin: Kombiglyze			Hypoglycaemia especially in older people	
Meglitinides Repaglinide Nataglitinide	0.5–16 mg	2–3 per day	Hypoglycaemia with other GLMs Weight gain GIT disturbance	

TABLE 26.2
Glucose-Lowering Medicines, Doses, Side Effects and Duration of Action – cont'd

Medicine	Usual Daily Dose	Frequency	Possible Side Effects	Duration of Action (DA)
Thiazolidinediones Reduce HbA1c by 0.5–1.4% Rosiglitazone: 4, 8 mg Pioglitazone: 15, 30, 45 mg	4–8 mg	Daily	Oedema, weight gain, CCF, heart failure Raised liver enzymes, Fractures Rosiglitazone: pregnancy risk in women with polycystic ovarian disease, increased LDL-C and MI risk Pioglitazone: might increase bladder cancer risk	
Alpha-glucosidase inhibitors Acarbose: 50, 100 mg Reduce HbA1c by 0.5–0.8%	50–100 mg	TDS with food	GIT problems, for example, flatulence, diarrhoea Hypoglycaemia	
Incretin Hormones Two types: DPP-4 and GLP-1 DPP-4 Inhibitors Reduce HbA1c 0.5–0.8% Sitagliptin Vildagliptin Saxagliptin Linaglyptin Alogliptin	100 mg per day in twice-daily regimen in combination with metformin, sulphonylurea or a TZD Moderate renal failure 50 mg Severe renal disease 25 mg	With or without food	Do not cause hypoglycaemia	
GLP-1 receptor agonists Reduce HbA1c by 0.5–1% Exenatide Bydureon Lixisenaride	1–3 times per day depending on the medicine: Lixisenatide is administered daily Bydureon is administered once per week		Flatulence and abdominal bloating	
Sodium-glucose cotransporter-2 (SGLT-2) Dapagliflozin Canagliflozin			Increased incidence of urinary tract and genital infections Possibility of polyuria in volume-sensitive people	

Not all brand names are shown. Refer also to the Australian Medicines Handbook, Therapeutic Guidelines Endocrinology and the National Prescribing Service website.

resistance to the insulin produced by their pancreas, which enhances the action of their insulin. People with type 2 DM frequently start on one injection of long-acting insulin per day with short-acting insulin being added before meals if the BGL is not within their target range.

Basal insulin is generally prescribed at either pre-supper or at bedtime. In clinical practice, insulin start doses are usually weight-related. While insulin-requiring people generally require large doses of insulin to achieve good glucose control (up to 2.0 units per kg per day), starting doses are usually much lower and may be as low as 0.1 unit per kilogram per day. For example, a 100 kg person may be prescribed 10 units of long-acting insulin at bedtime in addition to oral medications. Insulin doses in type 2 DM are adjusted according to the person's specific response.

If insulin therapy is introduced because there are contraindications to oral and other injectable GLMs, long-acting analogues are usually preferred because of their low risk of hypoglycaemia. However, twice-daily doses of premixed insulin are often prescribed. The choice of premixed insulin depends on the individual's blood glucose pattern. Start doses are usually estimated as 0.5 units per kilogram per day, with the total daily dose divided so that 60% is injected at breakfast and 40% is injected at the evening meal. Therapeutic adjustment of insulin depends on the individual's health status and may be as frequent as daily or according to 2-hourly BGLs if intravenous insulin infusions are used for people who are acutely ill in hospital and during surgery. Often dose adjustments are made weekly for people in the ambulatory or community settings when insulin is first commenced. A goal of diabetes education is to teach people to use their blood glucose patterns to adjust their own insulin doses.

Dietary Interventions
Type 1 diabetes
The development of type 1 DM is not associated with obesity or a sedentary lifestyle; however, that is not understood by many people, including health professionals. As a result, it is not unusual for children with type 1 diabetes and their parents to be blamed for contributing to the development of type 1 DM. Nurses need to understand the differences between the two types of diabetes and educate the community when they are aware of inaccurate perceptions.

Likewise, uninformed people, including clinicians, believe type 1 is 'genetic' and type 2 is caused by 'lifestyle'. In fact, type 2 possibly has a stronger genetic component than type 1. Fewer than 20% of people with type 1 have a close relative with the disease. Some genes predispose people to type 1, as they do with type 2. Unless various environmental stressors activate those genes, people do not develop diabetes.

While type 1 DM is not specifically associated with weight gain, it is particularly important that people with type 1 consider the type and quantity of carbohydrate they eat and the timing of meals relative to the administration of insulin to achieve optimal glycaemic control. People with type 1 DM are at particular risk of hyperglycaemia leading to DKA and hypoglycaemia, both of which can lead to loss of consciousness (addressed later in this chapter under Acute Complications). Dietary counselling and education will assist people with type 1 DM to prevent those acute complications and also slow down the development and progression of both micro- and macrovascular complications, which are invariably present to some degree in people who have had type 1 DM for more than 5 years (The DCCT Research Group 1993).

Type 2 diabetes
Obesity is increasing in all developed countries, and lifestyle modification, usually geared to weight management using both diet and exercise, is essential to achieve weight loss in those people who are overweight and obese. Research has unequivocally demonstrated that type 2 DM can be prevented, or at least delayed, by appropriate and timely lifestyle modification (Moore et al 2007).

Nutritional management and education are the cornerstones of DM care (Dietitians Association of Australia, New South Wales Branch Diabetes Interest Group 2006). Everybody, including clinicians and people with type 2 DM (and when possible those with IGT), should follow the Australian Dietary Guidelines. Specialist assessment and education from a dietitian is recommended for people with diabetes (see Case Study 26.1). The basic principles centre around regular meals, with an emphasis on low-fat, high-fibre and controlled carbohydrate intake, such as the Mediterranean diet, which is associated with lower risk for diabetes, cardiovascular disease and cancer (Perry 2016).

CASE STUDY 26.1
Issues for Dietary Management in Culturally Diverse Groups

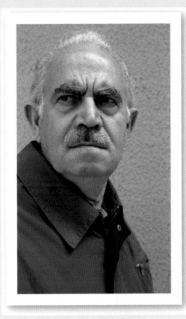

iStockphoto/okeyphotos.

Mr A is a 78-year-old man who was admitted to the stroke unit with a provisional diagnosis of TIAs or syncope. He has lived in Australia since 1995, but speaks only limited English. He was accompanied by his son. The medical history was taken in the emergency department. Clinical observations noted: radial pulse rate 125 bpm irregular; blood pressure (BP) 145/62; respiratory rate 28 bpm. Results of blood analysed for urea, electrolytes, creatinine (UECs) were within normal limits (plasma glucose was not ordered). Haematological profile was described as unremarkable. An electrocardiograph (ECG) identified acute inferior changes with ST-segment elevation.

A healthcare interpreter speaking Arabic was booked for the next day, when a full nursing assessment was conducted. During this assessment Mr A stated that he had diabetes in 2001, but after taking insulin injections for a couple of months he was started on tablets, but 'they ran out a few years ago'. Other medical history included essential hypertension and intermittent central chest pain associated with exercise for several months. Nursing staff noted his ECG, and troponin levels confirm AMI complicated by pulmonary oedema. Also, random capillary blood glucose estimation was attended with the post-breakfast result of 13.1 mmol/L. No formal measurements of blood glucose or HbA1c had been ordered on admission due to

the absence of history of DM being noted by ED medical staff. Mr A lives with his extended family and his daughter-in-law is his main carer.

The nursing staff notified the medical team and suggested investigations of formal blood glucose and HbA1c, in addition to ward-based capillary blood glucose levels pre-meals. A 'diabetic diet' was also ordered. Referrals were made to the diabetes educator, dietitian and cardiac rehabilitation nurse. The discharge planner was notified of admission as Mr A may require support post-discharge.

Mr A's general practitioner was contacted by the medical staff and a comprehensive list of prescribed medications was provided. The Arabic-speaking registrar discussed the prescribed medication list with Mr A. It was discovered that he was not taking any of the prescribed medications because he stated that there were just too many. The medical staff prescribed an ACE inhibiter for BP, Diamicron MR for diabetes and aspirin as an anticoagulant.

The following is a chart of the ward-based capillary BGL:

Before Breakfast	Before Lunch	Before Dinner	Before Bed
6.1	12.8	3.4	16.7
7.8	8.1	19.8	27.1
7.0	16.8	2.3	6.1
8.7			

The nursing staff noted that Mr A had been eating the food the family brought from home in addition to the food provided by the hospital. Mr A's carbohydrate intake could be twice that recommended by the dietitian. As a result, his BGL was variable. The family told the nursing staff they thought their father would prefer the food from home because he doesn't like 'Aussie food', and 'anyway we always bring food when people are ill'. Mr A was bored and hungry in hospital, so he ate the food provided by both the hospital and his family. Following a family discussion, Mr A decided to only eat the food from home and the family agreed to bring all his meals from home. His daughter needed to discuss Mr A's dietary requirements with the dietitian. Mr A's blood glucose levels became more stable when the diet was modified; however, the medical staff prescribed Diamicron MR 120 mg and a single dose of Glargine 10 units at 21:00 hrs.

The diabetes educator conducted family education sessions with the assistance of the Arabic-speaking healthcare interpreter. These sessions addressed self-management in diabetes. Topics included: what is diabetes?; the importance of controlling blood glucose levels for short- and long-term health; self-blood glucose monitoring; and the role of Diamicron MR and Glargine insulin as therapy.

Continued

CASE STUDY 26.1
Issues for Dietary Management in Culturally Diverse Groups – cont'd

A clear explanation that there was no cure for diabetes was emphasised. Techniques for self-injection using a Solostar device, basic principles regarding storage and supply of insulin, injection site selection and rotation and needle disposal were also explained.

The dietitian performed a full nutritional assessment, including preference in diet. Basic principles of the diet recommended for diabetes management including glycemic index (GI) were explained, with particular emphasis on the size of a meal, avoiding missing meals and only having one large meal each day. In Arabic culture it is usual for families to eat a large evening meal and many family members will not eat either breakfast or lunch. Mr A likes both Turkish-style coffee (highly sweetened with sugar) and Lebanese sweet pastries. Information about how these goods can be included in the diabetic diet, when eaten occasionally and in small servings, was also included in the education sessions.

Post-discharge from the ward Mr A has been attending his local diabetes centre for ongoing management and further education. He feels well and is now taking his prescribed medications regularly and his blood glucose control is classified as acceptable.

Weight loss might not be advisable in older people who lose muscle mass rather than fat, which predisposes them to sarcopaenia, functional decline and falls. In addition, many older people are under- or malnourished, even when they are overweight (McCulloch & Munshi 2016).

The introduction of regular physical activity to achieve weight loss is essential; however, recent studies have noted that resistance training provides the most overall benefit in the management of type 2 DM, especially for older people, where it is associated with greater strength and flexibility and reduced falls (Gillespie et al 2012).

The significance of dietary modification and weight loss in people who are at risk or have been diagnosed with type 2 DM cannot be over-emphasised. Obesity is the strongest known risk factor for type 2 DM and is associated with disturbed carbohydrate, fat (dyslipidaemia) and protein metabolism (Hossain et al 2007). The combination of dietary advice and exercise has been demonstrated to achieve a significant reduction of HbA1c within 6 months of commencing the program (Moore et al 2007).

Dietary advice for people with DM follows the *Australian Guide to Healthy Eating*, recommended for all people: food should be high in unrefined carbohydrate; there should be some protein and it should be low in saturated fat. For people with DM, the recommended diet is 25–30% of energy from fat and around 50% of the total energy from unrefined carbohydrate (Moore et al 2007; NHMRC 2013). These guidelines are consistent with those from the National Heart Foundation (National Vascular Disease Prevention Alliance [NVDPA] 2009).

In recent years, the significance of the GI of foods has attracted increasing attention from researchers and clinicians. The GI is the measure of the effect of different carbohydrate foods on BGLs. Foods with high GI are quickly digested and absorbed into the bloodstream, causing the BGL to rise rapidly and stimulating a corresponding release of insulin (Brand-Miller et al 2003; Gilbertson et al 2001). Foods with low GI are digested and absorbed slowly causing a slow rise in the BGL and a slower and reduced release of insulin. Low GI foods include legumes and dairy products, whereas potatoes, rice and white bread have a high GI.

Insulin has a growth factor-like effect and high levels are associated with weight gain. Current thinking is that a steady release of glucose into the blood may have an insulin-sparing effect, which, in conjunction with other interventions, contributes to optimal gylcaemic control for people with diabetes (Barclay et al 2008). However, the GI is not widely used outside Australia.

Exercise

While regular exercise is not an intervention per se for the management of type 1 DM, regular exercise is recommended for health and wellbeing of everybody with and without diabetes. As indicated, exercise, particularly when combined with healthy eating, plays a significant role in the prevention and progression of type 2 DM (Moore et al 2007) and is fundamental to preventing type 2 DM and obesity (Colagiuri et al 2009).

However, as all types of exercise require a readily available source of energy, adjustments in the patient's overall management strategy are required. People with type 1 DM and those with type 2 on insulin and/or a sulphonylurea need to take particular precautions before, during and after exercise. Prior to exercise, people with type 1 DM need to check their BGL and, if necessary, eat some rapidly digested carbohydrate.

Exercise increases the sensitivity of muscle cells to insulin, which is one reason it is encouraged in people with type 2 DM, particularly those with insulin resistance and hyperinsulinaemia, and it has a beneficial effect on cardiac risk factors (Chipkin et al 2001; Thomas et al 2007). Exercise assists the circulating insulin to enable circulating glucose to enter the muscle, where it is used for energy or stored for future use. The shift of glucose from the blood can result in hypoglycaemia during exercise or several hours after exercise finishes in people on insulin. If exercise is sustained, such as in a game of football or tennis, the person may need to take additional carbohydrate during exercise. Exercise reduces insulin requirements in the hours after physical activity, therefore the person on insulin should continue to monitor their BGL following exercise.

If there is too little insulin circulating at the time of exercise, the body will convert fat into ketone bodies to provide energy to the cells, despite the elevated circulating glucose, resulting in ketosis. Exercise also stimulates the release of glucose from the liver, which can result in hyperglycaemia. Therefore, people with hyperglycaemia are advised not to exercise until the cause is determined and treatment initiated. Education in self-management must include guidelines for dietary or insulin adjustment prior to, during and following exercise to decrease the risk of hypoglycaemia and hyperglycaemia with ketosis (Colagiuri et al 2009).

Many people with DM may find establishing an exercise program, including resistance training, challenging. Likewise, many older people and those with functional deficits are often unable to undertake some forms of exercise. The nurse should advise people to ask their doctor to perform a health assessment before they commence an exercise program. Generally they should begin with gentle exercise, such as a walking program or participating in gentle exercise classes, and encourage the person to progress to more strenuous forms of exercise as their fitness improves. People should discuss exercise with their clinicians prior to commencing an exercise program, especially if they are prone to hypoglycaemia, have foot problems or cardiovascular disease. Foot care and appropriate types of shoes should be discussed and education provided if necessary.

This section provided a brief background to the significance of healthy eating and appropriate exercise in the management of DM. Information describing specific nutrition and exercise interventions can be accessed in dietary guidelines for all Australians and for older Australians. Nurses in all practice settings play a key role in educating people with pre-diabetes and those with diagnosed diabetes, to enable them to effectively manage self-care. It is important that nurses establish a therapeutic relationship with people with diabetes and develop care plans with them to improve health outcomes. Negative and judgemental language has a significant impact on the way people with diabetes feel and their outcomes, for example, words such as 'diabetic', 'poor', 'control', 'regimen' and 'tests' (Diabetes Australia 2011; Dickinson 2017; Dunning et al 2017; Speight et al 2012).

DIABETES COMPLICATIONS

DM-related complications are briefly outlined in this section. The care of people with complications requires a comprehensive management plan that is beyond the scope of the chapter. References, such as recent editions of The Australian Diabetes Society, The American Diabetes Association, Standards of Medical Care, The UK NICE Guidelines, and the Scottish Intercollegiate Guidelines, which are revised regularly, provide more detailed information.

Acute Complications
Hypoglycaemia
Hypoglycaemia (also referred to as 'a hypo') occurs when the person has taken insulin or one of the sulfonylurea medicines and has eaten insufficient carbohydrate causing the BGL to fall to below 4.0 mmol/L. Other common causes of hypoglycaemia include excessive exercise without additional carbohydrate, medicine side effects and medicine interactions and rapid weight loss by people with type 2 DM without reducing their GLM doses. Overmedication is a less common cause, but may result from malfunctioning pen injecting devices, drawing up a larger dose because of poor eyesight or unintentional repeat doses of GLMs. Children may exhibit symptoms of hypoglycaemia at higher BGLs than adults.

Hypoglycaemia is very common among people with type 1 DM, and those who are poorly controlled may experience episodes of mild hypoglycaemia on most days. People with type 2 DM who inject insulin or take medications that stimulate insulin release, and those with renal and liver disease, are also at risk of hypoglycaemia. Annual rates of severe hypoglycaemia are 1.4–1.6 per 100 person years (Pathak et al 2016). The risk of serious hypoglycaemic episodes (hypos) is greater in high-risk groups; see Dunning and colleagues (2013) for a hypoglycaemia risk assessment tool. This can be used to plan care to reduce the risk of hypoglycaemia.

Hypos are frightening and embarrassing for people who experience them. It is common for the person to experience severe headache and difficulty concentrating after a hypo. Waking in the morning with a headache may be a sign of nocturnal hypoglycaemia.

Older people are prone to hypoglycaemia because they are not able to mount a counter-regulatory response to low glucose, because glucose and other counter-regulatory hormones such as glucagon production, decrease over time, and because they do not recognise the usual symptoms of hypoglycaemia. In fact, hypoglycaemia is associated with cognitive changes in the short term, which inhibits the person's ability to treat the hypo, and dementia in the longer term (Dunning et al 2013; IDF 2013). A hypo is also associated with significant cardiovascular changes that can result in sudden death (Hsu et al 2012). If the hypoglycaemia is caused by a sulphonylurea, the individual is at increased risk of readmission to hospital within 30 days (Emons et al 2016).

There are two major groups of signs and symptoms of hypoglycaemia:
- autonomic/sympathetic: weakness, sweating, tachycardia, palpitations, tremor, nervousness, irritability, tingling of the mouth and fingers and hunger
- neuroglucopaenic: headache, shivering, visual disturbances, mental dullness, confusion, amnesia, seizures and coma. It is important to realise that neuroglycopaenic symptoms are more common than autonomic symptoms in older people.

Hypoglycaemia may be managed quickly with little assistance if the person is able to recognise the symptoms and has a ready source of glucose available with a high (GI), such as glucose tablets, a third of a glass of regular soft drink or 5 to 7 jelly beans. This initial treatment is usually followed by one 15 g carbohydrate exchange of lower GI food, such as one slice of bread or two biscuits.

However, if the person requires assistance, it is recommended that medical assistance is summoned, usually by phoning for an ambulance. It is recommended that all people with type 1 DM and all older people have a family member or friend who is able and willing to administer a glucagon injection. Glucagon is a hormone, which is secreted from the alpha cells of the pancreas. Its action is the opposite of insulin: glucose is released from the liver to raise the blood glucose (Harmel & Mathur 2004). However, with long duration of diabetes the ability to produce glucagon declines, increasing the risk of serious consequences from hypoglycaemia (McCulloch & Munshi 2016).

Long-term Complications

The avoidance of both short- and long-term complications are among the goals of the management of DM. Long-term complications of DM are caused by the disturbance in metabolism triggered by the absolute or relative lack of insulin that leads to hyperglycaemia, which in turn leads to an inflammatory process that damages tissues and organs. DM is a leading cause of renal failure (nephropathy), blindness (retinopathy), coronary vascular disease and amputation of lower limbs (neuropathy). Some health professionals are reluctant to discuss the complications, particularly at the time of diagnosis. Nurses need to be familiar with the complications and have sufficient knowledge to discuss them with people with diabetes and their families.

Long-term complications may be categorised in three major groups:
- microvascular (small vessel disease), which includes retinopathy and nephropathy
- macrovascular (large vessel disease), which includes coronary artery disease, peripheral vascular disease and cerebrovascular disease
- neuropathy (both autonomic and peripheral nervous systems).

The specific pathophysiology for the formation of diabetic complications is not clear. However, chronically elevated BGLs appear to be a major factor in the development of diabetes complications (Brett & Holman 2008; Stratton et al 2000; The DCCT Research Group 1993; The United Kingdom Prospective Diabetes Study [UKPDS] 33 1996). Abnormalities in the connective tissues and in blood vessels are associated with elevated levels of complex compounds known as advanced glycosylation end-products (AGEs). These products may well be the key to the formation of both micro- and macrovascular complications (McDermott 2002). Neuropathic complications, however, appear to be more closely associated with the demyelination and axonal damage, possibly due to the accumulation of sorbitol in the nerve structures (McDermott 2002). As indicated earlier, glucose variability has been implicated in diabetes complications and may play a bigger role than HbA1c.

The landmark diabetes trials (The DCCT Research Group 1993; UKPDS 33 1996) noted the relationship between glucose control and a reduced risk of developing complications. Results of both trials stressed the importance of early diagnosis and treatment of all complications and associated conditions such as hypertension and mixed dyslipidaemia. Recent studies also demonstrated a 'legacy effect' of normoglycaemia (Brett & Holman 2008).

While screening for long-term complications is strongly recommended (American Diabetes Association 2016), the challenge may be persuading people with DM to attend for various tests which are often time-consuming, therefore a focus on secondary health promotion is needed. An explanation of the reasons for testing is essential. As wellness is the goal for management of all chronic diseases, the regimen of testing may be referred to as a 'wellness program' or 'cycle of care'. The recommended annual cycle of screening for complications is presented in Table 26.3 and is a key standard for primary care in Australia.

SELF-MANAGEMENT

Diabetes Education

Diabetes education is an essential component of diabetes management (Colagiuri et al 2009; Corser et al 2007). Diabetes requires a great deal of self-care and multiple daily decisions, which represents a lifetime of hard work that places a significant burden on the individual and often on their families. Consequently, the emphasis is on making decisions WITH the individual and personalising the education program as well as the management regimen. In the case of older people and children, parents and other relatives need to be involved and participate in the education.

Education is best provided by a multidisciplinary team comprising practitioners with specialist knowledge and skills in diabetes care, GPs and including the person with diabetes and their supporters/carer(s). Medical practitioners, nurses, dietitians, podiatrists and psychologists (when available) should collaborate to ensure the best outcomes for people with DM. Research in the fields of psychology, human behaviour, social learning theory and health education has improved our understanding of the problems that underlie relapse from self-care regimens in chronic disease (Colagiuri et al 2009; Corser et al 2007), and underpin the formal education programs for people with DM. It is essential that all people are familiar with the individual's care plan and goals and give consistent advice.

Over recent years there has been a change in the emphasis of and approaches to diabetes education, partly due to increased understanding of the complex relationship between adherence to treatment and glycaemic control (Seley & Weinger 2007; The DCCT Research Group 1993; UKPDS 33 1996). People with DM and their support people are required to make many decisions per day to balance diet, physical activity and medication to achieve their optimum level of control (Colagiuri et al 2009).

People with DM are required to comprehend and act on content covering an extensive list of topics, including the carbohydrate content of various foods and menu design, the action of oral and injectable GLMs and insulin, precautions related to exercise, managing DM during concomitant illness and screening for complications, signs of onset of complications and SBGM. Education sessions are most effective when they focus on developing skills that enable the person to proactively adjust their treatment to account for variations in their day-to-day routines and to identify potential causes of hypo- and hyperglycaemia.

In tandem with the changing emphasis on diabetes education, value outcomes have also changed (Bradshaw, Richardson & Kulkarni 2007; Bradshaw, Richardson, Kumpfer et al 2007). Adherence to treatments is no longer the only outcome measured. Teaching is no longer limited to a checklist of do's and don'ts on the assumption that giving information equates with people's understanding, awareness and confidence to make the necessary adjustments in their lives (Colagiuri et al 2009; Dunning 2014a, 2014b).

TABLE 26.3
Screening for Long-Term Complications: The Annual Cycle of Care

Test to be Conducted	Timing/ Frequency
HbA1c (average BGL for last 2–3 months)	3-monthly
Review of SBGM	3-monthly (compare to HbA1c)
Weight and height (BMI)	3-monthly
Blood pressure	3-monthly
Blood lipid profile	6-monthly
Feet examination	6-monthly
Microalbuminuria	Annually
Eye examination	Annually
Self-management skills	Annually
Healthy eating plan	Annually
General health status and vaccinations	Annually

The frequency of assessments needs to be individualised.

Nurses need to be familiar with the information that is provided to people with diabetes and to play a supporting and reinforcing role to assist people to make the necessary lifestyle changes. The challenge for nurses is to translate a treatment regimen into a plan of care that a person with DM and their support people can follow. While the role and functions of specialist diabetes educators have been described (Australian Diabetes Educators Association [ADEA] 2010; Seley & Weinger 2007) as well as standards of practice developed as a basis for professional accreditation and service provision (American Association of Diabetes Educators 2007; ADEA 2003), nurses working in all clinical settings will be required to provide care and, in the absence of specialist practitioners, provide education and ongoing follow-up to people with DM. The professional associations have developed resources that assist health professionals to provide care to people with DM. They are available on the websites developed by the Australian Diabetes Educators Association (ADEA) (www.adea.com.au) and Diabetes Australia (www.diabetesaustralia.com.au).

Self-Blood Glucose Monitoring

Self-blood glucose monitoring (SBGM) is important to the management of people with DM. Regular tests using home blood glucose monitoring (HBGM) assist the person with DM and their health professionals to maintain the balance between medications, diet and exercise on a day-to-day basis and identify trends over time (blood glucose pattern). People who inject insulin are particularly advised to perform regular monitoring and record results, which are used to guide insulin doses (ADEA 2010; Farmer et al 2007). The value of SBGM in management of people who are not taking insulin therapy has been questioned, and has led to changes to the National Diabetes Services Scheme (NDSS) eligibility for subsidised blood glucose test strips in July 2016 on recommendations from the Pharmaceutical Benefits Advisory Committee (PBAC). PBAC recommended continuing SBGM and access to subsidised test strips for people with type 1 DM, people with type 2 DM using insulin, women with GDM, people using medicines that could affect BGLs, such as corticosteroids and sulphonylureas, and people with intercurrent illnesses. It is too early to determine what impact these changes will have on people's blood glucose monitoring behaviours. People with diabetes can be referred to the Diabetes Australia helpline for more information (1300 637 700). However, most people with DM benefit from regular SBGM.

ADEA's Position Statement: Use of Blood Glucose Meters (ADEA 2010) recommended that people using insulin therapy be encouraged to perform SBGM. The ADEA position statement recommends that all people with diabetes using insulin therapy be encouraged to perform blood glucose monitoring. The testing regimen needs to be developed specifically for the individual, therefore the support of appropriately trained health professionals is recommended. Factors such as age, culture, dexterity and physical and intellectual capabilities, level of control required, current medication regimen and motivation, are taken into account by the health professional. People testing their blood for glucose also need to receive comprehensive education because effective SBGM requires more than an accurate technique. Effective self-management also requires the individual to understand and interpret their blood glucose levels in order to be able to apply the results as a part of their self-management (ADEA 2010).

The Role of the Nurse

The role of the nurse in diabetes care and education has been mentioned in several places in the chapter. Effective diabetes management requires interdisciplinary team care. Nurses are a key part of the team in all practice settings and their role depends on the setting to some extent as well as their knowledge, competence and experience. Nurses are involved in the following diabetes care and education activities:

- diabetes primary and secondary prevention programs
- educating people with diabetes, families, health professionals and the public
- developing care plans with the individual and the healthcare team
- providing acute, rehabilitation and palliative and end-of-life diabetes care
- managing acute complications such as hypoglycaemia and other causes of clinical deterioration
- managing medicines
- monitoring health and other outcomes
- engaging in diabetes research, e.g. implementing research findings, guidelines and policies and undertaking research.

CONCLUSION

DM, particularly type 2, affects the lives of many Australians. Type 1 and type 2 DM cause significant disability and premature death, and the prevalence is increasing globally (IDF 2019). DM is the fifth national health priority identified by the Australian

Government. It is associated with almost all the other national health priorities.

Management of DM is increasingly complex, reflecting advances in technology and approaches to management of all chronic disorders. While the management of DM has developed to be a specialty practice, and professional sub-groups have been established to support nurses (Australian Diabetes Educators Association), medical practitioners (Australian Diabetes Society), dietitians (Dietitians Association of Australia), and nurses working in all clinical settings will be caring for large numbers of people with diabetes in all practice settings.

Managing diabetes involves using a combination of medication, exercise and diet, and managing stress. Each person needs a diabetes care plan tailored to their health status and goals. Some people need to adopt substantial lifestyle changes and self-discipline to achieve their optimum BGL and other goals. Changing long-held practices, attitudes and priorities is difficult for most people; however, once diagnosed with diabetes, all activities need to be planned around the treatment. When a person is diagnosed with diabetes, particularly type 1, the opportunity for much of the spontaneity we take for granted is compromised.

The role of the nurse in the management of DM is considerably more complex than teaching people how to test blood glucose and inject insulin. As is the case in the management of other chronic disorders that require the person to change their lifestyle, nurses frequently adopt the roles of educator, coach and motivator. It is difficult to put yourself in the shoes of another person and there is a tendency for some clinicians to focus on the signs and overlook the underlying causes. For example, the reason a person with type 1 DM presents with a life-threatening episode of DKA could be as diverse as a malfunctioning insulin pen device through to an underlying psychiatric issue. The nature of nursing care enables nurses to talk with people and, in the process of doing that, they might identify the clues.

The purpose in writing this chapter was to provide an overview of DM and introduce the reader to the principles and goals of management. DM is a complex disorder. However, the management is well described in various textbooks and journal articles, including those in the recommended reading and reference sections of this chapter. We recommend that readers seek detailed information when they are caring for a person with DM to assist the team of health professionals and the person to work together to achieve the best outcomes.

Reflective Questions

1. How would you respond to the statement: 'I used to have diabetes, but now that I've lost some weight and follow the diet given to me by the dietitian, I am cured'?

2. Although John is only 5 years old, he is very familiar with his diabetes care regimen. His mother is very concerned about and does not understand why he ate a bag of lollies when he knows that sugar raises his blood glucose levels and makes him sick. How would you counsel her?

3. Mr Jones is prescribed insulin as part of his treatment for type 2 diabetes. He had three episodes of hypoglycaemia this week when he usually has one or two episodes each month. What questions should the nurse ask and what investigations could the nurse perform?

RECOMMENDED READING

Dunning T 2014a. Care of people with diabetes: a manual of nursing practice. Wiley Blackwell, Chichester.

Dunning T 2014b. Diabetes education: art, science and evidence. Wiley Blackwell, Chichester.

Malanda UL, Welschen LMC, Riphagen II et al 2012. Self-monitoring of blood glucose in patients with type 2 diabetes mellitus who are not using insulin. The Cochrane Database of Systematic Reviews (1), Art No: CD005060.

Renders CM, Valk GD, Griffin SJ et al 2009. Interventions to improve the management of diabetes mellitus in primary care, outpatient and community settings. The Cochrane Database of Systematic Reviews (4), Art No: CD001481.

USEFUL WEBSITES

Australian Medicines Handbook: www.nps.org.au/contact-us/medicines-line.

National Diabetes Services Scheme: www.ndss.com.au and https://www.ndss.com.au/older people.

Therapeutic Guidelines Endocrinology: www.nps.org.au/australian-prescriber/articles/therapeutic-guidelines-endocrinology-version-5.

REFERENCES

Aguilar-Salinas C, Rojas R, Gonzalez-Villalpando C et al 2006. Design and validation of a population-based definition of the metabolic syndrome. Diabetes Care 29(11), 2420–2426.

Alberti KGMM, Zimmet P, Shaw J et al 2004. Type 2 diabetes in the young: the evolving epidemic. Diabetes Care 27(7), 1798–1811.

American Association of Diabetes Educators 2007. National standards for diabetes self-management education. Diabetes Care 30, 1630–1637.

American Diabetes Association (ADA) 2019. Standards of medical care in diabetes – 2019 Abridged for Primary Care Providers. Clinical Diabetes 37(1), 11–34.

American Diabetes Association (ADA) 2016. Standards of medical care in diabetes – 2012. Diabetes Care 35(Suppl. 1), S11–S63.

American Diabetes Association (ADA) 2007. Diagnosis and classification of diabetes mellitus. Diabetes Care 30(Suppl. 1), S42–S47.

Australian Bureau of Statistics (ABS) 2019. National Aboriginal and Torres Strait Islander Health Survey: statistics about long-term health conditions, disability, lifestyle factors, physical harm and use of health services. Online. Available: www.abs.gov.au/statistics/people/aboriginal-and-torres-strait-islander-peoples/national-aboriginal-and-torres-strait-islander-health-survey/latest-release#diabetes.

Australian Bureau of Statistics (ABS) 2014. Australian Aboriginal and Torres Strait Islander Health Survey: Updated Results 2012–13. ABS, Canberra. Online. Available: www.abs.gov.au/ausstats/abs

Australian Bureau of Statistics (ABS) 2012. Year Book Australia 2012. ABS, Canberra.

Australian Diabetes Educators Association 2010. Position Statement. Use of Blood Glucose Meters. Australian Diabetes Educators Association, Canberra.

Australian Diabetes Educators Association 2003. National Standards of Practice for Diabetes Educators. Australian Diabetes Educators Association, Canberra.

Australian Diabetes In Pregnancy Study Groups (ADIPS) 2013. Consensus Guidelines for the Testing and Diagnosis of GDM. Online. Available: http://adips.org/downloads/ADIPSConsensusGuidelinesGDM-03.05.13VersionACCEPTEDFINAL.pdf.

Australian Diabetes Society (ADS) 2019. Consensus position statement on: utilising the Ambulatory Glucose Profile (AGP) combined with the Glucose Pattern Summary to support Clinical Decision Making in Diabetes Care. Online. Available: https://diabetessociety.com.au/downloads/20200626%20ADS%20AGP%20Consensus%20Statement%2024062020%20-%20FINAL.pdf

Australian Diabetes Society (ADS) 2017. Position Statements and Guidelines. Online. Available: diabetessociety.com.au/position-statements.asp.

Australian Institute of Health and Welfare (AIHW) 2019. Diabetes. Cat. no. CVD 82. AIHW, Canberra.

Australian Institute of Health and Welfare (AIHW) 2018. Australia's mothers and babies 2016—in brief. Perinatal statistics series no. 34. Cat. no. PER 97. AIHW, Canberra.

Australian Institute of Health and Welfare (AIHW) 2011. Diabetes Prevalence in Australia: Detailed Estimates for 2007–2008. AIHW, Canberra.

Australian Medicines Handbook (AMH) 2016. Online. Available: https://amhonline.amh.net.au/.

Australian Medicines Handbook (AMH) 2015. Online. Available: https://amhonline.amh.net.au/.

Barclay A, Petocz P, McMillan-Price J et al 2008. Glycemic index, glycemic load, and chronic disease risk – a meta-analysis of observational studies. American Journal of Clinical Nutrition 87(3), 627–637.

Bonadonna R, Cucinotta D, Fedele D, The Metascreen Writing Committee et al 2006. The metabolic syndrome is a risk indicator of macrovascular and macrovascular complications in diabetes. Diabetes Care 29(12), 2701–2707.

Bradshaw B, Richardson G, Kulkarni K 2007. Thriving with diabetes. An introduction to the resiliency approach for diabetes educators. The Diabetes Educator 33(4), 643–649.

Bradshaw B, Richardson G, Kumpfer K et al 2007. Determining the efficacy of a resiliency training approach in adults with type 2 diabetes. The Diabetes Educator 33(4), 650–659.

Brand-Miller J, Hayne S, Petocz P et al 2003. Low-glycemic index diets in the management of diabetes. A meta-analysis of randomized controlled trials. Diabetes Care 26(8), 2261–2267.

Brett A, Holman R 2008. 10-year follow-up of intensive glucose control in type 2 diabetes. New England Journal of Medicine 359(15), 1577–1589.

Care Quality Commission 2014/15 State of care. Online. Available: www.cqc.org.uk/sites/default/files/20151221_cqc_state_of_care_report_web_accessible_pdf.

Chipkin S, Klugh S, Chasan-Taber L 2001. Exercise and diabetes. Cardiology Clinics 19(3), 489–505.

Colagiuri R, Girgis S, Eigenmann C et al 2009. National evidence based guideline for patient education in type 2 diabetes. Diabetes Australia and the NHMRC, Canberra.

Corser W, Holmes-Rovner M, Lein C et al 2007. A shared decision-making primary care intervention for type 2 diabetes. The Diabetes Educator 33(4), 700–708.

Craig ME, Twigg SM, Donaghue KC et al 2011. For the Australian Type 1 Diabetes Guidelines Expert Advisory Group. National evidence-based clinical care guidelines for type 1 diabetes in children, adolescents and adults. Australian Government Department of Health and Ageing, Canberra.

Current Research into Cures for Type-1 Diabetes. Online. Available: http://cureresearch4type1diabetes.blogspot.com.au.

De Fronzo R, Ferrannini E, Keen H et al 2004. International textbook of diabetes mellitus, vol. 1. John Wiley & Sons, Chichester.

Diabetes Australia 2020. Gestational diabetes. Online. Available: www.diabetesaustralia.com.au/about-diabetes/gestational-diabetes

Diabetes Australia 2011. Position statement: A new language for diabetes. Online. Available: https://static.diabetesaustralia.com.au/s/fileassets/diabetes-australia/f4346fcb-511d-4500-9cd1-8a13068d5260.pdf.

Diabetes Victoria 2016. National Diabetes Week campaign. Online. Available: www.diabetesvic.org.au/.

Diabetes UK 2019. DESMOND – Diabetes education and self-management for ongoing and newly diagnosed. Online Available: www.diabetes.co.uk/education/desmond.html

Dietitians Association of Australia New South Wales Branch Diabetes Interest Group 2006. Evidence based practice guidelines for the nutritional management of type 2 diabetes mellitus for adults. Author, Sydney.

Dickinson JK, Guzman SJ, Maryniuk MD et al 2017. The use of language in diabetes care and education. Diabetes Care 40(12), 1790–1799.

Dunning T 2014a. Care of people with diabetes: a manual of nursing practice. Wiley Blackwell, Chichester.

Dunning T 2014b. Diabetes education: art, science and evidence. Wiley Blackwell, Chichester.

Dunning T, Savage S, Duggan N 2013. The McKellar guidelines for managing older people with diabetes. Online. Available: www.adma.org.au/clearinghouse/doc_details/133-the-mckellar-guidelines-for-managing-older-people-with-diabetes-in-residential-and-other-care-settings_9dec2013.html.

Emons M, Bae S, Hoogwerf B et al 2016. Risk factors for 30-day readmission following hypoglycaemia-related emergency room or in patient admission. BMJ Diabetes Research Care 4(1), e000160.

Fajans S, Bell G 2011. MODY: history, genetics, pathophysiology, and clinical decision making. Diabetes Care 34, 1878–1884.

Farmer A, Wade A, Goyder E et al 2007. Impact of self-monitoring of blood glucose in the management of patients with non-insulin treated diabetes: open parallel group randomized trial. British Medical Journal 335(7611), 132–139.

Fourlanos S, Harrison LC, Colman PG 2008. The accelerator hypothesis and increasing incidence of type 1 diabetes. Current Opinion in Endocrinology Diabetes and Obesity 15(4), 321–325.

Garber AJ, King AB, Prato SD et al 2012. Insulin degludec, an ultra-longacting basal insulin, versus insulin glargine in basal-bolus treatment with mealtime insulin aspart in type 2 diabetes (BEGIN Basal-Bolus Type 2): a phase 3, randomised, open-label, treat-to-target non-inferiority trial. The Lancet 379(9825), 1498–1507.

Gilbertson H, Brand-Miller J, Thorburn A et al 2001. The effect of flexible low glycemic index dietary advice versus measured carbohydrate exchange diets on glycemic control in children with type 1 diabetes. Diabetes Care 24(7), 1137–1143.

Gillespie L, Robertson M, Gillespie W et al 2012. Interventions for preventing falls in older people living in the community. Cochrane Database of Systematic Reviews 2012(9), Art. No. CDOO7146.

Harmel A, Mathur R 2004. Diabetes mellitus diagnosis and treatment, 5th ed. Saunders, Philadelphia.

Hermansen K, Madsbad S, Perrild H et al 2001. Comparison of the soluble basal insulin analog insulin detemir with nph insulin. Diabetes Care 24(2), 296–301.

Holst J, Gribble F 2016. Roles of the gut in glucose homeostasis. Diabetes Care 39, 884–892.

Hossain P, Kawar B, El Nahas M 2007. Obesity and diabetes in the developing world – a growing challenge. The New England Journal of Medicine 356(3), 213–216.

Hsu PF, Sung SH, Yeh JS et al 2012. The association between clinical symptomatic hypoglycemia with cardiovascular events in type 2 diabetes: a nested case control study in nation-wide representative population. European Heart Journal 33, 180–181.

International Diabetes Federation (IDF) 2019, Diabetes Atlas 2019. Online. Available: https://diabetesatlas.org/upload/resources/material/20200302_133351_IDFATLAS9e-final-web.pdf.

International Diabetes Federation (IDF) 2015. Diabetes Atlas 2015. Online. Available: www.diabetesatlas.org/resources/2015-atlas.html.

International Diabetes Federation (IDF) 2014. Language philosophy technical document and recommendations for communicating with and about people with diabetes. Online. Available: www.idf.org.

International Diabetes Federation (IDF) 2013. IDF global guideline for managing older people with type 2 diabetes. Online. Available: www.idf.org/guidelines-older-people-type-2-diabetes.

Inzucchi S, Berngenstal R, Buse J et al 2012. Management of hyperglycemia in type 2 diabetes: a patient-centered approach. Position statement of the American Diabetes Association (ADA) and the European Association for the Study of Diabetes (EASD). Diabetes Care 35(Suppl. 1), S11–S63.

Kamp M 2007. Oral medications and type 2 diabetes. Diabetes Management Journal 19, 28–29.

Karvonen M, Viik-Kajander M, Libman I et al 2000. Incidence of childhood type 1 diabetes worldwide. Diabetes Care 23(10), 1516–1526.

Katzmarzyk P, Church T, Janssen I et al 2005. Metabolic syndrome, obesity, and mortality. Diabetes Care 28, 391–397.

Kids Health 2016. Online. Available: kidshealth.org/en/parents/weight-diabetes.html.

Lalor E, Cass A, Chew D et al 2014. Cardiovascular disease, diabetes and chronic kidney disease: Australian facts – mortality. Australian Institute of Health and Welfare. Online. Available: www.aihw.gov.au/publication-detail/?id=60129549287.

Lee A, Hiscock R, Wein P et al 2007. Gestational diabetes mellitus: clinical predictors and long-term risk of developing type 2 diabetes. Diabetes Care 30(4), 878–883.

McCulloch D, Munshi M 2016. Treatment of type 2 diabetes in older patients. UpToDate. Online. Available: www.uptodate.com/contents/treatment-of-type-2-diabetes-mellitus-in-the-older-patient.

McDermott M 2002. Endocrine secrets. Hanley & Belfus, Philadelphia.

McElduff A, Yue D 2007. Inhaled insulin: where are we and where might we go? The Medical Journal of Australia 186(8), 390–391.

McIntyre HD 2006. DAFNE (Dose Adjustment For Normal Eating): structured education in insulin replacement therapy for type 1 diabetes. Medical Journal of Australia 108(7), 317–318.

Ministry of Health NZ 2019. Annual Health Reports 2019 Online. Available: https://moh.gov.om/en_US/web/statistics/annual-reports.

Monnier L, Colette C, Owens DR 2008. Glycaemic variability: the third component of the dysglycemia in diabetes. Is it important? How to measure it? Journal of Diabetes Science and Technology 2(6), 1094–1100.

Moore H, Summerbell C, Hooper L et al 2007. Dietary advice for treatment of type 2 diabetes mellitus in adults (Review). Cochrane Library CD004097.

National Health and Medical Research Council (NHMRC) 2014. National Guidelines Endocrinology version 5. Online. Available: www.clinicalguidelines.gov.au/node/3342.

National Health and Medical Research Council (NHMRC) 2013. Australian dietary guidelines. Australian Government, Canberra. Online. Available: www.nhmrc.gov.au/guidelines-publications/n55.

National Institute for Health and Clinical Excellence (NICE) 2011. rev. Continuous Subcutaneous Insulin Infusion for the Treatment of Diabetes Mellitus. Review of Technology Appraisal Guidance 57. Technology Appraisal Guidance 151. NICE, London (UK).

National Vascular Disease Prevention Alliance (NVDPA) 2009. Guidelines for the Assessment of Absolute Cardiovascular Disease Risk. National Health and Medical Research Council, Canberra.

Pathak R, Schroeder E, Seaquist E et al 2016. Severe hypoglycaemia requiring medical intervention in a large cohort of adults with diabetes receiving care in the US integrated health care delivery systems 2005–2011. Diabetes Care 39(3), 363–370.

Perry M 2016. Mediterranean diet cuts risk for CV events, cancer and diabetes. Archives of Internal Medicine Medscape 16 July. Online. Available: www.medscape.com/viewarticle/866254.

Pihoker C, Gillam L, Hampe C et al 2005. Autoantibodies in diabetes. Diabetes 54(Suppl. 2), S52–S61.

Ratner R, Hirsch I, Neifing J et al 2000. Less hypoglycaemia with insulin glargine in intensive insulin therapy for type 1 diabetes. Diabetes Care 23(5), 639–643.

Rewers M, Zaccaro D, D'Agostino R et al 2004. Insulin sensitivity, insulinaemia, and coronary artery disease. Diabetes Care 27(4), 781–787.

Richter B, Bandeira-Echtler E, Bergerhoff K et al 2008. Dipeptidyl peptidase-4 (DPP-4) inhibitors for type 2 diabetes mellitus. Cochrane Database Systematic Reviews 2008.

Riddle M, Karl D 2012. Individualizing targets and tactics for high-risk patients with type 2 diabetes. Practical lessons from ACCORD and other cardiovascular trials. Diabetes Care 35, 2100–2107.

Rosenstock J, Cappelleri J, Bolinder B et al 2004. Patient satisfaction and glycaemic control after 1 year with inhaled insulin (Exubera) in patients with type 1 or type 2 diabetes. Diabetes Care 27(6), 1318–1323.

Rosenstock J, Lorber DL, Gnudi L et al 2010. Prandial inhaled insulin plus basal insulin glargine versus twice daily biaspart insulin for type 2 diabetes: a multicentre randomised trial. The Lancet 375(9733), 2244–2253.

Saeedi P, Petersohn I, Salpea P et al 2019. Global and regional diabetes prevalence estimates for 2019 and projections for 2030 and 2045: results from the International Diabetes Federation Diabetes Atlas, 9th edition. Diabetes Research and Clinical Practice 157, 107843.

Seley J, Weinger K 2007. The state of the science on nursing best practices for diabetes self-management. The Diabetes Educator 33(4), 616–626.

Sinclair A, Gadsby R, Penfold S et al 2001. Prevalence of diabetes in care home residents. Diabetes Care 24(6), 1066–1068.

Skyler J, Cefalu W, Kourides I et al 2004. Efficacy of inhaled human insulin in type 1 diabetes mellitus: a randomised proof-of-concept study. The Lancet 357(9253), 331–335.

Speight J, Conn J, Dunning T et al 2012. Diabetes Australia position statement. A new language for diabetes: improving communications with and about people with diabetes. Diabetes Research and Clinical Practice 97(3), 25–431.

Stratton I, Adler A, Andrew H et al 2000. Association of glycaemia and macrovascular and microvascular complications of type 2 diabetes (UKPDS 35): prospective observational study. British Medical Journal 321, 405–412.

The Australian Type 2 Diabetes Risk Assessment Tool (AUSDRISK). Online. Available: https://static.diabetesaustralia.com.au/s/fileassets/diabetes-australia/6d252140-1ff0-47b2-a83f-3 cc3db348131.pdf.

The Diabetes Control and Complications Trial (DCCT) Research Group, 1993. The effect of intensive treatment of diabetes on the development and progression of long-term complications in insulin-dependent diabetes mellitus. The New England Journal of Medicine 329(14), 977–986.

The Diabetes Prevention Trial – Type 1 Study Group 2005. Effects of oral insulin in relatives of patients with type 1 diabetes. Diabetes Care 28(5), 1068–1076.

The United Kingdom Prospective Diabetes Study (UKPDS) 33, 1996. Intensive blood glucose control with sulphonylureas or insulin compared with conventional treatment and the risk of complications in patients with Type 2 Diabetes. The Lancet 352, 837–853.

Thomas D, Elliott E, Naughton G 2007. Exercise for type 2 diabetes mellitus. Online. Available: www.thecochranelibrary.com.

United Nations 2015. Sustainable Development Goals (SDGs) UNDP. Online. Available: www.undp.org/content/undp/en/home/sustainable-development-goals.html.

World Health Organization (WHO) 2019. Classification of diabetes mellitus 2019. Online. Available: https://www.who.int/publications/i/item/classification-of-diabetes-mellitus.

CHAPTER 27

Principles for Nursing Practice: HIV/AIDS

STEPHEN NEVILLE • JEFFERY ADAMS

LEARNING OBJECTIVES

When you have completed this chapter you will be able to:

- understand the history, presentation and the contemporary management of people living with HIV/AIDS
- restate health-promoting measures to reduce the transmission of HIV infection and to encourage risk reduction in people living with HIV
- be aware of the social and professional stigma associated with living and working with HIV/AIDS
- examine your own attitudes towards people living with HIV/AIDS
- be able to provide an appropriate basic health service to people with HIV/AIDS.

KEY WORDS

HIV prevention	opportunistic diseases
HIV testing	stigma
HIV transmission	

INTRODUCTION

There have been few modern diseases that have captured the public imagination in so short a period of time as human immunodeficiency virus (HIV) and its fulminate expression, acquired immune deficiency syndrome (AIDS). The way the disease appeared to emerge so suddenly in the developed world in the late 1970s – the severity of the symptoms; its disfiguring, wasting and painful impact on people diagnosed with the condition; and the inevitably fatal nature of the diagnosis – gave rise to a climate of fear. Yet we have discovered more about HIV/AIDS in a shorter period of time than for any other disease in history. HIV/AIDS is today recognised as a chronic, manageable condition, although still life-threatening.

Rather than attempting to provide a definitive and exhaustive overview of this complex disease, three case studies will focus on some key issues associated with living with HIV in Australasia. The chapter begins with an overview of HIV/AIDS and provides a context for the development of your knowledge and understanding about the disease and its prevention. Case Study 27.1 is about an older gay man living with HIV who has been admitted to hospital for treatment and stabilisation, before being discharged home. Case Study 27.2 is about a transgender sex worker who is a regular street drug user. Case Study 27.3 is about a young married African migrant woman with two young children. Each of these cases represents the types of people living with HIV/AIDS who you may come across in healthcare settings when working as a nurse in Australasia.

BACKGROUND

There is compelling evidence that the viral ancestor of HIV existed in humans from the early decades of the twentieth century. It probably crossed into a very small pool of humans in South Central Africa who were hunting species of monkeys infected with a related virus (Sahoo et al 2017). Once a viral reservoir was created in the human population, largely due to post-colonial healthcare practices and sex workers, what we now know is HIV appears to have travelled along major transportation routes throughout Africa, and from these networks to airports in major cities around the world, where it took hold in vulnerable populations. In many ways, HIV may be the first disease of modern transportation, and has served as a brutal reminder of how quickly infectious diseases can spread around an unprepared world.

Since 1984 AIDS has been understood to be caused by HIV, although even at the time of writing there are some researchers and politicians who continue to deny the role of HIV in AIDS. Since HIV disease is much more common and comprehensive than AIDS, we will mostly use the term 'HIV' in this chapter from now on. HIV has been associated from its earliest days with stigmatised communities and, tragically, in many countries and regions much of that stigma has remained (Emlet et al 2015). In the early days of the epidemic, populations that were most affected in developed nations – men who had sex with other men; injecting drug users; the poor; African migrants and refugees; and other communities of colour – were socially and politically marginalised. Children and people who were infected through infected blood products were referred to as 'innocent victims', implying that others were somehow 'guilty'. This contributed to the marginalisation of large groups of people living with HIV. Some religious and political leaders even spoke of AIDS as 'God's punishment'.

When an individual is infected with HIV, they must deal not only with the medical aspects of the condition, but also with the social dimensions. Gay men, for example, may have to endure homophobic (irrational fear of gay people) reactions, resulting in isolation from their families and friends (Neville et al 2015); while those from ethnic minority groups experience racism, sexism and classism (Jaiswal et al 2019). Consequently, HIV is as much a social diagnosis as it is a medical diagnosis. For some bisexual or gay men, a diagnosis with HIV may be the first time their families have had any idea about the sexual behaviours or identity of their son or husband or father.

STATISTICS, TRANSMISSION AND PREVENTION

Statistics

By the end of 2010, UNAIDS estimated that there were approximately 36 million people worldwide living with HIV (UNAIDS 2016). In Australia, at the end of 2017, an estimated 963 people were newly diagnosed with HIV (The Kirby Institute 2018). Figures for 2018 show that 178 people were diagnosed with HIV in New Zealand, which are low when compared to other Western countries

(AIDS Epidemiology Group 2019). It is important to remember that while overall population prevalence may be low, different groups, particularly those who are marginalised, may have relatively high prevalence and within some groups there may be high rates of unidentified infection (Neville & Adams 2016).

Transmission

HIV is an unstable and fragile virus that can only be transmitted through direct human-to-human contact. Its transmission is via infected blood, semen, vaginal secretions or breast milk (Neville et al 2016). HIV cannot be transmitted through kissing or hugging, insect bites or other casual, household or ordinary workplace contact. Unprotected sexual intercourse, whether anal or vaginal, is the most common method of transmitting the virus. Recent studies have found that circumcising men can reduce the rates of HIV infection, particularly in heterosexual populations (Sahoo et al 2017).

HIV can be transmitted through exposure to contaminated blood products or the use of contaminated syringes, needles and other street drug paraphernalia. Even microscopic amounts of blood left in drug-use equipment can transmit HIV if they are not thoroughly disinfected. Therefore, people who choose to inject drugs such as opiates (including heroin and morphine), amphetamine-type stimulants, so-called 'party drugs' and steroids (used by some body-builders and transgendered persons) must never share any of their injecting equipment with anyone else. Syringe exchange schemes encourage safer drug-use behaviours (Allen et al 2016). Both New Zealand (see www.needle.co.nz) and Australia have expanded needle access for drug users. In addition, the provision of supervised injecting centres is an opportunity to educate injecting drug users about reducing their risk of contracting blood-borne infections including HIV, if they are going to continue to inject drugs (Mitra et al 2019).

Injecting street drugs is also strongly associated with unsafe sexual practices (Cheng et al 2015), because not only may people begin to exchange sex for drugs when the money runs out, but their judgement about what is safe may be impaired. The relationship between substance use and sexual risk-taking is strongly supported in the literature. Bond and colleagues' (2019) study found a relationship between trading sex for illicit drugs, mental health issues and, as a consequence, having sex without using a condom.

Tattooing and cultural rituals, such as tatau and moko, may involve exposure to infected blood; practitioners and clients must be sure that they are both well protected from infection. Appropriate sterilisation of all equipment and the use of gloves and other personal protective equipment must be routine, even in these very traditional cultural activities. There is also a small risk to people receiving blood and blood products. However, in developed nations the routine screening of blood donors and blood products has made the risk for HIV transmission in this way negligible (Dodd et al 2020).

Needlestick injuries can also result in transmission of the virus, as can splash exposures of infected products on skin with an open lesion or into the eye (Lewis et al 2016). All healthcare organisations have prevention and post-exposure protocols, and all healthcare workers should be familiar with them. Institution specific guidelines for preventing healthcare-associated infections, including HIV, should be followed at all times.

Perinatal transmission of the HIV virus from mother to infant can occur prenatally, at the time of delivery or through breastfeeding. People who live in the same home as a person with HIV and/or visitors will need good information on how the virus is and is not transmitted; the website of the Centers for Disease Control and Prevention has good basic prevention information (www.cdc.gov/hiv/basics/transmission.html).

Prevention

People who choose to be sexually active can prevent infection with HIV or any of the other blood-borne, sexually transmitted diseases by putting a latex barrier between themselves and the virus. This means correctly using a fresh latex condom, together with a water-based lubricant, for penetrative sexual activity every time (see Box 27.1).

Risk-reduction messages can vary from one country to another, based on local circumstances, cultural norms and politics. For example, the New Zealand AIDS Foundation has historically advocated for the use of a condom and lubricant for every sexual encounter in all situations where men have sex with men. However, currently in Australasia, as well as other parts of the world, a broader suite of prevention approaches are now supported. HIV pre-exposure prophylaxis (PrEP) is a biomedical option for HIV negative that effectively eliminates the acquisition of HIV when approved treatment guidelines are followed (World Health Organization [WHO] 2019). For people with HIV who are taking HIV medicine as prescribed and are virally suppressed or undetectable, there is virtually no risk of HIV transmission to HIV negative partners (WHO 2020). Some studies have found, however, that people in relationships are likely to ignore safer sex guidelines and utilise monogamy as a way to manage the risk of being exposed to HIV

> ### BOX 27.1
> ### How to Use a Male Condom
>
> 1. Make sure the condom package is not broken or punctured. Check the 'use-by date' on the condom package to ensure that the condom has not passed its use-by date. Do not open it with any sharp object, or with your teeth. Do not use oil-based lubricants such as baby oil, petroleum jellies or moisturisers with the condom because they can degrade the latex. Do use purpose-formulated water-based lubricants.
> 2. When you remove the condom, ensure that it is not brittle, dried out or damaged in any way. Note which way the condom is rolled; if you start to put the condom on the penis and notice that the condom is backwards, do not simply turn it over; discard it and get a fresh one.
> 3. Place the condom at the end of the hard penis (if the penis is uncircumcised, pull back the foreskin first). Then pinch the tip of the condom to squeeze out the air and unroll the condom until it reaches the base of the penis. A drop of lubricant inside the condom can increase sensitivity, but too much lubricant may cause it to slip off.
> 4. Make sure the condom is secure and unbroken, and that there is room for the ejaculate (come) at the tip. Insert the penis into your partner.
> 5. After you have ejaculated (come), while the penis is still hard hold the condom at the base so it does not slip off as you withdraw. Remove the condom, being careful not to spill the fluid inside. Discard the condom.
> 6. Remember, with condoms, practice makes perfect. You can always ask your partner for help.

(Neville et al 2016); this puts both partners at risk. In some cultural groups, however, if a woman asks her male partner to use a condom, the request may be interpreted that the woman does not trust her partner, or that the woman herself is involved in other sexual relationships; this interpretation can even lead to partner violence (WHO 2013).

Every opportunity should be taken by nurses to reinforce safer sex and harm reduction messages about drug use, so that patients are not put at risk because of their behaviour, and they do not put themselves at increased risk for infection or re-infection from others. Great care must be taken, however, not to scold, judge or frighten clients who have difficulty adhering to treatments, safer sex or drug-use guidelines or medical appointments. It is much more efficient to spend some extra time listening to a patient and collaborating with them to plan their own solutions than it is to risk losing them altogether. A woman who is trading sex for drugs or for money to feed her child is not going to change her entire life simply because she has begun a new medication; HIV is probably quite a low priority for her, coming somewhere after housing, food, utility bills, clothing, transportation or mobile phone chargers. Only by carefully building a trusting relationship will the nurse encourage the person with HIV to make their health more of a priority.

An issue requiring consideration is HIV discrimination in the workplace. There is no reason that people with HIV cannot work as nurses; standard precautions protect nurses, patients and colleagues. As long as nurses are not having unprotected sex with their colleagues or sharing non-sterile injection equipment with them, there is no workplace risk for acquiring HIV from a colleague. Workplace stigma and discrimination is both unnecessary and illegal. Good information, mutual respect and an overall positive environment will prevent unnecessary difficulties in the healthcare workplace.

Testing for HIV

Testing for HIV has become much simpler over the past two decades. The 'HIV test' is actually a test for antibodies to HIV. Testing is usually done with blood, although tests using oral mucosa and so-called rapid tests using finger sticks are available in some regions. A negative test simply means that the analysis was unable to detect antibodies to HIV; a repeat test in 3 months is recommended for individuals at high risk for infection, and particularly when the last possible exposure was less than 12 weeks prior to the test.

HIV testing should always be linked to supportive risk-reduction education to help an individual reduce their risk of exposure to HIV, or to prevent transmitting HIV to someone else if they are already infected. For HIV-positive people it is not possible to determine who infected them simply through taking an HIV test.

PROGRESSION AND TREATMENT
Progression

HIV is a progressive condition with a predictable trajectory. Different clinical features appear, depending on the stage of disease. One marker of immune system functioning is CD4 cells. Since HIV attacks the immune system, a decrease in the number of functional CD4 cells can be used as a marker for the progression of the disease. Stages of HIV can be classified as:
- acute HIV infection (at the time of infection)
- early infection (CD4 > 500/microL of blood)

- early symptomatic disease (CD4 between 200 and 499/microL)
- a diagnosis of AIDS (CD4 < 200/microL).

Acute HIV infection is also called 'acute retroviral syndrome' or a 'seroconversion illness'. After exposure to the HIV virus it may take between 3 and 12 weeks for seroconversion to occur (Lewis et al 2016). People may present to health practitioners with flu-like viral symptoms and lymphadenopathy, or may be clinically asymptomatic and may only be diagnosed after formal HIV testing.

The early infection stage may last from several months to up to 10 years or more. During this time the person is infectious, but may be clinically asymptomatic, or only experience mild symptoms, which health professionals may put down to being viral in nature (Cooper & Gosnell 2015). However, because the virus continues to replicate during this period, without treatment the body's immune system can become increasingly impaired. This may cause early symptoms associated with being HIV-positive. Some examples of early symptoms include:
- persistent high temperatures
- night sweats
- diarrhoea
- fatigue
- headaches
- localised infections (e.g. oral or vaginal thrush)
- persistent and frequently generalised lymphadenopathy.

The transition from being HIV-positive to having a diagnosis of AIDS is marked by the presence of opportunistic infections and/or a CD4 count < 200/microL. A diagnosis of AIDS marks the transition to the final stage of the disease. The Centers for Disease Control in the United States have developed a useful set of diagnostic criteria that supports a diagnosis of AIDS (see www.cdc.gov/mmwr/preview/mmwrhtml/00018871.htm).

Treatments

In developed nations, the treatment and management of HIV is a relatively fast-moving environment, and new therapies, new drugs and new combinations of drugs are frequently becoming available. For a current and comprehensive list of drugs available for treatment and management of HIV disease in New Zealand, see the New Zealand AIDS Foundation website (www.nzaf.org.nz/life-with-hiv/treatments/#Medication).

Since the more HIV there is in the body ('viral load') the more damage the virus can do, the management of HIV infection is focused around preventing HIV from replicating itself. Because of the way it replicates, HIV is known as a 'retrovirus'; and the group of drugs that interfere with the replication process at various stages are called 'antiretrovirals' (ARVs; sometimes these are called 'highly active antiretroviral therapies', or HAART). The major classes of antiretroviral agents include the oldest class of such drugs, the nucleoside/nucleotide reverse transcriptase inhibitors (Sears & Daar 2015). The non-nucleoside reverse transcriptase inhibitors were the next class of drugs to be developed. Following that, the class of drugs called protease inhibitors and fusion inhibitors were developed, and these have been made available most recently. Combinations of antiretrovirals are usually used because HIV is very mutable, and can develop resistance to one or more of these drugs. Antiretrovirals must be taken exactly as prescribed, and care must be taken to follow instructions related to food intake (and the kinds of food), liquids and sleep habits, as diet can affect the way the body processes these drugs. These drugs can often have significant side effects, including psychotropic effects, such as vivid dreams. Patients should be encouraged to be highly adherent to prescribed medication regimens, as individuals can develop resistance to medications in a relatively short period of time if they miss doses, or take unplanned 'drug holidays'.

Strategies to support adherence to medication can include planning dosing around mealtimes, sleep routines or other regularly scheduled activities, such as regular television or radio programs. Cues, such as pillboxes or mobile phones with alarms, text message reminders and enlisting the support of partners or friends, may also help adherence. If the person with HIV continues to use non-prescribed drugs, street drugs or alcohol regularly, these may interfere with their medication routine and their awareness of time and mealtimes. If the person is having particular difficulty managing the side effects of a drug, which can be quite dramatic (e.g. a condition called lipodystrophy is the result of a redistribution of body fat, which can be very disfiguring), this should be brought to the attention of the doctor or nurse, so that these side effects can be medically managed, or alternative therapies considered.

CASE STUDY 27.1

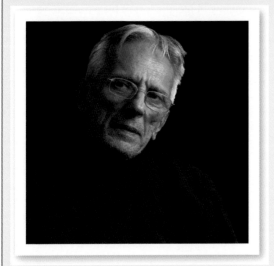

iStockphoto/VukasS.

Eric is a 68-year-old retired Caucasian male who has lived with a diagnosis of HIV for the last 15 years. He has no other significant health issues other than those related to his HIV status. Eric identifies as gay, has not been in a sexual relationship since his diagnosis and does not have good support networks from either family or friends. He lives alone with his pet budgie called 'Archie' and has one friend, Charles, who lives close by. Eric tells you that his long-term partner died of AIDS 10 years ago and over the years he has witnessed not only his partner, but a large number of his close friends die from the disease. He has few savings and is reliant on a government-funded benefit for income. Eric was admitted to hospital with flu-like symptoms, weight loss, dehydration, oral candidiasis, fatigue and decreased mobility. He is diagnosed with psittacosis (also called 'bird flu'), a bacterial infection caused by *Chlamydia psittaci*, an organism transmitted from birds to humans.

The psittacosis has responded well to antibiotic treatment and Eric is now being prepared to be discharged home. His hospital stay has coincided with your placement in the medical unit. The nurses you have been preceptored with have mainly been responsible for his care. Consequently, in conjunction with the registered nurses, you have been involved in the provision of nursing care to Eric and have a good understanding of issues that he faces as he struggles to adjust to living with this chronic and now debilitating illness.

In Case Study 27.1, as part of the nursing assessment, the key nursing issues are identified, as well as interventions to address these issues.

Fatigue

A key issue is Eric's fatigue, related to dehydration, malnutrition and the residual effects of having psittacosis. Constant tiredness is one of the common complaints associated with HIV, particularly in older adults, and it is known to cause anxiety, depression and sleep disturbance, which ultimately negatively impacts on quality of life (Barroso et al 2015). The nurse will need to work with Eric to identify the factors contributing to fatigue, plan activities and provide him with assistive devices. This is especially important, considering that he lives alone. For example:

- provide a shower stool and other occupational therapy aids
- develop a daily plan that includes regular rest periods
- include the involvement of an occupational therapist. Feeling constantly tired also affects Eric's ability to mobilise.

Activity intolerance

Another key issue is activity intolerance related to muscle atrophy, fatigue, peripheral neuropathy, decreased nutritional intake and the side effects of HIV-related medications. Peripheral neuropathy is an issue that specifically affects people with HIV, manifesting as either acute or chronic pain, and contributes to problems associated with maintaining activity levels (Tumusiime et al 2015). It is important in Eric's case to:

- administer pain medications as prescribed and monitor the effects
- ensure a physiotherapist is involved in Eric's care
- encourage the use of non-pharmacological treatments for pain, for example, the use of a transcutaneous electrical nerve stimulation (TENS) machine
- assess footwear to ensure it is comfortable and appropriate for exercise
- work with Eric to develop an exercise program that he enjoys and will increase his physical activity levels and endurance, and maintain lean muscle mass. Weight loss and malnutrition also limit Eric's ability to maintain lean muscle mass and remain active.

Weight loss

Eric's weight loss is related to a sore mouth as a result of having chronic oral candidiasis, dehydration and decreased nutritional intake. Weight loss remains a common consequence of HIV infection. Factors that contribute to weight loss include gastrointestinal issues, such as low food intake (due to side effects of drugs; opportunistic infections in the mouth, making eating painful; and digestive tract infections), poor nutrient absorption (due to HIV-related infections and the presence of diarrhoea) and altered metabolism (due to fever) (Santos et al 2016). One of the reasons for Eric's admission was that he had contracted psittacosis and presented with oral thrush. Oral thrush can lead to difficulties with eating and subsequently to weight loss. People with HIV therefore need more calories just to maintain their body weight. In Eric's case, the nurse should:

- encourage small, frequent meals that are highly nutritious and appetising
- if oral thrush remains, advise Eric to avoid spicy and acidic foods (such as citrus and fruit juices), replacing them with non-irritating foods (such as eggs, cream soups)
- encourage an adequate fluid intake and intake of foods high in potassium (such as bananas), especially if Eric experiences episodes of diarrhoea
- encourage Eric to weigh himself weekly, document his weight and inform his health practitioner of any significant changes
- ensure a dietitian works with Eric to assist with the establishment of appropriate nutritional principles to delay the progression of the disease and have a positive impact on his quality of life.

Coping with loss

A major issue for Eric is coping with loss related to reduced quality of life, the loss of his partner 10 years ago and having no family. As already identified, a diagnosis of HIV has transformed from one of terminal illness to one of chronic illness. In the 1980s people who had HIV might have asked the question, 'How am I going to live what little life I have left?'. This may have been the case for Eric's partner. However, Eric is faced with the question, 'Who am I to outlive my lover?'. Eric's partner was also his major source of social and emotional support. He watched the man he loved die and had to deal with the inevitable feelings of bereavement and grief. Eric's personal turmoil leaves him vulnerable to negative outcomes such as depression, loneliness, social isolation, hostility and lack of understanding from others (Bristowe et al 2016). In addition, Eric is going to have to find his pet bird, Archie, a new home. This is extremely distressing for Eric as Archie is a major source of social support. Consequently, the nurse should:

- reinforce the importance of consistently taking his medications and attending his appointments with his healthcare provider
- ensure the involvement of a social worker who works in the area of HIV to assess his psychosocial status and help provide links to the appropriate community services

- encourage participation in HIV support groups and contact with his local HIV organisation
- encourage involvement in other community organisations where Eric may be able to meet new people and expand his social network
- with Eric's permission, include his friend Charles in the discharge planning meetings
- work with Eric to find a suitable home for Archie and provide education to ensure he is not at risk of contracting psittacosis again
- offer appropriate referral to counselling, psychotherapy or other support workers.

As can be seen from Case Study 27.1, many of the issues associated with HIV are interrelated. For example, weight loss and dehydration contribute to Eric's fatigue, which concomitantly decreases mobility, leading to muscle atrophy and further weight loss. All these physiological disturbances affect his quality of life, an important concept for nurses to consider when working with people who have a chronic illness.

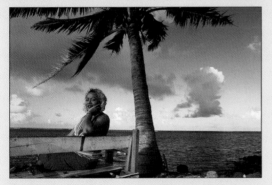

CASE STUDY 27.2

Getty Images/Olivier Chouchana/Gamma-Rapho.

Fa'atasi is a 23-year-old fa'afafine who now lives in Auckland. A fa'afafine is a Samoan cultural term for someone who was born a biological male, who embodies both male and female characteristics, but takes on the cultural role of a woman, and presents publicly and socially as a woman. Fa'atasi is unemployed, although she has worked casually as a street sex worker. She tested positive for HIV 4 years ago. She does not have a regular doctor, but sometimes turns up at the sexual health clinic when she suspects she may have an STI or is otherwise not feeling well. Fa'atasi uses cannabis, alcohol and amphetamine-type stimulants (ATS) when she is engaged in sex work. She has a strong support community within the Pacifica transgendered community.

In Case Study 27.2, as part of the nursing assessment, the key nursing issues are identified, as well as interventions to address these issues.

Sexually transmitted infections

Fa'atasi's repeated diagnosis with sexually transmitted infections is concerning because it means that she is not practising safer sex. Particularly concerning is the emergence of drug-resistant gonorrhoeae in Australasia and globally (Lewis 2015). Nursing interventions will include safe sex education and reinforcement of risk reduction plans already in place. It is important not to simply lecture Fa'atasi on safer sex or sex work, because she will have heard it all before. Rather, it would be more productive to help her identify ways in which she can take responsibility for reducing her own risks of STIs, and reducing her risks of transmitting STIs and HIV to others. Using aiga (family) as a model, and perhaps drawing on her own spiritual or religious beliefs, Fa'atasi can be assisted to develop a plan to reduce her sexual risk, even when she is engaged in sex work. Sex work can be very risky, so it is also important to ensure that Fa'atasi has a safety plan while on the streets and that she is aware of the resources available to her. Assessment for violence or rape may be necessary, as many street sex workers are victims of both. Her relationships with clinic staff and with her Pacifica community are strengths.

Substance use

Fa'atasi's substance use, particularly ATS, puts her and other users who may share her drug-using equipment at greatly increased risk of all blood-borne pathogens, including re-infection with HIV. Equally importantly, people who use ATS may make decisions about sexual activity which may increase their risk of disease transmission. The nurse will reinforce the importance of education on reducing the harms of substance use and consider a referral to a substance use treatment program.

Medical Appointments

Fa'atasi does not have regular medical appointments to monitor her HIV. While HIV does not appear to be the major presenting issue at the moment, it is important that she is monitored regularly in order to prevent opportunistic infections and to assess whether antiretroviral medication may be appropriate. In collaboration with Fa'atasi and the clinical team, the nurse will develop strategies to support her adherence to medical appointments, such as introducing her to the medical team, ensuring that she has access to transportation, encouraging her to bring a support person to appointments or ensuring that appointments are available at convenient times of the day. Incentives could be offered, such as meals or social events. The clinic staff must also be prepared for Fa'atasi by ensuring that all staff treat her respectfully from the moment she walks in the door. Respectful treatment can include things like ensuring that staff use female pronouns and learn respectful greetings in Samoan, or allowing her to use the female toilet.

There may be other significant social issues in Fa'atasi's life that should be considered and assessed. Working casually as a sex worker suggests that her financial resources are fragile, which may put her housing, food and other essentials at risk. Her legal residency status may need to be clarified, and she may have outstanding legal issues that will need to be addressed. Other issues that may need to be explored include income and/or employment alternatives to sex work; access to medications; and social and family supports. A referral to a social worker or case manager should be considered to assess these issues.

In Case Study 27.3, as part of the nursing assessment, the following key nursing issues are identified, as well as interventions to address these problems.

Medical presentation

Ruth needs to be assessed for progression of her HIV disease, including opportunistic diseases such as *cryptococcal meningitis*. The doctor may repeat her CD4 and viral load testing to determine the current state of her immune system. The nurse will provide or review education about HIV and HIV treatments and opportunistic infections.

Pregnancy testing

Ruth has missed her period. It is possible that a pregnant mother can transmit HIV to her baby either during gestation or during the birthing process. This is often called 'vertical' transmission. Although the risks of vertical transmission have been greatly reduced today with antiretroviral therapies, women with HIV should carefully consider the risks to themselves and

---

CASE STUDY 27.3

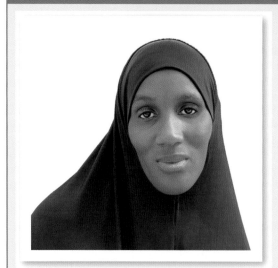

iStockphoto/valeriebarry.

Ruth is a 29-year-old migrant to New Zealand from Somalia. She has been married for 8 years and has two children, aged 3 and 7. Ruth and her husband are both Muslim. Ruth's husband came to New Zealand 5 years ago, almost

1 year before Ruth, in order to begin his new job and establish a home for Ruth and the children. During that time Ruth had a brief affair with another man in Somalia. Ruth works evenings as a care worker in a nursing home. About a year ago Ruth and her husband underwent routine health screening for her permanent residency visa. Ruth was told that she was HIV positive. She has also tested PPD+ for tuberculosis. Ruth's husband is HIV negative. They have no other family in New Zealand. Ruth sees her doctor, who has treated her for vaginal candidiasis and is prophylaxing her for tuberculosis.

Ruth has told no one except her husband about her HIV status. She tries to avoid other African migrants because she 'feels dirty inside her', and thinks that if anyone sees her they will know about her. She is keenly aware of how small immigrant African communities are, and knows how much everyone gossips. She feels overwhelmed by her diagnosis and is sure that she will die, because everyone she knew with AIDS in Somalia has died. She is deeply religious, however, and believes her disease is punishment for her brief affair. Nevertheless, she feels hurt and angry with her husband because she feels he does not understand her, although she understands his sense of anger and betrayal. She presents with fever, nausea and vomiting, headache and fatigue. She missed her last menstrual period.

to their babies before they become pregnant. Many countries follow World Health Organization (WHO) guidelines and routinely use rapid HIV tests at delivery for women with an unknown HIV status, and use antiretroviral therapy with HIV-infected women during pregnancy and infants after birth (Downie et al 2016). Ruth should be advised of these concerns and risks.

Partner education
Ruth's husband needs to be educated about HIV disease and risk reduction; and probably re-testing would be recommended for him if he has been sexually active with Ruth without a condom.

Testing of children
Although this case does not provide information about the children, the birth of at least one of them fell after the time when Ruth may have been infected with HIV. Therefore, assessing these children for HIV infection is important. We have not included a section on paediatric HIV disease in this chapter, as it is quite a different disease presentation and merits attention all on its own.

Social factors
In addition to these issues, it is apparent that there are a number of other social factors that are contributing to Ruth's current health and mental health status. These include:
- her apparent social isolation
- her perception of her disease, which will relate to her motivation to care for herself
- her relationship with her husband
- her legal and immigration status, which may affect her treatment options and her ability to stay in the country
- permanency planning for the children, should her health deteriorate rapidly.

INTERVENTIONS
Since HIV is a syndrome that may affect many body systems, people may present with a number of possible symptoms, conditions and opportunistic infections, each of which requires careful assessment, planning (including the person, their family and significant others) and intervention. This section will expand the above discussion on treatment of HIV to include:
- an overview of opportunistic diseases
- collaboration with other allied health professionals.

As you read the material presented in the following sections think about how some of these interventions have affected, or could affect, Eric, Fa'atasi and Ruth.

Opportunistic Infections
One of the ways in which HIV damages the body is by impairing the immune system that would normally protect the body against an array of pathogens. These are commonly referred to as opportunistic infections, which pose no problems for a person who does not have HIV, but are problematic for someone with HIV. These opportunistic infections can involve every body system. Both Eric and Ruth present with opportunistic infections; Eric with *Chlamydia psittaci* (bacterial) and oral candidiasis (fungal) and Ruth with vaginal candidiasis (fungal). Ruth is also taking antibiotics prophylactically to help prevent her from getting *mycobacterium tuberculosis* (bacterial), another opportunistic infection. Lewis and colleagues (2016) identify the following opportunistic infections that may occur in people with HIV in addition to those presented above:
- *Chlamydia psittaci* (bacterial)
- cryptococcosis (fungal)
- histoplasmosis (fungal)
- toxoplasmosis (protozoal)
- cryptosporidium organisms (protozoal)
- cytomegalovirus (viral)
- herpes simplex types 1 and 2 (virus)
- Kaposi's sarcoma (cancer).

All nurses need to have an extensive knowledge and understanding of the array of opportunistic infections that commonly present themselves in people who have HIV. Doing so will ensure that they are in a position to monitor, report and appropriately intervene in a timely manner. The early recognition of changes to a person's health status benefits the person and their family, or significant other, from further distress and hospitalisation. Healthcare occurs in an environment where health resources are scarce, fiscal restraint on healthcare delivery is a reality and hospitalisation is expensive (McLennan & Meyer 2019). Consequently, the early detection and treatment of health issues in people living with lifelong conditions such as HIV/AIDS to prevent hospital admissions is one way of ensuring the health dollar goes further.

Collaboration with Allied Health Professionals
As can be seen in the case studies, HIV impacts on all aspects of an individual's life. It is therefore important to take the broadest possible view of the disease process and involve allied health professionals as necessary – and

it is almost always necessary. For example, many clients may present with mental health issues, gender or sexual identity issues, or substance misuse or dependency. In such cases, psychologists, psychiatrists, social workers, counsellors or substance misuse professionals may be helpful. If a person is having legal, financial, immigration, employment, housing, relationship or childcare problems, those concerns may distract them from taking care of themselves, and may affect access to or adherence to treatments; a referral to a social services worker will be in order. Other allied health professionals that have been or may in the future be recommended to contribute to the care of Eric, Fa'atasi and Ruth include physiotherapists, occupational therapists, dietitians, podiatrists and pharmacists.

Much of the work centred around nursing and medicines for people living with HIV focuses on the psycho-physical aspects of the disease, keeping people alive as well as free from the harmful effects of HIV-related opportunistic infections. Many people with HIV use complementary and alternative medicine (CAM) in combination with biomedical (or 'allopathic') therapies to manage the effects of their chronic illness. For example, those who report chronic or unmanageable pain may find benefit from massage or acupuncture. In addition, some people with HIV may be either socially isolated or live with family or partners who may be afraid to touch them; therefore massage may provide the only opportunity for these people to be touched in a non-clinical or non-painful way. While there are many CAM therapies available (Shere-Wolfe 2019), below is a list of some of those more commonly used. As you read through these, identify those that might be useful to encourage Eric, Fa'atasi and Ruth to consider:

- acupuncture
- herbal medicine
- manipulative and body-based therapies
- homeopathy
- meditation
- chiropractic
- the use of oil or incense
- reflexology
- massage.

In summary, care for people with HIV must be understood as a team effort, with every person contributing their expertise.

Family and Carers

The role of families and carers in HIV disease management is complex because many people with HIV are socially isolated, either by choice or because they have been rejected by their families. In addition, families and carers themselves may be subject to stigma from their communities (Vreeman et al 2019). Fortunately, there are a number of HIV service organisations located throughout Australasia that can provide support to individuals living with HIV and their families (see Recommended reading at the end of this chapter and the Multimedia Resources section at the end of the book). It is also important to recognise that there are many different constellations of families. As reflected in the case studies, people with HIV may have same- or opposite-sex partners; they may have children or parents, or grandparents; they may have people who are very close friends who accompany them to medical appointments and who help out at home. All these people will bring their own understandings of disease and wellness, confusion and clarity, despair and hope.

The most important thing that people both infected and affected by HIV need is information. They need to know that their healthcare providers will provide care and information and not judgement. There is a social stigma attached to having HIV that permeates society, negatively affecting quality of life and manifesting as mental health issues including symptoms of loneliness, social isolation and depression (Gardiner 2018). The people represented in the case studies are all susceptible to negative social attitudes related to their HIV status and their sexual orientation (Eric and Fa'atasi), for being a sex worker as well as using drugs (Fa'atasi) and for being a member of an ethnic minority (Ruth).

Frequently, nurses are the first point of contact for people living with chronic illnesses such as HIV and are therefore pivotal to providing care to this group of people when compared to other health professional groups (Rouleau et al 2019). It is therefore vital that nurses develop therapeutic relationships with people living with HIV, their families and significant others that are non-judgemental and accepting. The development of a supportive relationship based on these principles is more likely to positively influence health and wellbeing, including the adherence to treatment regimens.

As demonstrated in the case studies, nurses need to have a sound understanding of the principles of chronic illness such as HIV, so they can reassure and support the family in the following ways:

- explaining that there will be good days and bad days as part of the illness experience
- providing education about the often complicated regimen of medications and the potential side effects of these medications

- reinforcing the importance of adhering to drug and treatment regimens – this is especially important in HIV/AIDS as lack of adherence can lead to drug resistance
- making sure the family understand the disease trajectory, so they can monitor and provide a useful source of information to the health professionals they come in contact with
- reinforcing that people respond differently to challenges associated with living with HIV; for example, some people become profoundly depressed, some may even be affected by primary HIV and secondary infections of the brain itself, which result in mood changes and thought disorders, affecting the individual's ability to self-care; some people, however, may find new meaning and purpose, or a renewed sense of spirituality in their lives
- encouraging families and carers to be mindful of the stressful and even exhausting nature of supporting someone living with HIV and advising them about who to call for help, respite care, advocacy or professional assistance when required – they should be encouraged to keep a directory of emergency phone numbers and phone numbers for community support agencies in an accessible location
- ensuring that families know that spiritual support is available for them and the person with HIV and where to access this support. The local AIDS service organisation will be an invaluable resource.

The provision of healthcare is highly political and nurses engage with the socio-political context of healthcare provision and the impact it has on consumers of healthcare services (Montalvo 2015). Consequently, HIV can be seen as a political diagnosis; the lives of people living with an HIV-related illness are directly affected by government or private sector decisions and policies about, for example, what medications will be available (and at what cost), what services will be funded and which clinical trials they may have access to. Nurses need to be able to support and prepare families and caregivers to face the various political challenges that impact on the health and wellbeing of their family member living with HIV.

CONCLUSION

HIV shares many of the attributes associated with other chronic illnesses, including tiredness, a decrease in quality of life, an inability to independently undertake activities of daily living and being dependent on others. People living with a chronic illness, no matter what disease it is, are likely to have contact with healthcare,

government and social service organisations. Most importantly, they will all come into contact with nurses at some stage of their illness experience. Nurses working in any area where they are likely to come in contact with people living with HIV need to have appropriate knowledge and skills in order to provide a quality and holistic healthcare experience for this group of people.

Reflective Questions

1. How can nurses ensure that people with HIV are provided with optimal care when engaging with health service organisations?
2. What areas of knowledge do you need to add to your skills in order to provide an appropriate health service for people living with HIV?
3. As a nurse what role do you have in preventing the spread of HIV?

RECOMMENDED READING

Hardy D 2019. Fundamentals of HIV medicine. Oxford University Press, New York.

Rouleau G, Richard L, Cote J et al 2019. Nursing practice to support people living with HIV with antiretroviral therapy adherence: a qualitative study. Journal of the Association of Nurses in AIDS Care 30(4), E20–E37.

Sahoo C, Sahoo, N, Rao S et al 2017. A review on prevention and treatment of AIDS. Pharmacy & Pharmacology International Journal 5(1), 9–17.

REFERENCES

AIDS Epidemiology Group 2019. AIDS – New Zealand: Issue 78. University of Otago, Dunedin.

Allen S, Ruiz M, Jones J et al 2016. Legal space for syringe exchange programs in hot spots of injection drug use-related crime. Harm Reduction Journal 13, 16.

Barroso J, Leserman J, Harmon J et al 2015. Fatigue in HIV-infected people: a three-year observational study. Journal of Pain and Symptom Management 50(1), 69–79.

Bond K, Yoon I, Houang S et al 2019. Transactional sex, substance use and sexual risk: comparing pay direction for an internet-based U.S. sample of men who have sex with men. Sexuality Research and Social Policy 16(3), 255–267.

Bristowe K, Marshall S, Harding R 2016. The bereavement experiences of lesbian, gay, bisexual and/or trans* people who have lost a partner: a systematic review, thematic synthesis and modelling of the literature. Palliative Medicine 30(8), 730–744.

Cheng T, Johnston C, Kerr T et al 2015. Substance use patterns and unprotected sex among street-involved youth in a Canadian setting: a prospective cohort study. BMC Public Health 16(4).

Cooper K, Gosnell K 2015. Foundations and adult health nursing, 7th edn. Elsevier, St Louis.

Dodd R, Crowder L, Haynes J 2020. Screening blood donors for HIV, HCV and HBV at the American Red Cross: ten-year trends in prevalence, incidence and residual risk 2007–2016. Transfusion Medicine Reviews 34(2), 81–93.

Downie J, Mactier H, Bland R 2016. Should pregnant women with unknown HIV status be offered rapid HIV testing in labour? Archives of Disease in Childhood. Fetal and Neonatal Edition 101(1), 79–84.

Emlet C, Brennan D, Brennenstuhl S et al 2015. The impact of HIV-related stigma on older and younger adults living with HIV disease: does age matter? AIDS Care 27(4), 520–528.

Gardiner B 2018. Grit and stigma: gay men ageing with HIV in regional Queensland. Journal of Sociology 54(2), 214–225.

Jaiswal J, Singer S, Siegel K et al 2019. HIV-related 'conspiracy beliefs': lived experiences of racism and socio-economic exclusion among people living with HIV in New York City. Culture, Health and Sexuality 21(4), 373–386.

Lewis D 2015. Will targeting oropharyngeal gonorrhoea delay the further emergence of drug-resistant Neisseria gonorrhoeae strains? Sexually Transmitted Infections 91(4), 234–237.

Lewis S, Bucher L, Heitkemper M et al (eds) 2016. Medical–surgical nursing: assessment and management of clinical problems, 10th edn. Elsevier, St Louis.

McLennan K, Meyer J 2019. Care and cost. Current issues in health policy. Routledge, New York.

Mitra S, Rachlis B, Krysowaty B et al 2019. Potential use of supervised injection services among people who inject drugs in a remote and mid-size Canadian setting. BMC Public Health 19, 284.

Montalvo W 2015. Political skill and its relevance to nursing: an integrative review. The Journal of Nursing Administration 45(7/8), 377–383.

Neville S, Adams J 2016. Views about HIV/STI and health promotion among gay and bisexual Chinese and South Asian men living in Auckland, New Zealand. International Journal Qualitative Studies on Health and Well-being, 11, 10.3402/qhw.v11.30764

Neville S, Adams J, Mooley C et al 2016. The condom imperative in anal sex – one size may not fit all: a qualitative descriptive study of men who have sex with men. Journal of Clinical Nursing 25, 3589–3596.

Neville S, Kushner B, Adams J 2015. Coming out narratives of older gay men living in New Zealand. Australasian Journal on Ageing 34(2), 29–33.

Rouleau G, Richard L, Cote J et al 2019. Nursing practice to support people living with HIV with antiretroviral therapy adherence: a qualitative study. Journal of the Association of Nurses in AIDS Care 30(4), E20–E37.

Sahoo C, Sahoo N, Rao S et al 2017. A review on prevention and treatment of AIDS. Pharmacy & Pharmacology International Journal 5(1), 9–17.

Santos A, Silveira E, Falco M 2016. Gastrointestinal symptoms in HIV-infected patients: female sex and smoking as risk factors in an outpatient cohort in Brazil. PloS One 11(10), e0164774.

Sears D, Daar E 2015. NRTIs. In: T Hope, M Stevenson, D Richman (eds), Encyclopedia of AIDS. Springer, New York.

Shere-Wolfe K 2019. Complementary and alternative medicine/integrative medicine approaches. In: D Hardy (ed.), Fundamentals of HIV medicine. Oxford University Press, New York.

The Kirby Institute 2018. HIV in Australia: annual surveillance short report 2018. The Kirby Institute, Sydney.

Tumusiime D, Stewart A, Venter F 2015. Effect of physiotherapeutic exercises on peripheral neuropathy, functional limitations of lower extremity and quality of life in people with HIV. Physiotherapy 101(1), 1547–1548.

UNAIDS 2016. Global AIDS update. United Nations, Geneva.

Vreeman R, Scanlon M, Wanzhu T et al 2019. Validation of an HIV/AIDS stigma measure for children living with HIV and their families. Journal of the International Association of Providers of AIDS Care 18, 1–11.

World Health Organization (WHO) 2020. www.cdc.gov/hiv/risk/art/index.html. WHO, Geneva.

World Health Organization (WHO) 2019. What's the 2+1+1? Event-driven oral pre-exposure prophylaxis to prevent HIV for men who have sex with men: update to WHO's recommendation on oral PrEP. WHO, Geneva.

World Health Organization (WHO) 2013. Responding to intimate partner violence and sexual violence against women: WHO clinical and policy guidelines. WHO, Geneva.

CHAPTER 28

Principles for Nursing Practice: Cancer

PATSY YATES

LEARNING OBJECTIVES

When you have completed this chapter you will be able to:
- appreciate the trajectory of cancer as a chronic disease and its implications for the physical and psychosocial well-being of people affected by cancer
- identify key principles for reducing the risk and identifying cancer early
- discuss factors influencing quality of life for people affected by cancer across the disease trajectory
- describe the information and support needs for people affected by cancer
- identify interventions to enhance quality of life for people at all stages of the cancer trajectory.

KEY WORDS

cancer	survivorship
quality of life (QOL)	treatment effects
supportive care	

INTRODUCTION

Cancer is a chronic and complex set of diseases. In Australia in 2019, 396 new cases of cancer were diagnosed each day, and over 1 million people were either living with or had lived with cancer (Australian Institute of Health and Welfare [AIHW] 2019b). While cancer continues to be one of the most common causes of death among adult Australians and New Zealanders, considerable progress has been made in controlling this disease in recent years. Over the last 30 years ago, 5-year survival has increased from about 5 in 10 people to be closer to 7 in 10 people today (AIHW 2019b). In New Zealand, 5-year relative survival rates are similarly increasing, currently at 63% (Ministry of Health NZ 2015). Such scientific advances mean that cancer today is considered a chronic disease for many diagnosed with this condition.

Cancer is a set of diseases which have a natural history and course of progression, treatments and outcomes in the short and long term, which vary markedly. This means that the experiences and needs of people at risk or affected by cancer will vary considerably. While it is a disease that does not have a series of well-marked events, critical points at which health professionals may intervene to improve cancer outcomes can be identified. For well communities, these critical points include opportunities for reducing the risk of cancer and detecting the cancer early. For those with a diagnosis of cancer, Optimal Cancer Care Pathways have been developed in Australia to improve outcomes by facilitating consistent, safe, high-quality and evidence-based care. The pathways map the key stages in a cancer patient's journey, from prevention and early detection to survivorship or end-of-life care and describe key principles for optimal care at critical points (National Cancer Expert Reference Group 2020). Responding effectively to meet the needs of the person affected by cancer at these critical intervention points requires an appreciation of cancer as a chronic disease, and the factors that can influence an individual's experiences and responses at key phases along this journey.

REDUCING RISK AND DETECTING CANCER EARLY

Behaviours Which Contribute to the Development of the Cancer

There are several modifiable factors which increase a person's risk of developing cancer. While exposure to a risk factor does not mean that a person will definitely develop cancer, reducing exposure to such risks is critical to cancer control (AIHW 2019b).

Evidence to support the implementation of public policy and behavioural strategies to prevent cancer is growing. The IARC claims that feasible, affordable and cost-effective interventions are available to reduce exposure to key causes and other risk factors for cancer (International Agency for Cancer Research [IACR] 2020).

The Cancer Council Australia (CCA) makes specific recommendations for national action by governments and non-government organisations, including programs and strategies to reduce the incidence of specific preventable cancer types, in areas including tobacco control, overweight, obesity, nutrition and physical activity, ultraviolet radiation, alcohol, and occupational exposure

(CCA 2020a). These recommendations relate to simple steps for individuals to reduce their risk of cancer:

- Quit smoking
- Eat for health
- Maintain a healthy weight
- Be SunSmart
- Limit alcohol
- Move your body
- Get checked – men and women (CCA 2020b).

A summary of additional recommended public policy and program actions to reduce the risk of cancer is presented in Box 28.1.

Participation in Cancer-Screening Programs

For the majority of cancers, outcomes are dramatically improved when the cancer is detected early. Promoting participation in early detection programs is a critical concern for health professionals in all areas of practice. In the context of cancer, early detection can be achieved through population screening programs (such as screening mammography, cervical cancer screening or faecal occult blood testing), opportunistic screening (such as through

---

BOX 28.1
Cancer Prevention Policy and Recommendations: Cancer Council Australia

TOBACCO

- Continue to reduce the affordability of tobacco products
- Strengthen mass media campaigns
- Eliminate remaining advertising, promotion and sponsorship of tobacco products
- Reduce exceptions to smoke-free environments
- Strengthen efforts to reduce smoking in disadvantaged populations
- Regulate the contents, product disclosure and supply of tobacco products
- Provide access to evidence-based smoking cessation services
- Research and evaluation

ULTRAVIOLET RADIATION

- Investment in national mass media campaigns to increase public awareness about skin cancer risk, sun protection and associated behaviour change
- Investment in population health research into sun protection behaviours to inform evidence-based policy and programs
- Establish a roadmap towards recognised early detection of melanoma

NUTRITION AND PHYSICAL ACTIVITY

- Implement a comprehensive national obesity prevention strategy
  - Strategies should prioritise high-risk groups especially Aboriginal and Torres Strait Islander peoples and lower socioeconomic groups
- Create environments that support healthy food choices
  - Develop national food and nutrition action plan to improve the availability, accessibility and affordability of healthy foods, consistent with Australian Dietary Guidelines
  - Improve Health Star Rating system and make it mandatory to facilitate healthier food choices
  - Restrict exposure of children to the marketing of unhealthy foods
- Create environments that support physical activity
  - Develop a national active transport strategy
- Develop economic interventions for preventive health
- Increase taxes on energy dense and nutrient poor food products, including introducing a 20% health levy on sugar-sweetened beverages

Cancer Council Australia 2020a.

informal health checks) and diagnostic screening (i.e. when a person presents with symptoms for investigation). While familial cancers that are caused by inherited genetic mutations account for only around 10% of cancers, advances in genomics have meant that more than 120 genes in which rare mutations can confer an increased risk of cancer have been identified (IARC 2020). This growth in understanding of many of the genes responsible for heritable mutations is also raising a range of issues in relation to cancer screening (IARC 2020).

Despite the importance of early detection, rates of participation in screening programs vary between different social demographic groups. For example, women from a non-English-speaking background and Aboriginal and Torres Strait Islander women have lower participation rates in mammographic screening programs (AIHW 2019a). Understanding barriers to cancer screening enables health professionals to implement targeted intervention strategies to promote participation. For example, barriers to cancer screening that are potentially amenable to intervention include financial concerns, embarrassment, poor access, anxiety about test results, inconvenience, forgetting or procrastination and discomfort associated with the screening test. The World Health Organization (WHO) has defined principles that should underpin cancer-screening programs. These principles are described in Box 28.2. They provide a framework for health professionals to help them consider areas in which they may intervene to ensure optimal outcomes from cancer screening at the population and individual level.

ENSURING BEST POSSIBLE TREATMENT AND SUPPORT DURING AND AFTER ACTIVE TREATMENT
Issues of Quality of Life in Relation to Cancer

The cancer disease process and contemporary cancer treatments present many challenges to an individual's quality of life (QOL). Cancer is a multi-system disease, and its treatments are typically multi-modal, including surgery, chemotherapy, radiotherapy, biotherapy and/ or hormone therapy. Cancer treatment programs also tend to be long term, often requiring several administrations or doses delivered over a period of many months. Each of these treatments is often associated with a range of short-term and longer-term effects on an individual's QOL.

The presence and severity of the effects will vary from individual to individual, although the factors underlying these differences are not completely understood. QOL concerns for the person affected by cancer thus include many physical, psychosocial and practical issues and, for some, end-of-life concerns. Box 28.3 provides a summary of the key psychosocial concerns that may be experienced by people affected by cancer, many of which persist during and after treatment for cancer.

With improvements in cancer treatment, survival from cancer has been extended. A growing body of research has highlighted that cancer survivors have a unique set of health and support needs. For the majority of people diagnosed with cancer, the disease and its

---

BOX 28.2
WHO Principles for Cancer Screening

- The target disease should be a common form of cancer, with high associated morbidity or mortality
- Effective treatment, capable of reducing morbidity and mortality, should be available
- Test procedures should be acceptable, safe, and relatively inexpensive.

World Health Organization (WHO) 2020.

BOX 28.3
Psychosocial Needs of People with Cancer

- Physical needs (e.g. physical comfort and freedom from pain and other symptoms, optimum nutrition, activities of daily living (ADLs); may include assessment of complications such as late effects of treatment)
- Informational needs (e.g. to reduce confusion, anxiety and fear, to inform patient and family decision-making, and to assist in skill acquisition related to treatment or disease, system orientation)
- Emotional needs (e.g. sense of comfort, safety, understanding and reassurance in dealing with sadness, grief and loss)
- Psychological needs (e.g. coping with illness experience and its consequences, personal control, self-esteem)
- Social needs (e.g. family relationships and social networks, community acceptance and involvement in one's relationships)
- Spiritual needs (e.g. hope, belonging, meaning and purpose of life, existential concerns)
- Practical needs (direct assistance to accomplish tasks or activities – e.g. homemaking services, financial assistance, system navigation)

Canadian Association of Psychosocial Oncology 2009.

effects thus become chronic in nature. The specific risk for recurrence or late effects experienced by an individual who has undergone treatment for cancer will usually depend on the specific site, histology of their disease, the treatments they received, when those treatments were delivered (since regimens and techniques change over time), the length of time that has elapsed since those exposures and underlying risk factors independent of their cancer or its treatment (Institute of Medicine [IOM] 2006). Moreover, as cancer is largely a disease of the elderly, determining the late effects of the cancer disease and treatment process from unrelated co-morbid conditions can be difficult (IOM 2006). While there is considerable heterogeneity in post-treatment experiences for people with cancer, the Clinical Oncology Society of Australia (COSA) has developed a framework to guide the promotion of wellness for cancer survivors. The key principles underpinning the framework include:

- Survivor (person)-centred, in that it is: enabling individuals to participate in decision-making that will positively influence their health and wellbeing; engaging individuals to motivate them to make positive health choices; and, empowering them to seek information and support from the services that are most suitable to their needs at any given time.
- Integrating care across all service levels at all time points to ensure survivors have access to the right care, at the right intensity, at the right time.
- Coordinating care across all services.
- Promoting wellbeing by emphasising behaviours and actions that support wellness rather than focus on illness.
- Preventing illness by supporting survivors to engage in lifestyle behaviours, self-care and preventative health checks that are appropriate to maintain health.
- Managing symptoms and problems.

Cancer is a life-threatening disease. Unfortunately, despite developments in cancer treatments, nearly 40% of those diagnosed with cancer will ultimately die from their disease, although survival rates vary considerably for different tumour sites. For those who have disease recurrence, or for those whose disease is progressing, some important and unique QOL concerns arise during end-of-life care. Some of these concerns include physical symptoms, as well as psychosocial, existential and spiritual distress.

Our review of QOL concerns for people affected by cancer as a chronic disease highlights the significant impact of this disease on day-to-day living, both during and following the treatment process. Indeed, many people asked about their experience of cancer can describe numerous examples of how the problems resulting from cancer or its treatment affect their daily activities in the short and longer term. Nurses are well placed to respond to these concerns, by assessment of the factors contributing to these problems, and applying evidence-based interventions relevant to the individual's needs.

NURSING RESPONSES TO KEY QOL CONCERNS FOR PEOPLE AFFECTED BY CANCER

Altered Mobility and Fatigue – Relationship to Activities of Daily Living

Fatigue is almost universally reported as a frequent and significant treatment side effect in people undergoing cancer treatment and it is a symptom that persists long after treatment ends (National Comprehensive Cancer Network [NCCN] 2020a). Qualitative studies have identified that people describe cancer-related fatigue as making them feel angry, frustrated and depressed, as it prevents them from doing some of the most basic day-to-day activities and has major impacts on social lives (Scott et al 2011). In contrast to healthy individuals, people with cancer have fatigue that is more persistent and distressing (Goedendorp et al 2012). The exact mechanisms of cancer-related fatigue are not well understood, but may involve pro-inflammatory cytokines, circadian rhythm de-synchronisation or skeletal muscle deregulation (NCCN 2020a). Box 28.4 presents a summary of the factors that may contribute to fatigue in people affected by cancer, highlighting the multidimensional nature of this problem.

Assessment of the factors contributing to an individual's fatigue is integral to effectively managing this problem. Recent research has highlighted a number of interventions that nurses can use to manage cancer-related fatigue, during treatment and in the post-treatment phase. These interventions include:

- patient/family education and counselling; for example, information about patterns of fatigue during and following treatment
- general strategies; for example, energy conservation, distraction
- non-pharmacological strategies; for example, activity enhancement; psychological interventions (stress management, relaxation); attention-restoring therapy; nutrition consultation; sleep therapy; family interaction (NCCN 2020a).

BOX 28.4
Factors Contributing to Fatigue

- Cancer treatment
- Anaemia
- Medications
- Cachexia/anorexia
- Metabolic disturbances
- Hormone deficiency or excess
- Psychological distress
- Physical deconditioning
- Sleep disturbances
- Excessive inactivity
- Pulmonary impairment
- Neuromuscular dysfunction
- Pain and other symptoms
- Proinflammatory cytokines
- Nutritional deficiencies
- Dehydration
- Infection
- Concomitant medical illness
- Cardiac impairment

National Cancer Institute 2020.

People with cancer may also experience altered mobility and function as a result of their disease or its treatment. This can be due to the impact of a primary cancer resulting in muscle weakness, paralysis, hemiparesis or ataxia (e.g. with some brain tumours or multiple myeloma) or the secondary effects of metastatic disease (e.g. spinal cord compression or other obstructions) (Waitman 2016). It may also be due to the impact of treatments (e.g. restrictions or nerve damage due to surgery, or alterations from the neurotoxic effects of cancer treatments that result in peripheral neuropathies). Other disease- and treatment-related symptoms, such as pain or fatigue, may also result in impaired mobility. Some patients experience a quantitative decline in muscle mass (sarcopenia) (Waitman 2016). Strategies for optimising function for the person affected by cancer will thus be influenced by the specific factors causing the impaired function. These strategies should focus on increasing physical function, promoting safety, and reducing the complications of immobility (Waitman 2016). There is also increasing evidence that exercise has a number of

physical and psychological benefits for people both during and following cancer treatment. A recent review identified that specific doses of aerobic, combined aerobic plus resistance training, and/or resistance training could improve common cancer-related health outcomes, including anxiety, depressive symptoms, fatigue, physical functioning, and health-related QOL (Campbell 2019).

Body Image – Impact for the Person and their Family Carers

Body image is a complex, multifaceted construct that involves perceptions, feelings and behaviours related to the body and its functioning (Fingeret et al 2014). Patients with cancer can experience a broad range of bodily changes that can affect body image, including alterations to appearance (e.g. hair loss, scarring, swelling), sensory changes (e.g. pain, numbness) and functional impairment (e.g. dysphagia, dysarthria, impotence) (Fingeret et al 2014). One systematic review identified that cancer survivors often have a more negative body image than healthy controls. The review identified key areas where cancer survivors reported greater concern when compared to controls, including appearance evaluation, sexual attractiveness, self-consciousness, and feelings towards the body (Lehmann et al 2015).

It is important for nurses to explore whether the patient has significant concerns about the impact of treatments on their body or sense of self. Possible questions to prompt discussions about these concerns include (National Breast Cancer Centre & National Cancer Control Initiative 2005, p. 87):

> We don't often talk about it, but cancer certainly changes how we feel about ourselves. Many people tell me that they do have concerns about how they will look, and how they will feel about themselves after treatment. Is this something that you feel you could discuss with me?

A range of practical prosthetic or rehabilitative devices or procedures may be suitable for some people affected by cancer. For example, reconstructive surgery for breast cancer can be offered to improve a woman's body image. Other supportive and educative interventions that may assist include programs such as the Look Good ... Feel Better program. The purpose of the program, which is widely available through Cancer Councils and specialist cancer settings, is to help people manage the appearance-related side effects of chemotherapy and radiotherapy, thereby helping to restore appearance and self-image.

Family and Carers of People Affected by Cancer

Cancer is a disease experienced by the whole family. Studies suggest that couples react to cancer as an 'emotional system', as the distress experienced by the person with cancer is closely linked to the emotional wellbeing of the family (Northouse 2012). Family members can also play an important role as caregivers, providing physical, practical and emotional support to meet the diverse needs of their relative. The needs and concerns of families are therefore considerable across all phases of the cancer journey. Studies suggest that common needs of caregivers include how to access information about physical needs, prognosis and financial support, as well as how to address practical concerns about the impact of cancer on working life and how to obtain best medical care (Heckel et al 2015). During this time, families also often have to adjust to different roles and deal with strains associated with changes to social functioning and interpersonal relationships.

Studies have reported that the majority of partners of people affected by cancer report supportive care needs post diagnosis. One recent review classified carers into three broad groups and highlighted key needs for these groups (Kim et al 2019). For former carers, needs often related to concerns about remission and the cancer coming back, as well as management of emotional and financial distress. For those who continue to provide care, concerns related to meeting complex patient needs, communication with members of the healthcare team, family and friends, maintaining intimacy, responding to uncertainty and ongoing challenges relating to the disease, and managing outside work. For bereaved carers, key concerns relate to managing psychological distress, reintegrating daily life, and managing losses.

The needs of family members at the end of life become of particular importance, as family caregivers often take on substantial caregiving roles, while at the same time having to deal with the distress associated with losing a loved one. Some unique family-related challenges for health professionals when caring for families at end of life include high symptom distress, strained family relationships, feelings of abandonment, competing outside demands (e.g. work), lack of financial and community support and poor self-care (exercise, diet) (Northouse 2012).

A range of interventions can be applied to support family caregivers throughout the cancer journey. These need to be based on a comprehensive assessment of family needs and fall into four categories: providing information; providing psychological support; providing physical support; and mobilising resources (Ferrall 2010). Such supportive interventions can be delivered through family conferences, skills training, problem-solving, caregiver training and information resources. Enabling access to additional support services, such as respite, home modification or community support groups to deal with the longer-term impact of cancer as a chronic disease, may also be helpful (Ferrall 2010). A systematic review of 128 intervention studies of carer interventions focused on reducing caregiver strain and burden identified that psychoeducation, supportive care/support interventions, and cognitive behavioural interventions are recommended to decrease burden and strain, and that caregiver skill training, couples therapy, decision support, mindfulness-based stress reduction, multicomponent interventions, and palliative care are also likely to be effective (Jadalla et al 2020).

Education and Support for the Person and Family Affected by Cancer

The emotional and support needs of people affected by cancer are wide-ranging and profound. These psychosocial needs are significant, and frequently go undetected and are unmet (NCCN 2020b). Early detection of distress can lead to better adherence to treatment, better communication, and reduced risk of anxiety and depression (NCCN 20206b). Screening all patients for supportive care needs is an essential component of nursing practice in all settings. A range of screening tools exist to identify distress and supportive care needs (see toolkit available at: www.petermac.org/sites/default/files/media-uploads/ACSC_Needs_assessment_Toolkit_Jan_2016.pdf).

As one example, the Supportive Care Screening Tool developed by Peter MacCallum Cancer Centre comprises a checklist covering aspects of the individual's health and wellbeing to enable identification of needs. These areas include:

- communication and understanding
- physical health
- emotional health
- ADLs
- support and coping
- use of support services
- information requirements.

Once needs have been identified, responses that are targeted and tailored to an individual's needs are required. A tiered model of care has been suggested as a stepped care approach that aims to match the patient's or family member's level of distress and expressed needs to an appropriate level of psychosocial intervention (Steginga et al 2006). Components in this tiered model include:

- universal care: information, brief emotional and practical support (e.g. healthcare team, Cancer Helpline)
- supportive care: emotional, practical, spiritual care, psycho-education, values-based decision support, peer support (e.g. social worker, peers, chaplain, Cancer Helpline)
- extended care: counselling, time-limited therapy, skills training (e.g. psychologist, social work, tele-based cancer counselling service)
- specialist care: specialised therapy for depression, anxiety, relationship problems (e.g. psychologist, psychiatrist, tele-based cancer counselling service)
- acute care: intensive or comprehensive therapy for acute and complex problems (e.g. mental health team, psychiatrist).

According to this model, services are provided according to the level of need. Importantly, as a minimum, all persons require access to the components of universal care, including information and brief emotional and social support. Such informational and supportive interventions are fundamental elements of nursing care for people affected by cancer at all stages of the journey.

Specifically, education for the person and family affected by cancer involves a series of structured or non-structured experiences designed to help the person and their family to develop knowledge and self-care abilities needed to manage the impact of cancer and its treatments on their wellbeing. For the nurse seeking to design an effective educational intervention for people with cancer, there appears to be an overwhelming number of considerations to be taken into account. For example, issues to be considered may include what type/s of educational process should be employed, what the focus (content, topics) of the educational intervention should be and what the ideal context and most appropriate methods are for delivering an intervention. Current evidence suggests that patient-specific information (i.e. information specific to the individual's actual clinical situation) should be provided to patients and that patient education should be structured and involve multiple teaching strategies (Cancer Care Ontario 2009). It is also recommended that patient education for minority groups should be culturally sensitive (Cancer Care Ontario 2009).

Issues related to the accessibility of an intervention to various groups, the responsiveness of an intervention to diverse contexts and needs, as well as the efficiency with which interventions can be delivered, are also important considerations for healthcare providers.

A key goal of education for patients with cancer is to develop the person's self-management abilities. This enables the patient to take greater control in managing the short- and longer-term effects of cancer. Specific elements of self-management education in cancer include the following. They should:

- be tailored to the needs, characteristics, and life circumstances of the patient (includes low health literacy and cultural diversity)
- facilitate mastery and the patient's confidence (self-efficacy), so that they can manage their illness and related symptoms
- support the patient in developing effective skills to communicate with healthcare providers
- facilitate the patient's understanding and confidence (self-efficacy) for managing their care (includes health and support services system navigation)
- be coached by a specially trained instructor
- be supported by collaboration and guidance from the healthcare team
- facilitate uptake of health behaviours through goal setting/action planning
- support development and practice of problem-solving skills to address barriers to behaviours (Cancer Care Ontario 2016).

CONCLUSION

A diagnosis of cancer is an enormously distressing and disruptive experience for the person diagnosed and their family. As a multi-system disease, which typically requires multiple systemic treatments over long periods of time, cancer is today a chronic disease. There are many points throughout the cancer journey where nurses can intervene to improve a person's QOL. In particular, nurses are well placed to provide information and supportive care to help promote a person's health and wellbeing and enhance the person's ability to prevent and manage disease- and treatment-related effects in the short and longer terms. Cancer is a chronic disease that can have long-lasting impacts for the person and their family. Applying best available evidence to manage these impacts has the potential to significantly reduce mortality and morbidity from the disease.

CASE STUDY 28.1

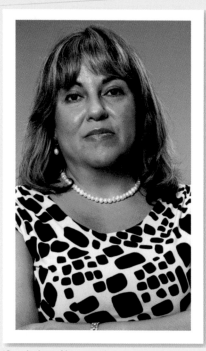

iStockphoto/Juanmonino.

Mrs Jones is a 58-year-old woman with three children and two grandchildren, who has just undergone routine screening mammography in the nearby breast screen service. Mrs Jones is accompanied by her husband as she returns to her GP for discussion of the results. Mrs Jones' GP explains that the mammography indicates she has evidence of breast cancer, and she will need to be referred to the breast clinic at the local hospital for follow-up. Mrs Jones and her husband are extremely distressed and shocked. While Mrs Jones is slightly overweight, she does not understand how she could have developed this cancer. She explains that she has not attended the routine screening mammography when she received reminder letters in recent years because she has been too busy with her new grandchildren and work commitments. Mrs Jones is anxious to find out more information about what is likely to happen, and searches the internet to find information to answer her questions. The practice nurse at the GP clinic spends some time talking with Mr and Mrs Jones about the planned visit to the breast clinic, and assists them to make an appointment at the centre. The nurse ensures all appropriate clinical information and diagnostic tests are forwarded to the clinic as part of the referral.

Mrs Jones is referred to a multidisciplinary team at the cancer centre for treatment planning. Following breast-conserving surgery for early stage breast cancer, she undergoes a course of adjuvant chemotherapy and radiotherapy. Her treatment goes well; however, she experiences a range of side effects including oral mucositis, persistent nausea and fatigue. The nurses in the treatment centre teach Mrs Jones and her husband how to prevent and treat her side effects. They provide a range of written resources so that they can manage at home, including information about what signs or symptoms should prompt Mrs Jones to return to her doctor or call the clinic for advice between treatments.

During the treatment program, Mr Jones also tells the nurse he is having trouble coping with his wife's diagnosis. He feels helpless, not knowing what he can do to help her. He also worries about their future and if the cancer will return. The nurses refer Mr Jones to information resources provided by the local Cancer Council and teach him some techniques to help him relax. Mr Jones also tells the nurse that he has convinced his wife to visit a naturopath to see if they can do anything to help her beat her cancer. The nurse provides information to Mr Jones from the local Cancer Council about the use of complementary and alternative medicines in cancer. The nurses encourage Mr and Mrs Jones to discuss any decisions with them and with the doctor.

Mrs Jones completes her treatment and talks with nurses about diet and exercise recommendations that would help her to maintain her health into the future. She says she has read lots of information on the internet, but is not sure what sources of information she should access to ensure it is reputable. She is also keen to establish an exercise program that fits with her busy schedule, including work and looking after her grandchildren.

Twelve months after completing her treatment, Mrs Jones returns for another routine check-up. She says the fatigue is still a problem, and still worries a lot about her cancer returning, and that these visits for check-ups are especially hard for her husband. She says her life is now very different as a result of her cancer. She is maintaining a regular exercise program and has lost a few kilos to be at a healthy weight. Mrs Jones admits her relationship with her husband has changed, as he seems to want to 'wrap her in cotton wool'. She also says it has been helpful to access a local support group, as she finds it helpful to be able to talk about what is worrying her and her fears about the future with others who are going through the same experience.

Reflective Questions

1. What are likely to be some of the major physical, psychological and social concerns of a person during and following treatment for cancer? How might these needs change for a person whose cancer recurs, and whose illness progresses?

2. How would you respond to questions from a person with cancer about what they can do to optimise their health during and following treatment for cancer? What community and information resources are available in your region to assist the person affected by cancer?

3. What actions can a nurse take to support the self-management abilities of a person affected by cancer and their family members?

RECOMMENDED READING

National Comprehensive Cancer Centre. Clinical practice guidelines: distress management. Online. Available: www.nccn.org/professionals/physician_gls/pdf/distress.pdf.

Olver I (ed.) 2011. The MASCC textbook of cancer supportive care and survivorship. Springer, New York.

Rodriguez M, Foxhall L 2018. Handbook of cancer survivorship care. Springer Publishing, New York.

REFERENCES

Australian Institute of Health and Welfare (AIHW) 2019a. BreastScreen Australia monitoring report 2019. Cancer series no. 127. Cat. no. CAN 128. AIHW, Canberra.

Australian Institute of Health and Welfare (AIHW) 2019b. Cancer in Australia 2019. Cancer series no.119. Cat. no. CAN 123. AIHW, Canberra.

Campbell W 2019. Exercise guidelines for cancer survivors: consensus statement from international multidisciplinary roundtable. Medicine and Science in Sports and Exercise 51(11), 2375–2390.

Canadian Association of Psychosocial Oncology 2009. A Pan Canadian clinical practice guideline: assessment of psychosocial health care needs of the adult cancer patient. Canadian. Online. Available: www.capo.ca/ENGLISH_Adult_Assessment_Guideline.pdf.

Cancer Care Ontario 2016. Self management education for patients with cancer. Online. Available: www.cancercare.on.ca/common/pages/UserFile.aspx?fileId=351865.

Cancer Care Ontario 2009. Effective teaching strategies and methods of delivery for patient education. Online. Available: www.cancercare.on.ca/common/pages/UserFile.aspx?fileId=60063.

Cancer Council Australia (CCA) 2020a. National Cancer Prevention Policy 2020. Online. Available: https://wiki.cancer.org.au/policy/.

Cancer Council Australia 2020. Resources on cancer prevention, screening and diagnosis 2020. Online. Available: www.cancer.org.au/health-professionals/patient-resources.

Ferrall S 2010. Caring for the family caregiver. In: R Carroll-Johnson, L Gorman, N Bush (eds), Psychosocial nursing care along the cancer continuum. Oncology Nursing Society, Pittsburgh.

Fingeret MC, Teo I, Epner DE 2014. Managing body image difficulties of adult cancer patients: lessons from available research. Cancer 120(5), 633–641.

Goedendorp M, Andrykowski M, Donovan K et al 2012. Prolonged impact of chemotherapy on fatigue in breast cancer survivors: a longitudinal comparison with radiotherapy-treated breast cancer survivors and non-cancer controls. Cancer 118(15), 3833–3841.

Heckel L, Fennell K, Reynolds J 2015. Unmet needs and depression among carers of people newly diagnosed with cancer. European Journal of Cancer 51, 2049–2057.

Institute of Medicine (IOM) 2006. Implementing cancer survivorship care planning. Washington, IOM.

International Agency for Cancer Research (IARC) 2020. World Cancer Report. IARC Press, Lyon.

Jadalla A, Page M, Ginex P et al 2020. Family caregiver strain and burden: a systematic review of evidence-based interventions when caring for patients with cancer. Clinical Journal of Oncology Nursing 24(1), 31–50.

Kim Y, Carver C, Ting A 2019. Family caregivers' unmet needs in long-term cancer survivorship. Seminars in Oncology Nursing 35(4), 380–383.

Lehmann V, Hagedoorn M, Tuinman MA 2015. Body image in cancer survivors: a systematic review of case-control studies. Journal of Cancer Survivorship 9(2), 339–348.

Ministry of Health NZ 2015. Cancer patient survival. Ministry of Health, Wellington.

National Breast Cancer Centre (NBCC) and National Cancer Control Initiative (NCCI) 2005. Clinical practice guidelines for the psychosocial care of adults with cancer. Camperdown, NSW, National Breast Cancer Centre.

National Cancer Expert Reference Group 2020. Framework for optimal cancer care pathways in practice. Online. Available: www1.health.gov.au/internet/main/publishing.nsf/Content/ocp-framework.

National Cancer Institute 2020. Fatigue (PDQ®) – Health Professional Version. Online. Available: www.cancer.gov/about-cancer/treatment/side-effects/fatigue/fatigue-hp-pdq#_12.

National Comprehensive Cancer Network, Inc (NCCN) 2020a. Clinical Practice Guidelines in Oncology (NCCN Guidelines). Cancer related fatigue Version 2.2020. Online. Available: NCCN.org.

National Comprehensive Cancer Network, Inc (NCCN) 2016b. Clinical Practice Guidelines in Oncology (NCCN Guidelines) National Comprehensive Cancer Centre Clinical Practice Guidelines, Distress Management. Online. Available: www.nccn.org/professionals/physician_gls/pdf/distress.pdf.

Northouse L 2012. The impact of caregiving on the psychological well-being of family caregivers and cancer patients. Seminars in Oncology Nursing 28(4), 236.

Scott J, Lasch K, Barsevick A et al 2011. Patients' experiences with cancer-related fatigue: a review and synthesis of qualitative research. Oncology Nursing Forum 38(3), E191–E203.

Steginga S, Hutchinson S, Turner J et al 2006. Translating psychosocial care: guidelines into action. Cancer Forum 31(1), 28–31.

Waitman K 2016. Alterations in musculoskeletal, integumentary,
and neurological functions. In: J Itano (ed.), Core curriculum for oncology nursing, 5th edn. Elsevier, Missouri.

World Health Organization (WHO) 2020. Screening for various
cancer. Online. Available: www.who.int/cancer/detection/
variouscancer/en/

Index

Page numbers followed by '*f*' indicate figures, '*t*' indicate tables, and '*b*' indicate boxes.